THE SYNAPTIC ORGANIZATION
OF THE BRAIN

THE
SYNAPTIC ORGANIZATION
OF THE BRAIN

Fourth Edition

Edited by
Gordon M. Shepherd

New York   Oxford
OXFORD UNIVERSITY PRESS
1998

Oxford University Press

Oxford   New York
Athens   Auckland   Bangkok   Bogota
Bombay   Buenos Aires   Calcutta   Cape Town
Dar es Salaam   Delhi   Florence   Hong Kong
Istanbul   Karachi   Kuala Lumpur   Madras
Madrid   Melbourne   Mexico City   Nairobi
Paris   Singapore   Taipei   Tokyo
Toronto   Warsaw
and associated companies in
Berlin   Ibadan

Copyright © 1998 by Oxford University Press, Inc.

Published by Oxford University Press, Inc.

198 Madison Avenue, New York, New York 10016

Oxford is a registered trademark of Oxford University Press

Library of Congress Cataloging-in-Publication Data
The synaptic organization of the brain/
edited by Gordon M. Shepherd.— 4th ed.
p.   cm.   , Includes bibliographical references and indexes.
ISBN 0-19-511823-5 (cloth)—0-19-511824-3 (pbk)
1. Brain.   2. Synapses.   3. Neural circuitry.
I. Shepherd, Gordon M., 1933-   .
[DNLM: 1. Brain—physiology.
2. Neurons—physiology.
3. Synapses.
WL 300 S992 1998]   QP376.S9   1998   612.8'2—dc21
DNLM/DLC   for Library of Congress   97-2176

1 3 5 7 9 8 6 4 2
Printed in the United States of America
on acid-free paper

PREFACE

Nearly a quarter of a century has passed since the first edition of this book appeared, and therefore, it is timely to consider the development of the field of synaptic organization during this period.

The first edition in 1974 was a synthesis of the newly emerging information concerning the organization of synapses into circuits within the most accessible regions of the brain. The aim was to identify principles that applied across regions and could serve in guiding the analysis of less accessible regions. The main methods were Golgi stains, electron microscopy, and electrophysiological recordings from in vivo neurons in anaesthetized animals. These methods provided the keys to opening up the brain: with them, one could identify basic circuits and see how they were adapted in different regions for different information-processing tasks.

By 1979 tools of neurochemical and pharmacological analysis had become sufficiently developed so that the basic circuits could be fleshed out with neurotransmitters and neuromodulators, and the second edition therefore added these findings. During the following decade the use of tissue slices for intracellular electrophysiological analysis became widespread, leading to an explosion in the field of synaptic organization, so much so that by 1990, when a third edition was needed, it was appropriate to ask colleagues working in different areas to take responsibility for writing the different chapters. These colleagues responded splendidly; they produced not only authoritative syntheses of synaptic organization for each region, but also, by agreeing to follow the same format in each chapter, a new level of integration of principles across regions.

These principles have stood the test of time well, but now the onrush of new methods and findings has led to the need for a new edition. The methods include improved light microscopy that has allowed clear visualization in tissue slices of dendrites and even dendritic spines; the routine use of single and double patch recordings from soma and dendrite of the same neuron as well as dual recordings from neuron pairs; use of Ca^{2+} imaging at these levels of resolution to map neuronal activity and second messenger actions; and application of new molecular engineering methods, including knockouts, knockins, site-directed mutagenesis, caged compounds, etc., in slices, cultured cells, and expression systems. From these have come new findings about how receptors and channels in different neurons are formed from different combinations of subunits with appropriate operational properties. Perhaps most significant for this book, whose aim from the start has been to emphasize dendritic properties and incorporate them into concepts of neuronal and circuit organization, has been the rediscovery of dendrites and their active properties; for example, the science media have declared that this is "The Year of the Dendrites." Readers of earlier editions know that this is a phenomenon that has repeated itself over the past half century, and that many of the present authors have played key roles, both then and now. Thus, with the new findings has come a renewed appreciation for many of the principles elucidated in earlier times, which can now be demonstrated more clearly and put on a molecular basis. Many of these principles were developed originally from experiments in living animals; there is renewed awareness that properties of neurons and synapses in culture and in the slice need constantly to be assessed against properties in the whole animal.

How significant is this progress in synaptic organization and related fields of brain function? One can argue that the progress over the past quarter of a century is leading toward a revolution equivalent to that in concepts of the physical world brought about by the quantum physicists in the 1920s and 1930s. Arnold Sommerfeld of Munich warned his physics students in the 1920s: "Caution! Dangerous structure! Temporarily closed for complete reconstruction!"[1] The present book contains the building materials and blueprints for an equivalent reconstruction of our concepts of the neural basis of brain function. However, the new structure will only arise when both experimentalists and theorists recognize that, just as mechanisms at the level of quantum physics are the basis for understanding the physical world, so mechanisms at the molecular, cellular, and circuit level are the basis for understanding brain function. As noted in the preface to the previous edition: "It is only by incorporating. . . properties at the synaptic circuit level that we can simulate fully and accurately the mechanisms underlying brain function at the systems level." When this is recognized; when neuroscientists and theorists working at the systems level accept that concepts about the functions of different regions and of different distributed brain systems must be built directly on the properties of synaptic organization, it will be possible to say that a fundamental reconstruction of neuroscience is underway. The authors of this book are leading the way in this effort, which for most regions is well begun.

The plan of this edition follows that of previous editions. The first chapter introduces principles of functional organization at different levels that apply to all of the regions. The second chapter summarizes the tremendous range of membrane properties, both receptors and voltage-gated channels, and some of the principles of how combinations of these properties underlie different input-output functions of different neurons. The remaining chapters consider in sequence many of the best understood regions of the brain. We welcome as the first of these a new region, the cochlear nucleus in the auditory pathway, which has become one of the best sites for working out structure–function correlations at the cellular and circuit level. The remaining chapters follow the sequence in previous editions. Special attention has been given to the hippocampus, where new coauthors provide authoritative summaries of their own and others' work on the anatomy of hippocampal circuits and the key roles of hippocampal neurons in studies of active dendrites and synaptic plasticity. An account of dendritic electrotonus and its relevance for synaptic integration has traditionally been a part of this book; however, this subject matter is now thoroughly integrated into experimental and theoretical neuroscience, as can be seen in each chapter of this book, and where relevant the reader is directed to several accounts that are now available elsewhere in the literature.

As in previous editions, each chapter considers the same topics: neural elements, synaptic connections, a basic canonical circuit summarizing the overall functional organization of the region, synaptic physiology, neurotransmitters and neuromodulators, membrane properties, dendritic properties underlying impulse generation and synaptic integration, and finally a synthesis of one or more specific information processing tasks of that region.

All references have been gathered in a common reference list. This turned out to be a tremendous editorial task, with the list running to over 2,000 entries. As in the previous edition, this reference list by itself should be a valuable resource for anyone interested in brain organization.

To make the material covered in the book more available as a resource, the main types of output neurons in these regions have been included in a database of neuronal properties, called NeuronDB, that is being constructed on the World Wide Web with support of the Human Brain Project. The address is http://senselab.med.yale.edu/neurondb. This site also has links to other relevant databases of neuronal properties.

My debts are numerous, first to my colleagues who agreed enthusiastically to do the new edition and were able to fit the writing of new chapters or the rewriting of previous chapters into their very busy schedules. I can assure the reader that these people, who are pioneers in their fields and can at the same time integrate multidisciplinary data for a given region, are a rare breed; my hope is that they are not an endangered species, but rather are serving as role models for encouraging new generations of neuroscientists to think in integrative terms. In combining and editing the reference lists I have been grateful for the assistance of Jason Mirsky and Jason Smith. I am grateful to Frank Zufall, Trese Leinders-Zufall, Wei Chen, Paul Kingston, Michael Singer, Emmanouil Skoufos, Changping Jia, Minghong Ma, in my laboratory for expert advice and for allowing me to divert energies to these editorial duties. Valuable support and advice have been provided by Thomas Hughes and Colin Barnstable in my current work, and by Charles Greer and Christof Koch in preparing this volume. Nancy Wolitzer has expertly coordinated the production of the book. It is a pleasure to thank once again Jeffrey House, my editor at Oxford University Press, who enthusiastically supported the first edition and, all these years later, has been just as enthusiastic about this one. Finally, to Grethe: tak.

G.M.S.
Hamden, Connecticut
June 14, 1997

1. Quoted in R. Jungk, Brighter Than a Thousand Stars. New York: Harcourt Brace,1958.

ACKNOWLEDGMENTS

Chapter 1. Gordon M. Shepherd is grateful for support from the National Institute on Deafness and Other Communication Disorders and the National Institute of Neurological Diseases and Stroke (National Institutes of Health), and the National Aeronautics and Space Agency, National Institute of Mental Health, and the National Institute on Deafness and Other Communication Disorders through the Human Brain Project. Christof Koch has been supported by research grants from the National Science Foundation and National Institute of Mental Health (National Institutes of Health).

Chapter 2. David A. McCormick's work has been supported by the National Institutes of Health, the National Science Foundation, and the Klingenstein Fund.

Chapter 3. Robert E. Burke's research support comes entirely from the Intramural Program of the National Institute of Neurological Disorders and Stroke (National Institutes of Health). He is grateful to his colleagues Michael O'Donovan, Jeffrey C. Smith, and William Marks for much stimulating discussion.

Chapter 4. Eric D. Young is grateful to Phyllis Taylor for help in preparing the figures and to Kevin Davis, Paul Manis, Roger Miller, David Ryugo, and Jane Yu for comments on the manuscript. The work has been supported by the National Institute on Deafness and Other Communication Disorders (National Institutes of Health).

Chapter 5. Gordon M. Shepherd and Charles A. Greer are grateful for support from the National Institute on Deafness and other Communication Disorders and the National Institute of Neurological Diseases and Stroke (National Institutes of Health). Dr. Shepherd is also grateful to the National Aeronautics and Space Agency, National Institute of Mental Health, and the National Institute on Deafness and other Communication Disorders (National Institutes of Health) for support through the Human Brain Project.

Chapter 6. Peter Sterling thanks Sharron Fina for preparing the manuscript, Christina Geuke for preparing the illustrations, and Michael Freed, Robert Smith, and Noga Vardi for critically reading the manuscript. He also thanks the many scientists who contributed illustrations to this chapter. His work has been supported by the National Eye Institute (National Institutes of Health).

Chapter 7. Rodolfo Llinás and Kerry D. Walton would like to thank Dean Hillman for furnishing the light and electronmicrographs in the chapter. The work upon which this chapter is based has been generously supported by the National Institute of Neurological Disorders and Stroke (National Institutes of Health).

Chapter 8. The laboratory of S. Murray Sherman has been supported by research grants from the National Eye Institute (National Institutes of Health), and that of Christof Koch from the National Science Foundation and the National Institute of Mental Health (National Institutes of Health).

Chapter 9. Charles Wilson is supported by the National Institute of Neurological Disorders and Stroke (National Institutes of Health).

Chapter 10. Much of the work described in this chapter was supported by the National Institute of Neurological Disorders and Stroke (National Institutes of Health).

Lewis Haberly would also like to acknowledge the contributions that many students and colleagues have made to the ideas that are presented.

Chapter 11. Dan Johnston and David G. Amaral have been supported by grants from the National Institute of Neurological Disorders and Stroke and the National Institute of Mental Health (National Institutes of Health), and by the Human Frontiers Science Program during the preparation of the manuscript. Dr. Johnston is grateful to Jeff Magee and Costa Colbert for feedback on the manuscript and to Rick Gray for assistance with the figures.

Chapter 12. Rodney J. Douglas and Kevan A.C. Martin are supported by generous grants from the Swiss National Science Foundation Schwerpunktprogramm for Biotechnology, and by grants from the Human Frontiers Science Program, the European Union, and the Office of Naval Research. We thank our colleagues for their encouragement and assistance.

Contents

CONTRIBUTORS

DAVID G. AMARAL, PH.D.
Center for Neuroscience
University of California
Davis, California

ROBERT E. BURKE, M.D.
Laboratory of Neural Control
National Institute of Neurological Disorders
  and Stroke
National Institutes of Health
Bethesda, Maryland

RODNEY DOUGLAS, M.D.
Institute of Neuroinformatics, ETH/UZ
Zurich, Switzerland
Computation and Neural Systems Program
California Institute of Technology
Pasadena, California

CHARLES A. GREER, PH.D.
Department of Neurosurgery
Yale University School of Medicine
New Haven, Connecticut

LEWIS B. HABERLY, PH.D.
Department of Anatomy
University of Wisconsin
Madison, Wisconsin

DANIEL JOHNSTON, PH.D.
Division of Neuroscience
Baylor College of Medicine
Houston, Texas

CHRISTOF KOCH, PH.D.
Computation and Neural Systems Program
California Institute of Technology
Pasadena, California

RODOLFO R. LLINÁS, M.D., PH.D.
Department of Physiology & Neuroscience
New York University Medical Center
New York City, New York

KEVAN A. C. MARTIN, D.PHIL.
Institute of Neuroinformatics, ETH/UZ
Zurich, Switzerland
Computation and Neural Systems Program
California Institute of Technology
Pasadena, California

DAVID A. MCCORMICK, PH.D.
Section of Neurobiology
Yale University School of Medicine
New Haven, Connecticut

GORDON M. SHEPHERD, M.D., D.PHIL.
Section of Neurobiology
Yale University School of Medicine
New Haven, Connecticut 06510

S. MURRAY SHERMAN, PH.D.
Department of Neurobiology
State University of New York
Stony Brook, New York

PETER STERLING, PH.D.
Department of Neuroscience
University of Pennsylvania
Philadelphia, Pennsylvania

KERRY D. WALTON, PH.D.
Department of Physiology & Neuroscience
New York University Medical Center
New York City, New York

CHARLES J. WILSON, PH.D.
Department of Anatomy and Neurobiology
University of Tennessee College of Medicine
Memphis, Tenessee

ERIC D. YOUNG, PH.D.
Department of Biomedical Engineering
Johns Hopkins University
Baltimore, Maryland

1

INTRODUCTION TO SYNAPTIC CIRCUITS

GORDON M. SHEPHERD AND CHRISTOF KOCH

Synapses are the contact sites that enable neurons to form connections between each other in order to transmit and process neural information. Synaptic organization is thus concerned with the principles by which neurons form circuits that mediate the specific functional operations of different brain regions.

Synaptic organization differs from other fields of study in several ways. First, it is *multidisciplinary*, requiring the integration of results from experimental work in molecular neurobiology, neuroanatomy, neurophysiology, neurochemistry, neuropharmacology, developmental neurobiology, and behavioral neuroscience. It is also a *multilevel* subject, beginning (from the "bottom up") with the properties of ions, transmitter molecules, and individual receptor and channel proteins, and building up through individual synapses, synaptic patterns, dendritic trees, and whole neurons to the multineuronal circuits that are characteristic of each brain region. Finally, it is increasingly a field with a *theoretical foundation*, building and testing its concepts within a framework of theoretical studies in biophysics, neuronal modeling, computation neuroscience, and neural networks.

A common lament in neuroscience is that there is a lack of basic principles for understanding the vast amount of information about the brain that is accumulating from experimental studies. One of the main aims of this book is to show that the study of synaptic organization—in its full multidisciplinary, multilevel, and theoretical dimensions—is a powerful means of integrating brain information to give clear insights into the neural basis of behavior.

In this chapter we introduce some of the basic principles underlying synaptic organization in different regions of the nervous system. These synaptic circuits form the elementary functional units (cf. Shepherd, 1972b; Koch and Poggio, 1987) of which the nervous system is constructed and with which it computes ("processes information"). We will describe some of the basic operations that all regions must perform, and provide an introduction to the adaptations for these operations that are unique for each of the regions considered in subsequent chapters.

THE TRIAD OF NEURONAL ELEMENTS

Figure 1.1 illustrates that the brain consists of many local regions, or centers, and many pathways between them. At each center, the *input fibers* make synapses onto the cell body (soma), and/or the branched processes (dendrites) emanating from the cell body of the nerve cells contained therein. Some of these neurons send out a long axon that in turn carries the signals to other centers. These are termed *principal*, *relay*, or *projection* neurons. Other cells are concerned only with local processing within the center. These are termed *intrinsic* neurons, *local* neurons, or *inter*neurons. An example of this latter type is shown in the cerebral cortex in Fig. 1.1. The distinction between a

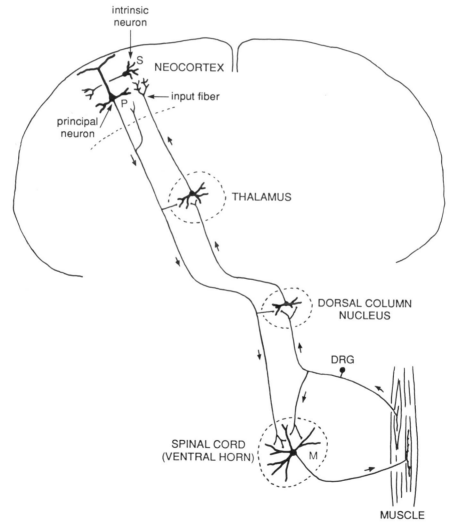

Fig. 1.1. Examples of local regions and some interregional pathways formed through the long axons of principal neurons. M, motoneuron; DRG, dorsal root ganglion cell; P, pyramidal (principal) neuron; S, stellate (intrinsic) neuron.

principal and an intrinsic neuron cannot be rigid, since principal neurons also take part in local interactions. It is nonetheless a useful way of characterizing nerve cells, which is used throughout this book.

The principal and intrinsic neurons, together with the incoming input fibers, are the three types of neuronal consituents common to most regions of the brain. We will refer to them as a *triad* of neuronal elements. The relations between the three elements vary in different regions of the brain, and these variations underlie the specific functional operations of each region.

THE SYNAPSE AS THE BASIC UNIT OF NEURAL CIRCUIT ORGANIZATION

Interactions between 13 neuronal elements are mediated by small, specialized junctions termed *synapses*. It follows that the synapse is the elementary structural and functional unit for constructing of neural circuits. Traditionally, most concepts of neural organization have assumed that a synapse is a simple connection that can impose either excitation or inhibition on a receptive neuron. Current experimental evidence indicates that this assumption needs to be replaced by an appreciation of the complexity of this functional unit. In this section we summarize briefly the properties of synapses; their physiological actions are discussed at greater length in Chap. 3.

Figure 1.2 summarizes the current view of the synapse. Most synapses involve the apposition of the plasma membranes of two neurons to form a *punctate junction*, also termed an *active zone*. Note that the junction has an orientation, thus defining the *pre*synaptic process and the *post*synaptic process. At a chemical synapse such as the one depicted in Fig. 1.2, the presynaptic process liberates a *transmitter* substance that acts on the postsynaptic process. From an operational point of view, a synapse converts a presynaptic electrical signal into a chemical signal and back into a postsynaptic electrical signal. In the language of the electrical engineer, such an element is a nonreciprocal two-port (Koch and Poggio, 1987).

THE SYNAPSE AS A MULTIFUNCTIONAL UNIT

The mechanism for the action of a synapse involves a series of steps, which are summarized in Fig. 1.2. These include depolarization of the presynaptic membrane (1); influx of Ca^{2+} ions into the presynaptic terminal (2); a series of steps (3–5) leading to fusion of a synaptic vesicle with the plasma membrane; released of a packet (quantum) of transmitter molecules (6); diffusion of the transmitter molecules across the narrow synaptic cleft separating the presynaptic and postsynaptic processes (7); and action of the transmitter molecules on receptor molecules in the postsynaptic membrane (9), leading in some cases to direct gating of the conductance at an ionotropic receptor (10). This changes the membrane potential (11) and hence the excitability of the postsynaptic process. The mechanisms mediated by ionotropic receptors are concerned primarily with rapid (1–20 msec) transmission of information, as in rapid sensory perception, reflexes, and voluntary movements (such as those we are using to type this text and you are using to read it).

The transmitter molecule may also activate a metabotropic receptor (10a) linked to a second-messenger pathway that modulates a membrane conductance or has other metabolic effects (11a, 12). The presynaptic process is itself a possible target, either

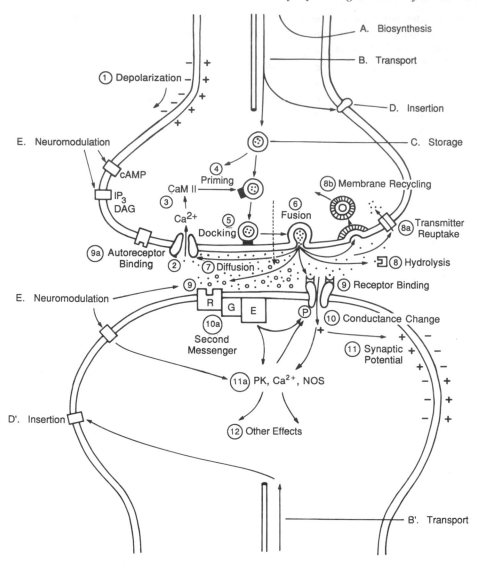

Fig. 1.2. A summary of some of the main mechanisms involved in immediate signaling at the synapse. Steps 1–12 are described in the text. Abbreviations: IP₃, inositol trisphosphate; CaM II, Ca/calmodulin-dependent protein kinase II; DAG, diacyglycerol; PK, protein kinase; R, receptor; G, G protein; E, effector enzyme; NOS, nitric oxide synthase. [Modified from Shepherd, 1994b, with permission.]

of the transmitter acting on autoreceptors (9a) or of diffusible second messengers such as nitric oxide, produced by nitric oxide synthase (NOS) in the postsynaptic process, which can modulate transmitter release in an activity-dependent manner (so-called retrograde messengers). The synapse is thus increasingly regarded not only as a one-way relay but as a more complicated bidirectional junction (Jessell and Kandel, 1993). However, whereas pre- to postsynaptic activation may take only a few thousandths of a millisecond, retrograde messengers are likely to act more slowly.

Activation of second messengers by either ionotropic or metabotropic receptors can have short- as well as long-term metabolic effects that lead to changes in synaptic efficacy. Of these activity-dependent changes, long-term potentiation (LTP) and long-term depression (LTD) are the most prominent. They will be discussed in the following chapters as prime candidates for the activity-dependent changes that may underlie learning and memory. More recently, short-term synaptic facilitation and depression have received much attention. Here, the synaptic weight of any one synapse can rapidly (10–100 msec) increase or decrease as a function of the previous history of usage of the synapse (Markram and Tsodyks, 1996; Abbott et al., 1997; for a review see Koch, 1997).

Many cellular mechanisms impinge on synaptic transmission over longer time periods. These include the steps involved in axonal and dendritic transport; storage of transmitters and peptides; co-release of peptides; and direct modulation of transmitter responses (see Neuromodulation in Fig. 1.2). These effects are slow (seconds to minutes) or very slow (hours and longer); the slowest processes merge with mechanisms of development, aging, and hormonal effects.

From these properties one can appreciate that the synapse is admirably suited as a unit for building circuits. The multiple steps of its mechanism confer a considerable flexibility of function by means of different transmitters and modulators, different types of receptors, and different second-messenger systems linked to the different kinds of machinery in the cell: electrical, mechanical, metabolic, and genetic. Several mechanisms, with different time courses, can exist at the same synapse, conferring on it the ability to coordinate rapid activity with the slower changes that maintain the behavioral stability of the organism over time.

TYPES OF SYNAPSES

In view of this tremendous potential for functional diversity, it is remarkable that synapses throughout the nervous system show such a high degree of morphological uniformity. One of the clearest differences has been the finding that synapses in the brain tend to fall into two groups, those with *asymmetrical* densification of their pre- and postsynaptic membranes, and those with *symmetrical* densification. Gray (1959) termed these *type 1* and *type 2*, respectively. Depending on the histological fixatives used, type 1 is usually associated with small, round, clear synaptic vesicles. In a number of cases, type 1 synapses have been implicated in excitatory actions. By contrast, type 2 is usually associated with small, clear, flattened, or pleomorphic vesicles, and is implicated in inhibitory synaptic actions.

Many examples of these types of synapses are shown throughout this book. There are well-recognized exceptions to these structure–function relations—for example, inhibitory actions by synapses that do not have type 2 morphology (cf. cerebellar basket cells, Chap. 7). Moreover, the physiological effect of a synapse may be dependent on the modulatory actions of different second-messenger systems. Thus, although the type 1 and type 2 designations are a useful working hypothesis and will be invoked often in later chapters, there is always the clear understanding that this is only a first step in classifying synaptic structure and function. For consistency in constructing the diagrams of synaptic connections in the different regions covered in this book, neurons making type 1 synapses and having primarily excitatory actions are depicted in open profiles, whereas those making type 2 synapses and having primarily inhibitory actions are depicted in filled profiles.

THE SYNAPSE AS A MICRO-UNIT

In addition to its ability to mediate different specific functions, an important property of the synapse is its small size. The area of contact has a diameter of 0.5–2.0 μm, and the presynaptic terminal (bouton) has a diameter that characteristically is only slightly larger. These small sizes mean that large numbers of synapses can be packed into the limited space available within the brain. For example, in the cat visual cortex, 1 mm^3 of gray matter contains approximately 50,000 neurons, each of which gives rise on average to some 6,000 synapses, making a total of 300 million (300×10^6) synapses (Beaulieu and Colonnier, 1983). It has been estimated that 84% of these are type 1 and 16% are type 2. Given an approximate density of 100,000 neurons below 1 mm^2 of cortical grey matter in primates and if assuming that the cortical area of one hemisphere in the human is approximately 100,000 mm^2, there must be 10 billion cells in the human cortex and 60 trillion (60×10^{12}) synapses. In humans, these packing densities can be as large as one billion synapses per cubic millimeter of cortical tissue!

Like the national debt, these numbers are so large that they lose meaning. The important point is that the number of synapses in the brain is several orders of magnitude larger that the number of neurons, providing a rich substrate for the construction of microcircuits within the packed confines of the brain. During early development an exuberance of synapses is generated throughout the nervous system. During this time, synapses are very dynamic and appear and disappear rapidly. When the animal reaches maturity, the final synaptic density is half the density present earlier on (yet the size of the brain has usually expanded considerably) (Rakic et al., 1986). Study of these kinds of mechanisms involved in the development of synaptic connections is important for understanding the strategy of construction of synaptic circuits, but in this book, we will be concerned primarily with the organization and functional operations of the mature nervous system.

LEVELS OF ORGANIZATION OF SYNAPTIC CIRCUITS

It might seem that one could simply connect neurons together by means of synapses and make networks that mediate behavior, but this is not the way nature does it. A general principle of biology is that any given behavior of an organism depends on a hierarchy of levels of organization, with spatial and temporal scales spanning many orders of magnitude. This is nowhere more apparent than in the construction of the brain. As applied to synaptic circuits, it means that one needs to identify the main levels of organization in order to provide a framework for understanding the principles underlying their construction and function.

The analysis of local regions over the past four decades has led to the recognition of several important levels of circuit organization (see Fig. 1.3). The most fundamental level is the information carried in the *genes*, which, interacting with the environment, read out the basic *protein* components in the different brain regions. These mol-

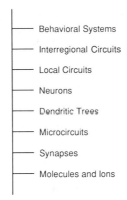

Fig. 1.3. Some of the main levels of organization in the nervous system. This book focuses on the levels from *Synapses* to *Local Circuits*, as a basis for understanding the expression of *Molecules and Ions* in an integrative context, and for understanding the circuit basis of *Behavioral Systems*.

ccular components are organized into organelles of the cell. For circuit formation, as we have seen, the most critical organelle is the *synapse*. Synaptic organization begins at the next level, with the organization of gene products into the synapse. The most local patterns of synaptic connection and interaction, involving small clusters of synapses, are termed *microcircuits* (Shepherd, 1978). The smallest microcircuits have sizes measured in microns; their fastest speed of operation is measured in milliseconds. These are grouped to form *dendritic subunits* (Shepherd, 1972b; Koch et al., 1982) within the *dendritic trees* of individual neurons. The whole *neuron*, containing its several dendritic subunits, is the next level of complexity. Interactions between neurons of similar or different properties constitute *local circuits* (Rakic, 1976); these perform the operations characteristic of a particular region. Above this level are the interregional *pathways*, columns, laminae, and topographical maps, involving multiple regions in different parts of the brain, that mediate specific types of behavior. These many interwoven levels of organization are a trait of the brain not shared by its closest artificial cousin, the digital computer, in which few intermediate modular structures exist between the individual transistor on the one hand, and a functional system, such as a random-access memory chip, on the other.

An important aim of the study of synaptic organization is to identify the types of circuits and the functional operations they perform at each of these organizational levels. In the rest of this chapter, we will consider examples at each of these levels. Subsequent chapters show how, in each region, the nervous system rings the changes on these basic themes, expressing variations of circuits exquisitely adapted for the specific operations and computations carried out by that region on its particular input information.

SYNAPTIC MICROCIRCUITS

Excitation and inhibition by single synapses usually have little behavioral significance by themselves; it is the assembly of synapses into patterns of connectivity during development that produces functionally significant operations. The process can be likened to the assembly of transistors onto chips to form microcircuits in computers. By analogy, we refer to these most local synaptic patterns as *neuronal microcircuits*. Let us consider several basic types.

SYNAPTIC DIVERGENCE

One of the simplest types of patterns provides for a divergence of output from a single terminal. In neural network terminology, this is called *fan-out*. As indicated in Fig. 1.4A, left, a presynaptic terminal (a) has excitatory synapses onto multiple dendrites (b–f). An action potential (ap) invading the presynaptic terminal can thus cause simultaneous excitatory postsynaptic potentials (EPSPs) in many postsynaptic dendrites. The advantage of this arrangement is that activity in a single axon is amplified into activity in many postsynaptic neurons, conferring a high gain upon the system. The activity is simultaneous, thus retaining the timing of the input, and it is of the same sign; excitation of the presynaptic terminal by the invading impulse leads to synaptic excitation of the postsynaptic cell.

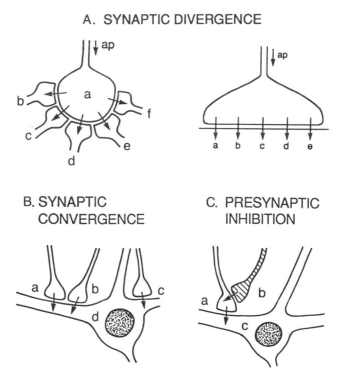

Fig. 1.4. The simplest types of microcircuits. **A:** Left, synaptic divergence from a single large axonal terminal (a) onto multiple postsynaptic dendrites (b–f). Synapses are indicated by arrows. ap, action potential. Right, synaptic divergence from multiple active zones of a single large terminal onto a single postsynaptic target (muscle cell). **B:** Synaptic convergence of several axons (a–c) onto a single postsynaptic neuron (d). **C:** Presynaptic inhibition by axon (b) onto axon (a), which is presynaptic to axon (c). See text.

Comparison of this arrangement with the well-known model of the neuromuscular junction (NMJ) is shown in Fig. 1.4A, right. The NMJ consists of a large presynaptic terminal with many release sites, in this case, made onto the muscle. It is known that of 1,000 or so release sites, only 100–200 are actually activated by invasion of a single impulse into the presynaptic terminal. This means that there is a probability of only 0.1–0.2 that a given site will release transmitter when depolarized by an impulse. The release sites of the NMJ are equivalent to the active zones of central synapses, each with its own release probability. Thus, in the example of Fig. 1.4A, presynaptic depolarization would cause some synapses to release transmitter (e.g., b,c) but not others (e.g., d). In summary, morphological studies can identify the pattern of synaptic connections, but their actual use is physiological and probabilistic (see Korn and Faber, 1987). The release probability can be up- or down-regulated by the amount and timing of pre- and post-synaptic activity, providing an effective mechanism for adjusting the effect that a synapse has on its postsynaptic target in an effective manner (Stevens and Wang, 1994; Abbott et al., 1997).

An important point to note is that, whereas all active zones at a NMJ connect to the same postsynaptic cell, in the example of Fig. 1.4A, left, they connect to different cells; in this way divergence leads to amplification at the level of a single terminal. Such an arrangement is found in many parts of the nervous system. A single mossy fiber terminal in the cerebellum, for example, may make synapses onto dendrites of as many as 100 or more granule cells (see Chap. 7). Single terminals with more modest divergence factors are made by sensory afferents in thalamic relay nuclei (Chap. 8) and the substantia gelatinosa of the dorsal horn. In addition to divergence from a single terminal, there is also divergence of axons as they branch to give rise to multiple terminals. This is a more common means of achieving multiple synaptic outputs, as exemplified by the several thousand synapses of a typical cortical cell mentioned above.

SYNAPTIC CONVERGENCE

The considerable divergence that characterizes the output of a neuron is matched by the convergence of many inputs onto a neuron. In neural network terminology, this is called *fan-in*. The essence of this convergence at the microcircuit level is depicted in Fig. 1.4C, where three terminals (a, b, and c) make synapses onto a postsynaptic dendrite (d).

Let us consider first the case in which terminals a and b are excitatory. Spread of an impulse into terminal (a) sets up an EPSP; slightly later, spread of an impulse into terminal (b) sets up an EPSP that summates with that of (a). This is termed *temporal summation*. Note that although the impulses in (a) and (b) may be asynchronous, their EPSPs nonetheless can summate. For relatively fast EPSPs, the prolongation that makes temporal summation possible is due mainly to the membrane capacitance, which slows the dissipation of charge across the postsynaptic membrane (cf. Johnston and Wu, 1995; Shepherd, 1998). For slower EPSPs, the time course is controlled by biochemical processes, such as second messengers.

Although it might appear that temporal summation involves simple addition of PSPs, in general this is not the case. This is because PSPs are generated by changes in membrane conductance to specific ions and not by current injection (see Chap. 2); the conductances act to shunt, or short-circuit each other, so that the combined amplitude of a PSP is less than the sum of its parts. This means that synaptic summation is essentially a nonlinear process (Rall, 1964, 1977; Johnston and Wu, 1995; Shepherd, 1998; see Chap. 2).

Synaptic convergence also involves summation of excitatory and inhibitory PSPs. This process lies at the heart of the integrative mechanisms of neurons. Consider, for example, that (b) in Fig. 1.4B is inhibitory. Activation sets up an inhibitory postsynaptic potential (IPSP) that opposes the EPSP set up by (a), and repolarizes the membrane toward the reversal potential for the inhibitory conductance (see Chap. 2). If the reversal potential is near the resting membrane potential, this is called *silent* or *shunting* inhibition. Obviously, integration of excitatory and inhibitory synaptic responses can be nonlinear even without the added complication of active membrane properties (Rall, 1964; Koch et al., 1983; Koch, 1997).

It remains to be noted that inputs are characteristically distributed over the entire dendritic surface of a neuron [see (c) in Fig. 1.4B]. This means that in addition to temporal summation there is *spatial summation* of responses arising in different parts of a dendrite, as well as in different parts of the whole dendritic tree. Spatial summation allows for the combining of many inputs into one integrated postsynaptic response. The separation of PSPs reduces some of the nonlinear interactions between synaptic conductances, making the summation more linear. However, it also increases the possibilities for local active mechanisms and the generation of nonlinear sequences of activation from one site in the dendritic tree to the next.

Presynaptic inhibition is a final type of simple synaptic combination involving convergence. In this arrangement (Fig. 1.4C), a presynaptic terminal (a) is itself postsynaptic to another terminal (b). The presynaptic action may involve a conventional type of IPSP produced by (b) in the presynaptic terminal (a). Alternatively, there may be a maintained depolarization of the presynaptic terminal, reducing the amplitude of an invading impulse and with it the amount of transmitter released from the terminal. The essential operating characteristic of this microcircuit is that the effect of an input (a) on a cell (c) can be reduced or abolished (by b) without there being any direct action (of b) on the cell (c) itself. Control of the input (a) to the dendrite or cell body can thus be much more specific.

Presynaptic control may be exerted by either axon terminals or presynaptic dendrites. Note that the effect is presynaptic only with regard to the response of the postsynaptic cell. From the point of view of the presynaptic terminal, the effect is postsynaptic. There are many situations in the nervous system, involving multiple synapses between axonal and/or dendritic processes, in which sequences of pre- and postsynaptic effects can occur (see Chaps. 3, 5, 6, and 8, on the spinal cord, olfactory bulb, retina, and thalamus).

INHIBITORY OPERATIONS

The patterns of synaptic connections considered thus far provide for elementary excitatory and inhibitory operations. Let us next consider arrangements that carry out operations that are building blocks for specific information processing functions.

Feedforward Inhibition. Sensory processing commonly involves an inhibitory "shaping" of excitatory events. A role in this shaping is played by a pattern of synaptic connections that mediates feedforward (afferent) inhibition. As illustrated in Fig. 1.5A, the arrangement consists of an afferent terminal (a) which makes synapses onto the dendrites of both a relay neuron (b) and an interneuron (c). The dendrites of both neurons respond by generating EPSPs. However, the interneuron also has inhibitory dendro-dendritic synapses onto the relay neuron; the EPSP activates these synapses, producing an inhibition of the relay neuron. The extra synapse in this pathway helps to delay the inhibitory input, so that the combined effect in (b) is an excitatory–inhibitory

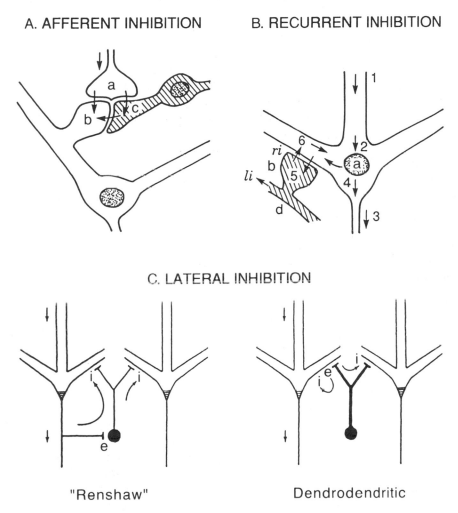

A. AFFERENT INHIBITION   B. RECURRENT INHIBITION

C. LATERAL INHIBITION

"Renshaw"   Dendrodendritic

Fig. 1.5. Microcircuits that mediate different types of postsynaptic inhibition. **A:** Feedforward inhibition: presynaptic axon (a) excites relay neuron dendrite (b) and interneuron dendrite (c), which feeds forward inhibition onto (b). **B:** Recurrent inhibition: a relay neuron (a) is both pre- and postsynaptic to the dendrite (d) of an inhibitory interneuron (b). This microcircuit mediates both recurrent (ri) and lateral inhibition (li) through the steps indicated by 1–6. **C:** Comparison between lateral inhibition mediated by axon collaterals and interneurons (left) and by dendro-dendritic connections (right). e, excitatory; i, inhibitory. See text.

sequence. This type of sequence is common in the thalamus (Chap. 8) and many sensory pathways. By restricting the excitation of relay neurons to the onset of an excitatory input, feedforward inhibition serves to enhance the sensitivity to changing stimulation and thus performs a kind of *temporal differentiation* of the sensory input (Koch, 1985). By spread of postsynaptic responses through dendritic trees, it may also contribute to the enhancement of spatial contrast through *lateral inhibition (see below)*.

Note that the microcircuit in Fig. 1.5A is built of all three elementary patterns discussed above and depicted in Fig. 1.4. Thus, it combines *divergence* from terminal (a) with *convergence* of (a) and (c) onto (b) and *presynaptic* control by (a) of (c). Many variations of this circuit occur throughout the CNS, the more common involving feedforward inhibition through more widely dispersed local circuits than those illustrated in Fig. 1.5A. Note that inhibition is sign inverting: excitation of the presynaptic terminal leads to inhibition of the postsynaptic cell.

Feedback Inhibition.   A very common type of operation in the nervous system is one in which the excitation of a neuron leads, sometime later, to inhibition of that neuron and/or of neighboring neurons. This is called *feedback* or *recurrent inhibition*. It can be mediated by several types of circuit, the most local type of which involves reciprocal dendrodendritic synapses.

This mechanism has been worked out at the synaptic level in the olfactory bulb, and is illustrated in Fig. 1.5B (Rall and Shepherd, 1968). The output neurons of the olfactory bulb are mitral and tufted cells (a). They are activated by EPSPs which spread through a primary dendrite (1) to the cell body (2) to set up an impulse that propagates into the axon (3). The impulse also backspreads into secondary dendrites (4), where it activates output synapses excitatory to spines of granule cell dendrites (5). The EPSP in the spine then activates a reciprocal inhibitory synapse back into the mitral cell dendrite (6); the IPSP spreads through the neuron to inhibit further impulse output.

Reciprocal synapses thus form an effective microcircuit module carrying out an elementary computation, in this case, for recurrent inhibitory feedback of an activated neuron. Reciprocal synapses are found in a number of regions of the nervous system; in addition to the olfactory bulb (Chap. 5), these include the dorsal horn of the spinal cord, the retina (Chap. 6), thalamus (Chapter 8), and suprachiasmatic nucleus. They appear to be largely absent from the basal ganglia and the different regions of cortex. It is interesting that although they are absent from the local circuits of the neocortex, their presence in the different nuclei of the thalamus means that they play a role in the interregional circuits that control the input to cortex (cf. Chap. 8). One may conclude that they are not special for a particular region or a particular modality. Rather, they are an excellent example of a microcircuit module that can perform several operations of information processing and can be assembled during development for that purpose wherever it is needed. At this local level of organization, full-blown action potentials in the dendrites may or may not be needed; synaptic output can be controlled by graded electrotonic spread of nearby EPSPs (as in the case of the granule cell) or by partial, voltage-dependent "boosting" effects (cf. Chap. 5).

Lateral inhibition.   In addition to recurrent inhibition, the same module may also mediate lateral inhibition: in Fig. 1.5B, the EPSP in the granule cell spine spreads through the dendritic branch to other spines, activating inhibitory output onto neighboring, less active, mitral cells. Lateral inhibition is a fundamental mechanism of neural processing. The most common implementation in the nervous system is through axon collaterals of an output neuron feeding back onto an interneuron, which inhibits other output neurons through axon connections. This was first described in the spinal cord, and was named *Renshaw inhibition* after its discoverer (see Chap. 3).

The two neural substrates for implementing lateral inhibition are compared in Fig. 1.5 C in relation to the axon hillock, which is the critical area for impulse initiation (see below). Dendrodendritic inhibition is activated by the backspreading impulse from the axon hillock and is therefore "prehillock" in location (Fig. 1.5, right). The activation threshold is set by the excitability of the axon hillock of that cell; the intensity and time course reflect the excitability of that neuron; and the pathway is local, limited to the dendritic tree of that neuron and its interactions with local subunits of the interneuronal dendrites. By contrast, Renshaw inhibition is due to the forward-propagating impulse from the axon hillock and is therefore "trans-hillock" in nature (Fig. 1.5, left). The activation threshold depends on the excitability of the axon hillock of both that cell and the interneurons; the intensity and time course can be amplified and modulated by the properties of the interneurons; and the final pathway back onto that cell consists of the global output of the axon branches of the interneurons. These properties have direct consequences for shaping recurrent and lateral inhibition in different regions of the brain (see later in this chapter, and in subsequent chapters). For example, different dendrodendritic local subunits mediate recurrent vs. lateral inhibition in the olfactory bulb, which is essential for the memory mechanism in that region (see Chapter 5).

DENDRITIC INTEGRATION AND DENDRITIC SUBUNITS

We take for granted that the extensive branching of neuronal dendrites increases their surface area for receiving synaptic inputs. If this were their only function, there would be some justification for reducing our representation of the neuron to a single node, with all inputs converging onto this node. This is a common practice in neuroanatomical textbooks, and it is the common assumption underlying the vast majority of neural network simulations, which consider individual nerve cells to be single-node, linear integration devices utilizing a simple, stationary threshold operation for triggering an output. In these cases, the effects of dendritic morphology and synaptic patterns on the functions of individual cells are totally neglected.

In fact, the patterns of dendritic branching, unique to different types of neurons, impose geometrical constraints which partially compartmentalize the activity in different branches. The geometry of the branches and the sites of specific inputs combine with the electrotonic properties to ensure that parts of a dendritic tree can function semi-independently of one another. If one adds the fact that voltage-gated channels can confer excitable properties onto local dendritic regions, it is clear that the dendrites, far from being functionally trivial appendages of a cell body, are the substrate for generating a rich repertoire of computation that contributes critically to the overall input–output functions of the neuron. It is thus evident that single-node network models ignore several levels of dendritic organization responsible for much of the computational complexity of the real nervous system.

Four factors—dendritic branching, synaptic placement, and passive and active membrane properties—must be taken into account in assessing the nature of the integrative activity of dendrites. Characterization of the electrotonic spread of potentials is difficult because of the complex branching patterns of many dendrites. An introduction to one-dimensional passive cable theory is provided in several accounts (Johnston and Wu, 1995; Segev, 1995; Shepherd, 1998). The ways that active conductances can contribute to dendritic activity are considered in Chap. 2. The functional role of dendritic activity in information processing within synaptic circuits is a common theme running through the accounts of most of the brain regions considered in this book. Here we provide a brief introduction to the nature of dendritic integration and the ways that functional compartments are created at several levels of dendritic organization.

DENDRITIC COMPUTATION

In assessing the nature of dendritic integration, it is increasingly fashionable to use computational metaphors. This obscures many functional roles of dendrites that are not strictly "computational" (e.g., mechanisms involved in development, maturation, activity-dependent changes, etc.). However, it has the advantage of providing a specific framework within which the capacity of dendrites to carry out well-characterized types of operations can be assessed.

The importance of the sites and types of synaptic inputs on a dendritic branch can be illustrated by using the paradigm of logic operations. In the diagram of Fig. 1.6A, alternating excitatory and inhibitory synapses are arranged along a dendritic branch. Given the nonlinear interactions between these synapses, as discussed above, an inhibitory synapse (i1, i2, i3) with a synaptic reversal potential close to the resting potential of the cell (*shunting* or *silent* synapse, Chap. 2) can effectively oppose (*veto*) the ability of a membrane-potential change due to any local or more distal excitatory synapses to spread to the soma and generate impulses there. By contrast, an inhibitory synapse has little effect in vetoing the voltage change initiated by more proximal excitatory synapses. This operation is an analog form of a digital AND-NOT gate (e *and not* more proximal i), and has been postulated to be a mechanism underlying various computations, such as direction selectivity in retinal ganglion cells (Koch et al., 1983).

This type of synaptic arrangement can also be found in more localized parts of dendritic trees. Figure 1.6B depicts a case in which a dendrite has numerous distal branches, each with an excitatory and an inhibitory synapse. The same "on-path" rule still applies: an inhibitory synapse effectively vetoes a more distal excitatory synapse on the same branch, but it has little effect in opposing excitatory responses originating anywhere else in the dendritic tree, which are effectively sited more proximally to the soma. Thus, the combination of dendritic morphology in conjunction with synaptic placement enables the cell to "synthesize" analog versions of logical, boolean operations.

DENDRITIC SPINE UNITS

The smallest compartment, structurally and functionally, within a dendritic tree is the dendritic spine, a small (1–2 μm), thornlike protuberance. It is already evident from Fig. 1.5 that spines are an important component in many kinds of microcircuits. An electron micrograph of a spine in the cerebral cortex is shown in Fig. 1.7. Spines are

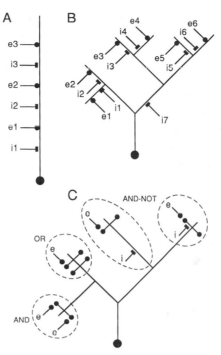

Fig. 1.6. Arrangements of synapses that could subserve logic operations. **A:** A single dendrite receives excitatory (e1–e3) and inhibitory (i1–i3) synapses. A shunting inhibitory input can veto only more distal excitatory responses; this approximates an AND-NOT logic operation, e.g., [e2 AND NOT i2]. **B:** Branching dendritic tree with arrangements of excitatory and inhibitory synapses. As in A, inhibitory inputs effectively veto only the excitatory response more distal to it, e.g., [[e5 AND NOT i5] AND NOT i7]. **C:** Branching dendritic tree with excitatory synapses on spines, and inhibitory synapses either on spine necks or on dendritic branches. Different types of logic operations arising out of these arrangements are indicated. In all cases (A–C), inhibition is of the shunting type. See text. [A, B from Koch et al., 1983; C based on Shepherd and Brayton, 1987, with permission.]

extremely numerous on many kinds of dendrites; in fact, they account for the majority of postsynaptic sites in the vertebrate brain. They are especially prominent in the cerebellar cortex (Chap. 7), basal ganglia (Chap. 9), and cerebral cortex (Chaps. 10–12). Within the cerebral cortex, about 79% of all excitatory synapses are made onto spines and the rest directly onto dendrites, whereas 31% of all inhibitory synapses are made onto spines. A spine with an inhibitory synapse always carries an excitatory synapse as well (Beaulieu and Colonnier, 1983). Given the dominance of excitatory synapses, about 15% of all dendritic spines carry both excitatory and inhibitory synaptic profiles. On dendrites of cortical pyramidal cells, spine densities may reach several spines per micrometer of dendrite.

Because spines are characteristically located on dendrites at some distance from the cell body, experimental evidence regarding their physiological properties is still limited. However, their obvious importance has stimulated considerable interest (reviewed in Harris and Kater, 1994; Shepherd, 1996). Some of the hypotheses that have been

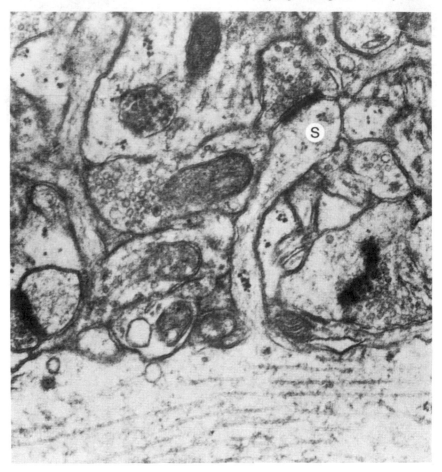

Fig. 1.7. The fine structure of a dendritic spine. This electron micrograph shows, at the bottom, a longitudinally cut dendrite from which a spine (s) arises. The spine is approximately 1.5 μm in length and 0.1 μm at its narrowest width. At its head it receives a synapse, which has the round vesicles and asymmetrical density characteristic of Gray's type 1. In the neck and head are small clumps of ribosomes; in the dendrite are longitudinally cut microtubules. [From Feldman, 1984, with permission.]

generated are listed in Table 1.1. The simplest view of spines is that they serve chiefly as sites for synaptic connections, which only raises many fundamental questions about the roles spines play in establishing synapses during development. Some spine properties are relatively obvious, such as increasing dendritic membrane area, but even this simple property can have a critical function in controlling neuronal excitability (cf. Chap. 9). Spines are especially associated with dendrites, where in most neurons they receive predominantly glutamatergic excitatory synapses. However, they are also found on the axon hillocks and initial axon segments of some neurons, where they receive predominantly inhibitory GABAergic synapses. This shows that spines have more gen-

Table 1.1. Functions That Have Been Ascribed To Spines

Site of synaptic connection
  Receives synaptic input
  Site of excitatory synaptic input
  Site of inhibitory synaptic input (axon initial segment)
  The spine only connects

Developmental synaptic target
  Increases dendritic surface area
  Makes synaptic connections tighter
  Critical for development of synaptic connections
  Matching of pre- and postsynaptic elements

Local dendritic input-output unit
  Mediates prolonged synaptic output
  Serves as dendrodendritic input-output unit

Passive synaptic potential modification
  Spine: dendrite impedance matching
  Synaptic potential attenuation
  Constant current device
  Large amplitude, rapid local responses (EPSP amplification)

Unit for synaptic plasticity
  Spine stem modulates synaptic spread into dendrite
  Spine stem involved in memory (EPSP amplitude modulation)
  Site of LTP/LTD
  Rapid mechanical changes: do spines twitch?

Active synaptic boosting unit
  Site of local impulse amplification
  Site of pseudosaltatory conduction

Information processing unit
  Thresholding operational unit
  Active logic gate: specific information processing in distal dendrites

Temporal processing unit
  Acts as coincidence detector

Biochemical compartment
  Absorbs nutrients
  Provides for biochemical isolation related to single synapse
  Site of local protein synthesis (polyribosomes)
  Site of local Ca^{2+} increase
  Neuroprotection: isolates the dendrite from toxic Ca^{2+} levels

Membrane surface shape properties
  Target for electrophoretic membrane migration
  Increases dendritic membrane capacitance
  Shortest wire in the nervous system
  Increases intersynaptic distance

For references, see text. EPSP, excitatory postsynaptic potential; LTP, long-term potentiation; LTD, long-term depression. [From Shepherd, 1996, with permission.]

eral functional properties than those related only to dendritic integration of excitatory inputs. The spines on most neurons appear to combine multiple and differing subsets of the functions listed in Table 1.1. In view of these multiple properties, the spine has been characterized as a "multifunctional integrative unit." Many of these possible properties and functions of spines are discussed in the different chapters of this book. Here we focus on one example, the possible significance of spines for rapid signal processing.

Specific information processing. The very small size of spines has important electrical and biochemical consequences. The narrow neck of the spine suggests that the spine head could function as a metabolic compartment (Shepherd, 1974). There is increasing theoretical and experimental evidence that the spine is a virtual biochemical compartment for calcium ions and other second-messenger molecules, isolated from the chemical environment present in the main dendritic compartment (Koch and Zador, 1993). At rest, two free calcium ions can be inferred to be present in the average dendritic spine head, owing to the low concentration of free calcium at rest and the small volume of the spine head. The small volume and correspondingly high surface-to-volume ratio means that internal concentrations of some metabolites and second messengers are likely to be high, and membrane ion fluxes are likely to have large and rapid consequences. Biochemically, therefore, the spine head appears to be suitable for rapid signal processing.

Electrically, a synapse on a spine head "sees" a much higher resistance than the same synapse on the dendritic branch (see Brown et al., 1988, and Johnston and Wu, 1995, for specific examples). This means that even with a purely passive membrane, "the amplitude of a synaptic potential on the spine head will be greater than if the same synaptic conductance change had occurred on the dendritic shaft" (Johnston and Wu, 1995). The small size of the spine head also means that the membrane capacitance is very small, so the synaptic potential also has a very rapid time course. The spine is thus well suited electrically for rapid local signal processing, even when sited on distal dendrites.

The signal-processing potential of spines is even more interesting in relation to the possibility that they contain voltage-sensitive membrane properties, such as active sodium or calcium channels (e.g., Denk et al., 1995). This encourages one to pursue the metaphor of logic operations in dendrites and to inquire to what extent it might apply to interactions between spines. The diagram in Fig. 1.6C represents a dendritic tree with its distal branches covered by spines. Assume that there are patches of active membrane in the distal dendrites and that these give rise to a regenerative membrane event if there is sufficient depolarization by an excitatory synaptic response. One possible arrangement is that the impulse would fire if any one of several spines in a cluster were to receive an excitatory input; this would be equivalent to an OR gate in the logic paradigm. Alternatively, two simultaneous inputs might be required; this would constitute an AND gate. Finally, one might have AND-NOT gates. Depending on the placement of the inhibition, the gate might be localized to an individual spine, or it might involve a dendritic branch containing a cluster of spines. These possibilities can all be traced in the diagram of Fig. 1.6C. Experimental studies suggest that these simple combinations of excitatory and inhibitory interactions do occur in natural activity, and computer simulations have shown that the logic operations arise readily out of these arrangements (Shepherd and Brayton, 1987; Shepherd et al., 1989).

The point of these studies is not to suggest that the brain is constructed like a digital computer based on binary logic. Rather, it is to explore the properties of interactions in the smallest compartments of the nervous system—terminal dendritic branches and dendritic spines—and show that they may be capable of powerful, rapid, and precise types of information processing. Of further interest is that, through sequential activation of active sites along branches within the dendritic tree, synaptic responses initiated in the most distal parts of the tree nonetheless can exert precise control over the generation of impulses in the cell body and initial axonal segment.

Associative Learning. Spine interactions may also be a mechanism for associative learning. Considerable attention has been focused on the possibility that long-term potentiation (LTP) of cortical neurons may underly learning and memory (reviewed in Nicoll and Malenka, 1995). This involves a long-term (hours to weeks) increase in synaptic efficiency in response to a presynaptic input volley. Following an initial hypothesis of Rall (1974a,b), there has been growing evidence of changes in the dendritic spines of these cells during LTP (reviewed in Harris and Kater, 1995), as well as in the presynaptic terminals. It has been shown, for example, that sufficient depolarization of a spine increases local calcium ion concentration; the calcium ions are then available to bring about biochemical and structural changes in the spine that could function in the storage of information (see Fig. 1.2 above; these mechanisms are discussed in detail in Chap. 11). To the extent that these changes involve thresholds and nonlinear properties, they can be incorporated into the logic paradigm of spine interactions illustrated in Fig. 1.6C.

DENDRITIC BRANCH SUBUNITS

Functional compartmentalization of dendrite trees can be created in various ways. The interactions between excitatory and inhibitory synaptic responses described above define relatively small functional subunits. At the other extreme are larger functional compartments built into the branching structure during development.

The mitral cell of the olfactory bulb provides a clear example of this level of organization. As shown in Fig. 1.8A, each mitral cell has a primary dendrite divided into two subunits: a terminal tuft (t) and a primary dendritic shaft (1°). The function of the terminal tuft is to receive the sensory input through the olfactory nerves and process the responses through dendrodendritic interactions (see insert). The function of the primary dendritic shaft is to pass on this integrated response to the cell body. The third dendritic subunit in this cell consists of the secondary (2°) dendrites, which take part in dendrodendritic interactions with the granule cells and thereby control the output from the cell body (these have been described above; see Fig. 1.5B). Thus, the mitral cell dendritic tree is fractionated into three large subunits, each with a distinct function that is carried out semi-independently of the others (see Chapter 5 for further details).

Another example of this level of organization is provided by the starburst amacrine cell of the retina. This cell (see Fig. 1.8B) has a widely radiating dendritic tree, which at first glance would seem to be diffusely arranged. Like olfactory granule cells,

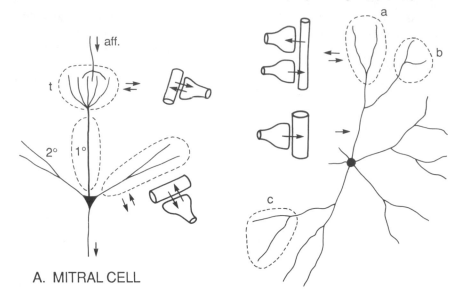

A. MITRAL CELL

B. STARBURST AMACRINE CELL

Fig. 1.8. Organization of subunits within dendritic trees. **A:** Mitral cell of the olfactory bulb, showing division of the dendritic tree into three main subunits. aff., afferent; t, dendritic tuft; 1°, 2°, primary and secondary dendrites. Synaptic microcircuits are indicated in insets. **B:** Starburst amacrine cell in the retina, showing division of dendritic tree into functional subunits, as exemplified by a–c. Microcircuits are indicated in the insets. [A after Shepherd, 1979; B based in part on Koch et al., 1982, with permission.]

amacrine cells lack axons; the distal dendritic branches are the sites of synaptic output, whereas synaptic inputs are present both distally and proximally (see inserts). Thus, each dendrite appears to function as a relatively independent input–output unit (Koch et al., 1982; Miller and Bloomfield, 1983). These dendritic subunits appear to be part of the circuitry for computing the direction of a moving stimulus in the vertebrate retina (see below, and Chap. 6 for further details).

The starburst cells synthesize and release acetylcholine (ACh), providing excitatory input to direction-selective ganglion cells. Pharmacological evidence suggests that the most common inhibitory neurotransmitter, gamma-aminobutyric acid (GABA), provides the inhibitory input in the cell's null direction. Thus, an excitatory bipolar cell input to the amacrine cell could, in conjunction with GABAergic input from inhibitory bipolar or other inhibitory amacrine cells, function as an AND-NOT gate, in analogy with the corresponding arrangement illustrated in Fig. 1.6B. However, paradoxically, starburst amacrine cells also appear to synthesize, store, and release GABA (see Chap. 6). Until recently, such a colocalization of two fast-acting neurotransmitters was thought not to exist. Its presence obviously increases the opportunities for more complex synaptic interactions at the local level.

In summary, there are skeptics who still maintain that we do not know what dendrites do. But we have seen in the examples of the dendrites of mitral cells and amacrine cells unambiguous evidence of their structural differentiation and specific functional operations. These are but two of many other examples throughout this book of the rich repertoire of operations that are mediated by different types of dendrites (for a recent review of this topic, see Koch, 1997).

A BIOPHYSICS OF COMPUTATION

We have seen that a neuron generally contains several levels of organization within it, starting with the synapse as the basic functional unit. Many different patterns of synapses, coupled with passive and active membrane properties and the geometry of the dendrites, provide a rich substrate for carrying out neuronal computations. The time scale of these computations varies greatly, from the fraction of a millisecond required for inhibition to suppress EPSPs in dendritic spines to many hundreds of milliseconds or seconds in the case of the slowly acting effects of neuropeptides on the electrical properties of neurons.

A detailed description of the way that different types of membrane conductances, each with a characteristic distribution in the cell body and dendrite, combine to control the flow of information through the neuron is given in Chap. 2. In Table 1.2, we provide a brief compendium of some elementary synaptic circuits and biophysical mechanisms underlying specific computation in the nervous system. In addition to their importance for neuroscience, these operations are of considerable potential relevance in computer science, where work on the "physics of computation" attempts to characterize the physical mechanisms that can be exploited to perform elementary information-processing operations in artificial neural systems (Mead and Conway, 1980). These mechanisms in turn constrain the types of operations that can be exploited for computing. We believe that a "biophysics of computation" is now needed for understanding the roles of membranes, synapses, neurons, and synaptic circuits in information processing in biological systems in order to bridge the gap between computational theories and neurobiological data (Koch and Poggio, 1987; Shepherd, 1990). This knowledge will also enable us to understand the fundamental limitations in terms of noise, accuracy, and irreversibility of neuronal information processing.

The vast majority of neural network simulations—in particular, connectionist models—consider individual nerve cells to be single-node, linear integration devices. They thus neglect the effect of dendritic, synaptic, and intrinsic membrane properties on the function of individual cells. An important goal of the study of synaptic organization is therefore to identify the specific operations (such as those summarized in Table 1.2) that arise from these properties and to incorporate them into more realistic network simulations of specific brain regions.

THE NEURON AS AN INTEGRATIVE UNIT

How are these different levels of dendritic functional units coordinated with the soma and initial segment of the axon to enable neurons to function as complex integrative units? The answer to this question requires an understanding of how synaptic responses in the dendrites are related to impulse generation in the axon hillock and initial axonal segment.

Table 1.2. Some Neuronal Operations and Their Underlying Biophysical Mechanisms

Biophysical mechanism	Neuronal operation	Example of computation	Time scale
Action potential initiation	Threshold, one-bit analog-to-digital converter		0.5–5 msec
Action potentials in dendritic spines	Binary OR, AND, AND-NOT gate	[a]	0.1–5 msec
Nonlinear interaction between excitatory and inhibitory synapses	Analog AND-NOT veto operation	Retinal directional selectivity[b]	2–20 msec
Spine–triadic synaptic circuit	Temporal differentiation high-pass filter	Contrast gain control in the LGN[c]	1–5 msec
Reciprocal synapses	Negative feedback	Lateral inhibition in olfactory bulb[d]	1–5 msec
Low, threshold calcium current (I_T)	Triggers oscillations	Gating of sensory information in thalamic cells[e]	5–15 Hz
NMDA receptor	AND-NOT gate	Associative LTP[f]	0.1–0.5 sec
Transient potassium current (I_A)	Temporal delay	Escape reflex circuit in Tritonia[g]	10–400 msec
Regulation of potassium currents (I_M, I_{AHP}) via neurotransmitter	Gain control	Spike frequency accommodation in sympathetic ganglion[h] and hippocampal pyramidal cells[f]	0.1–2 sec
Long-distance action of neurotransmitters	Routing and addressing of information	[j]	1–100 sec

Note: The time scales are only approximate. LGN, lateral geniculate nucleus; LTP, long-term potentiation; NMDA, N-methyl-D-aspartate.

Sources: Includes the chapter in which the mechanism is discussed and the original reference.

[a]Chap. 1; see also Shepherd and Brayton, 1987.

[b]Chap. 1; see also Koch et al., 1982, 1983.

[c]Chap. 8; see also Koch, 1985.

[d]Chap. 5; see also Rall and Shepherd, 1968.

[e]Chaps. 2 and 8; see also Jahnsen and Llinás, 1984a,b.

[f]Chap. 2; Jahr and Stevens, 1986.

[g]See Getting, 1983.

[h]Chap. 3; see also Adams et al., 1986.

[i]Chap. 11; see also Madison and Nicoll, 1982.

[j]See Koch and Poggio, 1987.

IMPULSE INITIATION IN THE INITIAL AXON SEGMENT

The first intracellular recordings from motoneurons in the 1950s showed that EPSPs generated in the dendrites spread through the soma to initiate the impulse in the axon hillock–initial segment. From there, the impulse propagates down the axon, but because electrotonic spread of current occurs in all directions, it also backspreads into the soma and dendrites. This backspread hypothesis was proposed by Fuortes et al (1957) and supported and popularized by Eccles and his collaborators (Eccles, 1957). One of the best classical models was the crayfish stretch receptor neuron, where it was shown that a receptor potential spreads all the way from the dendritic terminals through the dendrites and soma to initiate the impulse several hundred micrometers out in the axon (Edwards and Ottoson, 1958), a finding repeatedly confirmed (cf. Ringham, 1971). Adding to this picture was the evidence first obtained by Fatt in motoneurons but most clearly in hippocampal pyramidal neurons (Spencer and Kandel, 1961) and cerebellar Purkinje cells (Llinás and Nicholson, 1971) for active properties of the dendrites.

Since the 1970s there has thus been a consensus that synaptic responses in the dendrites are boosted by local active properties, leading to impulse generation in the axon hillock, impulse propagation through the axon, and variable degrees of impulse backspread into the soma–dendrites. One of the most explicit examples of this classical model and its functional organization has been the mitral cell of the olfactory bulb, by virtue of the restriction of its excitatory olfactory input to a primary dendritic tuft several hundred microns distant from the cell body. As described above (see Fig. 1.5), the sensory-evoked EPSP in the distal dendritic tuft spreads through the primary dendrite and soma and axon hillock to initiate the impulse, which both propagates into the axon and spreads back into the soma and dendrites. Computer simulations (Rall and Shepherd, 1968) first showed that, by either active or passive backspread, the impulse produces sufficient depolarization to activate the dendrodendritic circuit through the granule cells. Recently, double patch recordings (Chen et al., 1997a,b) under infrared microscopy in olfactory bulb slices have confirmed the classical model that, with weak synaptic excitation, full impulses are initiated at the soma-axon hillock region (Fig. 1.9A, $17 \mu A$). However, with strong synaptic excitation, the site of impulse initiation shifts to the dendritic tuft region, and a full active impulse propagates through the primary dendrite to the soma (Fig. 1.9B, $33 \mu A$). In either mode, the impulse backspreading into the secondary dendrites mediates the specific functions of self and lateral inhibition (cf. Fig. 1.5) as well as contributing to the generation of oscillatory firing of the mitral cell population and the implementation of a form of olfactory memory. These functions will be described further in Chap. 5.

The classical model has been confirmed and extended in several central neurons by the double and triple patch recording technique combined with infrared microscopy introduced by Stuart and Sakmann (1994). Impulse initiation in cortical pyramidal neurons appears to occur at the axon or axon hillock at all levels of synaptic excitation (Fig. 1.9B, right, bottom), with backpropagation of the action potentials supported by Na^+ channels in the dendrites (B, right top; cf. Stuart et al., 1997). The active dendritic response to synaptic input in these cells has been considered to be a form of synaptic amplification, as first suggested by Miller et al. (1985) and Perkel and Perkel (1985). However, active dendrites may generate impulses under some conditions, as in mitral cells (See Herraras, 1990; Turner et al, 1991; Mainen et al., 1996). With re-

A. Mitral Cell

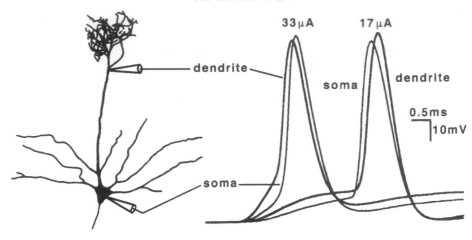

B. Pyramidal Cell

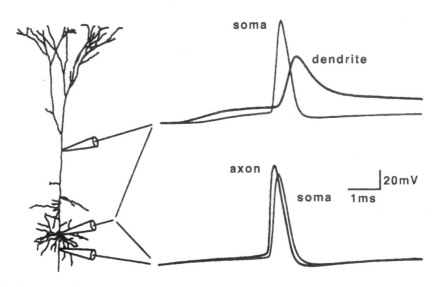

Fig. 1.9. **A:** Impulse initiation in a rat olfactory mitral cell. **Left:** Schematic view of recorded neuron and experimental setup. Synaptic excitation occurs in the distal tuft of the primary dendrite, approximately 400 microns from the cell body. Double patch recordings were made from the soma and distal dendrite near the tuft during synaptic excitation by a volley in the olfactory nerves. **Right:** With weak or moderate excitation ($17\,\mu A$), the EPSP spreads from the tuft through the primary dendrite to elicit the impulse first in the soma-axon hillock region, with backpropagation through the primary dendrite (and secondary dendrites as well). With strong excitation ($33\,\mu A$), the impulse arises first in the distal dendrite and forward propagates to generate the impulse at the soma. [Based on Chen et al., 1997a,b.] **B:** Impulse initiation in a rat neocortical pyramidal neuron. **Left:** Camera lucida drawing of a recorded layer 5 pyramidal neuron. **Right, top:** Patch recordings showing that impulse initiation in the soma precedes that in the dendrite during threshold synaptic excitation in the apical dendrite. **Right, bottom:** Impulse initiation in the axon precedes that in the soma. [From Stuart et al., 1997, with permission.]

gard to the backpropagating impulses, since pyramidal cell dendrites do not have output synapses like mitral cells, it has been necessary to consider other possible roles. First, they may function as "hot spots" to boost EPSPs in spreading from distal dendrites to the soma and axon hillock. Second, they may serve as sites of local integration and thresholding operations at dendritic branch points. Third, their boosting activity may contribute to synaptic plasticity and memory mechanisms. One such mechanism could be to implement Hebbian learning rules that are sensitive to the timing of presynaptic spike and postsynaptic backpropagated action potential. A recent experimental study (Markram et al., 1997) has provided direct evidence of how the difference in arrival times can influence synaptic weight increases or decreases. Finally, these voltage-dependent channels might enable the action potential to invade the entire dendritic tree and propagate to the postsynaptic site of the synapses, implementing a sort of "acknowledgment" to the synapse that the neuron just spiked. This sort of information could be crucial in the initiation and control of synaptic plasticity (see especially Chap. 8 [cerebellum], Chap. 11 [hippocampus], and Chap. 12 [neocortex]).

THE CONCEPT OF THE CANONICAL NEURON

If the neuron is a complex integrative unit as described above, a key question is how much of this complexity is necessary for building realistic neuronal and network models to simulate brain functions. The pyramidal neuron of the cerebral cortex is a prime example of this problem. Clearly, an understanding of the functional organization of this type of neuron is critical for an understanding of cognitive functions. Pyramidal neurons are the principal neuron in all three basic types of cortex: olfactory (Chap. 10), hippocampal (Chap. 11) and neocortex (Chap. 12). Although they vary in size and shape, one can identify a "canonical" pyramidal neuron in the same way that one identifies a gene family by certain shared characteristics. What we particularly need to know is the minimum architecture necessary to capture the integrative structure of the pyramidal neuron. An approach to this answer is illustrated by the simplified representation in Fig. 1.10A. It consists of (*1*) division of the dendritic tree into apical and basal parts; (*2*) dendritic spines on the apical and basal dendrites; and (*3*) different excitatory and inhibitory synaptic inputs to different levels of the apical and basal dendritic trees. (Only limited branching and four spines are depicted in the figure to keep it simple.) A final feature (*4*) is a long axon that gives off axon collaterals that make synapses on targets within the neighborhood of the cell and at different distances from the cell.

This canonical cell can be converted into a canonical model by representing it as a series of compartments, as in Fig. 1.10B. Each compartment can be seen to form a local subunit that can play a critical role in information processing within the neuron by virtue of its unique combination of synaptic inputs, active properties, anatomical structure, and relation to other subunits. Thus, the spines (A_1, A_2) are the principal sites of excitatory inputs; their interactions may generate *specific local information processing* and *local activity dependent changes*, as discussed earlier. The activity spreading in dendritic branches (B, C) is summed at the branch point (D), which acts as a *local decision point* for passing activity toward the soma. Whether this activity spreads effectively to the soma depends on *modulatory gating* by both excitatory and inhibitory inputs along the apical shaft (D). There is a further stage of summation between the activities spreading to the soma from the apical (D) and basal (E) fields. Finally, there

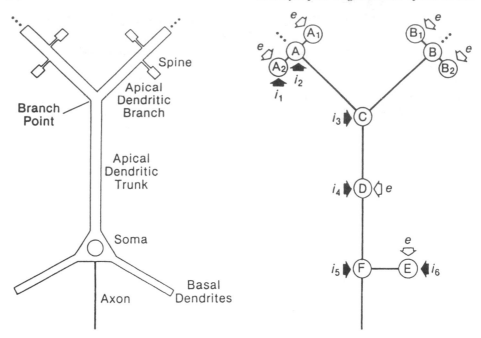

Fig. 1.10. **A.** Canonical representation of a cortical pyramidal neuron. **B.** Pyramidal neuron as a branching system of compartments. See text. [Modified from Shepherd, 1994.]

are direct inputs to the soma, many of them inhibitory, which provide for *global integration and modulation* of the neuronal output, in contrast to the local activities taking place within each dendritic branch and field. When the impulse is initiated in the axon hillock, in addition to propagating along the axon it backpropagates into the dendrites, thus sending a global signal that an output has occurred to the local subunits.

In summary, a logical parsing of the canonical structure indicates a sequence of functional operations, proceeding from the local to the global, that is likely to underlie the roles of pyramidal neurons in cortical functions. The diagram indicates the minimal structure necessary to capture the essential functional organization of the pyramidal neuron. One of the aims of this book is to provide the reader with a sense of the canonical structure and function of the key neurons in different regions so that they can be incorporated into more realistic simulations of the neural operations of those regions.

LOCAL CIRCUITS

No matter how complicated a single neuron may be, it cannot play a role in the processing of information without interacting with other neurons. The circuits that mediate interactions between neurons within a region are called *intrinsic*, or *local* circuits. They include all of the levels of organization we have considered previously, plus the longer-distance connections made by axons and axon collaterals within a given brain region. In turning our attention to these more extensive circuits, we will continue to distinguish between simple excitatory and inhibitory synaptic actions. Although the types of neurons and their circuits appear to be distinctive for each region, we will see that the operations they carry out can be grouped into several basic types.

EXCITATORY OPERATIONS

Excitatory operations can be grouped into two main types: feedforward excitation in input pathways, and feedback excitation through axon collaterals within the region. We will discuss these operations in relation to the organization of the cerebral cortex.

Feedforward Excitation. In many regions of the nervous system, the input fibers (arising from output cells in other regions) are excitatory. Thus all the long-range projections to, from, and within the cerebral cortex are excitatory, as are the projections to and from the specific thalamic nuclei. The rules of connectivity for the targets of these excitatory inputs vary, however, in different regions.

   A common pattern is that the input connects directly to the output neurons of that region. As shown in Fig. 1.11 in an area of cerebral cortex, the target may be the distal dendrites (AFF_1), or the proximal dendrites (AFF_2) of pyramidal output neurons (P_1). Although it is widely believed that the distal sites can provide only for weak, background modulation of more specific proximal responses, this is not generally true. There are many cortical regions, such as the olfactory cortex (Chap. 10), where specific inputs in fact preferentially and exclusively make connection only to the most distal dendrites. We have seen above that these distal sites provide a fertile ground for local signal processing. Furthermore, voltage-dependent sodium and calcium channels in

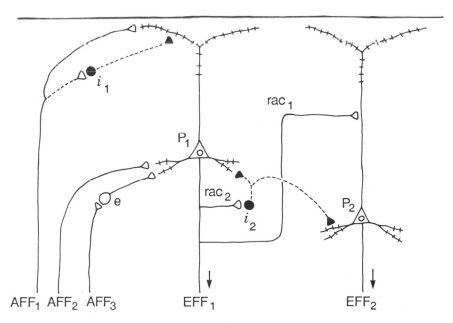

Fig. 1.11. Canonical representation of the synaptic organization of cerebral cortex. See text. [Modified from Shepherd, 1988b, with permission.]

the distal dendritic tree can act as amplifiers of the synaptic current, enabling it to modulate effectively the firing properties of the distant soma (Bernander et al., 1994).

Another common pattern is that input fibers also connect to interneurons that make excitatory connections within the region in question, providing circuits for feedforward excitation. In the cerebellar cortex, for example, mossy fibers make excitatory synapses onto granule cells, which then make excitatory connections onto Purkinje cells. The advantage of this arrangement is that it provides the opportunity for additional patterns of convergence and divergence. In the cerebellar cortex, these complex patterns through granule cells are in parallel with the direct access of excitatory climbing fiber inputs to the Purkinje cells (see Chap. 7).

In the cerebral cortex, excitatory interneurons in input pathways are exemplified by the spiny stellate cells of laminar IV found in sensory areas and association areas of granular cortex. As shown in Fig. 1.11 (AFF_3), this provides for an intracortical feedforward excitatory relay from the afferents onto the output neurons (P_1). This relay in turn can set up an additional step in the processing of afferent information, by convergence–divergence patterns of connections as mentioned above. In addition to serial sequences, there are also parallel input pathways, including direct afferent inputs to the pyramidal neurons, which contribute to the abstraction of receptive field properties. Inhibitory interactions also contribute to cortical operations, as described further below and in Chap. 12.

Feedback Excitation. Excitation fed back through axon collaterals of an excitatory output neuron onto that neuron and neighboring output neurons is a special property found only in certain regions of the brain. Recurrent excitation, where it exists, rarely is fed back through an excitatory interneuron. An obvious reason is that this would create a loop for amplifying positive feedback that would lead to powerful and widespread excessive excitation and seizure activity. Thus feedback excitation is usually limited to direct connections of the recurrent collaterals onto other principal neurons.

The clearest examples of this type of excitation are to be found in the vertebrate cerebral cortex. The simplest case is the olfactory cortex, where the pyramidal neurons give off recurrent collaterals that feed back excitation onto the basal dendrites of nearby pyramidal neurons (Chap. 10). Another example is the Schaffer collateral system of the hippocampus, in which recurrent collaterals from pyramidal neurons of CA3 make excitatory connections onto the apical shafts of pyramidal neurons in CA3 and CA1 (Chap. 11). Evidence for direct feedback excitation has also been obtained in reptilian dorsal general cortex, which has been regarded as a model for the evolutionary precursor of mammalian neocortex (Kriegstein and Connors, 1986). In the neocortex itself, pyramidal neurons have well-developed recurrent axon collateral systems, and there has long been evidence for excitatory actions attributable to them. In addition to this intraregional excitatory feedback, there is a massive interregional feedback system originating among the pyramidal cells in the lower layers of cortex which projects back to those specific thalamic nuclei providing the input to the cortex (Chap. 12).

The significance of the local feedback connections is that activated pyramidal neurons can respond to an initial excitatory input with subsequent waves of reexcitation. This has at least two significant functional consequences. First, it greatly amplifies the effect of the input on the cortical circuits. Second, the subset of activated pyramidal neurons imposes a subsequent pattern of activation onto an overlapping subset of pyramidal neurons in the same region. It is believed that this is a powerful mechanism for achieving combinatorial patterns of activation reflecting both the pattern of the input signal and the experience-dependent patterns stored within the distributed connections of the local circuits of the region in question (see Haberly, 1985; Granger et al., 1988; Wilson and Bower, 1988; Douglas et al., 1995).

A CANONICAL CIRCUIT FOR CORTICAL ORGANIZATION

Comparisons between the local circuits in the different types of cortex, as discussed above, give a perspective on cortical organization different from that derived from traditional views based on cortical cytoarchitectonics. From this new perspective, what is striking is the local circuit elements that are common to the different types. Thus far we have emphasized the pyramidal neuron and the intrinsic circuits for feedforward and feedback excitation. These are paralleled by circuits for feedforward and feedback inhibition, respectively. These circuits are largely implemented by GABAergic interneurons, which comprise some 20% of cortical neurons. They can be subdivided into a large number of subclasses according to their morphology, size, location, postsynaptic targets, and functions (Fitzpatrick et al., 1987). Thus, cortical inhibitory circuits are likely to subserve a number of different cortical operations, as will be discussed below.

Building on the concept of the canonical neuron, we can designate a basic "canonical circuit" for the cortex, which may be defined as *the minimum architecture necessary for capturing the most essential cortical input–output operations*. As depicted in Fig. 1.11, the elements comprising this basic circuit consist of (*1*) pyramidal (P) output neurons, with apical and basal dendrites; (*2*) differentiation of P cells into different laminar populations (i.e., superficial P_1 and deep P_2); (*3*) dendritic spines, which receive excitatory inputs; (*4*) input fibers which connect to P cells in specific ways—direct excitation (AFF_1 and AFF_2), feedward excitation (AFF_3, e), and feedforward inhibition (AFF_1, i_1; (*5*) intrinsic recurrent axon collaterals (rac) for feedback excitation of P cells (rac_2); (*6*) intrinsic recurrent axon collaterals (rac) for feedback and lateral inhibition of P cells (rac_2, i_2); (*7*) lamination of different inputs at different levels of the P cell dendritic tree for complex gating of input responses; and (*8*) different targets of different populations of P cells (EFF_1, EFF_2). Note how the properties of the canonical pyramidal neuron depicted in Fig. 1.11 are incorporated into the basic circuit which contains it. Typical of the very rich associational structure of the cerebral cortex is the fact that the vast majority of connections are intrinsic to the cortex, giving rise to massive excitatory and inhibitory feedback circuits (Braitenberg and Schultz, 1991).

The set of local circuits depicted in Fig. 1.11 can be considered a superfamily unique to the vertebrate cerebral cortex. It constitutes a basic canonical circuit for cerebral cortical organization, which is adapted and elaborated in the different types of cortex and the different cortical regions in order to carry out the set of operations characteristic of each (Shepherd, 1974, 1988a,b). The version depicted in Fig. 1.11 shares many common elements and properties with the canonical cortical circuit of Douglas and Martin in Chap. 12. A full exposition of these circuit elements and their roles in different cortical functions is given in Chaps. 10–12. The general properties of basic circuits will be discussed further after consideration of inhibitory local circuits.

INHIBITORY OPERATIONS

As is already clear, inhibitory circuits play large roles in determining the types of operations generated within a region. This is supported by studies showing that if synaptically mediated inhibition is blocked pharmacologically, cells lose most of their distinguishing features; an example is the loss of sensitivity of cortical neurons to bars of a certain orientation or moving in a particular direction (see Chap. 12).

We will examine here three examples of inhibitory local circuits. Our aim is first to show how inhibitory circuits can give rise to specific functions. A second aim is to consider these circuits within a comparative framework. This will allow us to see that each circuit employs an inhibitory neuron in a slightly different way, so that distinctly different operations can be generated by relatively fine tuning of the connections of a generic inhibitory interneuron.

Rhythmic Generation. Rhythmic activity can be generated by two main mechanisms: intrinsic membrane properties and synaptic circuits. Intrinsic membrane properties were first found in pacemaker neurons in central pattern generator circuits controlling breathing, walking, and other highly stereotyped behaviors in invertebrates. Since the early 1980s, research carried out on brain slices has shown that many types of neurons in the vertebrate central nervous system possess complex and highly nonlinear ionic conductances that endow these cells with the ability to respond to inputs with oscillations at various frequencies (Llinás, 1988). Thus, intrinsic oscillatory neurons may be far more common in the CNS than previously thought, enhancing the computational power of the system. An introduction to these ionic conductances is provided in Chap. 2, and examples will be described throughout this book (see especially those in the cerebellum [Chap. 7], thalamus, [Chap. 8], and the different types of cortex [Chaps. 10–12]).

Rhythmic activity can also be a property of local circuit interactions. A common model, shown in Fig. 1.12A, consists of output neurons (b) connected through axon collaterals to inhibitory neurons (*i*), which in turn connect back into the output neurons. When an input (a_1) activates the output neurons, they begin to generate impulses, which leads to activation of the interneurons. This activation leads to feedback inhibition of the output neurons, which now can no longer respond to the input and thus also deprives the interneurons of their source of activation; they are, in a sense, presynaptically inhibited by themselves. Both populations, therefore, are silent until the IPSPs in the output neurons wear off and the cycle is ready to be repeated. The degree of synchronization of a region will obviously depend on the extensiveness of the connections. The circuit could thus be laid down during development by a simple rule for the interneurons to make extensive random connections on the output cell populations.

Rhythmic activity can also be generated by dendrodendritic microcircuits, as discussed above (see Fig. 1.5B). Although the neural elements are different, the principles underlying the interactions are similar. This illustrates an important concept, namely that similar functions can be mediated by different neural substrates. Conversely, similar substrates can mediate different functions by specific adaptations of general mechanisms.

High-frequency oscillations (40–60 Hz) of a large proportion of the neuronal population in a given area appear to be a common occurrence in the awake, behaving animal. Evidence from the olfactory system of both invertebrates and vertebrates (Free-

A. RHYTHM GENERATION   C. DIRECTION SELECTIVITY

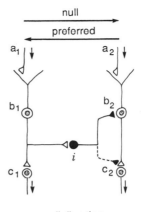

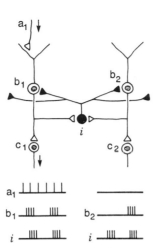

B. SPATIAL CONTRAST

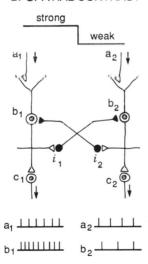

Fig. 1.12. Intrinsic inhibitory circuits are organized to mediate different types of functional operations characteristic of a given region. **A.** Rhythm generation (a_1, input; b_1, b_2, relay neurons; c_1, c_2, targets of relay neurons; i, inhibitory interneuron). Impulse firing patterns are shown below. **B.** Spatial contrast, mediated by lateral inhibition. Stimulation consists of strong and weak areas of stimulation with a sharp edge between them. **C.** Direction selectivity. Arrows indicate movement of a stimulus in the null and the preferred direction. See text.

man, 1983; Wehr and Laurent, 1996) as well as in the visual cortex and other neocortical areas relates these oscillations to perception and behavior. Thus, both at the single-cell and at the network level, neurons show very complex, dynamic patterns of neuronal excitability that are essential for the neural computations they carry out. This is another property of real neurons that needs to be incorporated into network simulation and connectionist models.

Receptive Field Organization. Concepts of circuit organization are further exemplified by the role of lateral inhibitory circuits in mediating spatial contrast, a common property of receptive field organization in many sensory systems. This property is illustrated in Fig. 1.12B, where there is strong stimulation of input (a_1) and all of the elements to the left in the diagram (not shown), and weaker stimulation of input (a_2) and all of the elements lying to the right. The responses of b_1 and b_2 would start out being proportional; however, the stronger inhibition by b_1 and i_1 suppresses b_2 more than the suppression of b_1 by b_2 and i_2, thereby enhancing the difference in firing rates of b_1 and b_2. This effect diminishes the further away the elements are from the border, thereby enhancing the contrast between strong and weak simulation at the border.

This is the basis for the classical description of Mach bands in the visual system, as first demonstrated in the *Limulus* eye (see Ratliff, 1965). It has turned out that the circuit for mediating this effect in *Limulus* appears to involve dendrodendritic connections without intervention of an inhibitory interneuron (Fahrenbach, 1985). In mammalian sensory systems, however, this operation characteristically involves inhibitory interneurons interacting with the output neurons through the types of local circuits indicated in Fig. 1.10B, or through dendrodendritic microcircuits.

Directional Selectivity. A third type of local circuit in which an inhibitory interneuron plays an essential role is in direction selectivity. The best known model is the retina, where ganglion cells in most vertebrate species show selective activation by stimuli moving in one direction. The proposed model is shown schematically in Fig. 1.12C. The essential element is an inhibitory interneuron whose connections are made in one direction that runs *opposite* to the preferred direction. This means that stimuli moving in that direction (called the *null* direction) activate the inhibitory connections in that direction, so that cells further along cannot respond. In the opposite, preferred direction, by contrast, the cells are free to respond.

Several types of circuit connections might mediate this selectivity. As is common in biology, direction selectivity in the retina appears to be computed in a redundant manner using a number of different mechanisms at a number of discrete anatomical sites. Prime candidates are synaptic interactions within the dendritic trees of retinal ganglion cells and of the starburst amacrine cells that provide the driving inputs to the ganglion cells (Amthor and Grzywacz, 1993; see Chap. 6). The organization of the starburst amacrine cell has been discussed above (see Fig. 1.8B). These cells synthesize, store, and release of the two common fast-acting excitatory (ACh) and inhibitory (GABA) neurotransmitters, which suggests that one and the same cell could potentially act as both an excitatory and an inhibitory circuit element.

Directional selectivity is also found in visual cortical cells, where it is mediated by a combination of excitatory inputs and inhibitory interneurons (Ferster and Koch, 1987;

see above) whose connections are mainly on cell bodies and proximal dendrites (solid line b_2 in Fig. 1.12C). This site is less selective but might be easier to target during development. Blocking the action of the inhibitory cells by an appropriate chemical substance leads to the almost total loss of direction selectivity (Sillito et al., 1980). Interestingly, interneurons, whether excitatory or inhibitory, appear to be absent or inoperant in the very young, immature cortex, and they begin to exert their specific effects only after the development of the extrinsic projection neurons (Jacobson, 1978).

COMPARING CANONICAL CIRCUITS

How can one represent the different excitatory and inhibitory local circuits, each with its underlying levels of functional units, in a way that is not merely a catalog, but gives insight into the functions of each region? As we have seen, a useful way to do this is by means of a *basic (canonical) circuit*, defined as a representation of the main patterns of synaptic connections and interactions most characteristic of a given region. Such a representation is useful in several ways: for identifying the principles of circuit organization of a region; for better understanding the relations between synaptic actions and dendritic properties; and finally, for identifying those aspects that must be included if a network simulation is to have validity as an accurate representation of that region.

An example of a canonical circuit has already been presented in Fig. 1.11, which represents the key elements and connections found in the cerebral cortex. This figure emphasizes those aspects that are common to different types of cortex, as discussed in the text. For closer examination of a given type, one could introduce the particular adaptations and elaborations that underlie its unique properties. The canonical circuit is thus a flexible tool that is not rigidly defined; its purpose is to represent the minimum of elements and connections that will capture the essence of the functional operations of a region.

Another important use of a canonical circuit is for making comparisons between the organizations of different regions. This is illustrated in Fig. 1.13, where a basic circuit of the retina (left) is compared with that of the olfactory bulb (right). Despite the fact that these regions process entirely different sensory modalities, the basic circuits are similar in outline and in several details. In each case, there are parallel vertical pathways for straight-through transmission of information. In addition, there are horizontal connections, arranged in two main levels, for the processing of information by lateral interactions. Within this framework are further similarities, such as reciprocal synapses and interneurons that lack axons.

The purpose of such a comparison is not, of course, to suggest that the two regions are identical; rather, it is to be able to identify more clearly the principles that are common across regions so that one can better analyze and understand the adaptations that make each region unique. Among the common principles is the notion that in each region there are three stages of information processing: an initial stage of *input processing*, a second stage of *intrinsic operations* within the synaptic circuits of the region, and a final stage of *output control*. These three levels can be seen most clearly in the basic circuits of tightly organized and highly laminar regions like the olfactory bulb and retina (see Fig. 1.13), but they are also evident in more spread-out regions

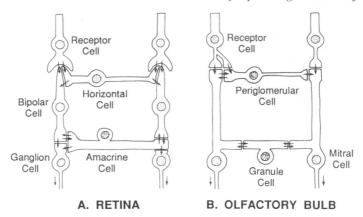

Fig. 1.13. Comparison between basic (canonical) circuits for the retina **(A)** and olfactory bulb **(B)**. [From Shepherd, 1974.]

like the cerebral cortex (Fig. 1.11). This approach thus provides a useful starting point for categorizing the overall organization of a region. In addition, it provides a rational framework for comparing the organization of disparate regions, a crucial step toward developing comprehensive theories of brain organization.

An objection to the idea of a basic (canonical) circuit is that it does not adequately represent the rich diversity of neural elements and synaptic connections that can be found in most brain regions. But the problem with this diversity is that it obscures the main issue of determining which properties are essential for which operations. This issue is critical not only for experimentalists attempting to analyze these operations but also for theorists who seek to incorporate these essential properties into network simulations.

FROM SYNAPTIC CIRCUITS TO NETWORK PROPERTIES

Now that we have examined the individual circuit components making up most brain regions and have studied some of the operations they can carry out, we are confronted with the challenge of understanding the resulting neural network within a given region consisting usually of hundreds of thousands of nerve cells interconnected by millions of synapses. These networks show emergent behaviors that may not be apparent or implied in their constituent elements. Furthermore, an understanding of the way the components are organized through their synaptic connections will be essential to understanding the functional properties and operating ranges of these behaviors.

An example of such an emergent property is shown in Fig. 1.14. Here three connection schemes are illustrated that possibly underly orientation selectivity in the mammalian visual cortex. Whereas cells in the lateral geniculate nucleus (LGN) have circular symmetrical receptive fields, their targets in the primary visual cortex (VI) have elongated receptive fields that respond best to an oriented bar (Fig. 1.14a). A large number of different wiring schemes have been proposed to explain this phenomenon, starting with the influential study of Hubel and Wiesel (1962). They postulated that a number of geniculate cells, with their receptive field centers arranged in a row, converge onto a cortical cell (Fig. 1.14b; for an overview, see Rose and Dobson, 1985; Ferster et al., 1996). Another class of models involves the use of the feedforward type of inhibition to prevent the cortical cell from firing if the visual stimulus falls on a neighboring region, outside the bar-shaped receptive field (Fig. 1.14c; *iso-orientation inhibition*; Sillito et al., 1980; Heggelund, 1981). So far, however, no significant population of nonoriented cells that could provide such inhibition has been reported in cat visual cortex. The same operation, however, can also be accomplished by a massively interconnected network of excitatory cortical cells, as indicated in Fig. 1.14d. The effect of such a network is that any preexisting bias for orientation in the lateral geniculate nucleus, even if weak, is amplified. Thus, in conjunction with inhibitory interconnections between cells, orientation selectivity is established by a collective network computation and not any one cell (Somers and Nelson, 1995). An important consequence is that no single neuron or biophysical mechanism is solely responsible for this orientation tuning, since the neurons act synergistically. If any one component fails, the overall system will perform, albeit at a somewhat reduced level of performance

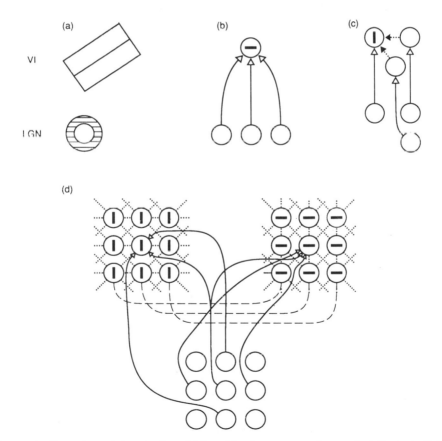

Fig. 1.14. Illustration of the way by which a selective response (e.g., orientation selectivity) arises as a network property. See text. [From Ferster and Koch, 1987, with permission.]

(referred to as *graceful degradation* in engineering terms). This will probably turn out to be a major feature of most biological computations. A further point is that even though all the different circuits in Fig. 1.14 lead to orientation selectivity, we cannot discover which ones are correct by mere theoretical considerations. Although many models have been proposed, all able in some measure to demonstrate orientation selectivity, it is only the experimental knowledge of the local synaptic circuits, the location and strength of inhibitory synapses, the detailed pharmacology, etc., which will enable us to identify the correct circuits underlying even this rather simple computation.

2

MEMBRANE PROPERTIES AND NEUROTRANSMITTER ACTIONS

DAVID A. McCORMICK

Information processing depends not only on the anatomical substrates of synaptic circuits but also on the electrophysiological properties of neurons and neuronal elements, and how these properties are altered and tuned by the plethora of neuroactive substances impinging upon them. Even if two neurons in different regions of the nervous system possess identical morphological features, they may respond to the same synaptic input in very different manners because of each cell's intrinsic properties. Understanding synaptic organization and function in different regions of the nervous system therefore requires an understanding of the electrophysiological and pharmacological properties of each of the constituent neuronal elements.

The electrophysiological behavior of a neuron is determined by the presence and distribution of different ionic currents in that cell, and by the ability of various neurotransmitters either to increase or decrease the amplitude or to modify the properties of these currents. This chapter will give a general overview of neuronal currents known to exist in brain cells, how they may be modulated by neurotransmitters, and how the interplay between the two can result in complicated patterns of activity in synaptic circuits. For a more detailed introduction to the biophysical mechanisms of ionic currents in neurons, the reader is referred to Hille, 1992; Nicholls et al., 1992; Huguenard and McCormick, 1994; and Johnston and Wu, 1995.

MEMBRANES AND IONIC CURRENTS

Neurons, like cells elsewhere in the body, are bounded by a lipid bilayer membrane that contains a large number of protein macromolecules. The lipid bilayer allows the composition of the medium on each side to be very different. Of particular importance for electrical signaling is the fact that certain key ions have different concentrations on the inside and outside of the neuron (Fig. 2.1). On the outside, Na^+, Ca^{2+}, and Cl^- exist in much higher concentrations; by contrast, K^+ ions and membrane-impermeant anions (denoted as A^-) are concentrated on the inside.

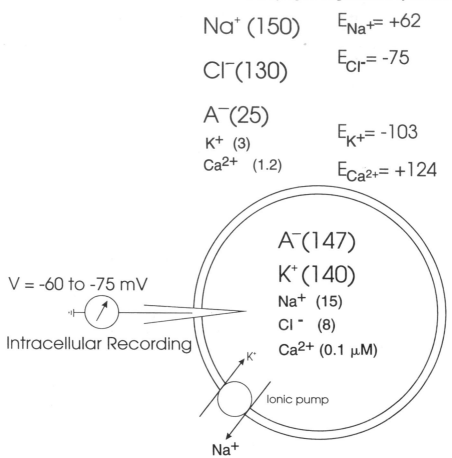

Fig. 2.1. Distribution of ions across neuronal membranes and their equilibrium potentials. At rest the cell membrane is permeable to K^+, Na^+, and Cl^- and exhibits a voltage difference (inside versus outside) of approximately -60 to -75 mV, as seen by an intracellular recording electrode.

Protein macromolecules in the membrane subserve a variety of functions. Those that underlie electrical signaling are large molecules that form ionic channels (see Ionic Channels, below). Membrane channels possess a number of important features, including the presence of a water-filled pore through which ions flow; selectivity for one or more types of ions (e.g., K^+, Na^+, Cl^-, Ca^{2+}); sensitivity to (i.e., opened or closed by) the electrical potential across the membrane or to a neurotransmitter substance, or both; and the ability to be modified by a variety of intracellular biochemical signals.

Because ions are unequally distributed across the membrane, they tend to diffuse down their concentration gradient through ionic channels. This tendency arises from the fact that the intrinsic movements of ions in a solution tend to disperse them from regions of higher to lower concentration. However, since ions are electrically charged molecules, their movements are dictated not only by concentration gradients but also by the voltage difference across the membrane. For example, if the membrane of a neuron were made permeable to K^+ ions by opening K^+ channels, the higher concentration of these ions on the inside versus the outside of the cell would make it more probable that K^+ ions would leave, rather than enter the cell. As K^+ ions exit the cell they carry positive charge with them, thereby leaving behind a net negative charge (made up in part of impermeant anions; Fig. 2.1). However, this negative charge (expressed as a *voltage difference*) on the inside versus the outside of the cell will attract the potassium ions and slow down the rate at which they leave. At some point, the tendency for K^+ to flow out of the cell will be offset exactly by the attraction of the negative charge left inside the cell. The voltage difference at which this occurs is known as the *equilibrium potential* (denoted as E) and is different for each ionic species (see Figs. 2.1 and 2.2). It will be seen later in this and other chapters that the equilibrium potential is important for determining the effect of activation (synaptic or intrinsic) of an ionic current.

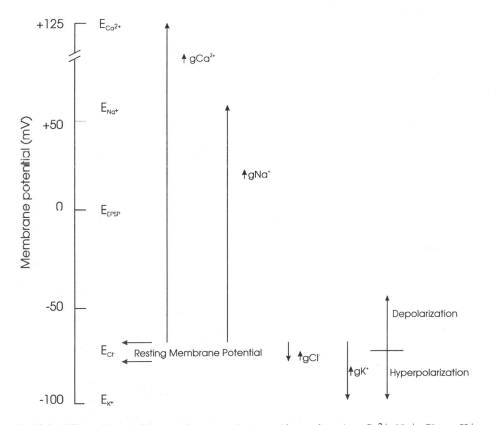

Fig. 2.2. Effect of increasing membrane conductance (denoted as g) to Ca^{2+}, Na^+, Cl^- or K^+. Increases in $g_{Ca^{2+}}$ or g_{Na^+} bring the membrane potential toward more positive values (depolarization), while increases in gCl^- or g_{K^+} brings it toward more negative values (hyperpolarization).

The flow of ions across the membrane obeys physical laws in a consistent and re-producible manner. Considering the basic forces involved in determining the passive distribution of ions (e.g., thermodynamic and electrical), it becomes clear that four of the important factors influencing the equilibrium potential are: *(1)* the concentration of the ion inside and outside the cell; *(2)* the temperature of the solution; *(3)* the valence of the ion; and *(4)* the amount of work associated with separating a given quantity of charge. A German physical chemist named Walter Nernst derived an equation in 1888 that related such factors, allowing for the calculation of the equilibrium potential (Nernst, 1888):

$$E_{Ion} = RT/zF \cdot \ln [Ion]_o/[Ion]_i \qquad (2.1)$$

where E_{Ion} is the membrane potential at which the ionic species under consideration (e.g., K^+, Na^+, Cl^-) is at equilibrium, R is the gas constant (8.315 Joules/Kelvin·mole), T is the temperature in degrees Kelvin ($T_{Kelvin} = 273.16 + T_{Celcius}$), F is Faraday's constant (96,485 Coulombs/mole), z is the valence of the ion (typically ± 1 or 2), and $[Ion]_o$ and $[Ion]_i$ are the concentrations of the ion in question on the outside and inside of the cell. Substituting the appropriate numbers as well as converting from natural log (ln) to log-base-10 ($\log_{10}$) results in the following equation at room temperature (20°C) for a monovalent, positively charged ion (cation):

$$E_{Ion} = 58.2 \log_{10} [Ion]_o/[Ion]_i \qquad (2.2)$$

and at a body temperature of 37°C the Nernst equation is:

$$E_{Ion} = 61.5 \log_{10} [Ion]_o/[Ion]_i \qquad (2.3)$$

As an example, consider the passive distribution of K^+ ions in the squid giant axon as studied by Alan Hodgkin and Andrew Huxley (1952 a–d). The squid giant axon is very large—approximately 1 mm in diameter—as its name implies, and is used by the squid for the generation of escape reflexes. The large size and robust nature of the squid giant axon allowed Hodgkin and Huxley in the 1940s and 50s to perform many different experiments, such as intracellular recording, that could not be performed at that time on mammalian neurons.

The inside of the squid giant axon has a concentration of K^+ of about 400 mM, while the outside of the axon is exposed to about 20 mM K^+. Since there are many more potassium ions on the inside versus the outside of this axon, they will tend to flow down their concentration gradient, taking positive charge with them as they do. The membrane potential at which the tendency for K^+ to flow down its concentration gradient will be exactly offset by the attraction for K^+ to enter the cell, because of the negative charge on the inside of the cell, at a room temperature of 20°C is:

$$E_K = 58.2 \log_{10} (20/400) = -76 \text{ mV} \qquad (2.4)$$

Therefore, at a membrane potential of -76 mV, there will be no net tendency for K^+ ions to flow either into or out of the axon.

The concentrations of K^+ experienced by mammalian neurons and glial cells are considerably different from that of the squid giant axon. In the mammalian brain the extracellular concentration of K^+ is approximately 3 mM whereas the intracellular concentration is approximately 140 mM (Fig. 2.1). Therefore, at a body temperature of 37°C, the equilibrium potential for K^+ in mammalian neurons is:

$$E_K = 61.5 \log_{10} (3.1/140) = -103 \text{ mV} \qquad (2.5)$$

At membrane potentials positive to -103 mV in mammalian cells, K^+ ions will tend to flow out of the cell, down their concentration gradient (Fig. 2.2). Therefore, at these membrane potentials, increasing the ability of K^+ ions to flow across the membrane, in other words, increasing the *conductance* of the membrane to K^+ (abbreviated as gK), will result in the membrane potential becoming more negative, or *hyperpolarizing*, because of the exiting of positively charged ions from the inside of the cell.

The ease with which an ion diffuses across the membrane is expressed as the ion's *permeability*. Increasing the permeability of the membrane to a particular ionic species (e.g., by increasing the probability that membrane channels which conduct that ion will be open) increases the electrical conductance and will bring the membrane potential of the cell closer to the equilibrium potential of that ion. This is true whether the membrane potential becomes more negative (i.e., hyperpolarized) or more positive (i.e., depolarized) towards the equilibrium potential. Of course, if the membrane potential is already at the equilibrium potential, then its value will not change in response to a further increase in conductance. In this circumstance, the most significant change will be that the ability of other currents to move the membrane potential away from its present potential will be diminished. For example, if the membrane were only slightly permeable to Cl^- ions, then increases in membrane conductance to other ionic species could easily move the membrane potential away from E_{Cl}. However, if the permeability to Cl^- were greatly increased, the membrane potential would be effectively "clamped" close to E_{Cl}. In this instance, movements of other ions into or out of the cell would now largely be offset by compensating movements of Cl^- ions, thereby keeping the membrane potential close to E_{Cl}.

For example, presume that the membrane is highly permeable to Cl^- and that the membrane potential is at E_{Cl}. If the membrane is now also made permeable to sodium, Na^+ ions will enter the cell. However, as the positive ions enter the cell and move the membrane potential away from E_{Cl}, Cl^- ions will also move into the cell, bringing the cell back towards E_{Cl} and negating some of the depolarizing influence of the increased permeability to Na^+. If the permeability to Cl^- is much higher than that to Na^+, then the membrane potential will stay close to E_{Cl}. As we shall see below, this type of "shunting" of the membrane potential near E_{Cl} is important in the actions of some types of inhibitory neurotransmitters.

RESTING MEMBRANE POTENTIAL

When there is no synaptic input, or the neuron is "at rest," the cellular membrane is dominated by its permeability to K^+. This permeability to potassium ions draws the membrane potential of the cell towards approximately -103 mV (see Figs. 2.1 and

2.2). If the membrane were only permeable to K^+, then the membrane potential would be equal to E_K. However, even at rest, neuronal membranes are also permeable to other ions, Na^+ and Cl^- in particular, so that the membrane potential is pulled towards E_{Na} (+62 mV) and E_{Cl} (−75 mV). The point at which the movements of these varied ions come into equilibrium such that there is no *net* current (denoted as *I*) flow across the membrane corresponds to the resting membrane potential and is typically between −60 and −75 mV (see Fig. 2.2).

The weighted mixture of all of the ionic currents flowing across the membrane determines the resting membrane potential, as well as the membrane potential during nearly all types of activity. This principle allows the calculation of the membrane potential at any given point in time by means of the *Goldman–Hodgkin–Katz* (GHK) equation, which is based upon the concentration gradient and membrane permeability (P) of each ion (Goldman, 1943; Hodgkin and Katz, 1949):

$$V_m = RT/F \cdot \ln \left((P_K[K^+]_o + P_{Na}[Na^+]_o + P_{Cl}[Cl^-]_i)/(P_K[K^+]_i + P_{Na}[Na^+]_i + P_{Cl}[Cl^-]_o) \right) \tag{2.6}$$

A consequence of this relationship of ionic currents and membrane potential is that, in general, the membrane potential of the cell will be closest to the equilibrium potential of the ion to which the membrane is most permeable (e.g., P_K, P_{Cl}, or P_{Na}). In this equation, each of the three different ions, K^+, Na^+, and Cl^- influence the membrane potential. The relative contribution of each is determined by the concentration differences across the membrane and the relative permeability (P_K, P_{Na}, P_{Cl}) of the membrane to each different type of ion. If the membrane were permeable to only one ion, for example K^+, then the GHK equation reduces to the Nernst equation. Experiments on the squid giant axon at resting membrane potential reveal permeability ratios of:

$$P_K:P_{Na}:P_{Cl} = 1/0.04/0.45 \tag{2.7}$$

In other words, the membrane of the squid giant axon at rest is most permeable to K^+ ions, followed by Cl^-, followed by a small permeability to Na^+. (Chloride appears to contribute considerably less to the determination of the resting potential of mammalian neurons.) These results indicate that the resting membrane potential is determined by the resting permeability of the membrane to K^+, Na^+, and Cl^-, and that this resting membrane potential may be, at least in theory, anywhere between E_K (e.g., −76 mV) and E_{Na} (+55 mV). Substituting in the values for the concentrations of Na^+, K^+, and Cl^- as well as their relative permeabilities into the GHK equation at a temperature of 20°C reveals:

$$V_m = 58.2 \log_{10} ((1 \cdot 20 + 0.04 \cdot 440 + 0.45 \cdot 40)/$$
$$(1 \cdot 400 + 0.04 \cdot 50 + 0.45 \cdot 560)) = -62 \text{ mV} \tag{2.8}$$

This suggests that the squid giant axon should have a resting membrane potential of −62 mV. In fact, the resting membrane potential may be a few millivolts hyperpolarized to this value through the operation of the electrogenic Na^+–K^+ pump (see below).

In the mammalian nervous system, the exact value of the resting membrane potential varies among different types of neurons and is very important in determining the manner in which a particular neuron behaves both spontaneously as well as in response to extrinsic inputs. For example, in the absence of synaptic input cortical pyramidal cells (Chap. 12) have a resting membrane potential of approximately -75 mV, thalamic relay neurons (Chap. 8) are at approximately -65 to -55 mV at rest in the waking animal, and retinal photoreceptor cells have a resting membrane potential of approximately -40 mV (Chap. 6). Some types of neurons do not have a true "resting" membrane potential in that they are spontaneously active even during the lack of all synaptic input (see below).

ACTION POTENTIAL

Rapid signaling in nerve cells is accomplished by brief changes in the membrane potential. Traditionally, the most characteristic type of signal has been considered to be the *action potential*, or *nerve impulse* (also referred to as a *spike*). Local action potentials in patches of dendritic membrane can also serve as boosters for the spread of synaptic potentials to the soma (as discussed in Chap. 1).

As with the resting membrane potential, the basic changes in membrane ionic permeability that underlie the action potential were first well characterized by Hodgkin and Huxley (1952a–d) using the squid giant axon preparation. The large size of the squid giant axon allowed Hodgkin and Huxley to thread a wire into the axon, giving them the ability to control accurately the membrane potential by a procedure known as *voltage clamp*. In this procedure, the amount of current injected into the cell is adjusted so that the voltage across the membrane is kept constant (i.e., the voltage is "clamped"). This technique not only allows one to observe directly the transmembrane currents responsible for the electrical behavior of the cell, but also to measure the current's kinetics and sensitivity to membrane potential. The isolation of the squid giant axon in vitro meant that Hodgkin and Huxley could also control the ionic composition of the medium on the outside as well as the inside of the axon. These experiments revealed that the rapid upswing of the action potential is mediated by a regenerative increase in a transient Na^+ current, denoted $I_{Na,t}$ (Fig. 2.3). Since $I_{Na,t}$ is rapidly activated by depolarization and is itself a depolarizing influence, it forms a positive feedback loop in the unclamped axon, as shown in Fig. 2.3A. Depolarization of the membrane causes a rapid increase in the number of Na^+ channels that are open, thereby allowing more Na^+ ions to enter the cell, resulting in even more depolarization of that portion of membrane, increased entry of Na^+, and so on.

Membrane currents that change their amplitude in response to changes in the membrane in a "nonlinear" manner, such as $I_{Na,t}$, are referred to as *voltage sensitive*, while the ionic channels that underlie these currents are said to be *voltage gated*. The depolarization caused by entry of Na^+ ions into the cell spreads to neighboring membrane by *electrotonic* current flow. The depolarization of one patch of membrane will also depolarize neighboring patches of membrane. The subsequent activation of the same

THE ACTION POTENTIAL

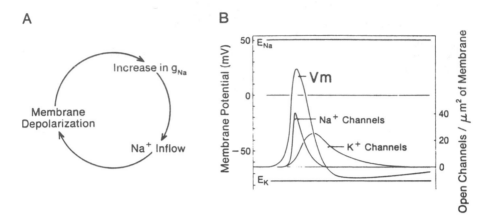

Fig. 2.3. **A:** Regenerative relation between membrane depolarization, increase in membrane conductance to Na^+ (gNa), and Na^+ current that underlies the action potential. **B:** Reconstruction of changes in ionic conductance underlying the action potential in squid giant axon; scale for the membrane potential (V_m) is shown on the left. The equilibrium potentials for Na (E_{Na}) and K^+ (E_K) are also indicated on the left. Changes in Na^+ and K^+ ionic conductances are scaled on the right in terms of calculated open channels per square micrometer of membrane. [Adapted from Hodgkin and Huxley, 1952d and Hille, 1992, with permission.]

regenerative mechanisms at these sites underlies the propagation of the action potential along the axon.

Repolarization of the action potential is very important not only because of the obvious need to be able to generate more than one action potential during the life of the cell, but also in determining the way the cell responds to repetitive inputs. Two processes are essential for the repolarization of the action potential in most neurons: the rapid inactivation of $I_{Na,t}$ and the activation of K currents. The rate of *inactivation* (termed *inactivation kinetics*) of $I_{Na,t}$ is only slightly slower than the rate of activation. Even during the rising phase of the action potential, the available Na^+ current becomes less and less because of inactivation. Simultaneously, but with a slower time course, a K^+ current, known as I_K, is activated by the membrane depolarization associated with the action potential, allowing K^+ to leave the cell. These two currents, flowing through their respective ionic channels, are indicated in Fig. 2.3B. At some point the hyperpolarizing influence of K^+ leaving overcomes the depolarizing influence of Na^+ entering, thereby terminating the action potential and repolarizing the membrane.

The triggering of an action potential occurs when the membrane potential of the neuron is depolarized sufficiently to reach action potential *threshold*. In many cells, this potential is approximately -50 to -55 mV. Action potential threshold is the membrane potential at which the regenerative activation of depolarizing currents (e.g., $I_{Na,t}$) is strong enough to overcome the inactivation of these currents as well as the activation of others that hyperpolarize the neuron back towards rest. At threshold, the generation of an action potential is an all-or-nothing event. If threshold is surpassed, an action potential is generated and the information is transferred down the axon to cause the release of neurotransmitter at synapses. If firing threshold is not reached by a depolarizing event, an action potential is not produced and the event is not relayed to other cells. However, as we shall see, the depolarization can still serve to modify the probability that other post-synaptic potentials in the neuron may cause the cell to discharge.

Since 1952, it has become apparent that $I_{Na,t}$ is the dominant current in the generation of action potentials in axons and cell bodies. However, in somatic and dendritic regions, voltage-gated Ca^{2+} currents are also involved, as documented below and in ensuing chapters (e.g., see Fig. 2.5B,C,E). In mammalian somata and dendrites, in contrast to squid giant axon, repolarization of action potentials is accomplished not only by I_K but also by a complicated array of different K currents (see sections on I_K, I_C, and I_A below).

IONIC CHANNELS

The generation of ionic currents useful for the propagation of action potentials requires the movement of significant numbers of ions across the membrane in a relatively short period of time. The rapid rate of ionic flow occurring during the generation of an action potential is far too high to be achieved by an active transport mechanism, but rather results from the opening of ion channels. Although the existence of ionic channels in the membrane has been postulated for decades, their properties and structure have only recently become known in detail. The development by Erwin Neher and Bert Sakmann of the patch clamp technique, in which a small patch of membrane containing a single or small number of ionic channel(s) is drawn up into a blunt microelectrode allowed for the miniscule (10^{-12} or picoamperes) currents flowing through single channels to be recorded in intact biological membranes for the first time (Neher and Sakmann, 1976, 1992; Hamill et al., 1981; Sakmann, 1992). In addition, the rapid advances made by molecular biology in the isolation, cloning, and sequencing of the proteins making up ionic channels have revealed much about their primary structure. The powerful combination of electrophysiological and molecular techniques together has yielded valuable insights into the structure–function relationships of ionic channels (see reviews by Miller, 1989; Anderson and Koeppe, 1992; Catterall, 1988, 1992, 1995; Salkoff et al., 1992).

Voltage-sensitive ionic channels appear to have several shared features. First, they are large proteins that span the 6–8 nm of the plasma membrane and are typically made up of subunits. Second, through protein folding, they form a cylinder surrounding a central water-filled pore that permits the passage of only certain classes of ions between the inside and outside of the cell. The selection of which ions are allowed to pass through each different type of ionic channel is based upon the size, charge, and degree of hydration of the different ions involved (see Hille, 1992). Finally, voltage-gated ion channels possess one or more "gates," or voltage-sensing regions within the ionic pore, and the flow of ions through the channels is regulated by these gates.

IONIC PUMPS

The quantity of ions that enter and exit the cell during electrical activity is actually very small in comparison with the number of ions present. For example, the generation of a single action potential in a hypothetical spherical cell 25 μm in diameter should result in an increase of intracellular concentration of Na^+ of only approximately 6 μM (from approximately 15 mM to 15.006 mM)! This means that the action potential is an electrical event that is generated by a change in the distribution of charge across the membrane and not by a marked change in intracellular or extracellular concentration of Na^+ or K^+.

However, even these small exchanges of ions across the membrane coupled with a constant "leak" at rest can eventually destroy the correct ionic distribution and thereby render a neuron nonfunctional. To compensate for this "rundown," neuronal membranes possess specialized protein macromolecules known as *ionic pumps*. Ionic pumps maintain the correct distribution of all of the ions involved in electrical activity by actively transporting these ions "upstream" against their concentration gradient. The energy required to perform this task is sometimes obtained through the hydrolysis of ATP (adenosine triphosphate). The ionic pump that has been best characterized is the electrogenic sodium-potassium pump (see Thomas, 1972; Skou, 1988). This ionic pump carries approximately three Na^+ ions out for every two K^+ ions it brings in, thereby generating an electric current (Fig. 2.1). The exact amplitude of this current depends upon the rate at which the pump is active, which is in turn related to the intracellular concentration of Na^+ and the extracellular concentration of K^+.

Besides the electrogenic Na^+–K^+ pump, neurons and glia also contain many other types of ionic pumps in their membranes (e.g., Pedersen and Carafoli, 1987; Läuger, 1991). Many of these pumps are operated by the Na^+ gradient across the cell, while others operate through a mechanism similar to the Na^+–K^+ pump (i.e., the hydrolysis of ATP). For example, the calcium concentration inside neurons is kept to very low levels (typically 50–100 nM) through the operation of both types of ionic pumps as well as special intracellular Ca^{2+}-buffering mechanisms. Ca^{2+} is extruded from neurons through both a Ca^{2+}–Mg^{2+} ATPase as well as a Na^+–Ca^{2+} exchanger. The Na^+–Ca^{2+} exchanger is driven by the Na^+ gradient across the membrane and extrudes one Ca^{2+} ion for each Na^+ ion allowed to enter the cell.

The Cl^- concentration in neurons is actively maintained at a low level through the operation of a chloride-bicarbonate exchanger, which brings in one ion of Na^+ and one ion of HCO_3^- for each ion of Cl^- extruded (e.g., Thompson et al., 1988; Reithmeier, 1994). Finally, intracellular pH can also have marked effects on neuronal excitability and therefore pH is also tightly regulated, in part through the efforts of a Na^+–H^+ exchanger which, again, extrudes one proton for each Na^+ that is allowed to enter the cell.

Ionic pumps are essential and important constituents of neurons and neuronal membranes. Their time scale of action is seconds to minutes and they are therefore thought of as being more involved in long-term rather than short-term neuronal processing.

TYPES OF IONIC CURRENTS

Neurons in the nervous system do not simply lie at rest and occasionally generate an action potential. Rather, neuronal membranes are in a constant state of flux because of the presence of a remarkable variety of different ionic currents (Table 2.1). These cur-

Table 2.1. Neuronal Ionic Currents

Current	Description	Function
Na⁺		
I_{Na} or $I_{Na,t}$	Transient; rapidly activating and inactivating	Action potentials
$I_{Na,p}$	Persistent; non-inactivating	Enhances depolarization; contributes to steady-state firing
Ca²⁺		
I_T, low threshold	Transient; rapidly inactivating; threshold negative to -65 mV	Underlies rhythmic burst firing
I_L, high threshold	Long-lasting; slowly inactivating; threshold around -20 mV	Underlies Ca²⁺ spikes that are prominent in dendrites; involved in synaptic transmission
I_N	Neither; rapidly inactivating; threshold around -20 mV	Underlies Ca²⁺ spikes that are prominent in dendrites; involved in synaptic transmission
I_P	Purkinje; threshold around -50 mV	Underlies Ca²⁺ spikes that are prominent in dendrites
K⁺		
I_K	Activated by strong depolarization	Repolarization of action potential
I_C	Activated by increases in $[Ca^{2+}]_i$	Action potential repolarization and interspike interval
I_{AHP}	Slow afterhyperpolarization; sensitive to increases in $[Ca^{2+}]_i$	Slow adaptation of action potential discharge; the block of this current by neuromodulators enhances neuronal excitability
I_A	Transient; inactivating	Delayed onset of firing; lengthens interspike interval; action potential repolarization
I_M	Muscarine sensitive; activated by depolarization; non-inactivating	Contributes to spike frequency adaptation; the block of this current by neuromodulators enhances neuronal excitability
I_h	Depolarizing (mixed cation) current that is activated by hyperpolarization	Contributes to rhythmic burst firing and other rhythmic activities
$I_{K,leak}$	Contributes to neuronal resting membrane potential	The block of this current by neuromodulators can result in a sustained change in membrane potential

rents are distinguished not only by the ions that they conduct (e.g., K^+, Na^+, Ca^{2+}, Cl^-) but also by their time course, sensitivity to membrane potential, and sensitivity to neurotransmitters and other chemical agents (for review see Llinás, 1988; Rudy, 1988; Storm, 1990; Hille, 1992; McCormick and Huguenard, 1992; Johnson and Wu, 1995; Stea et al., 1995). As the various ionic currents were discovered they were divided into two general categories: those that are sensitive to changes in membrane potential and those that are altered by neurotransmitters and internal messengers. However, with the recent discovery of a number of voltage-sensitive ionic channels they are also gated by neurotransmitters, and vice versa, it has become apparent that there is substantial overlap between these two groups. The currents that possess both voltage and neurotransmitter sensitivity have received much recent attention because of their ability to modulate the electrical behavior of neurons in unusual and interesting ways (see Chemical Synapses below).

Most currents that are sensitive to membrane potential are turned on (*activated*) by depolarization. The rate at which they activate as well as the membrane potential at which they start to become active (*threshold*) are important characteristics. Many voltage-dependent currents do not stay on once they are activated even during a constant shift in membrane potential. The process by which they turn off despite a stable level of membrane potential in their activation range is known as *inactivation*. Inactivation is a state of the current and ionic channels that is distinct from simple channel closure. Once a current becomes inactive, this inactivation must be removed before it can again be activated. *Removal of inactivation* is generally achieved by repolarization of the membrane potential. Like the process of activation, inactivation and removal of inactivation are time and membrane potential dependent. Together, all of these characteristics define the temporal and voltage domain over which the current influences the electrical activity of the neuron.

The names given to each ionic current often reflect one of the properties which distinguishes that current from the others. If the current is activated by relatively small deviations in the membrane potential (denoted as V_m) from rest, than it may be known as *low threshold* (for example, low-threshold Ca^{2+} current), whereas if the current is activated only at levels that are substantially positive (depolarized) from rest, the current may be known as *high threshold* (e.g., high-threshold Ca^{2+} current). In addition, if activation of the current through a constant and steady change in membrane potential (i.e., under voltage clamp conditions in which the membrane potential is held constant) leads to only a transient response, then it is known as *transient* or *rapidly inactivating* (examples are the A current and the T current). Likewise, a current that persists during constant activation (i.e., is noninactivating) is known as *sustained*, *persistent*, or *long lasting* (e.g., persistent Na^+ current and the L, or long-lasting, Ca^{2+} current).

The ionic currents that determine the neuronal firing behavior of neurons in different regions of the nervous system have been intensively investigated. To date, at least a dozen distinct neuronal currents, many of which are common to neurons at all levels of the neuraxis, have been identified (Table 2.1). We will briefly summarize these currents and the unique contribution that each makes to the firing behavior of neurons (see Fig. 2.4).

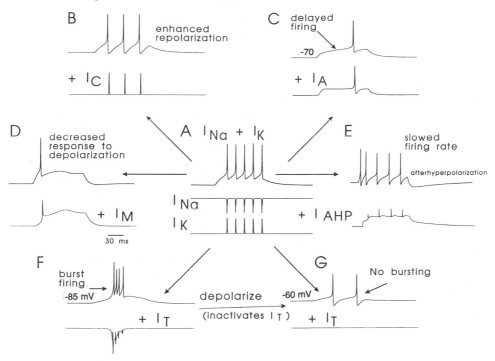

Fig. 2.4. A summary of different types of voltage-gated currents and the impulse firing patterns they produce in a neuron in response to steady injection of depolarizing current. At the center (**A**) is shown the repetitive impulse response of the classical Hodgkin-Huxley model (voltage recording above, current recordings below). Radiating out from this are changes in this pattern associated with the different types of ionic channels. **B**: Addition of the Ca^{2+}-activated K^+ current I_C (and the high-threshold Ca^{2+} current I_L) facilitates the repolarization of each action potential. **C**: Addition of the depolarization-activated but transient K^+ current I_A results in a delay to onset of action potential generation. **D**: Addition of the depolarization-activated but persistent K^+ current I_M results in a marked decrease in neuronal excitability. **E**: Addition of the slow Ca^{2+}-activated K^+ current I_{AHP} results in spike frequency adaptation and the generation of a slow hyperpolarization after the action potential train (afterhyperpolarization). **F**: Addition of the low-threshold and transient Ca^{2+} current I_T results in the generation of a burst of action potentials at -85 mV. **G**: Depolarization of the cell in F to -60 mV results in inactivation of I_T and now the cell generates a train of two action potentials. [Modified from Shepherd, 1994.] These traces are the result of computer simulations (Huguenard and McCormick, 1994).

SODIUM (NA) CURRENTS

Two sodium currents, $I_{Na,t}$ (transient) and $I_{Na,p}$ (persistent), are widely distributed in neurons from different regions of the nervous system. These two currents are distinguished from one another by their rate of inactivation, their threshold for activation, and their amplitude.

$I_{Na,t}$ Transient Sodium. As we have noted, the transient Na^+ ($I_{Na,t}$) current rapidly inactivates within a few milliseconds during steady depolarization. All central neurons stud-

ied to date possess a large $I_{Na,t}$, whereas $I_{Na,p}$ is considerably smaller in amplitude. The rapid activation and inactivation properties of $I_{Na,t}$ makes this current ideal for its role in the generation of action potentials (Fig. 2.4A).

$I_{Na,p}$ Persistent Sodium. In contrast to $I_{Na,t}$, the persistent Na^+ ($I_{Na,p}$) current shows little, if any, inactivation. This current is also rapidly activated by membrane depolarization, but its non-inactivating nature allows it to serve a very different role in neuronal function (Hotson et al., 1979; Llinás, 1981, 1988; Stafstrom et al., 1985). A large percentage of neuronal computations occur in a narrow range of membrane potential between approximately -75 and -50 mV. This range is between resting membrane potential and a level of depolarization at which the neuron is firing repeatedly at a high rate. The nature of $I_{Na,p}$ is such that it is activated by depolarizations, such as synaptic potentials, that bring the membrane potential from rest to near action potential firing threshold. The added depolarizing influence of the influx of Na^+ ions resulting from the activation of $I_{Na,p}$ serves to enhance markedly the response of the neuron to excitatory inputs. This may result in the generation of *plateau potentials* (Fig. 2.5C), which are prolonged depolarizations that persist despite the removal of all other depolarizing influences in the cell (such as a synaptic potential or the intracellular injection of current).

The amplitude and cellular distribution of $I_{Na,p}$ can therefore have an important role in determining the responsiveness of neurons. The persistent nature of $I_{Na,p}$ allows this current to participate in the determination of the baseline firing rate of neurons. $I_{Na,p}$ appears to be especially important to the ability of some neurons to maintain intrinsic "pacemaker" activity (e.g., the generation of action potentials in a repeated temporal pattern in the absence of synaptic input). In these cells, the steady influx of Na^+ ions into the neuron depolarizes the cell to above firing threshold, thereby triggering baseline activity. The membrane potential of these cells is in a state of constant change, cycling through the generation of an action potential to the repolarization of the cell (see Potassium (K) Currents below) to again the generation of an action potential. Examples of such neurons in the CNS are those of the locus coeruleus, dorsal raphe, and medial habenula (see Fig. 2.5F; Vandermaelen and Aghajanian, 1983; Williams et al., 1984; McCormick and Prince, 1987b).

CALCIUM (CA) CURRENTS

Ionic channels that conduct Ca^{2+} are present in all neurons. These channels are special in that they serve two important functions. First, Ca^{2+} channels are present throughout the different parts of the neuron (dendrites, soma, synaptic terminals) and contribute greatly to the electrophysiological properties of these processes (Llinás, 1988; Regehr and Tank, 1994; Markram et al., 1995). Second, Ca^{2+} channels are unique in that Ca^{2+} is an important second messenger in neurons and entry of Ca^{2+} into the cell can affect numerous physiological functions, including neurotransmitter release, synaptic plasticity, neurite outgrowth during development, and even gene expression.

Calcium currents have been separated into at least four separate categories based upon their voltage sensitivity and kinetics of activation and inactivation as well as their block by various pharmacological agents. Differences in the kinetics and pharmacology of three different categories of Ca^{2+} currents led Richard Tsien and col-

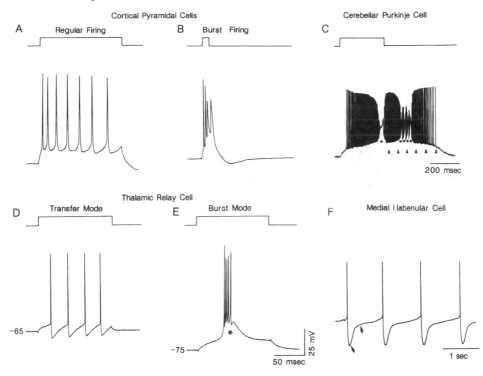

Fig. 2.5. Electrophysiological behavior of neurons in different regions of the mammalian brain.
A: Example of a "regular" firing cortical pyramidal neuron. Intracellular injection of a depolarizing current pulse (top trace) results in the generation of a train of action potentials that occur at progressively slower frequencies (spike frequency adaptation). **B:** By contrast, intracellular injection of depolarizing current pulses into a "burst" generating cortical pyramidal neuron results in the clustering of action potentials together on top of a slow potential. **C:** Electrical activity of a cerebellar Purkinje cell in response to intracellular injection of a depolarizing current pulse. The cell generates initially a high-frequency discharge of fast Na^+-dependent action potentials (generated in the soma). This discharge is modulated by the occurrence of dendritic Ca^{2+} spikes (asterisks). The discharge outlasts the duration of the intracellular depolarizing pulse (top trace) because of the presence of a plateau potential mediated by $I_{Na,p}$ and calcium currents (arrowheads). **D:** Depolarization of thalamic relay neuron results in the generation of a train of four action potentials if the membrane potential is positive to approximately -65 mV, but a burst of action potentials if the cell is at or negative to -75 mV (**E**). The low-threshold Ca^{2+} spike underlying this burst discharge is indicated by an asterisk. **F:** Example of a neuron in the medial habenula that generates intrinsic "pacemaker" discharge. Intracellular recording reveals the presence of large hyperpolarizations after each action potential which are complicated in time course and help determine the rate at which the neuron fires (arrows).

leagues (Nowycky et al., 1985) to name them I_T ("transient"), I_L ("long-lasting"), and I_N ("neither") (see also Carbonne and Lux, 1984). More recent experiments by Rodolfo Llinás and colleagues (reviewed in Llinás et al., 1992) demonstrated that Purkinje cells of the cerebellum, as well as many different cell types of the CNS, also possess another Ca^{2+} current termed I_P. Molecular biology has revealed a wide variety of genes involved in the production of Ca^{2+} channels, and it is certain that more Ca^{2+}

currents are yet to be characterized (e.g., see Tsien et al., 1991; Birnbaumer et al., 1994).

High-threshold Ca^{2+} Currents. Most Ca^{2+} channels are activated at membrane potentials positive to approximately -40 mV; these are termed *high-voltage activated* (HVA). These Ca^{2+} channels include at least those underlying the currents I_L, I_N, and I_P. These three different ionic currents are separable from one another through examination of their voltage dependence and kinetics of activation and inactivation, and through their sensitivity to various Ca^{2+} channel blockers and neural toxins. The Ca^{2+} channel antagonists known as dihydropyridines, which clinically are useful for their effects on the heart and vascular smooth muscle (e.g., for the treatment of arrhythmias, angina, and migraine headaches), selectively block the L-type Ca^{2+} channels (reviewed by Bean, 1989; Stea et al., 1995). L-type calcium currents exhibit a high threshold for activation (around -10 mV) and give rise to rather persistent, or long-lasting, ionic currents. In contrast to I_L, I_N is not blocked by dihydropyridines, but rather is selectively blocked by a toxin found in Pacific cone shells (ω-conotoxin-GVIA). N-type Ca^{2+} channels have a threshold for activation of around -20 mV, inactivate with maintained depolarization, and are modulated by a variety of neurotransmitters. In at least some cell types I_N is involved in the Ca^{2+}-dependent release of neurotransmitters at presynaptic terminals (e.g., Wheeler et al., 1994).

P-type calcium channels are distinct from N and L in that they are not blocked by either dihydropyridines or ω-conotoxin-GVIA but by a toxin (termed ω-Agatoxin-IVA) present in the venom of the Funnel web spider (Llinás et al., 1992; Stea et al., 1995). P-type calcium channels activate at relatively high thresholds and do not inactivate. This type of calcium channel appears to be prevalent in Purkinje cells, as well as in other cell types, and participates in the generation of dendritic Ca^{2+} spikes, which can strongly modulate the firing pattern of the neuron in which they occur (see Fig. 2.5C).

Collectively, the high threshold–activated Ca^{2+} channels also contribute to the generation of action potentials in mammalian neurons. The activation of these Ca^{2+} currents adds a bit to the depolarizing portion of the action potential, but more importantly, they allow Ca^{2+} to enter the cell and this has the secondary consequence of activation of various Ca^{2+}-activated K^+ currents (reviewed in Latorre et al., 1989). The activation of these K^+ currents then modifies the pattern of action potentials generated in the cell, as mentioned above (Fig. 2.4B,E).

Molecular biological studies have demonstrated that high-threshold Ca^{2+} channels are similar to the Na^+ channel in that they contain a central α_1 subunit that forms the aqueous pore and several regulatory or auxiliary subunits. As in the Na^+ channel, the primary structure of the α_1 subunits of Ca^{2+} channels consists of four homologous domains (I–IV), each of which contain six regions (S1–S6) that may generate transmembrane α-helices. The genes for at least five different Ca^{2+} channel α-subunits have been cloned (α_{1A-E}), and the properties of the different products of these genes indicate that I_L is likely to correspond to α_{1C} and α_{1D}, while I_N corresponds to α_{1B} and I_P may be related to α_{1A} (reviewed in Birnbaumer et al., 1994; Stea et al., 1995).

Low-threshold Ca^{2+} Currents. Low-threshold Ca^{2+} currents, also known as the *transient Ca^{2+} current I_T*, are also present in many different cell types in the nervous system and are often involved in the generation of rhythmic bursts of action potentials (Figs. 2.4F, 2.5E). The low-threshold Ca^{2+} current is characterized by a threshold for activation of around -65 mV, which is below the threshold for generation of typical Na^+/K^+-dependent action potentials (-55 mV). Another important feature of this current is that it inactivates with maintained depolarization. Owing to these properties, this Ca^{2+} current can perform a markedly different role in neurons from that of the high-threshold Ca^{2+} currents. Through activation and inactivation of the low-threshold Ca^{2+} current, neurons can generate slow (around 50–100 msec) Ca^{2+} spikes, which, because of their prolonged duration, can result in the generation of a high-frequency "burst" of short-duration Na^+/K^+ action potentials (Figs. 2.4F, 2.5E).

In the mammalian brain, this pattern is especially well exemplified by the activity of thalamic relay neurons, which in the visual system receive direct input from the retina and transmit this information to the visual cortex. During periods of slow-wave sleep, the membrane potential of these relay neurons is relatively hyperpolarized, resulting in the removal of inactivation (de-inactivation) of the low-threshold Ca^{2+} current. This allows these cells to spontaneously generate low-threshold Ca^{2+} "spikes" and bursts of 2 to 5 action potentials (Fig. 2.5E). The large number of thalamic relay cells bursting during sleep in part gives rise to the spontaneous synchronized activity that early investigators were so surprised to find upon recording activity in the brains of sleeping animals (reviewed in Steriade et al., 1993). It has even proved possible to maintain one of the sleep-related brain rhythms (spindle waves) intact in slices of thalamic tissue maintained in vitro, owing to the activation of low-threshold Ca^{2+} spikes and bursts of action potentials in networks of interacting thalamic cells (von Krosigk et al., 1993).

The transition to waking or the period of sleep when dreams are prevalent (rapid-eye-movement sleep) is associated with a maintained depolarization of thalamic relay cells to membrane potentials of around -60 to -55 mV. This maintained depolarization results in the inactivation of the low-threshold Ca^{2+} current and therefore an abolition of burst discharges in these neurons (see Figs. 2.4G, 2.5D). In this way, the properties of a single ionic current (I_T) help to explain in part the remarkable changes in brain activity occurring in the transition from sleep to waking!

Low-threshold Ca^{2+} channels have not yet been purified and sequenced, in part because of the lack of an agent that binds to these receptors with high affinity. Recent evidence suggests that some antiepileptic drugs may exert their therapeutic actions through a reduction in I_T. This is especially true of the drugs useful in the treatment of generalized absence (petit mal) seizures, which are known to rely upon the thalamus for their generation (see Coulter et al., 1990).

POTASSIUM (K) CURRENTS

Neuronal potassium currents form a large and diversified group. They are intimately involved in determining the pattern of activity generated by neurons. Because they are hyperpolarizing, they are responsible not only for the repolarization of the action potential, but also for the determination of the *probability* of generation of an action potential at any given point in time. As with other neuronal currents, potassium currents are distinguished by their voltage and time dependency, as well as by pharmacological techniques (reviewed in Jan and Jan, 1990; Storm, 1990; Salkoff et al., 1992; Johnston and Wu, 1995).

Recent molecular biological studies of voltage-sensitive K^+ channels, first done in *Drosophila* and later in mammals, have revealed the presence of four distinct gene families, *Shaker*, *Shab*, *Shaw*, and *Shal* (reviewed in Salkoff et al., 1992), that correspond to the newer nomenclature of Kv1, Kv2, Kv3, and Kv4 subfamilies (reviewed in Chandy and Gutman, 1995). These genes generate a wide variety of different K^+ channels through alternative RNA splicing and gene duplication. Functional expression of these different K^+ channels reveals remarkable variation in the rate of inactivation: *Shaker* channels are typically rapidly inactivating (A-current-like), *Shal* channels inactivate more slowly, *Shab* channels inactivate very slowly, and *Shaw* channels typically do not inactivate, in similarity with I_K. These studies indicate that each different type of neuron in the nervous system is likely to contain a unique set of functional voltage-sensitive K^+ channels, which are perhaps selected, modified, and placed in particular spatial locations in the cell in a manner to facilitate the unique role of that cell in neuronal processing.

I_K Delayed Rectifier. As we have seen, the early studies in the squid giant axon not only defined the role of the transient Na^+ current in the generation of the action potential but also identified an important outward potassium current known as the *delayed rectifier* or I_K. The activation kinetics of I_K are slower than those of the transient sodium current and therefore it appears somewhat "delayed" (Fig. 2.3B). This potassium current is voltage sensitive, being activated at membrane potentials positive to approximately -40 mV, and it only slowly inactivates. I_K is found in neurons throughout the nervous system and typically contributes to the repolarization of action potentials and the hyperpolarization that follows them (Figs. 2.3B and 2.4A).

Calcium-Activated Potassium Currents. An additional class of potassium currents that are important for determining the firing behavior of neurons are those that are Ca^{2+}-sensitive (denoted $I_{K,Ca}$). This family of potassium currents is activated by increases in the intracellular concentration of unbound Ca^{2+} ($[Ca^{2+}]_i$). Two $I_{K,Ca}$ currents have been widely identified in neurons: I_C and I_{AHP} (see Adams and Galvan, 1986; Rudy, 1988; Storm, 1990). I_C is not only sensitive to increases in $[Ca^{2+}]_i$ in the micromolar range but is also strongly voltage dependent, becoming larger with depolarization. I_C helps control the frequency of action potential generation during a steady depolarization by causing a marked hyperpolarization after the occurrence of each spike (Fig. 2.4B). I_C may even be important in some neurons in repolarization of the action potential. The voltage dependence of I_C results in its rapid inactivation once the membrane potential is repolarized. This inactivation constrains the influence of I_C in the temporal domain to tens of milliseconds or less.

I_{AHP}, in contrast to I_C, is much slower in time course and not very voltage dependent. Its influence on the membrane potential of the cell is best seen after the generation of a number of action potentials as a prolonged **afterhyper**polarization, for which it is named. This potassium current contributes significantly to the tendency of the firing frequency of some types of neurons (e.g., cortical and hippocampal pyramidal neurons) to decrease during maintained depolarizations, a process known as *spike frequency adaptation* (Fig. 2.4E; see below).

The generation of action potentials, by increasing $[Ca^{2+}]_i$ through L- or N-type Ca^{2+} channels, triggers I_C and I_{AHP}. The hyperpolarizations of the membrane potential resulting from K^+ leaving the cell during these currents regulate the rate at which the neuron fires. Due to its short time course, I_C contributes substantially to short interspike intervals. In contrast, because of its slow activation and prolonged time course, I_{AHP} contributes more to the overall pattern of spike activity. The relatively nonvoltage-dependent nature of I_{AHP} means that the influence of this current on the membrane potential is more closely related to changes in $[Ca^{2+}]_i$ than is I_C. Importantly, the amount of I_{AHP} appears to be under the control of putative neurotransmitters (see Decrease of I_{AHP} below).

Transient Potassium Currents. The first of a family of potassium currents that are activated by membrane depolarization and then undergo relatively rapid inactivation was discovered in molluscan neurons (Connor and Stevens, 1971; Neher, 1971) and termed I_A. The A current is a transient K current: after its activation by depolarization of the membrane potential positive to approximately −60 mV, it rapidly inactivates. Like other transient and voltage-activated currents (e.g., $I_{Na,t}$ and I_T), this inactivation is removed by repolarization of the membrane potential. I_A is involved in the response of neurons to a sudden depolarization from hyperpolarized membrane potentials and serves to delay the onset of the generation of the first action potential (Fig. 2.4C). I_A can also slow a neuron's firing frequency during a maintained depolarization and help to repolarize the action potential. For example, in a spontaneously active neuron, the hyperpolarization that occurs after the generation of an action potential will remove some of the inactivation of I_A. As the membrane potential depolarizes back towards firing threshold, I_A will be activated and slow down the rate of depolarization. Once firing threshold is reached and an action potential is generated, the rapid depolarization may activate more of I_A, which then helps to repolarize the cell. In this manner, I_A can be an important current in the determination of firing behavior of neurons.

Muscarine-Sensitive Potassium Currents. Another type of potassium current was discovered in sympathetic ganglion neurons of bullfrogs by David Brown and Paul Adams (1980). This potassium current is activated by depolarization of the membrane potential positive to approximately −65 mV, does not inactivate with time, and is blocked by stimulation of muscarinic cholinergic receptors (hence its name, I_M). I_M is found in neurons throughout the nervous system, including pyramidal cells of the cerebral cortex and hippocampus (reviewed in Brown, 1988; Nicoll et al., 1990; McCormick, 1992). Depolarizations that are large enough to result in the generation of action potentials also cause the activation of I_M. However, because of its relatively slow kinetics and modest amplitude, I_M probably does not affect substantially the waveform of a single action potential, but rather contributes to the slow adaptation of spike frequency seen during a maintained depolarization (Fig. 2.4D).

Currents activated by Hyperpolarization. Hyperpolarization of neurons in many regions of the nervous system results in the activation of a current that brings the membrane potential toward more positive values (e.g., back towards rest). This current, or family of currents, is generally referred to as I_h ("hyperpolarization-activated"), although it has also been given such lively names as I_Q ("queer") and I_f ("funny") (Halliwell and Adams, 1982; DiFrancesco, 1985; Crepel and Penit-Soria, 1986; McCormick and

Pape, 1990). The currents in this family are carried by both Na^+ and K^+ ions and are relatively slow in time course, although this varies widely between different cell types.

The activation of I_h has been demonstrated to be important in the generation of rhythmic oscillations in at least thalamic relay neurons and some types of cardiac cells (McCormick and Pape, 1990; DiFrancesco, 1985). The activation of the h current results in the slow depolarization of the cell, and in so doing, generates a "pacemaker" potential that can activate repetitive Na^+ and/or Ca^{2+} spikes (see Fig. 2.12B).

SUMMARY OF INTRINSIC MEMBRANE PROPERTIES

Neurons possess a virtual cornucopia of different ionic currents. The magnitude, cellular distribution, and sensitivity to pharmacological manipulation of each of these ionic currents is different for every major neuronal region in the central and peripheral nervous system. These differences result in widely varying electrophysiological properties and patterns of neuronal activity generated by cells in different parts of the brain. Each class of neuron is exquisitely "tuned" to do its particular task in the nervous system through its own special mixture of the basic ionic currents available and by the precise modulation of these currents by neuroactive substances. An analogy to this situation would be the "nature-versus-nurture" debate on determining human behavior. The cells are endowed with a particular mixture of ionic currents through genetic programming (nature) that can then be modified on either a short- or long-term basis through development or the actions of a number of substances impinging upon the cell (nurture).

Examples of the different electrophysiological "behaviors" of neurons due to different combinations of ionic currents are illustrated in Fig. 2.5. Cortical pyramidal neurons respond to a depolarizing current pulse with a train (Fig. 2.5A) or a burst (Fig. 2.5B) of action potentials (McCormick et al., 1985; Connors and Gutnick, 1990). The spike frequency adaptation of cortical pyramidal neurons (Fig. 2.5A) is due to the presence of I_{AHP} and I_M. In contrast to neocortical pyramidal neurons, the major output cell of the cerebellar cortex, the Purkinje cell, responds to a depolarizing current pulse with a high-frequency discharge of short-duration action potentials (Fig. 2.5C). This high-frequency discharge is modulated by dendritic calcium spikes (Fig. 2.5C, asterisks) as well as by prolonged sodium ($I_{Na,p}$) and calcium currents (I_P; Fig. 2.5C, arrowheads).

Thalamic relay neurons are unusual in that they possess two distinct modes of action potential generation: single spike activity when depolarized above -65 mV (Fig. 2.5D) and burst firing when depolarized at or negative to -75 mV (Fig. 2.5E). Thalamic neurons respond with a burst of action potentials at -75 mV because of the presence of a large I_T, which is completely inactivated at membrane potentials positive to -65 mV.

Some neurons display spontaneous activity in a regular and stereotyped manner, even in the lack of all synaptic input, such as the medial habenular neuron illustrated in Fig. 2.5F. These cells appear to possess prolonged and complicated spike afterhyperpolarizations (arrows) which help determine the rate at which the action potentials are generated.

Although the electrophysiological behavior of neurons can be markedly changed by the neurotransmitted "environment," they also remain distinct in that it generally is not possible to cause one class of neuron (e.g., cortical pyramidal neuron) to behave electrophysiologically identical to another (e.g., cerebellar Pukinje cell). However, substantial and interesting transformations take place in response to neuron-to-neuron communication.

TYPES OF NEURONAL COMMUNICATION

Communication from one neuron to another in the nervous system occurs through at least three different mechanisms: *(1)* gap junctions; *(2)* ephaptic interactions; and *(3)* the release of neuroactive substances.

GAP JUNCTIONS

Gap junctions are actual physical connections between neighboring neurons made by large macromolecules that extend through the membranes of both cells and contain water-filled pores (Fig. 2.6). Gap junctions allow for the direct exchange of ions and

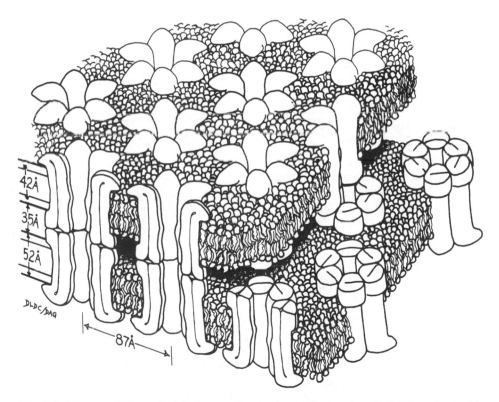

Fig. 2.6. Diagram of direct electrical connection between cells (gap junction). Channels provide for cell-to-cell exchange of low-molecular-weight substances and electric ionic current (in the form of ions). [From Makowski et al., 1977, with permission.]

other small molecules between cells. Ionic current through these channels directly couples the electrical activity of one cell to that of the other. Although in some cases gap junctions can be viewed as simple linearly conducting connections, in many other cases they are known to *rectify* (i.e., pass current in one direction much better than in the other). Gap junctions are known to be a prominent feature of neuron-to-neuron connections in many submammalian species, but in only a small number of regions in the mature mammalian nervous system (e.g., retina, inferior olive, vestibular nucleus, and the mesencephalic nucleus of the fifth cranial nerve). Gap junctions in these regions serve to synchronize the activity of individual elements with those of their neighbors. The ability of neurotransmitters to alter the conducting properties of gap junctions in some regions (e.g., retina) gives additional complexity to this system of communication.

EPHAPTIC INTERACTIONS

Ephaptic interactions refer to interactions between neurons based largely upon their close physical proximity (Fig. 2.7). The flow of ions into and out of one neuron will set up local electrical currents that can partially pass through neighboring neurons. The degree to which a neuron can be influenced by the activity of its neighbor is determined in part by the proximity of the cells and their processes (i.e., dendrites, cell bodies, and axons). In regions that possess closely spaced neuronal elements, such as the close packing of cell bodies in hippocampus and cerebellum or the bundling of dendrites in the cerebral cortex, there is the possibility of significant ephaptic interaction. Ephaptic interactions, like gap junctions, serve to synchronize local neuronal activity and may influence the general firing pattern of functionally related neurons (e.g., Taylor and Dudek, 1984).

CHEMICAL SYNAPSES

The release of neuroactive substances at the specialized connections called *synapses* is by far the most common method by which neurons influence other neurons. Some neuroactive substances can also diffuse over rather long distances to activate extrasynaptic sites, although it is not yet clear how common this type of transmission is.

As discussed in Chap. 1, neurotransmitters are released by neurons through exocytosis of packets (*vesicles*) of the substance from synaptic specializations into the space (*synaptic cleft*) between the cells. Examples of two of the most prevalent types of synapses are shown in Fig. 2.8. The release of transmitter is triggered by the entry of Ca^{2+} into the presynaptic terminal. This Ca^{2+} entry results from the depolarization associated with the arrival of the action potential. Once the neurotransmitter is released, it rapidly traverses the short distance between the neurons and binds to specific proteins (*receptor molecules*) on the postsynaptic cell. The activation of the receptors by the neurotransmitter may then cause a myriad of postsynaptic responses, many of which are expressed as an altering of the probability that a particular type of ionic channel will be open.

The actual receptor binding site may be part of, or separate from, the macromolecule making up the ionic channel. Examples of ionic channels to which the neurotransmitter directly binds include the glutamate and γ-aminobutyric acid (GABA)-activated channels (Fig. 2.8), and the nicotinic cholinergic receptor. The latter is acti-

Ephaptic Interactions

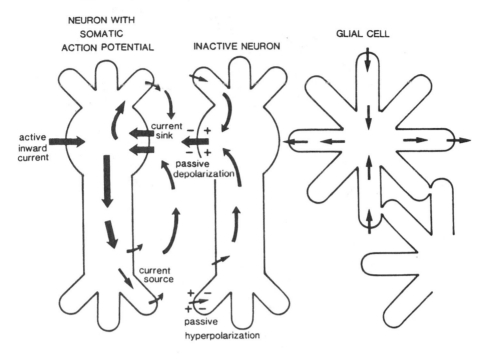

Fig. 2.7. Schematic diagram of current flow proposed to underlie excitatory electrical field effects between pyramidal neurons in the hippocampus (an example of ephaptic interactions). Arrows denote current flow of positive charges. The driving force of the ephaptic electrical field effect is the flow of positive current into somata produced by the synchronous firing if a population of hippocampal pyramidal cells (left). Positive current then flows passively out dendrites of active cells and returns through extracellular space. The relative decrease in positive charge in the extracellular space at the cell body layer causes the voltage on the inside of inactive cells (center) to appear relatively more positive (i.e., depolarized) than before. Likewise, the addition of positive current to the extracellular space at the levels of the dendrites by the neuronal activity causes the intracellular potentials of inactive dendrites to appear more negative (hyperpolarized) than before. Depolarization of the neuronal somata increases the probability that neighboring cells will generate action potentials in synchrony. Passive glial cell also develops transmembrane current flow within electrical field (right). [From Taylor and Dudek, 1984]

vated by acetylcholine (ACh) at the neuromuscular junction, in sympathetic ganglion neurons, and in many other regions of the nervous system. The binding of ACh to the nicotinic postsynaptic receptor induces a conformational change in the ionic channel, thereby opening the "gate" and allowing ions (in this case, Na^+, Ca^{2+}, and K^+) to flow through the pore (reviewed in Hille, 1992).

An example of a receptor site that appears to be separate from the channel molecule is the muscarinic receptor in the heart, which, when activated by acetylcholine, results in an increase in membrane potassium conductance. This response to ACh is associated with the receptor-mediated activation of an intracellular second messenger known as a *G-protein*. G-proteins are a class of molecule that require the binding of guanyl

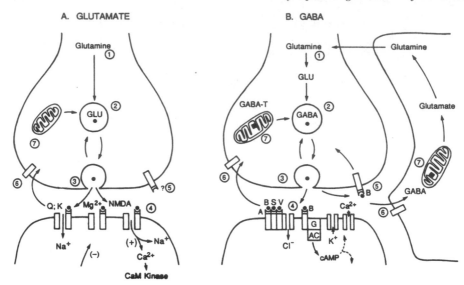

Fig. 2.8. Molecular mechanisms of ionotropic amino acid synapses. **A:** Glutaminergic synapses: (1) synthesis of glutamate (GLU) from glutamine; (2) transport and storage; (3) release of GLU by exocytosis; (4) binding of GLU to AMPA, kainate (K), and NMDA receptors. The Q (quisqualate or AMPA) and K receptors typically gate Na^+ and K^+ flux; the NMDA receptor also typically allows Ca^{2+} entry when the membrane potential is depolarized (+). When the membrane potential is hyperpolarized (−), Mg^{2+} blocks the channel. The release of glutamate may be regulated by presynaptic receptors (?5). Once GLU is released, it is removed from the synaptic cleft by re-uptake (6) and processed intracellularly (7). (From Shepherd, 1994; based on Cooper et al., 1987; Jahr and Stevens, 1987; Cull-Candy and Usowicz, 1987.) **B:** GABA-ergic synapse. (1) Synthesis of GABA from glutamine; (2) transport and storage of GABA; (3) release of GABA by exocytosis; (4) binding to a $GABA_A$ receptor that can be blocked by bicu-culline (B), picrotoxin or strychnine (S) and can also be modified by benzodiazepines, such as valium (V); $GABA_B$ receptors, by contrast, are linked via a G-protein to the opening of K^+ or the reduction of Ca^{2+} channels. (5) Release of GABA is under the control of presynaptic $GABA_B$ receptors; GABA is removed from the synaptic cleft by uptake into terminals or glia (6); (7) processing of GABA back to glutamine. [From Shepherd, 1994; modified from Cooper et al., 1987; Aghajanian and Rasmussen, 1987, Nicoll, 1982, with permission.]

nucleotides in order to be active. The active component (catalytic subunit) of the G-protein is then thought to act as an intermediary between the receptor molecule and the ionic channel (reviewed by Neer, 1995).

Once a neurotransmitter is released, the length of time that it is present in the synaptic cleft is controlled by either hydrolysis of the transmitter, reuptake into the presynaptic terminal, uptake into neighboring cells, or by diffusion out of the cleft.

NEUROTRANSMISSION VERSUS NEUROMODULATION

Neuroactive substances in the nervous system have often been classified as either "neurotransmitters" or "neuromodulators" according to the duration and the functional implications of their actions. Substances released by neurons that have typical neurotransmitter roles cause postsynaptic responses that are both quick in onset (e.g., <1 msec) and relatively short in duration (e.g., $<$tens of milliseconds). The summation of phasic excitatory and inhibitory postsynaptic potentials and the way they interact with the intrinsic electrophysiological and morphological properties of the neuron forms to a large extent the manner in which neuronal computations occur.

In contrast, modulatory actions of neuroactive substances are characterized by their prolonged duration and the ability to *modulate* the response of the neuron to other, perhaps more phasic, inputs. Although the distinction between these two types of neurotransmitter actions is not always easy, it is nonetheless useful. Receptors acted on directly by a neurotransmitter are called *ionotropic*, whereas those acted on indirectly by second messengers are sometimes referred to as *metabotropic*.

It is probably safe to say that most neurons in the brain are under the influence of as many as a dozen or more neuroactive substances (see Table 2.2). The wide range of cellular responses (ionic as well as biochemical) to these substances adds great depth and richness to the possible behavior or individual neurons and consequently to a neuronal circuit as a whole. For example, it is the job of neurotransmitters not only to al-

Table 2.2. Common Neurotransmitter Responses in the CNS

Response	Neurotransmitter	Receptor
$\uparrow I_{Na}$, $\uparrow I_K$	Glutamate	AMPA/kainate
$\uparrow I_{Na}$, $\uparrow I_K$, $\uparrow I_{Ca}$	Glutamate	N-methyl-D-aspartate (NMDA)
	Acetylcholine	Nicotinic
	Serotonin	5-HT$_3$
$\uparrow I_{Cl}$	γ-aminobutyric acid	GABA$_A$
	Glycine	
$\uparrow I_{K,IR}$	Acetylcholine	M$_2$
	Norepinephrine	α_2
	Serotonin	5-HT$_1$
	γ-aminobutric acid	GABA$_B$
	Dopamine	D$_2$
	Adenosine	A$_1$
	Somatostatin	
	Enkephalins	μ, δ
$\downarrow I_{AHP}$	Acetylcholine	Muscarinic
	Norepinephrine	β_1
	Serotonin	(?)
	Histamine	H$_2$
	Glutamate	Glu metabotropic
$\downarrow I_{K,leak}$	Acetylcholine	Muscarinic
	Norepinephrine	α_1
	Serotonin	(?)
	Glutamate	Glu metabotropic
$\downarrow I_{Ca}$	Multiple transmitters	

low neurons to communicate accurately and quickly the exact details of a complicated visual scene (e.g., the reading of this page), but also to control the proper level of arousal of the nervous system (e.g., awake and attentive) for efficient and accurate processing of the information, as well as to cause the generation of relatively permanent cellular changes (memory) through which the contents of the written page can be recalled. Considering the wide range of involvement of neurotransmitters in simple (e.g., reflexes) as well as complicated (e.g., emotions, psychiatric disorders) behavioral attributes, it is not surprising that one should find that there is an equally wide range of neurotransmitter actions on single neurons.

IONIC ACTIONS OF NEUROTRANSMITTERS

A large number of substances exist in the nervous system that are thought to be released by neurons in order to modify the electrophysiological properties of other neurons (Table 2.2). Many of these substances can cause more than one postsynaptic response. Most if not all of these various responses are mediated by pharmacologically distinct receptor molecules. In this manner, a neuroactive substance released onto a pyramidal neuron in the cerebral cortex may have a very different effect from the release of the same neurotransmitter onto a relay neuron in the thalamus (see below). Indeed, the same neurotransmitter may have very different, or even opposite, postsynaptic effects on neighboring neurons in the same neuronal region, depending upon the particular function of the neuron in the local circuit.

Many of the ionic currents in neurons are under the control of neuroactive substances. Recently, it has become apparent that different neurotransmitters, each acting through its own distinct class of receptor molecules, can modify the same ionic current. For this reason, I will review here the more common postsynaptic actions of neurotransmitters in terms of the physiological action rather than the type of neurotransmitter.

FAST POSTSYNAPTIC POTENTIALS

The classical postsynaptic potential (PSP) occurs through a temporally (e.g., milliseconds or less) and spatially (i.e., local) limited increase in membrane ionic conductance. The relatively brief time course of these postsynaptic potentials allows neurons to perform a large number of computations within short time periods, limiting the interactions between events that are widely separated in time. Synaptic potentials, especially those brief in duration, are usually classified by whether they increase (excitatory) or decrease (inhibitory) the probability of action potential discharge. However, it is always better to know the actual biophysical and biochemical actions of the neuroactive substance than to refer to them as being just "excitatory" or "inhibitory," especially when considering the *modulatory* actions of many putative neuroactive substances (see below).

Fast Excitatory Postsynaptic Potentials. Two main types of brief-duration PSPs have been identified in the nervous system: those due to the activation of nicotinic receptors by ACh, and those caused by the release of excitatory amino acids.

Nicotinic Cholinergic Responses. Fast nicotinic excitatory PSPs mediated by ACh have so far been shown to occur in the spinal cord, peripheral nervous system, and skeletal muscle. Nicotinic receptors are also located throughout the central nervous system (e.g., Albuquerque et al., 1995).

The activation of the nicotinic receptor-ionic channel complex by ACh results in a conformational change in the shape of critical portions of this macromolecule, thereby allowing ions to flow through. The nicotinic ionic channel is a "nonselective" cation channel, meaning that positively charged ions (e.g., Na^+, Ca^{2+}, and K^+) pass through the channel with about equal proficiency. Because of the mixed nature of the ions flowing through the nicotinic channel, the equilibrium (reversal) potential of the nicotinic response, approximately -5 mV, lies between the equilibrium potentials of the various cations (see Fig. 2.2).

The nicotinic receptor channel is a pentameric structure composed of, in order of mobility on SDS polyacrylamide gels, two α, one β, one γ (expressed in development; replaced by ϵ in adults) and one δ subunit surrounding a water-filled pore. Amino acid sequencing of α subunits, which contain the binding site for receptor activation, revealed the presence of at least eight distinct subtypes, termed $\alpha_1-\alpha_8$. These eight different α subunits (α_1, muscle; $\alpha_2-\alpha_8$, neural) differ not only in their primary structure, but also in their pharmacological properties and their distribution in the CNS.

The actions of ACh through nicotinic receptors in the nervous system is of particular interest, since nicotine, in the form of tobacco products, is still one of the most widely used drugs of addiction. Recent proposals suggest that the activation of dopaminergic neurons in the basal forebrain (ventral tegmental area) may be important in the pleasureful, and addictive, aspects of nicotine use (e.g., Calabresi et al., 1989).

Excitatory Amino Acid Responses. A substantial portion of the fast excitatory PSPs in the brain, particularly those in the cerebral cortex and hippocampus, are believed to be due to the release of an excitatory amino acid such as glutamate or aspartate. Postsynaptic ionotropic receptors for glutamate have been categorized according to their affinity for three different exogenous agonists: (RS)-α-amino-3-hydroxy-5-methyl-4-isoxazolepropionic acid (AMPA), kainate, and N-methyl-D-aspartate (NMDA) (reviewed by McLennan, 1983; Watkins and Olverman, 1987; Westbrook, 1994). More recent molecular biological studies of glutamate receptors have revealed that each of these three subgroups is encoded for by a number of different genes, including *GluR1–4* for AMPA receptors, *GluR5-7*, *KA1* and *KA2* for kainate receptors, and *NMDAR1* and *NMDAR2A-D* (also known as *NR1* and *NR2A-D*) for NMDA receptors (for review see Barnes and Henley, 1992; Hollmann and Heinemann, 1994; Schoepfer et al., 1994). Hetero-oligomers formed by the different subunits generated by these genes are of a wide variety and exhibit varying electrophysiological and pharmacological properties, depending upon the combinations of subunits expressed.

Activation of excitatory amino acid receptors underlies fast glutamatergic excitatory postsynaptic potentials (EPSPs). The postsynaptic potentials mediated by AMPA and kainate receptors, like those associated with nicotinic channels, are caused by an increase in a mixed cation conductance (mainly Na^+ and K^+, but sometimes Ca^{2+} as well) such that the reversal potential is approximately 0 mV (see MacDermott and Dale, 1987; Hollmann and Heinemann, 1994). These synaptic potentials have a very short delay from the arrival of the action potentials at the presynaptic terminal to the appearance of the postsynaptic potential, and a rapid rate of rise. The falling phase is much slower, being determined in large part by the membrane properties of the neuron (see Fig. 2.9B).

In contrast to the fast PSPs mediated by AMPA-kainate receptors, the action of glutamate through NMDA receptors is more complicated (reviewed by Ascher and Nowak, 1987). Stimulation of NMDA receptors results in the activation of a voltage-dependent current that is carried not only by Na^+ and K^+ but also importantly by Ca^{2+}. The voltage-dependent nature of this NMDA receptor–mediated current is due to the differential block of the ionic channel by magnesium ions (Mg^{2+}) at different membrane potentials (Mayer et al., 1984). At resting membrane potential (e.g., -75 mV) the driving force on Mg^{2+}, which is concentrated on the outside of the cell, to enter the neuron is quite high. Because of this, magnesium ions compete with Ca^{2+} and Na^+ ions for access to the pore of the channel. Since Mg^{2+} ions cannot flow through the pore, the channel is effectively blocked whenever one of the ions enters, thereby reducing the amount of time that the channel is open and conducting (see Fig. 2.9C).

When the cell is depolarized, the tendency for Mg^{2+} to fill the pore is substantially reduced, thereby lessening the block and allowing a larger $Na^+/Ca^{2+}/K^+$ current to flow. Because of this voltage dependence, activation of a glutaminergic synapse onto a neuron at resting membrane potentials may result in a fast EPSP mediated through the activation of kainate and AMPA (also known as quisqualate) receptors with little contribution of NMDA receptor mediated current, even though glutamate may be binding to these receptors (Fig. 2.9C). However, repetitive activation of the same synapse may cause a large depolarization of the cell through temporal summation of the unitary PSPs. The more these PSPs depolarize the cell, the more the degree of magnesium block will be removed, and thus the larger the activation of the NMDA current (Fig. 2.9D). Since NMDA channels conduct Ca^{2+} as well as Na^+ and K^+, calcium will flow into the postsynaptic cell and, by activating further biochemical mechanisms, can result in a *potentiation* of the strength of the unitary excitatory PSP. This enhancement of the PSP can last for prolonged periods (hours, days, longer?) and therefore is known as *long-term potentiation* (LTP) (see Collingridge and Bliss, 1987; Malenka and Nicoll, 1993; Nicoll and Malenka, 1995 for review). LTP is currently one of the leading models of the mechanisms by which synapses change their efficacy in order to participate in the encoding of memories in the nervous system (see Chap. 10, Olfactory Cortex; Chap. 11, Hippocampus; Chap. 12, Neocortex).

In addition to the activation of fast EPSPs, glutamate may also activate slow (seconds to minutes) EPSPs through the activation of glutamate "metabotropic" receptors (see below).

Fast Inhibitory Postsynaptic Potentials. Postsynaptic potentials that are quick in onset and inhibit the postsynaptic activity of the neuron are known to be mediated by two different neurotransmitters in the CNS: γ-aminobutyric acid (GABA) and glycine.

GABA-Mediated IPSPs. Gamma-aminobutyric acid is the major inhibitory neurotransmitter of the nervous system. GABA-releasing cells are present throughout all levels of the neuraxis. In the cerebral cortex and thalamus, they account for approximately 20–30% of all neurons. Neurons utilizing GABA as a neurotransmitter form a diverse

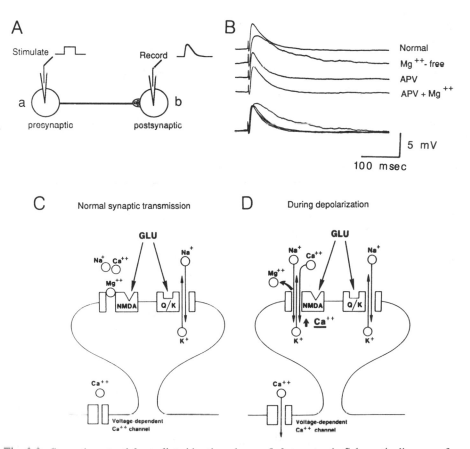

Fig. 2.9. Synaptic potentials mediated by the release of glutamate. **A:** Schematic diagram of experimental protocol in which the actions and pharmacology of monosynaptic connections between cultured cortical pyramidal cells is investigated. Intracellular recordings are used to stimulate a generator cell (a) that is monosynaptically connected to a follower cell (b). **B:** Activation of an action potential in the generator cell (a) causes a monosynaptic EPSP in the follower cell (b) through the stimulation of AMPA and kainate receptors (top trace, normal). Removal of Mg^{2+} from the medium bathing the cultures enhances the late components of this EPSP (second trace, Mg^{2+}-free). Addition of the NMDA receptor antagonist APV abolishes this late component indicating that it was due to the activation of NMDA receptors (third trace, APV). Returning Mg^{2+} to the bathing medium now has no additional effect on the EPSP (fourth trace, Mg^{2+}). At the bottom of B the traces are superimposed for comparison. These data illustrate that the release of glutamate can activate AMPA/kainate and NMDA receptors and that NMDA, but not AMPA/kainate, ionic channels can be blocked by Mg^{2+} ions. **C:** Schematic summary diagram illustrating that glutamate release from the presynaptic terminal at a low frequency (normal synaptic transmission) acts on both the NMDA and AMPA/kainate type of receptors. Na^+ and K^+ flow through the AMPA/kainate channel, but not through the NMDA receptor channel because of Mg^{2+} block. **D:** Depolarization of the membrane potential, or activation of the glutamatergic inputs at a high frequency, relieves the Mg^{2+} block of the NMDA channel, thereby allowing Na^+, K^+, and importantly, Ca^{2+} to flow through the channel. Depolarization due to the synaptic potential now also activates other voltage-dependent channels, such as those that conduct Ca^{2+}. [B from Huettner and Baughman, 1988; C and D from Nicoll et al., 1988, with permission.]

group, with several different morphologies specific for their own role in neuronal processing. They are instrumental in defining and confining the response properties not only of single neurons but also of large neuronal circuits. They figure prominently as interneurons in the types of inhibitory circuits illustrated previously in Chapter 1. It would be fair to say that without GABAergic neurons, the nervous system would not function in any logical manner.

There are three major types of GABA receptor, which are referred to as $GABA_A$, $GABA_B$, and $GABA_C$ (Bowery et al., 1987; Bormann and Feigenspan, 1995). Here we consider only the $GABA_A$ receptor ($GABA_B$- and $GABA_C$-mediated responses are discussed below). Many fast inhibitory PSPs in the brain are believed to result from the release of GABA acting upon the $GABA_A$ subclass of receptor (see early IPSP, Fig. 2.10). Binding of GABA to this class of receptor opens ion channels that are selective for Cl^- ions, and therefore the reversal potential of $GABA_A$-mediated responses is at the equilibrium potential for chloride (i.e., approximately -75 mV). Like the fast EPSPs in the nervous system, fast $GABA_A$-mediated inhibitory postsynaptic potentials (IPSPs) possess a rapid rising phase and a slower decay. These IPSPs are only tens of milliseconds in duration and are involved in rapid computations by neuronal networks (see Chap. 1).

$GABA_C$ receptors also conduct Cl^- ions and are most pronounced in the retina, although it is likely that they will be found in other parts of the CNS (see Bormann and Feigenspan, 1995).

Glycine-Mediated IPSPs. Glycinergic interneurons were first identified in the spinal cord and the brainstem. Glycine inhibits neuronal activity by increasing a Cl^- conductance similar to that activated by GABA (reviewed in Hamill et al., 1983; Kuhse et al., 1995). Indeed, it has been proposed that the glycine and GABA receptors may couple to the same Cl^- ionic channels (Hamill et al., 1983). Recent evidence suggests that glycine also serves as a classical neurotransmitter function in the forebrain (Betz, 1991; Trombley and Shepherd, 1994). Very low doses of glycine can greatly potentiate the actions of glutamate at NMDA receptors (Johnson and Ascher, 1987). This potentiating action occurs at low enough doses that even the concentrations of glycine occurring in the extracellular fluid are large enough to have a significant effect.

SLOW SYNAPTIC POTENTIALS

Like fast PSPs, slow PSPs are found at all levels of the nervous system. They have a large variety of sizes, shapes, and effects on the functional properties of neurons and neuronal circuits. Because of their delayed onset and prolonged duration, these PSPs are probably more involved in the regulation of the *excitability* of single neurons and neuronal circuits as opposed to underlying the relatively high frequency transfer of information (see Hartzell, 1981; Adams and Galvan, 1986).

Increase in Potassium Conductance. Applications onto neurons of a large variety of putative neurotransmitters, including acetylcholine, adenosine, norepinephrine, serotonin, γ-aminobutyric acid, dopamine, and various peptides, have been found to cause an increase in membrane potassium conductance (g_K; Fig. 2.10, and Table 2.2) (reviewed by North, 1987; Nicoll, 1988; Nicoll et al., 1990; McCormick, 1992). This occurs

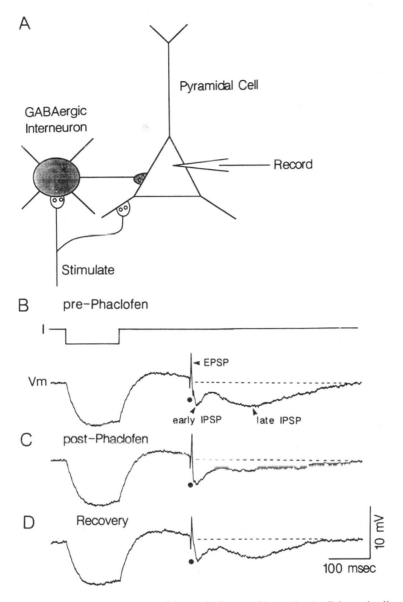

Fig. 2.10. Synaptic potentials generated in cortical pyramidal cells. **A:** Schematic diagram of stimulation and recording situation. Stimulation of afferent fibers activates both pyramidal cells and GABAergic interneurons that subsequently inhibit pyramidal cells. **B:** Intracellular recording from a human cortical pyramidal cell during stimulation of ascending axons. Injection of a hyperpolarizing current pulse (I) is used to investigate the apparent input resistance of the neuron. Electrical stimulation (dot) results in the generation of a fast EPSP followed by an early (fast) and late (slow) IPSP. Activation of the axons excites local GABAergic interneurons that subsequently release GABA onto the recorded pyramidal cell. GABA then activates both GABA$_A$ and GABA$_B$ receptors. Activation of GABA$_A$ receptors causes an increase in Cl$^-$ conductance and underlies the early IPSP, while activation of GABA$_B$ receptors causes an increase in K$^+$ conductance and is responsible for the generation of the late IPSP. **C:** Local application of the GABA$_B$-specific antagonist phaclofen substantially reduces the late IPSP, confirming that this PSP is due to the activation of GABA$_B$ receptors. The effect of phaclofen is reversible **(D).**

through a specific subtype of neuronal receptor for each neuroactive substance. Although all of these substances have the ability to increase potassium conductance in some region of the nervous system, the nonhomogeneous distribution of receptors that mediate this response means that some neurons exhibit it and others do not. For example, application of acetylcholine to GABAergic interneurons in the feline thalamus results in an *increase* in g_K, whereas in neighboring thalamocortical relay cells this putative neurotransmitter causes a *decrease* in g_K (McCormick and Prince, 1987a; Pape and McCormick, 1995; see Chap. 8). Furthermore, in many regions of the nervous system there is convergence of different neuroactive substances with each one generating an increase in g_K in the same postsynaptic neuron. For example, hippocampal pyramidal cells respond to serotonin, GABA (through $GABA_B$ receptors), and adenosine with an increase in the same potassium conductance (Nicoll et al., 1990; see Chap. 11). In this manner, a variety of neuroactive substances can activate or inactivate the same ionic currents in a given neuron and perhaps even converge onto the same ionic channel.

Functionally, an increase in membrane potassium conductance is considered inhibitory in that it usually decreases the probability of action potential discharge, and this can have important functional consequences. For example, GABA can increase both g_{Cl} (through $GABA_A$ or $GABA_C$ receptors) and g_K (through $GABA_B$ receptors); the result is a fast $GABA_A$-mediated increase in g_{Cl} followed by a slow $GABA_B$-mediated increase in g_K in the postsynaptic neuron (see late IPSP, Fig. 2.10; Newberry and Nicoll, 1985; Dutar and Nicoll, 1988a,b; McCormick, 1989b). In addition, there are many differences between the fast and slow GABA-mediated IPSPs other than just their time course. The conductance increase associated with the late IPSP is much smaller than that associated with the fast IPSP even though the amplitude of the voltage deviation associated with each may be similar. Indeed, if the membrane potential is negative to E_{Cl}, the fast IPSP will be *depolarizing* (although it is still inhibitory), while the late IPSP will still be hyperpolarizing. In addition, the GABA-activated late IPSP is mediated through a second messenger system (G-proteins) while the fast IPSP is the result of GABA binding to a receptor located directly on the ion channel.

These physiological differences make fast IPSPs more of a shunting inhibition (i.e., the membrane potential of the cell is held close to E_{Cl} and the input resistance of the cell is "shunted"), whereas the late IPSP operates more through the hyperpolarization of the neuron. Fast IPSPs are useful for local (e.g., particular subparts of the cell) "yes-no" decisions, whereas the late IPSP is useful for the modulation of the overall excitability of the neuron. The restricted time and space domains of the fast IPSPs allow them to participate in relatively high-frequency neuronal processing, whereas the slow IPSP is important for setting a particular level of excitability in the neuron for more prolonged periods of time.

The postsynaptic morphological locations of IPSPs are also very important in determining their consequences for processing within synaptic circuits. Many types of GABAergic neurons form synaptic contacts at specific locations of the postsynaptic neuron. For example, *chandelier cells* of the cerebral cortex give rise to chains of synaptic terminals on the axon hillocks of cortical pyramidal cells (see Chap. 12), while *basket cells* give rise to a "basket" or "pericellular nest" of terminals around the cell bodies of pyramidal neurons. In this way both of these inputs have powerful effects on the output of the entire neuron. It may even be possible for the chandelier cell to prevent the propagation of an action potential down the axon after its generation in the cell body and/or dendrite, or to determine the precise timing of action potential generation.

The opposite extreme of the above two examples of a rather global inhibition by GABA of the output of the neuron is found in the very localized synaptic processing in dendritic microcircuits (see Chap. 1). At this level of organization, individual GABAergic terminals may have effects that are relatively independent of one another, as well as independent of the output activity of the neuron itself. In these situations, the GABAergic process may affect only a particular portion of the postsynaptic dendritic tree, or perhaps, only particular synaptic terminals. Numerous examples of GABAergic contributions to processing in synaptic glomeruli, dendritic trees, and other types of microcircuits will be discussed in subsequent chapters.

Decrease in Potassium Currents. Neuroactive substances can decrease as well as increase neuronal potassium currents. To date, there are four different potassium currents that can be decreased in amplitude in response to various neurotransmitters: I_{AHP}, I_M, I_A, and a resting "leak" potassium current which I shall denote as $I_{K,leak}$.

Decrease in I_{AHP}. I_{AHP} has been shown to be decreased by a number of putative neurotransmitters (norepinephrine, acetylcholine, serotonin, histamine, glutamate, etc.) (Charpak et al., 1990; reviewed in Nicoll et al., 1990; McCormick, 1992). In the case of norepinpehrine, the decrease in I_{AHP} is achieved through an increase in the intracellular activity of a second messenger, cyclic adenosine monophosphate (cAMP) (Madison and Nicoll, 1986b; Pedarzani and Storm, 1993).

As stated previously, I_{AHP} contributes substantially to spike frequency adaptation. Therefore, block of this current greatly reduces the tendency for cells to slow down their firing rate during maintained depolarization (Fig. 2.11). This is an important effect, for it allows a neurotransmitter to increase the response of a cell to barrages of excitatory PSPs with little or no change in the resting membrane potential, or the response to inhibitory PSPs. Indeed, if the putative neurotransmitter simultaneously increases membrane conductance to K^+ or Cl^- while blocking I_{AHP}, the result may actually be an increase in "signal-to-noise" ratio. The baseline spontaneous firing of the cell will be reduced by the increase in potassium and/or chloride currents, while the response of the cell to barrages of large EPSPs may actually be enhanced by the decrease in I_{AHP} (see below).

Decrease in I_M. As stated above, I_M is a potassium current that is slowly (tens of milliseconds) activated by depolarization of the membrane potential above approximately -65 mV (Brown and Adams, 1980; Brown, 1988). This current has been shown to be potently reduced by stimulation of muscarinic receptors by acetylcholine. Like I_{AHP}, I_M contributes to spike frequency adaptation; blocking it subsequently increases the response of a neuron to barrages of excitatory PSPs. Because I_M is active only at depolarized potentials, its blockade may have little effect on the cell's resting membrane potential or response to IPSPs.

The M current may be reduced following the activation of a variety of receptors, including serotoninergic and glutamatergic receptors, and some types of peptide

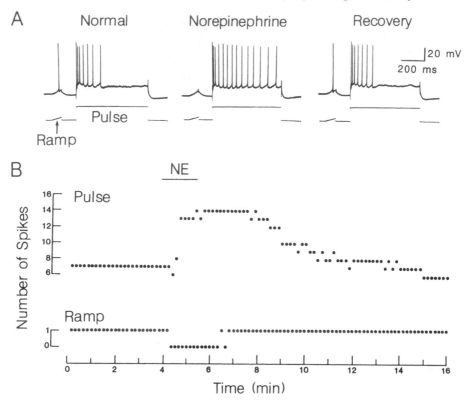

Fig. 2.11. Effect of norepinephrine on the excitability of cortical pyramidal neurons. The response of this hippocampal pyramidal neuron to two different types of input was examined: a small depolarizing ramp (to mimic weak EPSPs) and a prolonged depolarization (to mimic a train of strong EPSPs). **A:** In normal conditions, the small ramp input causes the generation of a single action potential while the prolonged depolarization results in a train of action potentials that show strong spike frequency adaptation (A, left). Addition of norepinephrine to the bathing medium results in a small hyperpolarization of the membrane potential (not shown). During the hyperpolarization the small depolarizing input no longer generates an action potential while the response to the prolonged input is actually potentiated because of the block of spike frequency adaptation (A, norepinephrine). The reduction in spike frequency adaptation is a secondary effect due to the block of I_{AHP} (not shown). This effect of norepinephrine is fully reversible (A, recovery). **B:** Graphic representation of the data in A. The generation of an action potential by the small ramp input is blocked, while the response to the prolonged input is greatly enhanced. In this manner, norepinephrine can increase the "signal-to-noise" ratio of the cell. [From Madison and Nicoll, 1986a, with permission.]

receptors (McCormick and Williamson, 1989; Charpak et al., 1990; Nicoll et al., 1990).

Decrease in I_A. Many of the different K^+ currents in neurons are differentiated by different rates of activation and inactivation. One of these, the A current, and probably others, can be modulated by the application of neurotransmitters (Aghajanian, 1985). Since I_A contributes to an increase in the interval between action potentials during certain types of neuronal activity, the blocking of I_A will enhance the response of the neuron by increasing the frequency of action potential discharge.

Decrease in calcium currents. Numerous putative neurotransmitters, including acetylcholine, norepinephrine, serotonin, and GABA, can reduce the flow of Ca^{2+} across the membrane (see Tsien et al., 1988; Stea et al., 1995). The functional consequences of neurotransmitter suppression of calcium currents has not been well studied in the CNS. One possible effect is related to the actions of neurotransmitters at presynaptic terminals. The amount of transmitter that is released after the invasion of the terminal by an action potential is under the control of neuroactive agents binding to receptors located on these terminals. In most (perhaps all) systems, the binding of the transmitter that is released by the terminal *reduces* the quantity released by subsequent action potentials. This *auto-inhibition* then forms a negative feedback loop that is useful for regulating the concentration of transmitter in the area of the synaptic cleft. The ionic mechanisms of this negative feedback are not known. However, since neurotransmitter release is highly dependent upon Ca^{2+} entry, transmitter-mediated decreases in Ca^{2+} currents may be involved.

Possible Gating Actions of Neurotransmitters. As discussed previously, many different types of neurons in the nervous system possess two intrinsic and physiologically distinct firing modes: single-spike and burst activity (e.g., Llinás and Yarom, 1981a,b; Jahnsen and Llinás, 1984a,b; Llinás, 1988). The cell's membrane potential determines in part which of these two firing patterns the neuron will exhibit. Burst firing occurs in response to excitatory inputs whenever the membrane potential is negative to approximately −65 mV, whereas single-spike activity occurs at membrane potentials positive to approximately −55 mV (Fig. 2.5D,E). Therefore, a neuroactive substance that activates a potassium conductance can actually increase the probability of a neuron firing by hyperpolarizing the cell into the burst firing mode of action potential generation (e.g., from −60 to −70 mV). In this situation, the increase in membrane conductance is acting more as a "switching" or modulatory mechanism than as a strict "yes-no" inhibition (McCormick, 1992). Likewise, decreasing resting conductance to K^+ is an effective mechanism by which a neuron can be tonically depolarized out of the burst firing mode and brought closer to threshold for generation of the more unmodulated single-spike discharge (Fig. 2.12). Such changes in membrane potential have been found to occur during shifts in arousal (Hirsch et al., 1983) and may underlie the well-known shift in the characteristics of the electroencephalogram (EEG) from synchronized slow waves to desynchronized, higher frequencies during increases in arousal (e.g., Moruzzi and Magoun, 1949; Steriade et al., 1993).

INTRINSIC AND SYNAPTIC CURRENTS: PUTTING IT ALL TOGETHER

With our new armament of knowledge of the intrinsic properties of neurons and how they may be affected by neurotransmitters we can proceed (with due caution) to propose a scenario of how synaptic computations may be implemented and modulated in a representative neuron. We take as our example one of the most abundant and important neuronal cell types in the human brain: the cerebral cortical pyramidal cell (see Chaps. 1, 10–12).

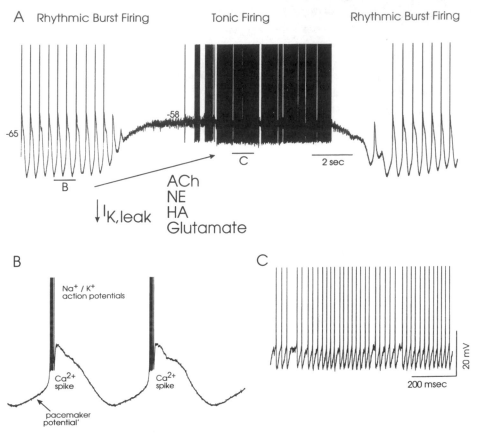

Fig. 2.12. Neurotransmitters control the firing mode in thalamic relay neurons. **A:** Thalamic re-lay neurons can spontaneously generate rhythmic bursts of action potentials (rhythmic burst fir-ing) through the generation of repetitive low-threshold Ca^{2+} spikes (see B). Application of a va-riety of neurotransmitters, including acetylcholine (ACh), norepinephrine (NE), histamine (HA), and glutamate, can reduce a "leak" K^+ current, $I_{K,leak}$, and therefore depolarize the thalamic cell. This depolarization inactivates the low-threshold Ca^{2+} current and therefore blocks rhythmic burst firing. Now the cell generates tonic trains of action potentials. Once the block of $I_{K,leak}$ wears off, the cell returns to rhythmic burst firing. **B:** Expansion of the rhythmic burst firing in A illustrating the rhythmic Ca^{2+} spikes interspersed by a "pacemaker potential" generated by the activation of I_h. **C:** Expansion of part of the tonic firing in A. [Modified from McCormick and Pape, 1990, with permission.]

Cortical pyramidal cells, like neurons in most other parts of the brain, receive exci-tatory, inhibitory, and modulatory inputs from a variety of sources. Putative *gluta-matergic* synapses, which have typical fast excitatory actions, are found on the spines of apical and basilar dendrites (Fig. 2.13). Notable sources of excitatory inputs are other pyramidal cells (located in neighboring or distant cortical regions), spiny stellate neu-rons of layer IV, and inputs from the thalamus (see Chap. 12). In contrast to excita-tory inputs, *GABAergic* inhibitory synapses are found on the soma, proximal and dis-tal dendrites, and initial segment of the axon; they arise largely from intrinsic cortical

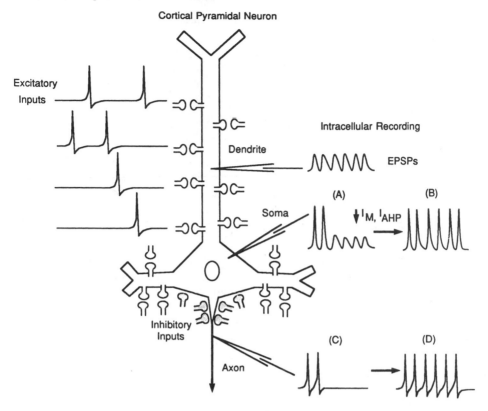

Fig. 2.13. Effect of activation of excitatory inputs to a cortical pyramidal cell. A train of action potentials arriving at different synaptic endings on the apical dendrite of the pyramidal cell results in the generation of a train of EPSPs. The first two EPSPs generate action potentials in the somatic region, while the last four fail because of activation of I_M and I_{AHP} (**A**). This is further reflected in the axonal output of the neuron (**C**). Block of these two currents reduced spike frequency adaptation and allows all six EPSPs to generate action potentials (**B** and **D**). See text for details.

interneurons, which are morphologically and functionally heterogeneous. Putative *neuromodulatory* substances arrive from a variety of subcortical (cholinergic, noradrenergic, serotonergic) and intracortical (cholinergic and peptidergic) neurons. Their synaptic contacts on pyramidal neurons are found largely on dendrites. Some types of GABAergic neurons also contain, and may release, one or more peptides. The ionic actions of these peptides and how they interact with the actions of GABA are not yet known.

Let us imagine that our cortical pyramidal cell is in the visual cortex and that, although the animal is awake and attentive, the cell is not yet receiving any specific visual input. The resting potential of our hypothetical cell will probably be somewhere around -65 mV, depending upon the state of input from the slowly acting neurotransmitters, especially those (e.g., acetylcholine) that can alter the level of resting potassium conductance. This resting potential is about 10 mV below (more hyperpolarized than) the threshold of around -55 mV for the generation of action potentials by a cortical pyramidal neuron.

Now let us stimulate the visual receptive field of our cell with an adequately adjusted light stimulus to the retina (for example, a moving bar of light). This input will first cause excitation of the thalamic neurons (see Chap. 8). Since the animal is awake and attentive, the thalamic neurons respond to the input in a one-spike-out-per-spike-in fashion (e.g., Fig. 2.5D) and in turn give rise to a train of action potentials that reach some of the presynaptic terminals onto our cell. Each action potential causes an increase in $[Ca^{2+}]_i$ in the presynaptic terminal that in turn causes the release of excitatory transmitter from a variable number of synaptic vesicles in a probabilistic manner (see Chaps. 1 and 3). The transmitter travels across the synaptic cleft and binds to specific receptor molecules on the postsynaptic spine, increasing the probability that certain ionic channels (assume they conduct Na^+ and K^+ ions) will be in the open and conducting state. In this manner, each presynaptic spike will cause an EPSP in the postsynaptic dendrite (Fig. 2.13). The exact amplitude–time course of each EPSP depends upon a large number of factors, including the amount of transmitter released, the density of postsynaptic receptor molecules, the sensitivity of the postsynaptic element to the transmitter, the size and shape of the postsynaptic element, and finally, the amplitude and distribution of active currents that the postsynaptic element possesses. Indeed, the "efficacy" of each synaptic connection is not a static number, since it is probably modified during the acquisition of new information, as well as new strategies to analyze that information, perhaps through a process similar to LTP (see Fast excitatory postsynaptic potentials above).

In order for the barrage of EPSPs generated by the train of inputs from the thalamus to cause our cell to fire, it must cause the output decision point of the cell (the cell body and *axon hillock* in this case) to rise above firing threshold (e.g., -55 mV). To do this, the EPSPs must spread from their points of generation in the dendrites, through the cell body, to the axon hillock. What happens to these EPSPs as they make this trip is determined by the intrinsic properties of our cell and the state of other neuroactive substances impinging upon it. The dendritic EPSPs will probably be large enough to activate $I_{Na,p}$, or a Ca^{2+} current and thereby receive an extra "boost" from these depolarizing currents. This enhancement is needed to help overcome the fact that cell membranes are not perfect insulators and some of the current will leak out, thereby reducing the size of the EPSP as it travels toward the cell body. If the train of EPSPs comes at a high enough frequency, they will exhibit temporal summation, while EPSPs that arise from more than one point in the cell will also exhibit spatial summation. If the summated EPSP is large enough, it may be capable of causing the generation of a dendritic Na^+/Ca^{2+}-mediated action potential that will, of course, greatly enhance and transform the response of the cell to the synaptic input (Fig. 2.5C). However, for simplicity, assume that the threshold for the generation of a dendritic Na^+/Ca^{2+} spike is not reached.

Now consider the situation in which many of the EPSPs in the train are large enough to cause the generation of an action potential in the cell body and axon hillock. In this circumstance, the initial EPSPs in the train will be more likely to cause the generation of spikes than the latter ones because of the progressive activation of I_{AHP} and I_M, both of which contribute to spike frequency adaptation (Fig. 2.13A,C). Thus, although the cell may fire to the initial few EPSPs, the later ones will not reach firing threshold and the cell's firing will cease. This is where our modulatory transmitters come into play. If we were to arouse our animal such that there were an increase in the release of, for example, norepinephrine and acetylcholine, then I_{AHP} and I_M (and perhaps $I_{K,1}$) would be reduced. Reduction of these potassium currents would enhance the response of the neuron by reducing spike frequency adaptation as well as by moving the cell's membrane potential closer to firing threshold (Fig. 2.13B,D).

As the visual stimulus moves out of the cell's excitatory receptive field and into those of neighboring cortical neurons, our pyramidal cell may now be actively inhibited through the connections of intrinsic GABAergic neurons. These barrages of IPSPs will meet with many of the constraints as did the previous EPSPs, although they may occur in a more "linear" portion of the membrane potential (i.e., between -65 and -75 mV). The fast GABAergic IPSPs will be important in terminating the residual excitation from the previous barrage of EPSPs by causing an increase in Cl^- conductance. The influential position of the IPSPs on or near the soma and initial portion of the axon (axon hillock) make them particularly effective.

Now let's consider the situation when the animal or person falls to sleep. As drowsiness sets in, the rate of release of the ascending modulatory neurotransmitters, such as acetylcholine, norepinephrine, and histamine, will decrease. The decreased release of these modulatory transmitters will result in a hyperpolarization of many cell types owing to increases in various K^+ conductances. For example, thalamocortical neurons in the thalamus (Chap. 8) may hyperpolarize by up to 20 mV because of the increase in a resting K^+ conductance that is normally reduced by the release of these agents. This hyperpolarization of neurons in the CNS and the increase in amplitude of various K^+ currents results in a decreased excitability of these cells. In addition, the hyperpolarization also results in the removal of inactivation of some ionic currents, most notably, the low-threshold Ca^{2+} current I_T. The removal of inactivation of I_T allows for the generation of low-threshold Ca^{2+} spikes, and the activation of these in thalamocortical networks results in the generation of the spontaneous rhythms of sleep (Steriade et al., 1993).

The presentation of a visual (or other sensory) stimulus to our drowsy or sleeping friend will now result in a reduced response in the visual cortex: his or her brain will be less responsive and less able to respond quickly. This reduction in responsiveness becomes more and more pronounced as the person falls deeper and deeper to sleep.

Many of the properties outlined for our hypothetical cortical pyramidal and thalamic neurons can be generalized to neurons in all regions of the nervous system. However, each type of neuron is unique, and generalizations must be used with caution so as not to neglect the important features of each neuronal type that allow it to perform its own brand of cellular processing and thereby make its specific contributions to the synaptic circuits of which it is a part.

3

SPINAL CORD: VENTRAL HORN

ROBERT E. BURKE

The spinal cord is a remarkably complex system of neurons that subserves sensory, motor, and autonomic functions. A great deal of detailed information about synaptic organization within the mammalian central nervous system has emerged from studies of the spinal cord. Indeed, modern neurophysiology began in the 19th century with work, notably by Sir Charles Sherrington, on spinal reflexes (Creed et al., 1932). Many of these stereotyped motor responses to particular sensory stimuli are the same in reduced preparations and intact animals, so that the underlying mechanisms can be studied in the laboratory. In addition, sensory inputs to and motor outputs from the spinal cord are physically accessible and functionally meaningful, so that it is possible to attach behavioral significance to the organization of the synaptic linkages between them—an elusive goal in most other parts of the central nervous system (CNS). This chapter will focus on the organization of neuronal elements and synaptic interconnections in the ventral horn which are relevant to the control of movement.

NEURONAL ELEMENTS

There are three major categories of neuronal elements in the spinal cord: *(1)* neurons with cell bodies outside the spinal cord but axons that carry information into it (primary sensory afferents and descending fiber systems that bring in signals from the supraspinal brain); *(2)* spinal neurons with axons that leave the cord to innervate skeletal muscle fibers (motoneurons) or autonomic ganglia (preganglionic neurons); and *(3)* spinal neurons with axons that terminate exclusively within the CNS, either locally or in distant spinal segments (interneurons), or that leave the spinal cord to project to supraspinal targets (tract cells).

The diagram in Fig. 3.1 illustrates some aspects of the structure of the spinal cord, viewed in cross-section. Unlike the rest of the brain, the outermost part of the spinal cord, the white matter, consists of the axons of spinal and supraspinal neurons running parallel to the long axis of the cord. The inner gray-matter core contains the cell bodies of spinal neurons and most of the synaptic neuropil in which they interact. The two major gray-matter divisions, the dorsal and ventral horns, can be subdivided into lay-

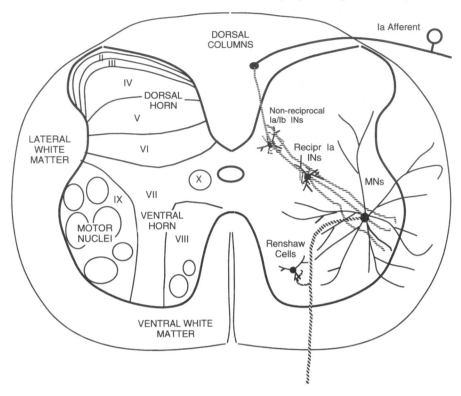

Fig. 3.1. Cross-section diagram of the spinal cord to show (left) the gray matter divisions and lamination determined by neuron densities and sizes (*cytoarchitectonics*; Rexed, 1952). The right half shows the trajectory of a group Ia afferent, the approximate extent of motoneuron dendrites, and the location of certain identified groups of interneurons discussed in the text.

ers, numbered I–X, on the basis of neuron sizes and densities (*cytoarchitectonic* divisions; left half of Fig. 3.1; Rexed, 1952). Identifiable classes of spinal interneurons (Ia/Ib INs, Ia INs, Renshaw cells) and motoneurons (MNs) occupy particular parts of the ventral-horn gray matter, as indicated on the right half of Fig. 3.1. The synaptic interactions among these neurons will be the main topic of this chapter.

PRIMARY AFFERENTS

A wide variety of primary afferent types has been identified on anatomical and functional grounds. The classification of afferents depends on the tissue innervated (muscle, skin, joints and other deep tissues, or the viscera) and the characteristics of the receptor organ giving rise to them, which governs an afferent's response to various types of natural stimulation. The axonal size (diameter) and the presence or absence of myelin control the speed with which its information can be conducted to the spinal cord. As might be expected, there are systematic interrelations between these characteristics and the type of peripheral receptor (for reviews see Darian-Smith, 1984; Fyffe, 1984). There is also evidence that different classes of afferent neurons exhibit distinctive intrinsic membrane properties (Koerber et al., 1988). Brown (1981) has provided detailed descriptions of the morphology and physiology of the central projections of a wide variety of primary afferents.

Primary afferents entering the spinal cord are often considered in terms of two functional classes, called *exteroceptive* and *proprioceptive*. Exteroceptors are viewed as primarily responsive to events in the external environment as sensed by the skin (touch, temperature, pain, etc.). Proprioceptors (from the Latin, *proprius*, meaning "one's own") are viewed as activated mainly by the animal's own movements, as signalled by sensory structures in muscles, joints, and deep tissues of the trunk and limb. An example would be the group Ia afferents, to be discussed later (see also Fig. 3.1). This dichotomy is useful and well entrenched, but it is important to remember that movements can, and do, activate many kinds of skin afferents as well as those from muscle and deep tissues. Still other systems group sensory afferents according to the type of response they produce when activated. An example of this is the *flexor reflex afferents* (FRA), an assortment of skin, joint, and muscle afferents with relatively high electrical thresholds that tend to activate flexor muscles and inhibit extensors (i.e., the *flexor reflex*; Eccles and Lundberg, 1959; reviewed in Baldissera et al., 1981). The FRA are likely to be an important source of proprioceptive information.

MOTONEURONS

Motoneurons (or motor neurons) are the only CNS neurons that make synaptic contacts on non-neuronal tissue (i.e., skeletal muscle fibers). They are also one of the relatively few classes of CNS neurons with a precisely defined functional role: to activate muscle. Motoneuron cell bodies and their dendritic extensions lie within the ventrolateral gray matter of the spinal cord (Fig. 3.1) and in certain cranial nerve nuclei in the brainstem. The cells that innervate a given muscle in the limbs or trunk lie clustered together in circumscribed *motor nuclei*, which are elongated, cigar-shaped collections of cell bodies spreading along the rostrocaudal axis of the ventral horn (Burke et al., 1977). The relative positions of the motor nuclei that innervate functionally related muscles exhibit fundamental similarities throughout the vertebrate series, from amphibia to humans (Romanes, 1951; Sharrard, 1955; Landmesser, 1978; Fetcho, 1987). The dendrites of motoneurons can extend more than 1–1.5 mm away from the cell body (Fig. 3.2; Cullheim et al., 1987), well outside of the motor nucleus. Within the gray matter they intertwine in an intricate feltwork where they receive synaptic contacts over their entire length (Brännström, 1993), including the distal parts that project into the white matter (Rose and Richmond, 1981).

There are two distinct types of motoneurons in mammals, α and γ motoneurons. These names were applied because α motoneuron axons have faster conduction velocities (generally >60 m/s, in the alpha peak of the compound action potential recorded from muscle nerves) than the γ motoneurons (conduction velocities <40 m/s, in the gamma peak; Matthews, 1972, 1981). The α motoneurons innervate the large *extrafusal* striated muscle fibers that make up the major bulk of muscles and produce output force. In contrast, the two subspecies of γ motoneurons (*static* and *dynamic*) exclusively innervate one or more of the three kinds of small, highly specialized *intrafusal* muscle fibers that exist only within the muscle spindle stretch receptors. Their action is to modulate the sensitivity of the two types of muscle spindle afferents, group Ia and

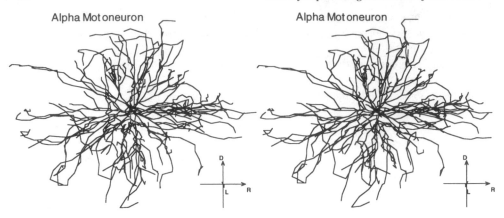

Fig. 3.2. Computer-generated stereoscopic drawing of a reconstructed cat α motoneuron, as viewed in the sagittal plane. The line thicknesses do not accurately depict the actual diameters of the dendritic branches, which are mostly much thinner than can be drawn. The calibration arrows are 500 μm in length.

group II, to changes in muscle length or to static length, respectively. The details of the operation of this remarkable sensory system can be found elsewhere (Matthews, 1981; Hasan and Stuart, 1984).

The somata of α motoneurons are larger and their dendritic trees are more numerous and highly branched (Cullheim et al., 1987) than those of γ-cells (Moschovakis et al., 1991a). Although the two neuron types are quite thoroughly intermixed within motor nuclei (Burke et al., 1977), they do not receive identical synaptic inputs. The most striking difference is that γ motoneurons receive no monosynaptic excitation from group Ia muscle spindle afferents (see below), while virtually all α motoneurons do (reviewed in Burke and Rudomin, 1977). The lack of direct excitation of γ motoneurons by spindle afferents presumably prevents a "positive feedback" loop which might produce instability in the spindle servo-control system.

This simple dichotomy became more complicated when Emonet-Denand and co-workers (1975) showed that some motoneurons in cats innervate both extrafusal and intrafusal muscle fibers. Such β motoneurons are quite common in certain limb muscles in cats (Jami et al., 1982) and they can also be found in primates (Murthy et al., 1982). In contrast to their γ motoneuron half-brothers, it is probable that most, if not all, β motoneurons receive monosynaptic excitation from group Ia afferents (Burke and Tsairis, 1977). This would appear to form a positive feedback system with still unknown functional consequences.

MOTOR UNITS

Motoneurons are, anatomically and functionally, inseparable from the muscle fibers that they innervate. Among the many key concepts that we owe to Sherrington is that of the motor unit—the combination of a motoneuron (α or β; see above) and the group of muscle fibers that it innervates (Liddell and Sherrington, 1925). Most limb and trunk muscles in mammals contain two fundamental motor unit types: fast twitch (type F) and slow twitch (type S); these are based primarily on the morphology, biochemistry, and mechanical properties of the innervated muscle fibers (the *muscle unit*; Burke et al., 1973). The type F population can be further divided into two major subtypes, one relatively fatigable (type FF) and the other much more resistant to fatigue (type FR), and one minor subtype intermediate between the two (type FI). All of the muscle fibers in a muscle unit share the same morphology, chemistry, and presumably, mechanical characteristics.

There is a long list of intrinsic motoneuron properties that are systematically related to motor unit type, as defined by the innervated muscle unit (Burke, 1981; Gustafsson and Pinter, 1984; Zengel et al., 1985). A further extension of interrelations has been found in the quantitative and even qualitative organization of synaptic inputs to the various motor unit types, which will be discussed later. Some of these interrelations, as illustrated in the multidimensional plot shown in Fig. 3.3, almost certainly represent functional specializations that enable the different types of motor units to play particular roles during reflex and voluntary movements. These points will be discussed later.

INTERNEURONS

Strictly speaking, all neurons with axons confined entirely within the CNS are interneurons. Most spinal cord interneurons are considerably smaller than motoneurons but a few are almost as large and complex as α motoneurons. It is useful to define three subgroups of spinal interneurons on the basis of the location of their main axonal trajectories. *Segmental*, or *local* interneurons project to spinal-cord regions relatively close to the parent cell body, i.e., within the same spinal segment or in nearby segments. Segmental interneurons participate in reflexes to coordinate the action of motoneuron groups within a given limb. Interneurons with axons that end at greater distances but still within the spinal cord itself are referred to as *propriospinal cells*. Propriospinal neurons have obvious utility in coordinating activities in many spinal segments, such as ensuring correct movements of fore- and hindlimbs in four-footed animals and, perhaps less obviously, the actions of widely distributed trunk muscles in maintaining balance and posture while providing a stable platform for limb movements. Spinal interneurons that send their axons primarily to supraspinal destinations can be conveniently distinguished as *tract cells*. Examples include the various divisions of the spinocerebellar tracts that end as mossy fibers in the cerebellar cortex and neurons of the spinothalamic tract that end within the thalamus. The most obvious role for tract neurons is to deliver information to supraspinal regions of the brain that are specifically associated with movement control or sensory perception.

Of course, as with most biological systems, these neat categories are oversimplifications because they are not mutually exclusive (Jankowska, 1992). For example, some tract cells also have axon collaterals that end locally within the spinal cord (Brown et al., 1977). Such neurons may therefore also participate as local interneurons in reflex actions. As information about the structure and function of spinal interneurons improves, it seems quite likely that many of these neurons will be shown to have multiple sites of action, and therefore multiple functional roles.

There are at present relatively few morphological clues to guide a functional taxonomy of spinal cord interneurons and tract cells, other than a few cell groups with characteristic morphology. One example of the latter is Clarke's column in the upper lum-

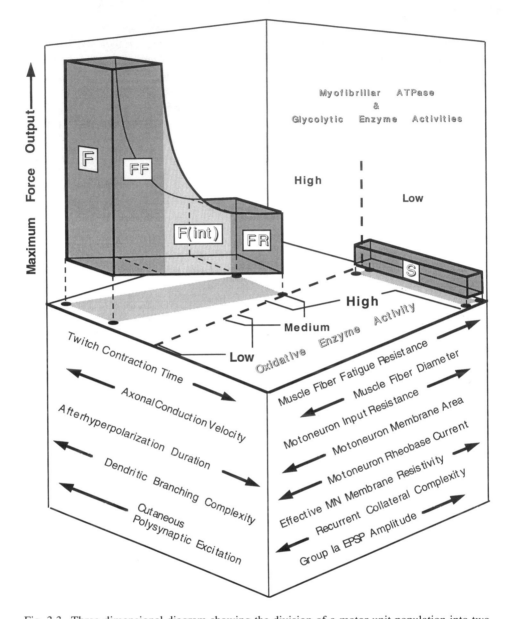

Fig. 3.3. Three-dimensional diagram showing the division of a motor unit population into two basic clusters, fast twitch (type F) and slow twitch (type S), according to properties of the muscle unit. The type F cluster is subdivided into types FF, F(int), and FR, on the basis of relative resistance to fatigue. The box outlines denote the loci of data points for individual motor units (see text-fig. 5 in Burke et al., 1973) plotted against maximum tetanic force (vertical ordinate), twitch contraction time (left horizontal abscissa), and muscle fiber resistance to fatigue (right abscissa). Histochemical enzyme activities characteristic of each muscle unit type are given on the main diagram. The two abscissae also show other properties of muscle units (twitch contraction time, etc.), motoneurons (motor axon conduction velocity, etc.), and quantitative characteristics of synaptic organization (group Ia EPSP amplitude, etc.), with arrows to indicate increasing magnitudes. Most of the actual distributions of these characteristics are not discontinuous, as implied by this summary diagram. Data for the graph is taken from Burke, 1967, 1968; Burke et al., 1970, 1971, 1973, 1976b; Cullheim and Kellerth, 1978a; Fleshman et al., 1981b; Friedman et al., 1981; and Cullheim et al., 1987.

bar spinal segments, which contains neurons that project to the cerebellum in the dorsal spinocerebellar tract (DSCT). The laminae present in the dorsal horn (Rexed's laminae I–IV) have been shown to contain neuronal organizations that process incoming afferent information, especially from cutaneous sources, in orderly dorsal-to-ventral sequences that also display topographical relations to the receptive field of particular afferent species (Brown, 1981; Darian-Smith, 1984). However, the functional identities of the many interneurons in the more ventral regions of the spinal gray (Rexed's laminae V–VIII) are much less clearly delineated by spatial location or morphology alone.

SYNAPTIC TYPES AND TRANSMITTERS

There are three basic types of synaptic boutons found in electron microscopic studies of the ventral horn (Fig. 3.4; see Brännström, 1993): (*1*) type S synaptic boutons that range from 0.5 to 8 μm in average diameter and contain spherical synaptic vesicles; (*2*) type F boutons that range from 0.5 to 7 μm in diameter but contain vesicles that appear irregular (pleomorphic) or flattened with many types of fixation; and (*3*) type P (presynaptic) boutons that are small (0.5–1.5 μm in diameter) and contain flat or pleomorphic vesicles. The S and F boutons contact the somata and dendrites of neurons with synaptic specializations, or *active zones*, at which the vesicles congregate. The P boutons end on type S boutons with synaptic specializations that indicate functional synaptic connections onto the larger type S that they contact. Such axo-axonic contacts are believed to modulate the release of transmitter from the recipient boutons, producing presynaptic inhibition (which will be discussed later). A subtype of large type-S bouton that exhibits a postsynaptic "cistern," called the *C type*, has also been recognized (Conradi et al., 1979).

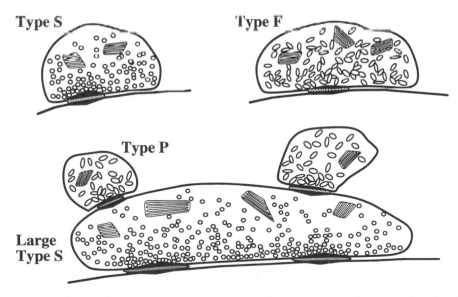

Fig. 3.4. Drawings of the ultrastructural appearance of the major types of synapses found in the ventral horn of the spinal cord. Type S boutons also receive axo-axonic (type P) synapses. [Adapted from Fig. 2 in Conradi et al., 1979, with permission.]

There is evidence that vesicle shape indicates whether a given synaptic bouton exerts excitatory or inhibitory action on its postsynaptic target; type S boutons are excitatory in nature whereas the F and P boutons with flat vesicles are inhibitory (see Chapter 1). It is likely that most of the excitatory synaptic transmission in the ventral horn is due to release of glutamate (Shupliakov et al., 1993). Results of immunocytochemical studies show that synaptic boutons with pleomorphic vesicles on and near the somata of large ventral horn neurons (presumably motoneurons) are immunopositive for the inhibitory transmitter, glycine (Destombes et al., 1992). Glycine immunoreactivity has also been described in the boutons of functionally identified inhibitory interneurons (Fyffe, 1991a). Synaptic boutons that are immunopositive for the other major inhibitory neurotransmitter γ-aminobutyric acid (GABA), are also found on motoneuron somata (Shupliakov et al., 1993). In fact, a substantial proportion of boutons immunopositive for GABA is also reactive for glycine, suggesting that some inhibitory synapses may liberate both neurotransmitters (Örnung et al., 1994). In addition, there are synaptic boutons in the ventral horn that contain 5-hydroxytryptamine (5-HT), thyrotropin-releasing hormone (TRH), and substance P, which are sometimes colocalized in various patterns (Ulfhake et al., 1987). The 5-HT immunoreactivity disappears after spinal cord section, indicating supraspinal origin of the 5-HT system (Arvidsson et al., 1990).

The graph in Fig. 3.5 shows the total percentage of motoneuron membrane covered by S and F boutons in the cat ventral horn (data from Brännström, 1993). The densest synaptic coverage is found on the most proximal parts of the motoneuron dendrites and there is a gradual decline in more distal regions. Although the curves for S and F boutons follow the same general pattern, there is some excess of F boutons on and near

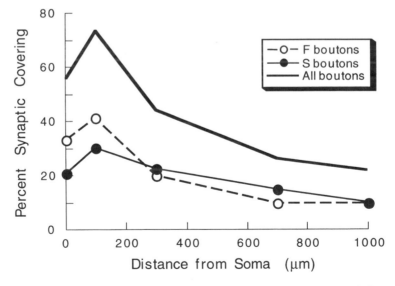

Fig. 3.5. Graph showing the percentage of membrane covered by F and S synaptic boutons, and their sum, as functions of anatomical distance from the soma (abscissa). Data from Brännström (1993).

the motoneuron somata, suggesting that inhibitory synapses outweigh excitatory synapses on the proximal regions of motoneuron membrane. Taken together with the distribution of membrane area in these cells, Brännström's data suggest that cat α motoneurons receive on average about 50,000 synapses from all sources.

Although the direct dendrodendritic synaptic arrangements that are found in some specialized CNS regions (see Chapters 5 and 6) are not present in the spinal ventral horn, there is some evidence for types of nonsynaptic cell-to-cell interactions beyond those associated with "plain vanilla" synapses. For example, there is evidence (Nelson, 1966; Gogan et al., 1977) for a weak electrical (*ephaptic*) interaction between motoneurons in the cat spinal cord. This phenomenon is much more potent in the frog, where there are many gap junction contacts between motoneuron dendrites (Sonnhof et al., 1977). There are sites of apparent close apposition, without membrane specializations, between cat motoneuron dendrites, especially in regions where dendrites are bundled closely together (Matthews et al., 1971). Electrical coupling between motoneurons has been demonstrated to produce sharply timed, synchronous discharge of motoneurons in electric fish (Bennett, 1977), and this might also be of use to frogs. However, there is little evidence of, nor much functional reason for, this type of tight coupling among mammalian spinal motoneurons.

Oddly enough, however, motoneurons apparently also interact directly via synaptic connections from recurrent collaterals that arise from the motoneuron axons before they leave the spinal cord. Such recurrent synaptic contacts have been shown to end monosynaptically on motoneurons as well as on Renshaw interneurons (Cullheim et al., 1977; see below). It has been difficult to demonstrate any clear synaptic effects that can be attributed to such direct motoneuron-to-motoneuron contacts (Gogan et al., 1977), and it seems possible that such direct intermotoneuron connections might have some other function.

SYNAPTIC ACTION IN THE SPINAL CORD

POSTSYNAPTIC EXCITATION: GROUP IA AFFERENTS

Anatomy. The *group Ia*, or primary, muscle spindle afferents are of special significance to this chapter because they make direct, or monosynaptic, excitatory synaptic connections with α motoneurons. The organization and function of this synaptic system has been extensively studied because Ia afferents can be selectively activated in the laboratory and the resulting excitatory postsynaptic potentials (EPSPs) can be easily recorded in motoneurons using intracellular electrodes. Group Ia afferents arise from specialized annulospiral end organs in muscle spindles that are activated by muscle stretch, producing the familiar stretch reflex (Matthews, 1972). Many of our fundamental ideas about synaptic organization within the CNS are based on studies of this monosynaptic system.

The intraspinal anatomy of group Ia afferents is important to an understanding of their synaptic action on motoneurons. In mammals, group Ia afferents are among the largest-diameter and fastest-conducting primary afferents that enter the spinal cord. The Ia afferents from a given muscle enter the cord in the same spinal segments that contain their target motoneurons, which are the motoneurons that innervate the muscle from which the afferents originated and those of its mechanical and functional synergists (Eccles et al., 1957). As shown in Fig. 3.6A, each Ia afferent divides into a large ascending (*rostral*) and a smaller descending (*caudal*) branch, which travel in the ipsilateral dorsal column and give off collateral branches at roughly 0.5 to 2 mm intervals at right angles from the parent. Each Ia collateral then descends into the gray matter (Ishizuka et al., 1979) to give rise to preterminal arborizations, and associated synaptic boutons, in three definable locations: (*1*) the intermediate nucleus (the medial part of Rexed laminae V and VI, where they contact a variety of spinal interneurons [Czarkowska et al., 1981]); (*2*) in lamina VII, just dorsomedial to lamina IX, where they make contact with a more specific group of inhibitory interneurons (Jankowska and Lindström, 1972; see below); and (*3*) in lamina IX, where they intersect with and form contacts on the somata and dendrites of α motoneurons (Jankowska and Lindström, 1972; Brown and Fyffe, 1981; Burke and Glenn, 1996; see also Fig. 3.1).

The monosynaptic contacts on α motoneurons arise from these elaborate arborizations of the Ia collateral axons, either as *en passant* boutons (simple swellings along the course of a collateral where the myelin sheath disappears) or as terminal boutons, where a fine collateral branch ends in a synaptic swelling (Fig. 3.6B). There are about 70 group Ia afferents in the cat medial gastrocnemius muscle nerve (Boyd and Davey, 1968), so one can envision the interstices between collaterals from any given afferent as filled in by the collaterals of others (Burke and Glenn, 1996). The terminal fields of Ia synapses from a given muscle in the ventral horn can be viewed as longitudinal

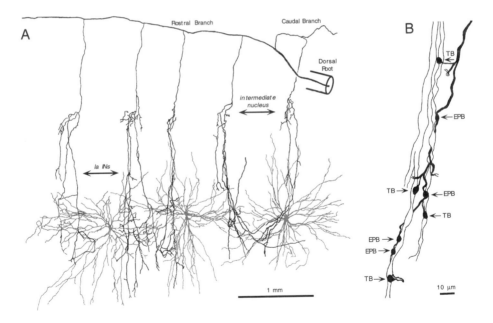

Fig. 3.6. **A:** Low-magnification reconstruction of a soleus group-Ia afferent (black lines) which made synaptic contacts on three triceps surae α motoneurons (stippled lines). All structures were functionally identified and injected with horseradish peroxidase. [Adapted from Burke and Glenn, 1996, with permission] **B:** High-magnification drawing of a small part of one of the Ia collateral arborizations (filled black; same preparation as in A), showing *en passant* (EBP) and terminal boutons (TB) on two dendritic branches of a soleus motoneuron (open outlines).

clouds of synaptic boutons in these three gray matter loci. Ultrastructural studies of synaptic boutons belonging to group Ia afferents show them to be medium to large in size, with spherical vesicles, and they often receive contacts from presynaptic P boutons (Conradi et al., 1983; Fyffe and Light, 1984). Pierce and Mendell (1993) have recently shown that there are systematic relations between bouton size and their positions within the group Ia afferent arborization, which may have relevance to variations in synaptic efficacy.

Motoneurons in a given motor nucleus receive functional Ia contacts from nearly all of the group Ia afferents originating in the innervated muscle (the *homonymous connection*; Mendell and Henneman, 1971; Fleshman et al., 1981a). The projection frequency is somewhat smaller but still considerable to motoneurons that innervate muscles that act synergistically at the same joint (*heteronymous connections*). Group Ia connections can also occur between muscles acting at different joints (for example, from the knee extensor, quadriceps, to the ankle extensor, soleus; Eccles et al., 1957). Presumably, such Ia connections facilitate the coordinated action of different muscles during movement (Eccles and Lundberg, 1958). Muscles that are linked by Ia interconnections are sometimes referred to as a *myotatic unit* (Lloyd, 1960) because they participate together in stretch (or myotatic) reflexes. Muscles in a myotatic unit often act together in a variety of movements but there are some interesting exceptions to this rule (Fleshman et al., 1984).

Intracellular injection of the tracer horseradish peroxidase (HRP) into Ia afferents and their postsynaptic motoneuron targets has shown that individual afferents can contribute as many as 35 boutons to a given motoneuron (average about 10), and these boutons often exhibit wide spatial dispersion in the dendritic tree. In fact, two and sometime three neighboring collaterals from the same afferent can make contact in different parts of the dendritic tree of a single motoneuron (Burke and Glenn, 1996). This recent anatomical evidence has confirmed earlier inferences about Ia synapse distribution that were based purely on electrophysiological information (Rall et al., 1967; Jack et al., 1971). The total number of group Ia boutons on a lumbosacral cat motoneuron is probably between 500 and 1000, or roughly 1 to 2% of the approximately 50,000 total synaptic boutons that end on these cells.

Physiology. The anatomy of Ia afferents defines a functional hierarchy in the group Ia synaptic action on motoneurons: (*1*) *single bouton* EPSPs produced by an individual Ia synaptic bouton; (*2*) *single fiber* EPSPs produced by all of the boutons belonging to an individual Ia afferent; and (*3*) *composite* EPSPs produced by synchronous action in multiple Ia afferents. This hierarchy (see Fig. 3.7) is fundamental for understanding synaptic organization throughout the central nervous system, where a given postsynaptic cell receives synaptic connections from multiple presynaptic neurons. The important point about the group Ia input to motoneurons is that it represents the only mammalian system (given current technology) in which this hierarchy can be studied in functionally defined pre- and postsynaptic neurons.

Using relatively simple but ingenious methods, David Lloyd (1960) was able to show that the stretch reflex is generated by the fastest-conducting (i.e., group Ia) afferents from muscle spindles and that the time delay (*central latency*) between the arrival of a volley of action potentials in group Ia afferents at the spinal cord and the activation

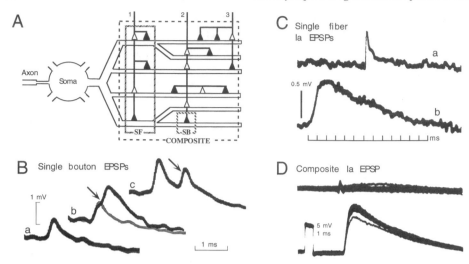

Fig. 3.7. **A:** Cartoon showing the anatomical hierarchy of synapses from group Ia afferents onto a motoneuron dendrite. Three group Ia axons make contact at various locations in the dendritic tree, some as *en passant* boutons (open triangles) and others as terminal boutons (filled triangles). The anatomical substrates of single-bouton (SB), single-afferent (SF), and multi-afferent (composite) PSPs discussed in the text are indicated by dashed lines. **B:** Three intracellular records of single-fiber Ia EPSPs in which unusually large, all-or-none single-bouton components are evident because of latency jitter (arrows). The gray trace in b is trace a, superimposed on another response in which two equal amplitude components exhibited a small latency shift (arrow). Record c shows a late component with the same amplitude. **C:** Single-fiber Ia EPSPs in a motoneuron produced by two different Ia afferents during controlled muscle stretch. The difference in shape is accounted for by differences in the spatial location of each afferent's synapses; the brief EPSP (a) had synapses concentrated much closer to the soma than the slower one (b). **D:** Intracellular multiple sweep records (note variable peak amplitudes) of a typical composite group-Ia EPSP (lower trace) in the same triceps surae motoneuron (same time scale but 10-fold greater amplification) from which the two SF components in C were recorded. The upper trace shows the Ia afferent volley immediately preceding it, recorded on the dorsal surface of the spinal cord. [Records in B, C, and D are adapted from Burke, 1967, with permission.]

of motoneurons is so short (<1.0 ms) that the connection between Ia afferents and motoneurons must be direct. The earliest intracellular recordings of synaptic potentials within the CNS were of composite Ia EPSPs in α motoneurons (Fig. 3.7D shows an example) following electrical stimulation of a muscle nerve (Brock et al., 1952). Intracellular recording provided great precision in measuring the time from the entry of the fastest-conducting afferent fibers at the dorsal root entry into the spinal cord, the arrival of the Ia volley in the ventral horn about 0.2 ms later (signaled by a small deflection known as the *terminal potential*; Fig. 3.8, record B, arrow), and the subsequent appearance of the intracellular EPSP after an additional synaptic delay of about 0.5 ms. The total central latency for Ia EPSPs ranges from 0.6 to 1.0 ms (Eccles, 1964).

More than a decade after the first intracellular experiments, Kuno (1964) and others (Burke, 1967; Jack et al., 1971; Mendell and Henneman, 1971) described single-

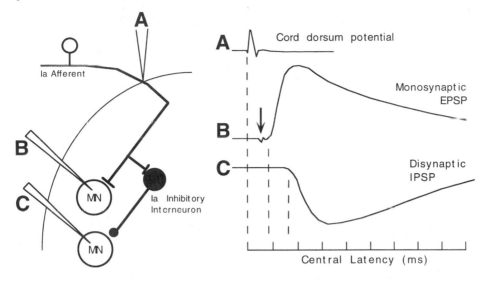

Fig. 3.8. The cartoon on the left shows the direct, monosynaptic group-Ia projection to a synergist motoneuron (B) and an indirect, disynaptic projection to an antagonist motoneuron (C) operating through an inhibitory interneuron (filled circle). The potentials that would be found at recording site A (on the dorsal surface of the spinal cord), and intracellularly in motoneurons B and C, are shown on the right. The arrival of the group Ia volley in the ventral horn arborization is indicated by the arrow in trace B. The synaptic delay between this arrival and the onset of the EPSP is about 0.2 ms. Note that the disynaptic Ia IPSP (trace C) has a central latency almost 1 ms longer than the monosynaptic EPSP.

fiber EPSPs produced in motoneurons by individual Ia afferents. The varying shapes of single-fiber EPSPs (Fig. 3.7C; Burke, 1967) fit theoretical predictions made by Rall (Rall et al., 1967) for synapses that are widely dispersed throughout the dendritic tree. As discussed above, this conclusion has now been confirmed directly by anatomical studies of HRP-labeled Ia afferents ending on labeled motoneurons (reviewed in Burke and Glenn, 1996). Synaptic potentials produced in motoneurons by individual group-Ia boutons (Fig. 3.7B) have only rarely been observed in isolation (Burke, 1967; see also Kuno, 1964), because their amplitudes in most motoneurons are usually much smaller than the average background synaptic "noise" from other sources. As will be discussed below, the characteristics of single-bouton PSPs have largely been inferred from statistical analysis of single-fiber EPSPs (Redman, 1990).

Quantization of Synaptic Action. Single-fiber group Ia EPSPs fluctuate in amplitude and sometimes apparently fail to occur during repetitive activation (Kuno, 1964; Jack et al., 1981a; Redman and Walmsley, 1983; Redman, 1990). Given that group Ia afferents contribute more than one synaptic bouton to each motoneuron (Fig. 3.6; Burke and Glenn, 1996), there are two potential explanations for such fluctuations. It is possible that action potentials arriving at the spinal cord might at times fail to invade some branches within the complex Ia collateral arborizations and thus fail to activate some boutons (*branch point failure*; reviewed in Burke and Rudomin, 1977; Lüscher and

Clamann, 1992). Alternatively, fully activated synaptic boutons might sometimes fail to liberate transmitter (*release failure*), as occurs at the peripheral neuromuscular synapse (Katz, 1966). Indeed, these mechanisms are not mutually exclusive. The weight of evidence available at this time favors a release failure mechanism (Katz, 1966; Lev-Tov et al., 1983b; Burke and Glenn, 1996) but some contribution from branch point failure has not been ruled out. In either case, it seems safe to say that the all-or-none EPSP components that make up a single-fiber Ia EPSP must represent events that are generated at the individual boutons belonging to that afferent.

A variety of statistical approaches has been used to infer that the amplitude fluctuations of single-fiber Ia EPSPs occur in standard size, or *quantal*, increments (reviews in Redman, 1990; Walmsley, 1991). One problem with evaluating this inference is that most statistical approaches assume at the start that the amplitude increments are the same, introducing a certain circularity into the argument. When the boutons from a single Ia afferent are scattered at different distances from the motoneuron soma, one would not expect them to generate equal voltages there. Nevertheless, in the few cases studied both physiologically and morphologically, the maximum numbers of quantal components in single-fiber Ia EPSPs pretty well match the numbers of HRP-labeled boutons observed anatomically for single Ia afferents (Redman and Walmsley, 1983). It is, of course, possible that quantal increments are in fact associated with active release sites in the synaptic boutons. Some large boutons contain multiple active zones (Walmsley et al., 1985), complicating the interpretation of quantal analysis statistics (Walmsley and Edwards, 1988). Thus, the mechanism (or mechanisms) underlying Ia EPSP fluctuations remains to be defined with certainty.

Mechanisms of Excitatory Transmission. Despite some early enthusiasm for the idea that Ia EPSPs result from direct transmission of the electrical currents from the presynaptic action potentials into the postsynaptic neurons (electrical synapses; see Chap. 1 in Eccles, 1964), it has been accepted for many years that, in mammals, the group Ia synapse operates by an exclusively chemical mechanism (see Chap. 2). The synapses between muscle afferents and motoneurons in amphibians, however, have both electrical and chemical components—a very useful combination for some research purposes (Shapovalov and Shiraev, 1980). The chemical component of amphibian Ia EPSPs can be blocked by increasing the external concentration of Mg^{2+} ions, leaving the initial electrical component unaffected. In mammals, however, the entire Ia EPSP behaves as expected for a purely chemically mediated event.

"As expected" means that composite Ia EPSPs exhibit an equilibrium potential ($E_{eq,syn}$; see Chap. 2) near 0 mV and reverse to hyperpolarizing polarity at more positive membrane potentials (Engberg and Marshall, 1979). This synaptic E_{eq} suggests that Na^{2+} ($E_{eq,Na}$ of about +40 mV), K^+ ($E_{eq,K}$ of about −90 mV), and possibly Ca^{2+} ($E_{eq,Ca}$ of about +145 mV) pass through the activated channels, since the observed $E_{eq,syn}$ depends on the net balance of the equilibrium potentials of relevant ions and their respective conductivities (see Puil, 1984 and Chap. 2). The reversal potential of Ia EPSPs is very difficult to demonstrate experimentally (Smith et al., 1967), which is due in part to the dendritic location of a majority of Ia boutons, where they are electrically isolated from current injected into the soma (Rall, 1967). An additional problem is the fact that motoneurons can exhibit sudden changes in membrane resistivity when strongly depolarized (Engberg and Marshall, 1979), limiting the ability of injected currents to alter the membrane potential further. Similar problems have been encountered in other parts of the CNS (e.g., the spiny neuron of the neostriatum; see Chap. 9).

For some time, the excitatory amino acid (EAA) glutamate has been the leading candidate as the neurotransmitter substance released at group Ia synapses in the mammalian spinal cord (Krnjevic, 1981; Puil, 1983). Identified group Ia synapses in the cat spinal cord exhibit immunoreactivity to glutamate (Maxwell et al., 1990a). With respect to the postsynaptic glutamate receptors involved, monosynaptic EPSPs produced by muscle afferent stimulation in the neonatal rat can be blocked by the AMPA receptor antagonist kynurenate but not by 2-amino-5-phosphovalerate (APV), a potent inhibitor of receptors for the other major EAA, *N*-methyl-D-aspartate (NMDA; Jahr and Yoshioka, 1986). On the other hand, more recent studies of monosynaptic EPSPs after dorsal root stimulation show a substantial NMDA component in neonatal rats, in addition to a larger non-NMDA EPSP (Pinco and Lev-Tov, 1993).

Recently, Walmsley and Bolton (1994) showed in adult cats that local perfusion with the AMPA antagonists CNQX and NBQX near the soma of intracellularly recorded α motoneurons produces partial or complete blockade of composite and single-fiber Ia EPSPs. Complete blockade was obtained with short-duration single-fiber EPSPs, as expected if most of the boutons were relatively close to the soma, where the drugs were applied. When blockade was incomplete, the remaining Ia EPSP was markedly slowed as well as reduced in amplitude, as expected for unaffected synapses in the distal dendrites. There was no evidence for a slow NMDA component in these adult animals. These observations provide evidence that the postsynaptic receptor involved in group Ia transmission in mature animals is largely, if not exclusively, due to non-NMDA (i.e., AMPA) glutamate receptors (see Chap. 2). They also fit very well with the anatomical evidence for dendritic distribution of Ia synapses discussed above.

Modulation of Transmitter Release at Ia Synapses. Whatever the transmitter involved, it is clear that the probability of transmitter release at any given Ia synaptic bouton can vary between 0 and 1. Such probabilities are not fixed but vary with time (Henneman et al., 1984; Lüscher and Clamann, 1992), with interesting consequences. If the probabilities of release at all 500 or so Ia boutons ending on an average motoneuron varied independently, then the amplitude of the resulting composite Ia EPSPs would change very little from moment to moment because the random changes at individual boutons would cancel each other. However, composite Ia EPSPs, as well as the monosynaptic reflexes produced by them, exhibit large, correlated fluctuations from trial to trial (Gossard et al., 1994). In addition, when composite Ia EPSPs are recorded simultaneously in two motoneurons in the same motor nucleus, their amplitude fluctuations are correlated (Rudomin et al., 1975). These observations indicate the existence of a mechanism that can produce synchronized changes in transmitter release among many group Ia boutons on many motoneurons. This mechanism, called *presynaptic inhibition*, will be discussed in the next section.

The average amplitude of composite group Ia EPSPs can also be changed systematically by the history of activation of the Ia afferents. For example, during repetitive activation of Ia afferents at moderate to high frequencies (>50 Hz), Ia EPSP amplitudes are depressed (Curtis and Eccles, 1960) because of an apparent depletion of the amount of transmitter immediately available for release by the active synapses (Barrett and Magleby, 1976). However, when tested *after* a prolonged high-frequency tetanus, Ia EPSPs are usually considerably larger than pretetanic control responses (Curtis and Eccles, 1960). This *post-tetanic potentiation* (PTP) ordinarily rises slowly over several tens of seconds and then decays to control amplitudes over a period of tens of minutes. The time course of PTP is complicated by the fact that EPSPs that occur immediately after the end of a tetanus are often transiently *smaller* than control values (*post-tetanic depression*, PTD). Note that these forms of synaptic potentiation and depression are quite different from the sustained long-term potentiation (LTP) and long-term depression (LTD) that are found in other areas of the brain (see Chaps. 2 and 11). Neither LTP nor LTD seem to occur in motoneurons.

The coexistence of simultaneous PTD and PTP can be revealed by the administration of the drug 1-baclofen, which activates $GABA_B$ receptors (see Chap. 2). Among its several effects, 1-baclofen reduces Ca^{2+} entry into synaptic terminals (Dunlap and Fischbach, 1981; Dolphin and Scott, 1986). This reduction in turn reduces the total transmitter output and consequently eliminates PTD, which results from short-term depletion of releasable transmitter (Lev-Tov et al., 1988). The net effect is to reveal uncontaminated PTP, in which EPSPs *immediately* after the end of the conditioning tetanus can be up to six times larger than the pretetanic EPSPs. The drug 4-aminopyridine, which prolongs the afferent action potential and allows greater influx of Ca^{2+}, also produces marked enhancement of Ia EPSP amplitudes (Jankowska et al., 1977) and increases the average probability of single-fiber quantal Ia EPSPs without changing their size (Jack et al., 1981b). In all of the above cases, the behavior of group Ia EPSPs within the CNS closely resembles that of cholinergic end-plate potentials at neuromuscular junction (Barrett and Magleby, 1976; Martin, 1977). Despite the great anatomical differences between the consolidated neuromuscular junction and the distributed, individual synaptic boutons belonging to a single Ia afferent, these results strongly suggest that the basic mechanism of transmitter release is the same at both synapses—increased intrasynaptic $[Ca^{2+}]_i$ secondary to the entry of Ca^{2+} during synaptic depolarization (see also Chap. 1).

Presynaptic Inhibition. In 1957, Frank and Fuortes reported that stimulating certain muscle nerves reduced group Ia EPSPs in extensor motoneurons without producing detectable IPSPs or changing the resistance of the postsynaptic cell. Frank (1959) later suggested two possible explanations for this observations, one of which he called *remote inhibition* and the other, *presynaptic inhibition*. Remote inhibition of an EPSP would be produced by local interactions between excitatory and inhibitory conductances generated by neighboring synapses in distal, electrotonically remote dendrites. As an alternative, Frank suggested that release of transmitter at Ia boutons might be modulated by some then-undefined mechanism operating presynaptically, that is, directly on the synaptic boutons themselves. A great deal of subsequent work has shown that *both* mechanisms are in fact present in the spinal cord, and it is possible to observe them separately (Burke and Rudomin, 1977).

Conditioning stimuli that produce presynaptic inhibition are invariably associated with signs of depolarization (*primary afferent depolarization*, PAD) in the intraspinal arborizations of the target primary afferents. The anatomical substrate necessary for selective depolarization of particular afferent terminals is found in the axo-axonic synapses that indeed end on group Ia and other primary afferent synapses that are subject to presynaptic inhibition (Fig. 3.4). There is little doubt that GABA is the neurotransmitter released by these axo-axonic synapses (Nistri, 1983; Rudomin, 1990). Direct application of GABA onto primary afferents in the spinal ventral horn depolarizes them, and PAD and presynaptic inhibition in several systems can be blocked by local application of picrotoxin or bicuculline, both of which block $GABA_A$ receptors (Peng and Frank, 1989b). Axo-axonic P boutons apposed to identified group Ia afferent terminals have been shown to contain GABA (Maxwell et al., 1990b). The depolarizing action of GABA on primary afferent terminals may seem somewhat odd because, when applied to motoneurons and many other types of neurons, GABA usually produces hyperpolarization by increasing Cl^- conductance. However, the Cl^- equilibrium potential in primary afferent terminals is more positive than the resting membrane potential, as is true also in frog motoneurons (Bührle and Sonnhof, 1985), so that an increased Cl^- conductance generates depolarizing potentials in these cells.

There are three possible mechanisms by which GABA could decrease presynaptic release of transmitter. The first two hypothesize that presynaptic inhibition is a direct result of PAD, while the third postulates a mechanism independent of PAD. First, PAD could decrease voltage-dependent Ca^{2+} entry into the depolarized synaptic boutons by reducing the voltage swing during incoming action potentials. Second, the invasion of action potentials into the fine-terminal arborizations of group Ia afferents might be blocked by PAD. Third, activation of $GABA_B$ receptors, which can also block Ca^{2+} entry, might reduce transmitter output independent of PAD. These mechanisms are not mutually exclusive.

There is a good deal of evidence that favors a causal association between PAD and presynaptic inhibition. Indeed, the existence of presynaptic inhibition in a given situation is often inferred by the presence of PAD in the target afferent population. There is a very close quantitative association between the magnitude and time course of PAD and presynaptic inhibition of group Ia EPSPs (Eccles, 1964; Lev-Tov et al., 1983a), leading many investigators to conclude that the relation represents cause and effect. Graham and Redman (1994) have used detailed models of the propagation of action potentials into group Ia afferent arborizations to infer that PAD-induced blockade of action-potential invasion into these arborizations probably plays no role in the phenomenon. Their model also suggested that very large Cl^- conductances would be necessary to reduce transmitter release significantly. Large conductance increases in Ia-terminal arborizations have recently been inferred during PAD using direct threshold measurement techniques (Curtis et al., 1995).

The presence of $GABA_B$ receptors on primary-afferent terminations certainly complicates this story. Activation of $GABA_B$ receptors (see Chap. 2), which are also present on primary afferent terminals (Bowery et al., 1987), can powerfully reduce transmitter output when activated (Shapovalov and Shiraev, 1982; Lev-Tov et al., 1988). Selective activation of $GABA_B$ receptors by the drug 1-baclofen generates little or no detectable change in primary afferent polarization or excitability (Fox et al., 1978; Curtis et al., 1981) but nevertheless markedly depresses transmitter release from spinal afferent synapses (Peng and Frank, 1989a), presumably by depressing the voltage-dependent influx of Ca^{2+} on which liberation of chemical transmitters depends (Dolphin and Scott, 1986; Mintz and Bean, 1993). Although this evidence suggests that presynaptic inhibition and PAD may not in fact be causally linked, Stuart and Redman (Stuart and Redman, 1992) used the $GABA_B$ blocker saclofen to conclude that $GABA_B$ activation, although clearly present during presynaptic inhibition, plays a subsidiary role in its production. It is likely, therefore, that PAD and $GABA_B$ receptor activation act cooperatively to modulate Ca^{2+} entry into afferent terminals, with additive effects on net transmitter output.

OTHER EXCITATORY SYSTEMS

The group Ia afferent system is obviously only one of many synaptic systems that control activity within the spinal cord ventral horn. Many segmental interneurons make excitatory synapses on one another as well as on motoneurons, but these synaptic systems are not well characterized because they are very difficult to study in isolation. However, some functionally defined systems that descend from the brain have been studied with experimental methods analogous to those applied to the group Ia system. Perhaps the best known are the corticospinal and rubrospinal tracts, which contain fibers that make direct, monosynaptic excitatory contact with certain species of α motoneurons in primates (see reviews by Phillips, 1969; Porter, 1987). Anatomical studies have shown that corticomotoneuronal afferents have terminal arborizations within motor nuclei in the cervical spinal cord of monkeys that are quite different from those of Ia afferents (Lawrence et al., 1985). Corticomotoneuronal collaterals are more widely spaced than Ia collaterals in the cat, and their arborizations within the gray matter tend to spread in a rostrocaudal direction for several millimeters, making fewer bouton contacts on individual motoneurons than do Ia afferents.

Corticospinal EPSPs recorded in primate motoneurons also differ from group Ia EPSPs, in that they tend to be smaller in amplitude and they exhibit remarkable intratetanic facilitation during double-pulse or short-train repetitive activation (Muir and Porter, 1973). This is not characteristic of all descending systems, however, since the vestibulospinal tract produces monosynaptic EPSPs in motoneurons that behave much like those of Ia afferents during repetitive activation (reviewed in Burke and Rudomin, 1977). The morphology of vestibulospinal fibers is also more like that of group Ia afferents (Shinoda et al., 1986). The evidence at hand suggests that the transmitter and/or receptor kinetics may be different for these various species of spinal afferent systems. The identities of the transmitter substances for these descending systems remain unknown. It should be noted that electrical stimulation of descending tracts is much less easily controlled than that of afferents in peripheral nerves and there is much less assurance that one is activating fibers with similar physiological roles.

POSTSYNAPTIC INHIBITION: DISYNAPTIC Ia RECIPROCAL INHIBITION

Inhibitory synaptic mechanisms are extremely important in controlling neural activity throughout the CNS. In the spinal cord, all of the various types of primary afferents make excitatory synapses with first-order spinal neurons. This is also true of the majority of long axonal systems that descend into the spinal cord from the brain. Thus, inhibition in the spinal ventral horn is largely produced by segmental interneurons, which are much more difficult to identify and activate in isolation than the afferent systems that feed them. Thus the information about specific inhibitory systems is much less abundant than is the case with group Ia excitation, as discussed above.

The first inhibitory postsynaptic potentials (IPSPs) to be recorded from the mammalian CNS were found by Eccles and colleagues in α motoneurons after stimulation of group Ia afferents (Brock et al., 1952) from antagonist group Ia afferents. The central latency of these reciprocal Ia IPSPs is sufficiently long (1.2–1.8 ms) to indicate the presence of one layer of interposed interneurons (Fig. 3.8; Eccles et al., 1956). Reciprocal Ia inhibition is thus referred to as *disynaptic* because there are two synaptic layers (and one layer of interneurons) interposed between the afferents and the target motoneurons. The identification and elucidation of the functional organization of the inhibitory interneurons in this pathway came much later and will be discussed below.

At normal motoneuron resting potentials (about -70 mV), group Ia disynaptic IPSPs are hyperpolarizing, indicating that the equilibrium potential for the process is more negative than the resting potential. The IPSPs can be reversed into depolarizing synaptic potentials when the transmembrane potential is more negative than E_{eq} (usually about -75 mV to -80 mV), as can be accomplished by injecting hyperpolarizing current. Injection of Cl^- ions into the motoneuron also produces rapid and marked changes in Ia IPSPs, reversing them to depolarizing events at normal resting potential (Coombs et al., 1955). It is generally accepted that Cl^- is the major ionic species involved in this inhibition (see Bührle and Sonnhof, 1985; see also Chap. 2). Because group Ia IPSPs are so readily influenced by injection of electrical current or small amounts of Cl^- ions into the motoneuron soma, it seems likely that the synapses of Ia inhibitory interneurons are located on and near the cell soma (Burke et al., 1971). Motoneuron responses to direct application of the amino acid glycine behave in exactly the same manner as Ia IPSPs, since they have the same reversal potential and sensitivity to changes in intracellular Cl^- (reviewed by Young and Macdonald, 1983). Group Ia IPSPs are blocked by the convulsant drug, strychnine, which also blocks postsynaptic glycine receptors. Thus it is accepted that glycine is the transmitter at this synapse.

DENDRITIC FUNCTION

The importance of dendrites to neuronal function is obvious when one considers that they contain over 95% of the cell membrane that receives synapses (i.e., excluding the axon; Cullheim et al., 1987). The dendrites thus dominate the electrical properties of the neuron, even when evaluated by a microelectrode in the soma. The distribution of synapses to motoneuron dendrites has already been discussed.

The pioneering work of Wilfrid Rall on the flow of subthreshold electrical signals that spread through the cell interior passively (i.e., without action potentials; these signals are known as *electrotonic potentials*) was based on data about the structure and electrophysiological properties of spinal cord motoneurons (Rall, 1959a,b, 1960, 1977; see collected papers in Segev et al., 1995). The early experimental work on the functional significance of synaptic inputs on dendrites was also done in motoneurons (Fadiga and Brookhart, 1960; Burke, 1967; Rall et al., 1967; Jack et al., 1971). One might expect that after more than three decades of work, the electrophysiological properties of motoneuron dendrites would be well understood. In some respects they are, but work on this problem also illustrates how difficult it is to extract fundamental information about dendritic membrane properties from real neurons in situ within the CNS.

DETERMINATION OF SPECIFIC MEMBRANE PROPERTIES

The specific resistivity and capacitance of the neuron membrane (R_m and C_m, respectively), and the resistivity of its cytoplasm (R_i), are critical values to any discussion of the electrotonic properties of neural dendrites. In order to estimate these key parameters in individual neurons, one needs to know the anatomy of the whole neuron in considerable detail, which is accomplished by injecting it with a tracer substance (e.g., Fig. 3.2). One also needs, at minimum, an estimate of the steady-state input resistance of the cell (R_N) and records of the cell's dynamic response to short and/or long pulses of current in the same cell. Work of this sort has taught us a great deal about how dendrites work, but we still do not have solid values for R_m, C_m and R_i. The generally accepted value for C_m is 1.0 μF/cm^2 in most biological membranes (Cole, 1968), although estimates as low as 0.7 μF/cm^2 have been obtained recently for hippocampal pyramidal neurons studied in tissue slices (Major et al., 1994). For cat motoneurons, estimates for R_i are about 70 Ω cm in cat motoneurons (Barrett and Crill, 1974; Burke et al., 1994), although here again values as high as 390 Ω cm have been found for hippocampal neurons (Major et al., 1994). Relatively small changes in both of these parameters have significant influence on estimates of R_m, particularly when C_m is allowed to be less than 1.0 μF/cm^2 (Burke et al., 1994).

The impediments to progress on this problem have been discussed at length in a recent review (Rall et al., 1992). For example, the anatomy of real neurons is very different from the requirements for ideal, mathematically tractable cable models. Rall showed that branched dendritic trees can be lumped together and represented electrically by a single, constant diameter membrane cylinder under certain conditions: (*1*) the sum of the 3/2 power of the daughter branch diameters at each branch point equals the 3/2 power of the parent branch (sometimes called the *three-halves power rule*); (*2*) the electrotonic lengths of all dendritic paths are the same; and (*3*) the boundary conditions at all dendritic terminations are the same (Rall, 1977). Although the three-halves power rule is reasonably well fulfilled in motoneuron dendrites, the individual paths within a dendritic tree terminate at widely varying anatomical distances (Fleshman et al., 1988b). If one assumes the same values for R_m and R_i through the dendritic tree, the electrotonic paths are also disparate, as shown in the branched tree in Fig. 3.9. For real neurons, the actual lumped electrotonic cable that represents the dendritic tree of an individual motoneuron is roughly cylindrical only in its proximal half, while the distal half tapers. This is apparent in the model neuron shown in Fig. 3.9, where 10 of the cell's 11 dendrites were lumped into one equivalent cable (see Fleshman et al., 1988b for details). It is usually easier to simulate such complex neuronal morphologies using compartmental models implemented in digital computers (Segev et al., 1989).

The second problem in parameter estimation is that one is forced to make a rather large number of assumptions, some little more than educated guesses and others, clearly oversimplifications. For example, the initial estimation of R_m, C_m and R_i requires that we assume that the neuron membrane is passive, i.e., that R_m is linear and invariant with time and voltage under the conditions tested. However, motoneurons generate action potentials in the initial axon segment, and these active responses propagate an-

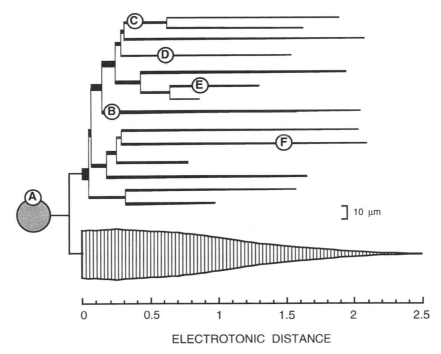

Fig. 3.9. A neuron model that includes a soma (stippled circle), one fully branched dendrite, and a tapered cable structure representing the other ten dendrites, based on morphology and electrophysiological parameter estimates from a cat type FR motoneuron (cell 43/5 in Fleshman et al., 1988). The dendrograms are plotted against electrotonic distance from the soma, calculated from the cell morphology and estimates of the specific electrical properties of the cell membrane and cytoplasm ($R_{m,s} = 225 \, \Omega \, cm^2, R_{m,d} = 11,000 \, \Omega \, cm^2, R_i = 70 \, \Omega \, cm, C_m = 1 \, \mu F/cm^2$). The diameters of dendritic branches are plotted according to the 10 μm scale shown. The model was used to simulate the EPSPs that would be produced by synapses located in positions typical of group-Ia synaptic boutons (open circles; see Fig. 3.10).

tidromically to involve the soma and proximal dendritic membrane. As discussed in Chap. 1, this indicates that active, voltage-dependent conductance channels must be distributed nonuniformly throughout these membrane regions. Modeling studies in motoneurons have illustrated the consequences of such nonuniform channel distributions (Traub and Llinás, 1977; Dodge, 1979). The use of in vitro slice preparations of spinal cord has provided direct evidence for the existence of variable densities of active channels on dendrites, which support variable penetration of action potentials from the soma (Larkum et al., 1996).

These active channels in the soma and dendritic membrane presumably contribute to net membrane conductivity at rest. They can also respond to the voltage perturbations that are used experimentally to measure cell input resistance and transient responses (Fleshman et al., 1988b). To the extent that active and/or passive conductance channels are distributed nonuniformly in the neuronal membrane, the effective net conductivity of the membrane, G_m, and its inverse, R_m, will also be spatially nonuniform. Unfortunately, there is little experimental data to constrain the choices about the location and nature of the active conductances that may be present in motoneurons. Thus, one begins by assuming that the membrane is passive and linear. Despite this simplification, conceptual and computer models that embody only passive membrane properties have provided very useful first approximations for understanding the role of dendritic electrotonus (Rall et al., 1992). They are the essential foundation upon which to build more realistic formulations that include the wealth of active conductances that are present in real neurons (Llinás, 1990; Midtgaard, 1994).

A second important assumption is whether or not the R_m can vary from place to place. Relaxation of the assumption that R_m is spatially uniform makes it even more difficult to obtain good estimates of the key parameters because it makes an already poorly constrained problem even worse. Nevertheless, a number of studies suggest that α and γ motoneurons exhibit spatially nonuniform R_m (Barrett and Crill, 1974; Durand, 1984; Fleshman et al., 1988b; Burke et al., 1994), with effective membrane resistivity much smaller in the soma ($R_{m,s}$) than in the dendrites ($R_{m,d}$). This "leaky soma" situation reduces the cell input resistance and affects the membrane responses to voltage perturbations, the former more than the latter. In particular, the cell no longer has a valid membrane time constant, τ_m, because there is no unique value for R_m (recall that $\tau_m = R_m C_m$). "Leaky" somata may well be an artifact of penetration by a sharp micropipette (Jack, 1979; Staley et al., 1992). However, there is no a priori reason to exclude the possibility that spatially nonuniform membrane may be present even in uninjured neurons. Estimates of the specific resistivity in α motoneuron dendrites ($R_{m,d}$) are relatively high (11,000–20,000 $\Omega - cm^2$) and 10-fold to more than 100-fold lower on and near the soma ($R_{m,s}$; see Fleshman et al., 1988b). Estimates of $R_{m,d}$ in γ motoneurons are even higher (about 30,000–60,000 $\Omega - cm^2$; Burke et al., 1994), so that their dendrites are electrotonically relatively short, despite being quite long and thin.

MODELING DENDRITIC SYNAPTIC POTENTIALS

The neuron model shown in Fig. 3.9 illustrates how passive membrane models can be used to gain insight into the processing of synaptic information in neuronal dendrites. The model is based on morphological and physiological measurements from a particular cat motoneuron. This representation of the neuron includes a spherical soma, a fully branched dendrite as obtained from the original cell reconstruction, and a tapered electrotonic cable that represents the other 10 dendrites belonging to this cell (see Fleshman et al., 1988b for details). The circles with letters indicate positions of simulated synapses on the soma (A) and at various electrotonic distances from it, with a distribution similar to that found for group Ia boutons (Burke and Glenn, 1996). The shape and amplitude for simulating single-bouton group Ia synaptic currents were based on voltage clamp data of Finkel and Redman (1983). This conductance (5 nS peaking at 200 μs) produced a rapidly rising and falling EPSP of about 100 μV when applied across the soma membrane (A), and slower and smaller EPSPs when applied at progressively greater electrotonic distances (B → F), when recorded at the soma (Fig. 3.10A).

The inset graph in Fig. 3.10A shows that fall-off of peak amplitude with increasing electrotonic distance from the soma (open diamonds) was much faster than the decline in integral of voltage over a relatively long time (20 ms in this case; filled diamonds). This integral reflects the electrical charge delivered by the synapses to the soma (Edwards et al., 1976). By this measure of synaptic efficacy, boutons at almost one λ from the soma are about half as effective as a bouton directly on the soma.

The lower large graph (Fig. 3.10B) shows that the peak amplitudes of *local* EPSPs, recorded at the site of generation, *increase* markedly with progressively more distant sites of generation (from B to F) and are manyfold larger than their somatic reflections (almost 3000-fold larger for F). These large local EPSPs result from the fact that the local input resistances at the sites of generation in branched dendritic trees can be very high (Rinzel and Rall, 1974). The local EPSPs in the dendrites are sufficiently large that they can influence the magnitude of synaptic current generated by the constant conductance used in this simulation. The inset graph in Fig. 3.10B shows that the peak inward current (hence negative polarity) at synapse F was only about 85% of that at the somatic bouton (A) and fell more rapidly. This can be understood by the fact that synaptic current, I_{syn}, depends not only on the conductance, g_{syn}, that produces it but also on the instantaneous difference between the local transmembrane voltage, $V(t)$, and the constant synaptic equilibrium potential, E_{syn}, for the ionic species involved (see also Chapter 2):

$$I_{syn}(t) = g_{syn}(t) \cdot (V(t) - E_{syn}) \qquad (3.1)$$

In the case of Ia EPSPs, E_{syn} is near 0 mV, so that the rising phases of the local EPSPs at synapses E and F cause a substantial reduction in the EPSP driving potential during the conductance transient, despite the latter's brevity.

BASIC CIRCUITS: REFLEXES AND BEYOND

The central nervous system is a vast assemblage of neurons with highly complex but quite specific patterns of interconnection. As mentioned at the beginning of this chapter, one of the great advantages of the spinal cord for functional analysis is the fact that primary afferents and motoneurons, the two linchpins of functional identification in the motor system, are both locally present, separately accessible, and readily identifiable. A set of interneurons that receives direct (monosynaptic) input from a particular afferent system and projects, directly or indirectly, to motoneurons can be defined in terms of spinal cord circuitry and probable function. Such aggregates form the reflex pathways.

REFLEX PATHWAYS

What we now call neuroscience began with studies of reflexes—the predictable output patterns in muscles or autonomic effector organs that are produced by particular inputs. The simplest example, as noted already, is the contraction of a muscle (and sometimes of its synergists) when it is suddenly stretched (the monosynaptic *stretch reflex*). Another classic example is the withdrawal of a limb away from a painful stimulus (the *flexion reflex*), which can be accompanied by autonomic effects such as constriction of arterioles and pupillary dilation. Elaborate reflexes can involve precisely coordinated action of many muscles, such as the rhythmic scratching movements in a dog's hindleg in response to tickling its ear (the *scratch reflex*). These and other reflexes have been used for the past two hundred years to elucidate the neuronal circuits

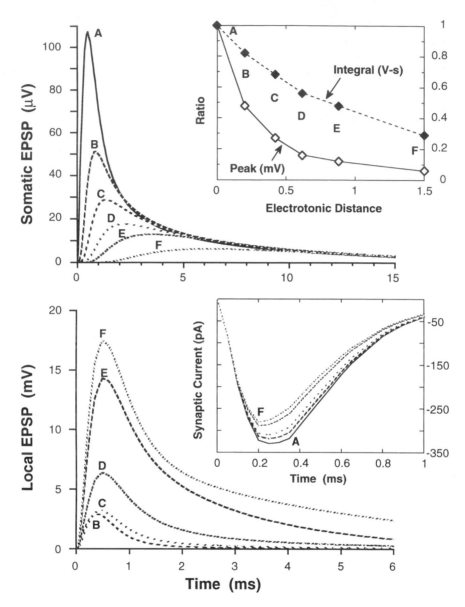

Fig. 3.10. The large graphs show calculated EPSPs produced by model synapses A through F (open circles) in the model shown in Fig. 3.9 when each synapse is individually activated. The upper graph plots EPSPs recorded in the cell soma while the lower graph shows the local EPSPs recorded in the dendritic compartments containing the active synapses. The upper inset graph shows the fall-off in peak EPSP amplitude and the integral of voltage over the initial 20 ms for the somatic EPSPs, both as functions of the electrotonic distance of the respective synapses. The lower inset shows the time course of synaptic current injected into the local compartments receiving the active synapses. See full discussion in the text.

and synaptic interactions that produce them. One cannot overstate the importance of reflexes in the development of ideas about CNS function that we now take for granted (Brazier, 1960).

Until relatively recently, the various reflexes have usually been regarded as distinct entities, resulting from the operation of separate bits of neural machinery. In addition, these *automatic* responses were viewed as qualitatively different from *voluntary* motor acts, with separate sets of neuronal machinery for each. However, over the past three decades, research on the synaptic organization of the spinal cord has revealed that the *same* spinal neuronal circuits can participate in both reflex and voluntary actions. The ventral horn of the spinal cord is a region in which incoming sensory information is integrated with motor command signals descending from supraspinal brain regions, making an efficient control system. The following section stresses two points: (*1*) the spinal pathways of nominally different reflexes in fact interact extensively, often by sharing common interneurons; and (*2*) control of movement (i.e., of motoneurons) by the supraspinal brain is mediated mainly through interneurons in reflex pathways. This is likely to be true even in primates, including humans, despite the existence of the direct corticospinal pathway to motoneurons.

DIRECT ACTION OF AFFERENTS ON MOTONEURONS: THE STRETCH REFLEX

The simplest reflex is the contraction of a muscle after sudden stretch, which depends on the monosynaptic excitation of motoneurons by group Ia afferents, already discussed in detail. The monosynaptic projections of group Ia afferents are directed not only to the muscle from which those afferents arise (the *homonymous* muscle) but also to its functional synergists (*heteronymous* muscles). These synergists can be at the same joint, as with the potent heteronymous Ia connections exhibited between the ankle extensor muscles soleus and medial and lateral gastrocnemius (Eccles et al., 1957). There are examples, however, of monosynaptic group Ia interconnections between muscles acting at different joints, such as gluteus (hip extensor) and soleus (ankle extensor; Eccles et al., 1957). In general, the heteronymous composite EPSPs are smaller than the homonymous ones, which is in keeping with evidence that a smaller proportion of heteronymous Ia afferents reach synergist motoneurons than their homonymous targets. It is now known that the slower-conducting group II muscle-spindle afferents also produce monosynaptic excitation in many motoneurons, albeit weaker than that produced by Ia afferents (Sypert and Munson, 1984). The only primary afferent systems that make direct connections onto motoneurons are thus the muscle spindle afferents of groups Ia and II.

Although the monosynaptic stretch reflex is obviously designed for speed it is important to recognize that it is also reliable, in the sense that a monosynaptic connection cannot be completely interrupted, because presynaptic inhibition (see above) does not cause monosynaptic PSPs to disappear. There is a great deal of debate over what stretch reflexes are good for, but one function seems clear: to facilitate muscle activity to resist externally imposed stretch, which tends to restore the muscle to its original length (a length-servo function; Houk and Rymer, 1981). The apparent simplicity of the monosynaptic pathway is deceptive, however, since the sensitivity of stretch receptor afferents can be controlled by the CNS through the γ motoneurons. In addition, both group Ia and II spindle afferents exert significant effects on motoneurons indirectly through interneuron pathways (Lundberg et al., 1987; Jankowska, 1992). This subject continues to be a matter of intense research interest.

MULTISYNAPTIC REFLEX ARCS: INTERNEURONS

The fact that a monosynaptic reflex arc cannot be completely disabled is a weakness as well as a strength. When at least one layer of interneurons is interposed between an afferent system and the target motoneurons, two significant advantages accrue. First, the sign of the effect at motoneurons can be changed. So far as is known, all primary afferents excite the neurons to which they project, but an interposed interneuron can produce an inhibitory synaptic effect (Fig. 3.8). Second, transmission in a multisynaptic reflex pathway can vary from zero to considerable amplification, by virtue of the other excitatory and inhibitory effects that converge onto the interposed interneurons that regulate their excitability. Multisynaptic circuits can thus function as logical elements (in effect, digital gates of any configuration) and as signal amplifiers. In addition, the same interneurons can be used in a variety of functions, depending on circuit organization. The spinal cord provides some of the most compelling examples of these points.

Disynaptic Recurrent Inhibition: Renshaw Cells. The first spinal interneurons to be functionally identified using microelectrodes were the *Renshaw cells*, as termed by John Eccles and co-workers (Eccles et al., 1954) in honor of Birdsey Renshaw, an American neurophysiologist who first described inhibition of motoneurons following antidromic activation of motor axons (*recurrent inhibition*). Renshaw cells are monosynaptically excited by synapses from collaterals that arise along the course of motoneuron axons toward the ventral spinal roots. In turn, they project back to the same and related motoneurons (for reviews, see Burke and Rudomin, 1977; Baldissera et al., 1981). The central latency of onset for recurrent inhibitory postsynaptic potentials (IPSPs; central latency about 1.5 ms) in motoneurons indicated a disynaptic connection.

The key to functional identification of Renshaw interneurons was that the input and output sources were clearly identified; indeed, they were the same cells (i.e., motoneurons). Individual Renshaw cells are identifiable in microelectrode recordings because the excitatory postsynaptic potentials (EPSPs) produced in them by motor axon collaterals are powerful and of relatively long duration (Walmsley and Tracey, 1981), and they generate distinctive, very high-frequency (up to 1000 Hz) repetitive action potentials when activated by stimulating a ventral root (Fig. 3.11A). Thus Renshaw cells can be easily identified in microelectrode recordings, without the considerable difficulty of proving that an individual cell indeed projects monosynaptically to motoneurons (Van Keulen, 1981).

Individual Renshaw cells have been studied morphologically and their projections confirmed directly (Lagerbäck and Kellerth, 1985; Fyffe, 1991b). Although Renshaw cells are located deep in Rexed's lamina VII, ventromedially adjacent to the motor nuclei to which they project (Fig. 3.1), their axons do not take the shortest route to the adjacent motor nuclei. Rather, the axons enter the ventral and lateral white matter and then drop finer collaterals back into the gray matter. This funicular pattern of axonal trajectory appears to be a common trait among the spinal interneurons that have been studied morphologically.

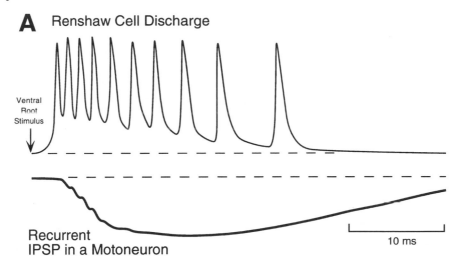

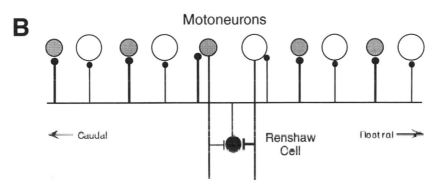

Fig. 3.11. **A:** Drawing of intracellular potential from a Renshaw interneuron (upper trace) during the powerful EPSP and high-frequency, repetitive firing produced by antidromic stimulation of motor axons (ventral root stimulus). The corresponding IPSP produced by Renshaw cells in many motoneurons (lower trace) has a prolonged time course due to the repetitive firing of the Renshaw cells responsible for it. **B:** Diagram showing the restricted spatial distribution of input to a Renshaw cell from local motoneuron collaterals and the much wider longitudinal distribution of its output. The larger motoneurons of fast-twitch motor units (open circles) tend to produce more powerful excitation of Renshaw cells than the smaller motoneurons of slow-twitch units (stippled circles), while the synaptic efficacy of the Renshaw cells on motoneurons is just the reverse (denoted by the width of the lines).

The recurrent IPSPs produced in motoneurons after ventral root stimulation are longer and less sharply peaked (Fig. 3.11A) than the group Ia IPSPs discussed above (Fig. 3.8) because they are produced by high-frequency bursts from the Renshaw cells. Recurrent IPSPs can often exhibit more or less synchronous wavelets, each generated by the relatively synchronized spikes in the multiple Renshaw cells that converge onto the motoneuron. The reversal potential for recurrent IPSPs is similar to that of disynaptic Ia IPSPs, indicating that increased Cl^- conductance is responsible. However, it has been reported that recurrent IPSPs are only partially blocked by the glycine antagonist, strychnine (Cullheim and Kellerth, 1981; Schneider and Fyffe, 1992). The strychnine-resistant remnant is instead blocked by the $GABA_A$ receptor blocker, picrotoxin. There may be two populations of Renshaw interneurons—one that secretes glycine and the other GABA (Fyffe, 1990)—although it is quite possible that individual Renshaw interneurons may secrete both inhibitory transmitters (Örnung et al., 1994).

Interestingly, recurrent IPSPs in motoneurons are less readily reversed by small injections of Cl^- into the motoneuron soma than are Ia IPSPs, even though both are about equally affected by current injected at the soma (Burke et al., 1971). This suggests that Renshaw cell synapses end mainly on proximal motoneuron dendrites, where they are relatively isolated from small alterations of intrasomatic Cl^- concentration but not from voltage perturbations. This conclusion was recently confirmed by direct anatomical reconstructions (Fyffe, 1991b). If Renshaw cell synapses are located on some proximal motoneuron dendrites and not others, it is possible that they might strategically reduce the effects of synapses located more distally on just those dendrites by mechanisms illustrated in Chap. 1.

The basic circuit diagram of the Renshaw system (Figs. 3.11B) is relatively simple but one must appreciate that many neurons are symbolized by the single element labeled "Renshaw cell." Many Renshaw cells may be interposed between the axon collaterals from a given motor nucleus and the motoneurons that receive recurrent inhibition. It is also clear that a given Renshaw cell receives input from many motoneurons (*input convergence*) and almost certainly projects to many individual motoneurons (*output divergence*; see Baldissera et al., 1981). Recurrent inhibition obviously provides negative feedback from active motoneurons to the same and other motoneurons, but there are a few interesting complexities in their synaptic organization that lend spice to this apparently simple circuit.

The collaterals of motoneuron axons spread for only about 1 mm in the rostrocaudal direction from their point of origin, so that a given Renshaw interneuron is activated only by collaterals of nearby motoneurons (Cullheim and Kellerth, 1978a). Since most motor nuclei in the cat spinal cord are 7–10 mm in length, this means that only a fraction of the motoneurons belonging to a given nucleus can contribute input to any local group of Renshaw cells. Indeed, some distal motor nuclei do not have recurrent axon collaterals at all (Cullheim and Kellerth, 1978b; McCurdy and Hamm, 1992). However, Renshaw cell axons can project over 12 mm rostrocaudally, thus extending their influence to large fractions of the motor nuclei (Jankowska and Smith, 1973; Fig. 3.11B).

In addition, recurrent collaterals from the motoneurons that innervate fast contracting muscle units (most notably, those of type FF motor units; see above) are more luxuriant than those of cells innervating slow-twitch muscle units (type S; Cullheim and Kellerth, 1978b) and appear to have greater functional input to Renshaw cells than that from type S motoneurons (Hultborn et al., 1988b). On the output side, by contrast, recurrent IPSPs are largest among type S motoneurons and smallest in type FF (Friedman et al., 1981; Hultborn et al., 1988a). Thus the motoneurons that excite Renshaw cells most strongly receive the weakest recurrent inhibition, and vice versa.

There are other rather clear patterns in the distribution of recurrent inhibition. Particular motor nuclei can be joined as input–output partners in recurrent inhibition even though separated by considerable distances, while near neighbors may not be. As a general rule, recurrent inhibition is not found between motor nuclei of muscles that are strict functional antagonists at a particular joint (Baldissera et al., 1981). Finally, motor axon collaterals are not the only source of synaptic input to Renshaw cells; they receive both excitatory and inhibitory input from a variety of other sources, including both muscle and skin afferents, and from a variety of supraspinal regions as well. Thus it is clear that Renshaw cells do not constitute a private pathway exclusive to motor axon collaterals.

On the output side, Renshaw cells can also inhibit one another, accounting for the phenomenon of *recurrent excitation* (Ryall et al., 1971). Renshaw cells also inhibit interneurons in the reciprocal disynaptic pathway between group Ia afferents and motoneurons. All of this evidence clearly suggests that Renshaw interneurons probably subserve functions that go well beyond simple negative feedback. The existence of supraspinal projections onto Renshaw cells suggests that recurrent inhibition can be modulated by descending motor commands. Thus what appears to be at first glance a rather simple neuronal organization has, on closer inspection, remarkable complexity, with functional implications that remain to be clarified.

Disynaptic Group Ia Reciprocal Inhibition. The complex nature of neuronal organization can be amplified by considering the synaptic organization found in disynaptic reciprocal Ia inhibitory interneurons introduced previously. Although the physiological characteristics of group Ia reciprocal inhibition clearly indicate its disynaptic nature, identification of individual interneurons in the reciprocal Ia inhibitory pathway was not as simple as in the case of Renshaw cells. Many spinal interneurons receive monosynaptic group Ia excitation (Eccles et al., 1960), and it was not clear how one could prove that any particular cell also directly inhibits antagonist motoneurons.

The key to this problem was found by Hultborn and co-workers (Hultborn et al., 1971a), who found that of all the inhibitory reflex pathways tested, disynaptic reciprocal Ia inhibition alone is subject to recurrent inhibition by Renshaw cells. Thus, if an individual interneuron is both monosynaptically excited by group Ia afferents and disynaptically inhibited after ventral root stimulation, it can be inferred that it belongs to the reciprocal Ia inhibitory reflex pathway (Hultborn et al., 1971b). Subsequent elegant work by Jankowska and Roberts (1972a,b) showed through the technique of spike-triggered averaging (the action potentials of a single interneuron were used to trigger a computer to average intracellular potentials) that such interneurons indeed directly inhibit the appropriate motoneurons. The Ia inhibitory interneurons have also been studied morphologically by intracellular injection of tracer substances (Jankowska and Lindström, 1972). Like Renshaw cells, Ia inhibitory interneurons have axons that travel in the white matter, dropping collaterals back into the gray matter to make synaptic contacts with both α and γ motoneurons.

Convergence of Control in Reciprocal Ia Inhibitory Interneurons. The disynaptic reciprocal Ia inhibitory pathway provides a striking example of the potential complexity of CNS control of interneurons in a reflex pathway that seems simple at first glance. The synaptic organization of this pathway was worked out largely through the technique of *spatial facilitation* of synaptic potentials recorded intracellularly from motoneurons. This powerful method enables inferences about the organization of synaptic input to interneurons in many spinal reflex pathways (Lundberg, 1975; Jankowska and Lundberg, 1981). It relies on the observation that stimulation of a two-input system (a test and a conditioning input) can either enhance or diminish, in a nonlinear manner, the amplitude of the EPSPs or IPSPs produced by the test reflex pathway in motoneurons (Fig. 3.12). With appropriate controls, it is possible to infer from such observations that both the test and conditioning input pathways both converge onto interneurons in the test pathway.

Using spatial facilitation and direct interneuron recordings, Hultborn, Jankowska, and their colleagues (for reviews, see Baldissera et al., 1981) have shown that the reciprocal Ia inhibitory interneurons receive input from a wide variety of input systems in addition to Ia afferents and Renshaw cells (Fig. 3.13). These other input sources include other primary afferent systems, such as ipsilateral group Ib muscle afferents, and high-threshold muscle, cutaneous and joint afferents from both sides of the body (the FRA; see above), as well as a variety of identifiable systems that descend to the spinal cord from supraspinal centers (e.g., the corticospinal, rubrospinal, vestibulospinal, and reticulospinal tracts). Most of these systems excite the pathway interneurons but it is important to note that they are inhibited by other groups of Ia inhibitory interneurons.

Although seemingly bewildering in complexity, the synaptic organization of reciprocal Ia inhibitory interneurons displays patterns that suggest important functional correlates. For example, descending systems like the vestibulospinal tract directly excite certain extensor motoneurons as well as Ia inhibitory interneurons that receive Ia input from the same muscle and then project to its flexor antagonists. These same *ex-*

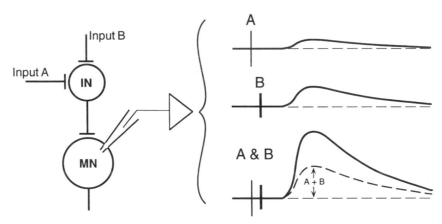

Fig. 3.12. Diagram showing the method of spatial facilitation that has been used to investigate synaptic organization in spinal reflex pathways, using PSPs recorded intracellularly from a motoneuron (MN) produced by two inputs (A and B) that converge onto common interneurons (IN) that then project to the motoneuron. In this hypothetical example, both inputs A and B generate a small EPSP when stimulated alone. However, when both A and B are stimulated such that their effects arrive synchronously at the interneuron, an EPSP is recorded in the motoneuron (A & B) that is much larger than the algebraic sum of A and B individually (A + B). [Adapted from Fig. 1 in Lundberg, 1975, with permission.]

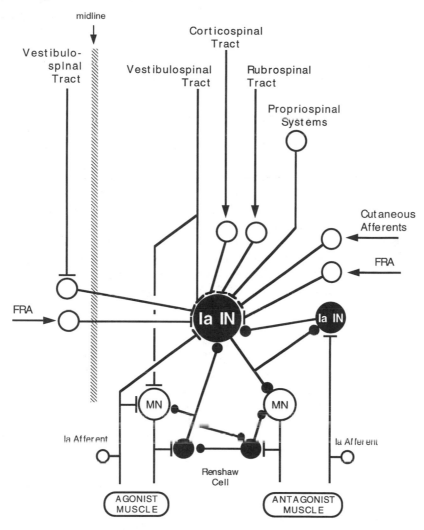

Fig. 3.13. Schematic diagram showing the organization of descending and afferent synaptic input to interneurons (Ia IN) in the disynaptic reciprocal inhibitory pathway between group Ia afferents and antagonist motoneurons (MN). The organization of Renshaw interneurons in the recurrent inhibitory pathway is also partially diagrammed. By convention, excitatory interneurons are denoted by open circles and excitatory synapses by bars, while inhibitory cells and synapses are indicated as filled circles. [Adapted from Fig. 11 in Baldissera et al., 1981, with permission.]

tensor Ia inhibitory interneurons also inhibit the Ia inhibitory interneurons that receive flexor Ia input and inhibit the extensor motoneurons (Fig. 3.11; Baldissera et al., 1981; Jankowska, 1992). Working through this organization, it becomes apparent that activation of an extensor muscle by, for example, descending vestibulospinal commands would at the same time reduce any ongoing extensor inhibition due to *flexor* Ia interneurons and increase inhibition of the antagonist flexor nucleus. If the flexor muscle were passively stretched by extensor contraction, the usual central effects of the resulting flexor Ia afferent input (activation of flexor motoneurons and disynaptic inhibition of extensors) would thus tend to be suppressed. This antagonist suppression presumably can be kept within bounds, at least to some extent, by the organization of the recurrent inhibition. Activation of the agonist (extensor) motor nucleus would, through recurrent inhibition, suppress its Ia interneurons and remove the antagonist suppression. This is, of course, only one possible scenario. Given the variety of inputs present, reciprocal Ia inhibitory interneurons can presumably participate in a wide variety of actions in addition to their simple reflex function. One important additional example—their participation in locomotion—will be discussed later.

The extensive convergence of multiple input systems onto Renshaw cells and reciprocal Ia inhibitory interneurons illustrates a critical point about spinal reflex pathways in mammals: few if any of them are "private" to a particular category of input or output (Lundberg, 1969, 1975; Baldissera et al., 1981). It seems quite likely that the spinal interneurons that are interposed in the long-recognized spinal reflex pathways and dominated by a particular kind of primary afferent under some conditions may under other conditions subserve quite different functions and obey other masters (Jankowska and Lundberg, 1981; Jankowska, 1992).

OTHER REFLEX SYSTEMS

A great many other spinal reflex organizations have been identified, some dominated by muscle afferent input and others by cutaneous or deep afferent systems. For example, group Ia and group II afferents from muscle spindles can also produce di- and multisynaptic excitation of some motoneurons. The Golgi tendon organ afferents that sense muscle tension also generate a wide variety of excitatory and inhibitory reflex effects (see Baldissera et al., 1981). There are also disynaptic excitatory pathways from skin afferents to some motoneurons (Illert et al., 1976; Fleshman et al., 1988a), although most cutaneous reflexes operate through at least two levels of interneurons (referred to simply as *multisynaptic*). These pathways are also subject to a variety of other control systems (see below). It is very difficult to make inferences about the synaptic organization in multisynaptic reflex pathways using the spatial facilitation approach because the neurons that receive direct afferent input are not the same as those that project to the output motoneurons. Nevertheless, many of these more complex pathways appear to exhibit the same kind of convergent control that is characteristic of the disynaptic systems discussed above.

THE SYNAPTIC ORGANIZATION OF ASCENDING TRACTS

The basic function of some ascending tract neurons is clearly to relay sensory information from primary afferents to regions of the brain where the information produces conscious sensation and/or guides the formation of appropriate actions. There is a great deal of information about such systems which, being located in the dorsal horn, are beyond the scope of this chapter. However, there are some ascending systems that appear to reflect a more integrative function at the spinal cord level that complements the organizations found in the reflex interneuron pathways discussed above.

The contrast between relay and integrative functions is apparent when comparing the synaptic organization of two major spinocerebellar systems that project from the lumbosacral enlargements of carnivores and primates to the cerebellar cortex and certain brainstem nuclei. The dorsal spinocerebellar tract (DSCT) originates from cells in Clarke's column, one of the few anatomically distinct groups of neurons in the upper lumber segments of the cord. Individual DSCT neurons receive powerful input from particular afferent species, either from muscle afferents (e.g., group Ia afferents from one muscle or a functionally related group of muscles) or from cutaneous and some high-threshold muscle afferents (for review, see Bloedel and Courville, 1981). The firing of a given DSCT cell is tightly coupled to, and relays with reasonable accuracy, the input from the afferents that project to it (Kröller and Grüsser, 1983). As always in nature, the relay analogy is not perfect because there is evidence that DSCT neurons also receive input from segmental reflex pathway interneurons (Hongo et al., 1983) and therefore can sometimes act to integrate sensory information from complex sources (Osborn and Poppele, 1993). Nevertheless, DSCT neurons appear generally to provide the cerebellar cortex with a relatively unprocessed version of information from particular kinds of primary afferents.

By contrast, individual neurons of the ventral spinocerebellar tract (VSCT) receive a complex mixture of inputs, some directly from primary afferents and some indirectly via segmental interneurons (Lundberg and Weight, 1971). Unlike DSCT neurons, there is often convergence of a complex mixture of mono- and polysynaptic effects from muscle and cutaneous afferent systems onto individual VSCT cells, resulting in inhibition as well as excitation. In general, no individual input system dominates the synaptic inputs to individual VSCT cells, which appear to be sufficiently diverse so that each VSCT cell appears to be unique in the constellation of information that it conveys.

What use can the cerebellum make of the output of VSCT neurons that receive such diverse inputs? Lundberg (1971) has suggested an intriguing hypothesis based in part on the observation that some VSCT cells receive monosynaptic excitation from group Ia afferents from a particular muscle nerve and, at the same time, disynaptic inhibition apparently produced by the same Ia afferents (Fig. 3.14; Lundberg and Weight, 1971). The probability of discharge from such cells would thus be increased by direct Ia excitation and simultaneously reduced by disynaptic Ia inhibition from the same source, depending on the degree to which the disynaptic inhibitory interneurons in fact responded to the initial Ia excitation. VSCT neurons with this organization could thus function as comparators, to signal the level of transmission through the disynaptic Ia inhibitory pathway.

When looking at Fig. 3.14, recall the complexity of input to the reciprocal Ia inhibitory interneurons shown in Fig. 3.13. It would seem important to the supraspinal brain, including the cerebellum, to have some reflection of the state of affairs at the segmental level, when so many of the reflex pathways discussed above are subject to complex control from many sources. It seems quite plausible that at least some elements of the VSCT inform the cerebellar cortex about the activity in spinal reflex pathways that are subject to descending control (Lundberg, 1971). The fact that the DSCT relay provides the cerebellum with a much more accurate, unprocessed version of Ia (for example) input would give the opportunity to make additional comparisons of input to, and output from, particular spinal interneuron pathways. Although much work is required to validate this hypothesis, it is in principle testable and suggests a further

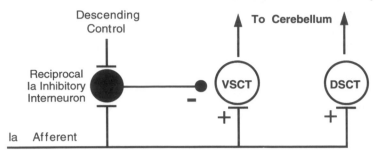

Fig. 3.14. Diagram showing contrasting organization of synaptic input found in some neurons of the dorsal (DSCT) and ventral spinocerebellar (VSCT) tracts. Full discussion is in the text. [Adapted from Fig. 1 in Lundberg, 1971, with permission.]

rationale for the remarkable complexity of synaptic organization at the spinal cord level (see Baldissera et al., 1981 for further discussion).

CONCLUDING COMMENT

The synaptic organization found in spinal interneuronal pathways implies great functional flexibility in the spinal cord. This phylogenetically old part of the CNS evidently retains mechanisms capable of sophisticated integration of sensory information with descending motor commands. The convergence of control on reflex pathway interneurons enables descending motor commands to take advantage of the fact that these cells have immediate access to the sensory information that signal, for example, current limb position, muscle lengths and tensions, and the existence of external objects. By operating through interneurons of segmental reflex pathways, descending motor commands can be effectively filtered according to the existing state of affairs in the limb and trunk before they reach the motoneurons. The filter is updated continuously as conditions change. This organization can operate in an efficient, predictive way, in contrast to feed-back mechanisms that depend on sensory signals about the *results* of a movement, which are inherently slower and quite unsuited to control movements of even modest speed (Rack, 1981). There is evidence that this type of organization is present in humans, where it appears to operate during voluntary movements (Nielsen et al., 1993; Pierrot-Deseillegny, 1996).

FUNCTIONAL CONSIDERATIONS: THE SPINAL CORD IN ACTION

Aspects of the synaptic organization of the ventral spinal cord have been discussed above at the level of individual synapses, recipient neurons, and simple neuronal circuits. This section is concerned with the influence of synaptic organization on two important aspects of dynamic spinal cord function: (*1*) the recruitment of motor units during a variety of movements; and (*2*) the operation of some interneuronal circuits during the generation of rhythmic motoneuron activity that resembles the patterns found in locomotion (called *fictive locomotion*).

RECRUITMENT: THE SIZE PRINCIPLE

Force output from a muscle is modulated by activating and de-activating its motor units (*recruitment* and *de-recruitment*, respectively), as well as by controlling the firing frequency of the active units (a process often referred to as *rate coding*; see Burke, 1981). Because of the systematic interrelations among individual motor unit properties (Fig. 3.3), an understanding of the recruitment process requires that the identities as well as the numbers of active motor units be taken into consideration. The process of motor unit recruitment is critical to the neural control of movement, but it has even wider significance. It is obvious that the motoneurons that innervate a given muscle (called a *motor unit pool*) form a group with a precise functional role. In the mammalian CNS, with its many millions of neurons, there must be many such functionally defined sets of neurons, but only in the spinal cord can they be identified with any precision. Thus, information about the process of motoneuron recruitment is relevant to understanding the operation of neural circuits throughout the mammalian CNS.

It has been known for over half a century that recruitment is usually a stereotyped and orderly process (Denny-Brown, 1929, 1949; Henneman et al., 1965, 1974). For example, recruitment in the stretch reflex begins with small, slow-twitch units and ends with very large force, fast units. De-recruitment proceeds in the reverse order. Henneman coined the term *size principle* to describe the recruitment sequence: the process depends on intrinsic motoneuron properties that are closely related to the anatomical size of the cells, irrespective of synaptic input source (Henneman et al., 1965).

Intrinsic Motoneuron Properties Related to Recruitment. There are quantitative variations in intrinsic motoneuron properties among the cells that belong to a given motor pool that are relevant to the control of cell excitability (Fig. 3.3). For example, the rheobase current (the depolarizing current necessary to bring a motoneuron to its firing threshold), when adjusted for differences in cell input resistance, increases systematically in the sequence type S < type FR < type FF (Fleshman et al., 1981b; Zengel et al., 1985). This implies that type S motoneurons are intrinsically more excitable than type FR, which are in turn more excitable than type FF cells. An intrinsic membrane process called *accommodation* also tends to limit the responsiveness of some type F motoneurons to injected current much more strongly than in type S cells (Burke and Nelson, 1971). The overall passive membrane resistivity in cat motoneurons, when adjusted for the influence of spatial nonuniformity, also increases in the sequence FF < FR < S (Fleshman et al., 1988b), which together with differences in total cell membrane (Burke et al., 1982) accounts for the fact that total cell input resistance increases in the same sequence. Such intercell differences are presumably accounted for by quantitative and qualititative differences in the voltage-sensitive conductance channels discussed in Chap. 2. All of these intrinsic motoneuron properties are organized to produce a recruitment sequence that begins with type S motor units, progresses to type FR, and ends with type FF, in general accord with the original size principle.

Motoneurons also exhibit what has been called *bistable behavior*, with sustained depolarizations (also called *plateau potentials*) that can be triggered in the decerebrate state by a short burst of excitatory synaptic input and reset by a short burst of inhibition (Crone et al., 1988). This bistable change in cell excitability appears to depend on the action of serotonin (5-HT) liberated by descending raphe-spinal axons because it disappears after spinal cord section but can be renewed by intravenous injection of 5-HT (Hounsgaard et al., 1988). Under these conditions, sustained firing at moderate frequencies can also be triggered in motoneurons by injecting short-lasting depolarizing currents; such firing continues until curtailed by a sudden membrane hyperpolarization. Bistable membrane behavior appears to depend on activation of an intrinsic Ca^{2+} membrane conductance, which then affects the slow Ca^{2+}-dependent K^+ conductance involved in the post-spike afterhyperpolarization (Hounsgaard and Kiehn, 1989). This direct action of neurotransmitters on membrane properties is an example of neuromodulation in the mammalian spinal cord (see Chap. 2) and it may well play an important role in such actions as locomotion (Brownstone et al., 1994). It is not known whether there is a systematic difference in this property that is related to motor unit type, but voltage clamp data suggest that the tendency toward self-sustained firing may be more characteristic of the cells with relatively high input resistance, as found in type S motoneurons (Schwindt and Crill, 1977).

Unlike many types of CNS neurons (see Chap. 2), motoneurons have a limited range of firing frequency, largely because of their well-developed, post-spike afterhyperpolarizing potentials of relatively long duration (AHPs; Kernell, 1965b; Calvin and Schwindt, 1972) that follow action potentials and that depend largely on Ca^{2+}-dependent K^+ conductances (Barrett and Barrett, 1976). The AHP conductance increases during repetitive firing (Baldissera and Gustafsson, 1974), which acts as a powerful brake on sustained firing frequency. On the other hand, motoneurons can fire at short intervals (10–20 ms) when they begin firing. Both features make excellent physiological sense with regard to the mechanical properties of the innervated muscle units. Muscle units produce virtually their full range of force output modulation over a relatively limited range of input frequencies (10–50 Hz in most limb muscles) during sustained firing but, at any sustained frequency, force output can be maximized by a single short interval at the onset of firing (Burke et al., 1976a).

Synaptic Organization Underlying Recruitment. Although intrinsic motoneuron properties play a role in recruitment control, a great deal of evidence has substantiated the early suggestion of Denny-Brown (1929) that the organization of synaptic input is also crucial. The recruitment sequence within a given motor unit population is not immutable, as would be the case if it depended on motoneuron properties alone, but rather can vary with the nature of the synaptic system driving the action and the movement in question (Burke, 1981, 1991; Binder et al., 1993). Indeed, there are differential fluctuations in the excitability of individual motoneurons responding to group Ia input that can only be explained by synaptic drives that regulate the relative excitability of individual motoneurons on a moment-to-moment basis (Gossard et al., 1994). This suggests that the CNS has some flexibility to produce recruitment patterns that are biomechanically and metabolically tailored to meet the enormous range of functional demand presented to the musculoskeletal system.

Monosynaptic group Ia EPSPs provide a good example of the importance of synaptic organization to recruitment control. The average amplitudes of EPSPs produced by group Ia afferents increase in the sequence FF < FR < S (Fig. 3.3; see Burke et al., 1976b; Fleshman et al., 1981a) and there is a clear correlation between Ia EPSP amplitude and the functional thresholds of individual motor units in the stretch reflex (Burke, 1968), as predicted by Henneman and Olson (1965). Moreover, assessment of the effective synaptic current delivered to the spike generation zone from group Ia synapses reveals the same ordering (Heckman and Binder, 1988). The factors that can produce this ordering of synaptic efficacy are discussed below. If all synaptic systems were organized like Ia afferents, one would expect an essentially invariant recruitment process under all conditions (Heckman and Binder, 1993). However, departures from this expectation have been observed.

Stimulation of distal skin regions can alter the ordering of relative thresholds among motor units responding to stretch reflexes in animals (Kanda et al., 1977) and during voluntary activation in humans (Garnett and Stephens, 1981; Nardone et al., 1989; Nielsen and Kagamihara, 1993). Under these conditions, normally high-threshold motor units can sometimes be activated before those with otherwise low-functional thresholds, some of which may in fact be inhibited. It seems quite possible that such observations can be linked to the finding that low-threshold afferents from distal skin regions in the cat hindlimb produce polysynaptic excitation that is ordered quite differently from Ia input (Fig. 3.3; *cutaneous polysynaptic excitation*). Polysynaptic EPSPs are small or even undetectable in many type S motoneurons but are present and sometimes quite powerful in motoneurons of FR and FF units (Burke et al., 1970). The responsible pathway in the cat includes at least two levels of interneurons between the afferent and the motoneuron and receives convergent supraspinal excitation (Pinter et al., 1982).

The two proposed patterns of synaptic input organization to motoneurons are illustrated schematically in the upper panel of Fig. 3.15 (Burke, 1991). The existence of even two different orderings of synaptic efficacy provides the CNS with at least three options: (*1*) a size-ordered recruitment sequence; (*2*) essentially synchronous activation of all pool motor units; and (*3*) selective recruitment of otherwise high-threshold motor units (see also the lower graph in Fig. 3.15). Input system A has greatest efficacy (denoted by line width) in type S motoneurons but has progressively less efficacy in FR and FF cells. The same set of motoneurons also receives another input, B, which (for simplicity) is organized to excite only FF and FR units. Activation of the pool by system A would generate the size-principle recruitment sequence, especially when combined with the intrinsic properties discussed above ("A alone" in the lower graph). If the pool were activated by *both* inputs A and B simultaneously ("A + B" in the lower graph), one would expect a narrowing, or compression, in the net range of functional thresholds (Heckman and Binder, 1993). In contrast, activation of the pool by an excitatory synaptic system organized like input B could produce selective activation of the large force, rapidly contracting muscle units alone ("B alone??" in the lower graph). The question marks are intended to convey that the evidence for this possibility remains controversial.

Functional Consequences. In the size-ordered recruitment sequence, the first-activated motor units produce small forces and are resistant to fatigue (i.e., type S). These features are advantageous to motor units that are likely to be used a good deal of the time (high duty-cycle units). The second advantage is that the small force outputs of the individual type S motor units permit precise incremental control of output force. Both features are important for the maintenance of posture, which requires only small to modest total forces (Walmsley et al., 1978). As force demand increases, size-ordered

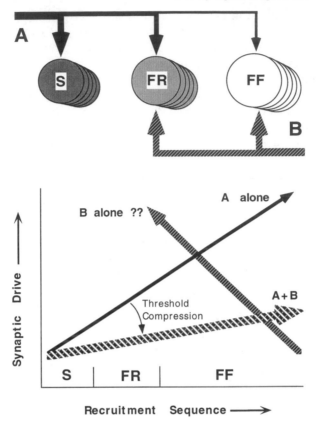

Fig. 3.15. The upper diagram shows two patterns of synaptic organization that have been found in cat motoneurons of different motor unit types. The relative efficacies of each input system is denoted by the width of the arrows. The lower diagram shows a much simplified view of the relation between recruitment sequence (abscissa) and intensity of synaptic drive (ordinate), given motor pool activation by input A alone, by a combination of A + B (resulting in threshold compression), or by B alone (resulting in possible reversal of the usual recruitment sequence). [Adapted from Fig. 1 in Burke, 1991, with permission.]

recruitment results in activation of increasingly forceful but less fatigue-resistant motor units. Motor units with the highest functional thresholds are likely to be recruited infrequently (low duty-cycle units), presumably in actions that require large force outputs but, being only occasional, need little resistance to fatigue. There is a long list of additional biomechanical and metabolic reasons why this ordering of motor unit recruitment is advantageous for many, but not all, motor acts (Burke, 1981; Henneman and Mendell, 1981).

Given that size-ordered recruitment is so well optimized, why should the CNS need an alternative synaptic organization at all? Garnett and Stephens (1981) demonstrated a compression of recruitment thresholds in human subjects when skin stimulation was superimposed on voluntary contractions. Threshold compression, which can be generated by activation of the pool via both of the alternative input systems (Fig. 3.15,

A + B), clearly facilitates virtually synchronous activation of the motor unit pool, which has been found in very rapid and forceful (ballistic) movements (Desmedt and Godaux, 1977) that presumably demand activation of all of the available motor units. However, whether such synchronous activation *requires* alternative synaptic organizations remains unknown.

The possible existence of selective recruitment of type FF units at the high-threshold end of the motor unit spectrum is more controversial. Perhaps the clearest evidence for such selective recruitment has been found by Nardone and co-workers in human subjects during controlled lengthening of an active muscle (Nardone et al., 1989). These authors speculated that rapid relaxation of motor units might be the reason for such selective recruitment of large, fast-twitch motor units, an argument that has also been made in connection with the apparent selective recruitment that occurs in very rapidly alternating movements (Smith et al., 1980). Clearly, much more needs to be done in this area before the issue is settled.

Factors That Control Synaptic Efficacy. One measure of synaptic strength, or efficacy (denoted by the width of the arrows in Fig. 3.15) is the peak amplitude of synaptic potentials measured by an intracellular electrode in the cell soma (Burke et al., 1976b). Other definitions are also possible (Heckman and Binder, 1988). The factors that can account for the large variation in Ia EPSP amplitude among homonymous motoneurons are surprisingly numerous and difficult to assess (Table 3.1). Systematic variations in any or all of them can, in principle, produce the experimentally observed difference in group Ia synaptic efficacy.

Table 3.1 includes three levels of synaptic organization at which interactions between presynaptic and postsynaptic factors can affect the efficacy of group Ia synapses in motoneurons. At the level of *single synaptic boutons*, one must consider the amount of transmitter (presumably glutamate; see above) released presynaptically, and the sensitivity and density of postsynaptic receptors for it. The interaction between these pre- and postsynaptic factors results in the transmembrane conductance change that gener-

Table 3.1. Factors that Control Synaptic Potential Amplitude at Chemical Synapses

Presynaptic Factors	Interaction	Postsynaptic Factors
	Single bouton level	
Amount of transmitter liberated	Conductance change per synapse	Receptor sensitivity, density, and kinetics
	Synaptic system level	
Number of active synapses	Synaptic density	Postsynaptic membrane area
	Electrotonic interaction level	
	Local PSP amplitudes	Dendritic morphology
Spatial distribution of active synapses	Nonlinear interactions between different synapses	PSP driving potential
	Electrotonic attenuation	Electrotonic parameters (R_m, C_m, and R_i)

ates a single bouton EPSP (Fig. 3.7). There is some evidence that variations at this level may be systematically related to motoneuron type (Honig et al., 1983; Lev-Tov et al., 1983b).

The next level of analysis is the *synaptic system*, including all of the Ia synapses that impinge on a given motoneuron. Effective synaptic strength can vary from cell to cell as a function of the total number of Ia synapses that release transmitter during any given presynaptic action potential (see above). However, synaptic number alone has little meaning without considering the total size of the postsynaptic cell over which they are distributed. The latter is best evaluated in terms of total cell membrane area. The ratio between synaptic number and membrane area is synaptic density. When all other things are equal, increasing synaptic density should result in increasing synaptic efficacy.

The last level of analysis concerns *electrotonic interactions* that depend on the spatial distribution of the active boutons and the electrotonic characteristics of the cell (soma and dendrites) on which they are distributed. Such spatial dispersion profoundly affects the amplitude and shape of synaptic potentials arriving at the cell soma, where they are integrated to produce, or fail to produce, action potentials (Rall, 1964). For example, if most of the Ia synapses to motoneuron A were electrotonically near the soma while those in cell B were most more distant, an equal density would still result in larger and faster EPSPs in A than in B. Equivalent spatial distributions of the same number of synapses to cells with very different electrotonic architectures could in principle give the same result. The electrotonic factor is of somewhat less consequence if EPSPs are measured by the electrical charge injected into the soma (Heckman and Binder, 1988), rather than peak voltage, because there is much less attenuation of the electrical charge injected by synapses on the dendritic tree than in PSP peak amplitudes (Fig. 3.10; see also Redman, 1973). In addition, synaptic inputs operate normally in repetitive sequences, so that the voltage changes at the spike generation site in the axon initial segment depend on timing and frequency of input, as well as on spatial location. Of course, all of this would occur with passive neuronal membranes. The existence of time- and voltage-dependent conductances in the dendritic membrane introduces a panoply of additional interesting complications (Mel, 1993; Midtgaard, 1994).

The problem for the physiologist is to sort out, to the extent possible with current techniques, which of this array of factors in fact accounts for the observed variation in Ia EPSP efficacy found among motoneurons within a single motor nucleus. A definitive answer is not yet available for this or any other synaptic system. However, a combination of electrophysiological, morphological, and computer modeling studies suggests that variations in the density of active Ia synapses (i.e., synaptic system level) can account for much of the experimental data (Segev et al., 1990). In particular, it is now known that the spatial distribution of group Ia boutons is the same on all three types of motoneurons, so this cannot explain the observed variations in EPSP efficacy (Burke and Glenn, 1996). In principle, the second and third levels of interactions noted in Table 3.1 can be attacked with available technologies in the intact spinal cord of mammals but the single-bouton level remains inaccessible in the intact CNS. Perhaps future refinement of experimental techniques and the use of more accessible preparations such as those afforded by tissue culture and spinal cord slice preparations will permit more concrete answers.

DYNAMIC CONTROL OF SPINAL INTERNEURONS: FICTIVE LOCOMOTION

The section on organization of reflex circuits dealt with the often complex patterns of synaptic organization among interneurons in reflex pathways. As described there, these patterns suggest that these spinal interneurons participate in the control of voluntary movement, in addition to their obvious role as mediators of reflex action. It is very difficult to obtain direct information to validate this suggestion in animal experiments. However, there is indirect evidence in humans that supports it (Nielsen et al., 1993; Pierrot-Deseillegny, 1996). Nevertheless, there are experimental preparations that allow recording from individual spinal neurons during the generation of patterns of rhythmic motoneuron discharge that resemble those found during locomotion. These preparations permit a look at motoneuron and interneuron function during dynamic action that can reveal important state-dependent properties that are not observed under any other conditions.

The basic pattern of coordinated motoneuron activations in locomotion is produced by a system of spinal interneurons organized into what is called the *central pattern generator* (CPG) for locomotion (reviews in Grillner, 1981; Rossignol and Dubuc, 1994). Patterned activity that closely resembles actual stepping can occur spontaneously in decerebrate, unanesthetized animals, or during low-frequency stimulation of a region in the midbrain known as the *mesencephalic locomotor region* (MLR; Grillner, 1981). There is some evidence that a CPG for locomotion is also present in the human spinal cord (Calancie et al., 1994). Coordinated motoneuron firing can be produced in animals that are paralyzed with neuromuscular junction blockading drugs without any rhythmic sensory input at all. Rhythmic firing of motoneurons is then recorded from muscle nerves; the activity is called *fictive locomotion* because the animal is immobile. It is then possible to record synaptic potentials intracellularly from individual motoneurons while stimulating skin or muscle nerves to examine changes in the resulting PSPs as a function of the step cycle (Fig. 3.16A).

Experiments in such preparations have shown that the locomotor CPG controls interneurons in reflex pathways. For example, the group Ia reciprocal inhibitory interneurons discussed earlier receive input from the locomotor CPG that modulates their excitability, thus regulating the transmission of information through them from antagonist group Ia afferents (Pratt and Jordan, 1987). Moreover, the centrally generated rhythm produced by the CPG can drive Ia inhibitory interneurons to rhythmic discharge in the absence of any phasic contribution from Ia afferents themselves (Feldman and Orlovsky, 1975)—as it were, co-opting them to generate locomotor inhibition rather than stretch reflex inhibition. In this situation, they might be called *CPG inhibitory interneurons*. What if, say, the descending rubrospinal system could also activate them without help from primary afferents? How would we then categorize the same set of interneurons? It is worth remembering that the neat pigeonholes produced by our need to organize and communicate information do not always fit the flexibility evident in reality.

Studies of modulation of transmission through other reflex pathways during fictive locomotion also provide examples of the precision and elegance of synaptic organization in the spinal cord. The flexor digitorum longus (FDL) muscle plantar flexes the hindpaw toes in the cat. Motoneurons that innervate the FDL receive di- and trisynaptic EPSPs from afferents that innervate the skin on the dorsal surface of the toes via the

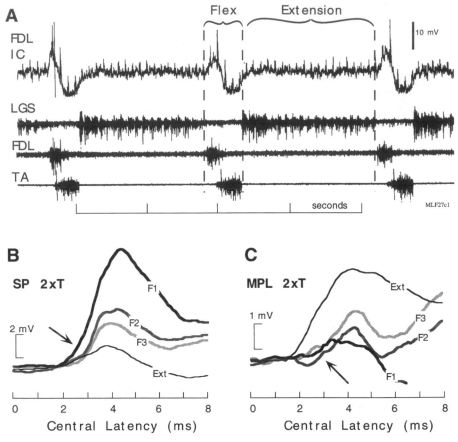

Fig. 3.16. **A:** Recordings made during spontaneous fictive locomotion in a decerebrate cat show-ing (from above downward) the intracellular potential in an flexor digitorum longus (FDL) mo-toneuron (FDL IC) and electrical recordings from an extensor muscle nerve (LGS) and two flexor muscle nerves (FDL and TA). During the flexion phase, the FDL membrane potential was first depolarized and then hyperpolarized, compared to the extension phase. Through the locomotor period, the skin nerve's superficial peroneal (SP) and medial plantar (MPL) were repeatedly stim-ulated electrically at 10 Hz (note small upward deflections in the IC trace), so that the effect of each phase of stepping on the resulting synaptic potentials was eventually sampled many times. Computer averages of the SP and MPL PSPs, sorted by step-cycle phase, are in panels **B** and **C**. During the first third of the flexion phase (F1), there was a marked increase in the amplitude of the SP EPSP and the appearance of a disynaptic component (arrow). In contrast, the disy-naptic EPSP evident in the MPL response during extension (Ext) was suppressed throughout the flexion period (arrow). (From experiments reported in Degtyarenko et al., 1996).

superficial peroneal (SP) nerve, and similar disynaptic EPSPs from medial plantar (MPL) nerve afferents that innervate the ventral (plantar) skin of the toes (Moschovakis et al., 1991b). The prevalence of disynaptic cutaneous PSPs in these two sets of mo-toneurons suggests that these are functionally specialized pathways, because cutaneous afferents produce only trisynaptic PSPs in most hindlimb motoneurons (see above). The possible nature of these functional specializations becomes apparent when the path-ways are examined during fictive locomotion.

Figure 3.16A illustrates an example in which SP and MPL PSPs were generated at regular intervals of 100 ms, superimposed on rhythmic bursting in extensor and flexor muscle nerve. With sufficiently long periods of rhythmic stepping, cutaneous PSPs were generated during all phases of the step cycle and were then averaged together, using special purpose computer programs (Moschovakis et al., 1991b; Degtyarenko et al., 1996). The intracellular record in Fig. 3.16 (FDL IC) shows that the FDL motoneuron was depolarized during the early part of the flexion phase of locomotion, at the same time as the FDL nerve showed a short burst of firing. When SP EPSPs were produced during early flexion (F1), a remarkable amplification of their amplitudes occurred, especially in the earliest component that had disynaptic central latency (<2 ms; Fig. 3.16B, arrow). This amplification, or facilitation, lessened during the later flexion phases (F2 and F3) and the EPSP returned to its control amplitude during the extension phase (Ext). In marked contrast, the MPL EPSP was suppressed during the entire flexion phase. This differential modulation clearly shows that the SP and MPL EPSPs, although both disynaptic, are produced by entirely separate sets of last-order interneurons (Moschovakis et al., 1991b). These data also demonstrate that the two sets of interneurons receive powerful control from the locomotor CPG, in one case excitatory and the other, inhibitory. This experiment demonstrates another use of the spatial facilitation technique to reveal aspects of synaptic organization in last-order interneurons.

The extensor digitorum longus (EDL) muscle is the antagonist to the FDL, causing plantar extension of the toes. EDL motoneurons also receive disynaptic excitation from the MPL nerve and these are suppressed during the flexion phase, just as in FDL cells. However, the SP nerve produces disynaptic IPSPs in EDL motoneurons, just the opposite of the EPSPs generated in FDL cells. The pattern of IPSP modulation in EDL motoneurons during locomotion is virtually identical to that in the antagonist FDL cells, in that the IPSP is maximally facilitated during early flexion and in fact disappears during extension (Degtyarenko et al., 1996).

A possible circuit diagram to explain these observations is shown in Fig. 3.17. The locomotor CPG is represented by two interacting half-centers (flexion and extension) but in the cases discussed, only the output from the flexion half-center affects the interneuronal pathways. This supplies excitatory drive during flexion that converges on interneurons in the SP to motoneuron pathways, both excitatory (to FDL) and inhibitory (to EDL). At the same time, this output line from the CPG also drives a set of inhibitory interneurons that in turn inhibit the disynaptic excitation from the MPL nerve to both FDL and EDL motoneurons. Note that the same MPL interneurons are shown projecting to both FDL and EDL motoneurons. The fact that MPL disynaptic EPSPs are suppressed in both kinds of motoneuron is compatible with, but does not prove that, the same interneurons actually do project to both sets of motoneurons. That is an interesting possibility because FDL and EDL motoneurons are antagonistic in function. The differential control of the SP and MPL pathways is remarkable because the areas of skin that are innervated by these two cutaneous nerves are immediately adjacent to one another at the tip of the hindpaw. This illustrates the precision with which some reflex systems are organized.

What could be the functional meaning of this precisely organized set of connections? The possible meaning of the suppression of MPL excitation during flexion is not obvious but the enhancement of SP effects during flexion does make sense. It is known

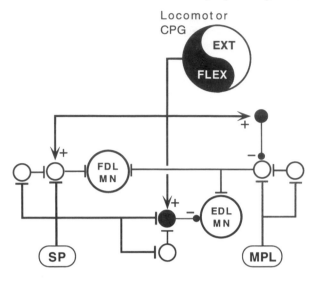

Fig. 3.17. Circuit diagram of the control of the SP and MPL disynaptic cutaneous reflex pathways to FDL and EDL (extensor digitorum longus) motoneurons, based in part on data such as shown in Fig. 3.16. See Degtyarenko et al., 1996, for full discussion.

that, when the dorsal surface of a cat's hindpaw encounters an obstacle during the early swing (flexion) phase of locomotion, the entire hindlimb undergoes an exaggerated flexion to lift the limb over the obstacle (the *stumbling corrective reaction*; Forssberg, 1979). This is, of course, the area of skin innervated by the SP nerve. The locomotor CPG evidently turns up the gain of excitatory input from this skin region as the foot begins to move forward in actual locomotion, just when the foot is most likely to meet an obstacle. The resulting activation of the FDL muscle and pronounced curling of the toes would contribute to lifting the foot over the obstacle. At the same time, EDL motoneurons would be maximally inhibited by the same stimulus. Why? It is known that coactivation of both FDL and EDL muscles produce claw protrusion in the cat. One possible reason for the powerful inhibition of EDL motoneurons might be to prevent this action, which would presumably interfere with the corrective movement. Thus the spinal cord appears to contain a precisely organized neural circuit to control fine details of the stumbling corrective reaction as part of the basic CPG for locomotion.

SUMMARY

This chapter has attempted to present an overview of the neuron types present in the ventral spinal cord, some features of their cellular and synaptic neurobiology, and some of the more significant circuit interactions between them, in order to provide the reader with an overview of synaptic organization in this part of the CNS. The spinal cord has been studied systematically from the earliest days of scientific investigation of brain function, but it still has much to teach us. It remains one of the few parts of the CNS in which the investigator has access to inputs and outputs with clearly defined functional roles. Given sufficient energy and time, these linchpins permit definition of neuronal properties and synaptic circuits that can be directly linked to behavior.

4

COCHLEAR NUCLEUS

ERIC D. YOUNG

The cochlear nucleus is the terminal zone of the auditory nerve; it consists of several groups of second-order auditory neurons whose axons initiate at least four different parallel pathways through the brainstem auditory system. The principal cells of the cochlear nucleus provide widely divergent examples of neural integration, ranging from very simple synapses that are specialized to preserve details of the temporal patterns of the input spike trains, to neurons embedded in intricate local circuits that generate sharp selectivity for features of the frequency content of sounds. The parallel pathways initiated by the principal cells each contribute a different form of analysis of the auditory signal. Thus calculations such as the location of a sound in space or the identification of a sound based on its frequency content are to some extent separated in the cochlear nucleus and conveyed through the brainstem auditory system by parallel pathways.

The basic auditory sensory map is generated in the cochlea, shown schematically in Fig. 4.1. Sound causes a traveling-wave of displacement on the basilar membrane, as drawn in this figure. The location of the largest displacement depends on the frequency of the sound, with low-frequency sounds causing displacement at one end (the apex) and high frequencies at the other (the base). There is a mapping of stimulus frequency into place along the basilar membrane, as shown by the scale at left of Fig. 4.1, for the cat cochlea (for a description of cochlear anatomy and physiology, see Pickles, 1988). What this means is that the location of the largest basilar membrane displacement moves from apex to base as sound frequency changes from low to high. Transduction of basilar membrane motion occurs in sensory cells, called *hair cells* (Pickles, 1988). Hair cells are contacted by the dendrites of *auditory-nerve fibers* (ANFs), and ANFs are driven to respond to sound in proportion to the degree of basilar membrane motion at the point on the membrane where the fiber's hair cell is located. As a result of this arrangement, each ANF responds to a limited range of sound frequencies. The frequency to which a fiber is most sensitive is its *best frequency* (BF) and a fiber's BF is determined by the location of the hair cell innervated by that fiber along the basilar membrane. ANFs, then, carry information about the sound arriving at the ear in the form of a *tonotopic map*. This mapping of a nonspatial modality (frequency) into neural space in the cochlea may be compared with the mapping of another nonspatial modality (odor molecular structure) into neural space in the olfactory bulb (Chap. 5). Per-

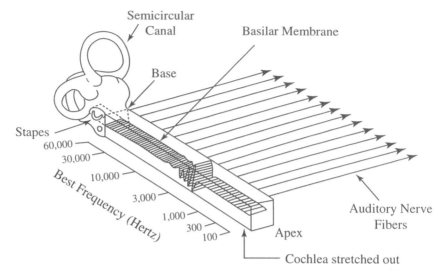

Fig. 4.1. Schematic of the cochlea illustrating the analysis of sound according to frequency on the basilar membrane. The cochlea is actually coiled like a snail, but is shown unrolled for clarity. Sound energy is coupled into the cochlea at the stapes and causes a traveling-wave of displacement of the basilar membrane; the traveling wave peaks at a particular place which depends on the frequency of the sound. Shown is a traveling wave for an ≈3000 Hz sound. The mapping of sound frequency into place is shown for the cat cochlea (Liberman, 1982) by the scale running along the basilar membrane. Type I auditory-nerve fibers are indicated schematically by the parallel lines. Each fiber innervates one inner hair cell and thereby samples the basilar membrane displacement at that hair cell's location. The result is a tonotopic representation of sound, in which each fiber conveys information primarily about frequencies near the best frequency of the point on the basilar membrane innervated by the fiber.

ceptually, position along the tonotopic map, or frequency of sound, corresponds to the sense of highness or lowness of the sound, which is like its position along a musical scale (Moore, 1989).

There are two groups of hair cells and ANFs (Spoendlin, 1973; Kiang et al., 1982; Ryugo, 1992). *Inner hair cells* and *type I ANFs* form the major afferent pathway to the cochlear nucleus; each type I fiber innervates one inner hair cell. Type I fibers are myelinated, constitute about 90–95% of the fibers in the auditory nerve, and are the afferent input to most of the cell types in the cochlear nucleus. *Outer hair cells* are innervated by *type II fibers*, which are unmyelinated and project to the granule-cell regions of the cochlear nucleus, as described below (Brown et al., 1988). To date, responses to sound have not been recorded from type II fibers and it is not clear what role they play. Outer hair cells appear to participate in generating the mechanical response of the organ of Corti; loss of outer hair cells leads to a loss of sensitivity to soft sounds and a decrease in the sharpness of tuning (i.e., the frequency selectivity) of the basilar membrane (Patuzzi, 1996). In the rest of this chapter, the term "auditory nerve fiber" will refer to type I fibers only, unless otherwise stated.

NEURONAL ELEMENTS AND THEIR SYNAPTIC CONNECTIONS

Because of the close correlations that have been made between neuronal types and their synaptic connections, these aspects will be discussed together in introducing the organization of the cochlear nucleus.

OVERVIEW

The modern definition of the cell types in the cochlear nucleus was developed by Kirsten Osen on the basis of cytoarchitecture (Osen, 1969) and modified by Morest and colleagues (Brawer et al., 1974; Cant and Morest, 1984) on the basis of Golgi material. Figure 4.2 shows the distribution of cell types in the cochlear nucleus of the cat in a roughly sagittal view of the nucleus. The organization of the cochlear nucleus is usually defined in terms of the projection pattern of the incoming auditory nerve. ANFs enter the nucleus at its ventral edge. Fibers bifurcate in the central region of the *ventral cochlear nucleus* (VCN) and send an ascending branch (a.b.) rostrally to the *anterior division* of the VCN (AVCN) and a descending branch (d.b.) caudally to the *posterior division* of the VCN (PVCN); the descending branch curves back rostrally to innervate the *dorsal cochlear nucleus* (DCN). The arrangement of fibers in the cochlear nucleus recapitulates the tonotopic organization created in the cochlea: low-

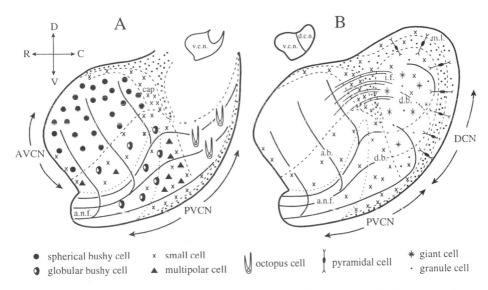

Fig. 4.2. Schematic showing the distribution of eight cell types in sagittal views of the cat cochlear nucleus. **A:** The ventral cochlear nucleus (VCN) by itself. **B:** The VCN partly covered by the dorsal cochlear nucleus (DCN). Lines marked *a.n.f.* show auditory nerve fibers with their ascending branches (a.b.) projecting to the anteroventral cochlear nucleus (AVCN) and descending branches (d.b.) projecting to the posteroventral (PVCN) and dorsal cochlear nucleus (DCN). Fibers are shown at three points on the tonotopic scale, with the lowest-frequency fiber in the most ventral position at the point where the fibers enter the nucleus. Cell types are indicated by symbols and are defined in more detail in later figures. Lines marked i.f. in B are axons interconnecting the VCN and DCN. m.l., molecular layer of the DCN; cap, small-cell cap. (Modified from Osen, 1970a with permission.)

BF fibers bifurcate first and innervate the most ventral and lateral portions of the nucleus whereas high-BF fibers innervate more dorsal and medial portions of the nucleus (Osen, 1970a; Bourk et al., 1981).

The symbols in Fig. 4.2 show the distribution of eight cell types that can be defined on the basis of cytoarchitecture. These are all principal cells except for the granule cells and some of the small cells. Note that the principal cells are arranged in such a way that each type receives ANFs over the whole tonotopic range. In this sense, each principal cell type constitutes a separate but complete parallel representation of the sound coming in the ear. Each cell type has its own unique pattern of response to sound, suggesting that each type is involved in a different aspect of analysis of the information in the auditory nerve. The diversity of these patterns can be explained by three features that vary among the principal cell types: (*1*) the nature of the innervation of the cell by ANFs, e.g., whether the synapses are located on the soma or dendrites, the size of the auditory-nerve terminals, and the number of fibers that converge on each cell; (*2*) the postsynaptic membrane properties of the cells, which determine the pattern of response of the cell and the degree of temporal integration performed by the cell; and (*3*) the interneuronal circuitry associated with the cell. In the following sections, the synaptic arrangements of the principal cell types are described and related to the cells' responses to sound.

The principal cell types project to different targets in the brainstem auditory system. Figure 4.3 shows the projection patterns of six of the cell types from Fig. 4.2. Figure 4.3A is a drawing of frontal-plane cross sections of the cat brainstem at two levels, through the AVCN (left side) and PVCN/DCN (right side). This figure shows the two major fiber bundles that leave the cochlear nucleus in relation to other structures in the brainstem. Figure 4.3B shows a wiring diagram for some of the auditory circuits of the cochlear nucleus. At the output of the cochlear nucleus, spherical and globular bushy cells (SBC and GBC, solid lines) project to the nuclei of the superior olive, the lateral (LSO) and medial (MSO) superior olivary nuclei and the medial nucleus of the trapezoid body (MnTB). The MSO and LSO are structures unique to the auditory system which receive an equally strong innervation from the two ears and perform the initial computations necessary for sound localization (Irvine, 1986). A number of unusual characteristics of cochlear-nucleus bushy cells are described below; these will be interpreted in terms of the needs of this sound localization system.

Multipolar (M), giant (Gi), and pyramidal (Py) cells bypass the MSO and LSO and project directly to the inferior colliculus (IC); the octopus cells (O) project to small nuclei scattered around the superior olive (the periolivary nuclei, PON). In addition to the structures shown in Fig. 4.3, there are other cell groups, called the *nuclei of the lateral lemniscus* (nLL), located between the superior olive and IC; these receive collateral projections from most of the cells shown, including the octopus cells. The IC is the final prethalamic structure in the auditory system. It receives direct projections from the cochlear nucleus and superior olive, as shown in Fig. 4.3, and also projections from periolivary nuclei (PON) and from the nLL. The axons of most subcollicular projections end in banded patterns within the colliculus, which suggests that there is selective interaction of inputs from different sources at this level (Oliver and Huerta, 1992).

Two nonprincipal cell regions of the cochlear nucleus are shown in Fig. 4.2, the

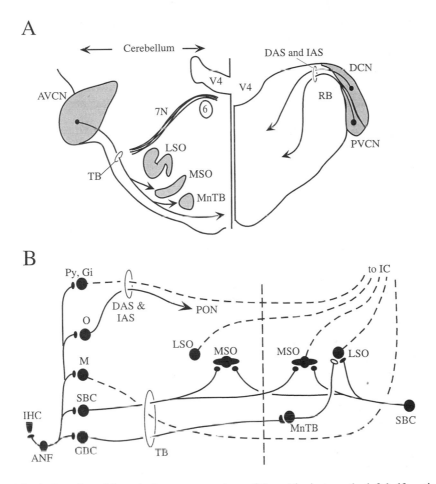

Fig. 4.3. **A:** Drawing of frontal-plane cross sections of the cat brainstem: the left half section is at the level of the anteroventral cochlear nucleus (AVCN) and superior olive; the right half section is slightly caudal, at the level of the dorsal (DCN) and posteroventral cochlear nucleus (PVCN). The auditory nerve enters the nucleus between these two planes of section. Efferent paths from the cochlear nucleus (trapezoid body [TB] and dorsal and intermediate acoustic striae [DAS and IAS]) are shown as arrows. V4, fourth ventricle; 6, abducens nerve nucleus; 7N, seventh (facial) nerve. **B:** Some of the cochlear-nucleus principal cell types with their projections to the nuclei of the superior olivary complex and the inferior colliculus (IC). The auditory pathway begins in the transducer cell, the inner hair cell (IHC), which is connected to the cochlear nucleus by auditory-nerve fibers (ANF). From the VCN, bushy cells (SBC and GBC) innervate the medial (MSO) and lateral (LSO) superior olivary nuclei. The innervation is bilateral, as illustrated on the right side (the midline of the brainstem is shown by the dashed vertical line). The contralateral projection to the LSO is via an inhibitory interneuron in the medial nucleus of the trapezoid body (MnTB). Multipolar cells (M) from the VCN and pyramidal (Py) and giant (Gi) cells from the DCN project through the TB and DAS, respectively, to the contralateral IC. From the PVCN, octopus cells (O) project via the IAS to the peri-olivary nuclei (PON), which are scattered nuclei surrounding the MSO and LSO, and to the nuclei of the lateral lemniscus (not shown).

granule-cell areas (dotted) and the small cell cap. The granule cells resemble those in the cerebellum (Mugnaini et al., 1980b) and are associated with the superficial, or molecular, layer of the DCN (m.l. in Fig. 4.2); they are discussed later with the DCN. The small cell cap is a collection of small multipolar cells that lies between the principal cell regions of the VCN and the granule cells (Osen, 1969; Cant, 1993). The synaptic connections of the cells in the cap are not known, except that this region receives collaterals of auditory-nerve fibers (Liberman, 1991) and collaterals of an efferent projection from the superior olive to the cochlea (Benson and Brown, 1990).

VENTRAL COCHLEAR NUCLEUS

The response characteristics of VCN cells are largely determined by their membrane properties and by the properties of their auditory-nerve innervation. This section describes the morphologies of VCN principal cell types and the number, size, and location of the auditory-nerve, and other, synapses that they receive. Figure 4.4A–D shows a montage of horseradish peroxidase (HRP)-filled examples of four VCN principal cell types. These are taken from studies in which intracellular recordings were done to identify cells' response properties. The bottom part of the figure shows sketches of the synaptic terminals on the somata of four VCN cell types to illustrate differences in their innervation.

SYNAPTIC CONNECTIONS

Most of the synaptic terminals in the cochlear nucleus fall into four types (Cant, 1992). (*1*) Terminals from ANFs contain large spherical synaptic vesicles (LS) and make asymmetric synaptic contacts; these terminals range in size from small boutons to large endbulbs (Rouiller et al., 1986) and appear on all of the cell types in the nucleus except the cells of the superficial layer of the DCN and those in the granule cell regions. Most of the unfilled terminals in Fig. 4.4G–J are of type LS. A variety of evidence shows that the auditory nerve neurotransmitter is glutamate (Wenthold, 1991; Hunter et al., 1993). (*2*) A second group of excitatory-type terminals makes bouton synapses containing small spherical vesicles (SS); these are diverse in size and several sources of SS terminals have been identified within the cochlear nucleus, including granule cells (Smith and Rhode, 1985), pyramidal cells (Smith and Rhode, 1985), and one type

---

Fig. 4.4. **A–E:** Camera lucida drawings of horseradish peroxidase (HRP)-filled cochlear-nucleus principal cells illustrating characteristic features of each type. **A:** Spherical bushy cell (Ostapoff et al., 1994); **B:** globular bushy cell (Smith and Rhode, 1987); **C:** multipolar cell (Rhode et al., 1983a); **D:** octopus cell (Rhode et al., 1983a); **E:** pyramidal cell (Rhode et al., 1983b). Part of the apical dendritic tree is shown separately in E; the trees should join at the arrows. The scale bars are equal, except for the spherical bushy cell in A. All cells are from cat except the spherical bushy cell, which is from a gerbil. In B–E, axons are indicated by a. **F:** Drawing of an endbulb of Held terminal of an auditory nerve fiber on a spherical bushy cell soma (Sento and Ryugo, 1989). **G–J:** Schematic drawings of cross sections of the somata of VCN principal cells showing the distribution of excitatory-type (unfilled, mainly LS) and inhibitory type (filled, PL and FL) terminals. Scale bar in F applies to F–J. **G:** Spherical bushy cell, the large terminal (arrow) is a portion of an endbulb; **H:** Globular bushy cell; **I,J:** Multipolar cells of two types (bushy cells from Cant, 1992; multipolar cells from Smith and Rhode, 1989). (A–J taken from the sources listed, with permission; A-F, I, V reprinted permission of Wiley-Liss)

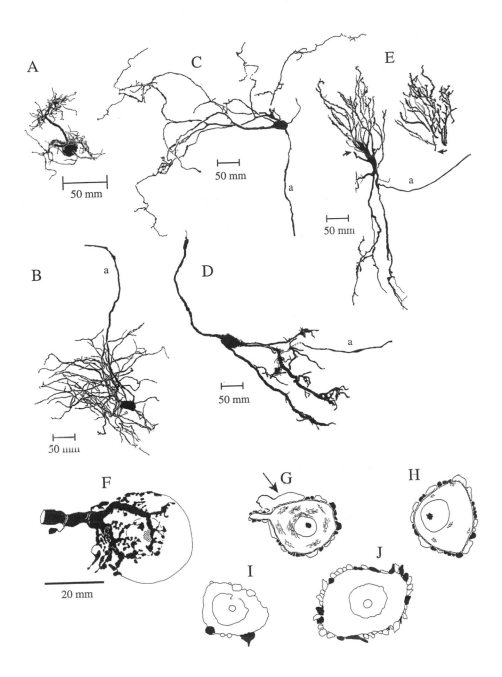

A

50 mm

C

50 mm

a

E

a

B

a

50 ᴍᴍ

D

a

50 mm

F

20 mm

G

H

I

J

127

of multipolar cell in the VCN (Smith and Rhode, 1989). The neurotransmitter used by granule cells is also glutamate (Hunter et al., 1993; Osen et al., 1995; Manis and Molitor, 1996), but the transmitters used at other SS synapses are unknown. (*3,4*) A diverse group of inhibitory-type terminals is seen, with either pleomorphic (PL) or flattened (FL) vesicles; these are shown as filled terminals in Fig. 4.4G–J. There are several known inhibitory interneurons in the cochlear nucleus, of both glycinergic and GABAergic variety; these are found mainly in the DCN and are discussed later (Osen et al., 1990; Wenthold, 1991).

NEURONAL TYPES

Spherical bushy cells (SBCs; Fig. 4.4A) are characterized by a spherical soma with one or a few thick dendrites that branch profusely into a bush-like structure near the cell body (Brawer et al., 1974). SBCs receive large auditory-nerve terminals, called *endbulbs of Held*, on their somata (Fig. 4.4F); these terminals consist of many finger-like processes and smaller branches that form a network over the postsynaptic cell (Ryugo and Fekete, 1982). In cross sections (Fig. 4.4G), endbulbs (arrow) contact the soma over significant distances and contain multiple synaptic contacts (Lenn and Reese, 1966; Cant and Morest, 1979b). Typically, an SBC receives endbulbs from only 1–3 ANFs (Lorente de Nó, 1981; Sento and Ryugo, 1989). In addition to the endbulbs, SBCs receive presumably inhibitory bouton terminals of both FL and PL types on their somata (Fig. 4.4G). By contrast to their heavy somatic innervation, SBCs receive few synaptic terminals on their dendritic trees. Given the massive nature of the somatic auditory-nerve innervation of SBCs, it is not surprising that their responses to sound are essentially identical to those of ANFs (see below).

Globular bushy cells (GBCs) are similar in appearance to SBCs except that GBCs have a more extensive dendritic tree with longer branches (Fig. 4.4B) and a more ovoid soma (Tolbert and Morest, 1982; Smith and Rhode, 1987). Synaptic terminals from ANFs are again mainly on the soma, but the terminals are smaller, modified endbulbs. As in the SBC, the soma has both excitatory-type and inhibitory-type terminals (Fig. 4.4H). The number of ANFs that converge on a GBC is larger than for a SBC. In one study, all the synapses on six Golgi-labeled GBCs were counted in electron-microscopic reconstructions (Ostapoff and Morest, 1991). LS-type terminals predominate on the soma and initial segment of the axon (27 LS endings out of 52 terminals on the soma and initial segment), but are less common in the dendrites (7.7/38 endings). The SS endings were infrequent everywhere on the cell (3.7 total endings per cell on average). Inhibitory-type terminals made up the remainder of the terminals and were the predominant terminal type in the dendrites (27/38 endings). Thus the GBC is like the SBC in having a heavy auditory-nerve input to the soma, but the input probably originates from many fibers instead of only from 1–3. The number of independent ANFs terminating on a GBC is an important parameter in determining GBC response characteristics (Rothman et al., 1993); unfortunately, the terminal counts quoted above do not translate directly into independent fiber counts, because fibers sometimes make multiple synaptic contacts on cells in VCN (Rouiller et al., 1986).

Multipolar cells are characterized by large dendrites that extend away from the soma in several directions (Fig. 4.4C; Brawer et al., 1974; Cant and Morest, 1979a); this cell type is called both *multipolar* and *stellate* in the cochlear-nucleus literature. Dendrites may be either smooth or covered with small spines; they generally branch sparsely but sometimes end in small sprays of dendritic branches. Two major classes of multipolar cells have been described and correlated with differences in responses to sound (Cant, 1981, 1982; Smith and Rhode, 1989; Oertel et al., 1990; Doucet et al., 1996). The cells of one group have a stellate morphology with dendrites spreading within a plane that tends to be aligned with the direction of travel of ANFs, which suggests that they receive input over a restricted range of frequencies. These cells have few synaptic terminals on their somas (Fig. 4.4I); their axons leave the nucleus through the trapezoid body and project to the contralateral IC (cell M in Fig. 4.3B); they will be referred to below as *T-multipolars* (for trapezoid body, Oertel et al., 1990). Cells of the second group (*D-multipolars*) have an elongate morphology with more bipolar dendritic fields that are arranged perpendicular to the ANFs. These cells have their somata densely covered with synaptic terminals including both LS-type terminals and inhibitory-type terminals (Fig. 4.4J). Their axons probably leave the nucleus through the intermediate acoustic stria, but multipolar cells of this type do not seem to project to the IC and their targets are unknown (Adams, 1983; Smith and Rhode, 1989; Oertel et al., 1990). The axons of both multipolar types have collaterals that terminate locally near the cell body and in the DCN to form intrinsic circuits, which are discussed later.

Multipolar cells receive small bouton endings from ANFs. In D-multipolars, 43% of the terminals on the soma are of the LS type, probably from ANFs; on T-multipolars, only 10.5% of the small number of somatic terminals are of the LS type (Smith and Rhode, 1989). In the proximal dendrites, 59% and 29% of the synapses on D- and T-multipolars, respectively, are LS type and in distal dendrites, the percentages are 7.5% and 12%. The remaining synapses are a mixture of the inhibitory PL and FL types. The number of independent ANFs contacting a multipolar cell has not been estimated and the same uncertainty as applies to GBCs applies here; however, given that most bouton terminals of ANFs are scattered in the neuropil (Liberman, 1991; Ryugo, 1992), it is likely that multipolar cells receive inputs from many ANFs. Thus the multipolar and bushy cells provide a continuum of synaptic input patterns, ranging from strong somatic input in bushy cells to primarily dendritic input in T-multipolars. D-multipolars are somewhere in between, with a mixed pattern of input.

Octopus cells, the final principal cell type in the VCN (Fig. 4.4D), lie in a concentrated group in the posterior PVCN (Fig. 4.2). They have 4–6 large dendritic trunks which usually emerge on the same side of the cell, giving the dendritic tree an oriented appearance (Kane, 1973; Oertel et al., 1990); the cell in Fig. 4.4D has an additional dendrite extending away in the opposite direction, but otherwise has the oriented dendrites typical of octopus cells. Octopus cells are similar to D-multipolar cells in that they have a dense auditory-nerve innervation of their somata and their dendrites are oriented perpendicular to the ANFs, so that they receive input from fibers with a relatively wide range of BFs.

DORSAL COCHLEAR NUCLEUS

In contrast to the VCN, the DCN contains a substantial interneuronal neuropil which is important in generating its responses to sound. Figure 4.5 is a drawing of a Golgi preparation showing the neural elements of the DCN (Osen et al., 1990). The DCN contains four layers, as indicated on the left in Fig. 4.5; layers 3 and 4 are frequently

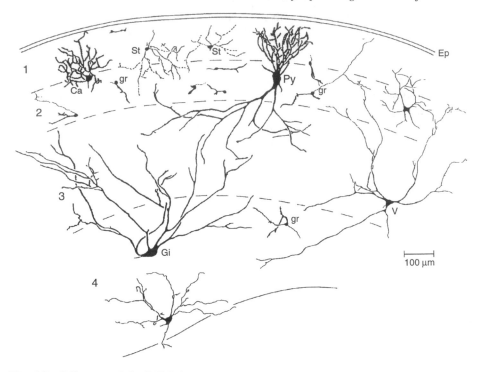

Fig. 4.5. Cell types of the DCN shown according to the layered structure of the nucleus in a plane approximately parallel to an isofrequency sheet; granule cell axons would run perpendicular to the page in layer 1 and ANFs would run within the page mainly in layer 3. The free surface of the DCN is at the top (Ep); layers are numbered at left. Abbreviations: Ca, cartwheel cell; Gi, giant cell; gr, granule cell; Py, pyramidal cell; St, stellate cell; V, vertical cell, also called *tuberculoventral* or *corn cell*. Some unidentified cell types are shown unlabeled. (From Osen et al., 1990 with permission.)

lumped together and called the *deep DCN*. The second layer is defined by the cell bodies of the pyramidal cells (Py), one of the DCN's principal cell types. The first layer, called the *superficial* or *molecular layer*, contains the axons of granule cells, along with several populations of small interneurons.

Pyramidal neurons are bipolar (Figs. 4.4E and 4.5), with an apical dendritic tree in the superficial layer (layer 1) and a basal dendritic tree in layer 3. Figure 4.5 shows only one pyramidal cell; in fact, pyramidal cells are lined up in the DCN with their cell bodies in layer 2 and their dendrites arranged in parallel. The apical and basal dendrites of pyramidal cells contact two very different sets of circuitry in the superficial and deep players.

The basal dendrites of pyramidal cells extend into layer 3 with few branches and occasional spines (Kane, 1974; Rhode et al., 1983b; Smith and Rhode, 1985). The apical dendrites branch profusely in the superficial layer and are densely covered with spines. The spines receive SS terminals from unmyelinated granule-cell axons; the non-spine surface of the apical dendrites are densely packed with inhibitory-type terminals (Smith and Rhode, 1985). The proximal dendrites and soma receive mainly FL and PL terminals with a few SS terminals. LS terminals, presumably from ANFs, are found on the basal dendrites where they form 10% of the terminals on the proximal dendrites and 38% of the distal dendrites. The remainder of the basal dendritic terminals are PL and FL.

The deep layers receive ANFs and collaterals of the axons of VCN multipolar cells (Osen, 1970a; Oertel et al., 1990). As shown in Fig. 4.2 for the ANFs, these axons form terminals within spatially confined sheets that run across the nucleus. Within each sheet, fibers have approximately the same BF, making them isofrequency sheets. Figure 4.5 is drawn in a plane approximately parallel to the isofrequency sheets. In addition to ANFs and the basal dendrites of pyramidal neurons, the deep layers contain large multipolar cells (*giant cells*, Gi), which are the second principal neuron type of the DCN (Kane et al., 1981). Giant cells have large dendritic trees that branch sparsely and are smooth; these dendrites run both within and across the isofrequency sheets, and are mostly confined to the deep layers. There seems to be several kinds of giant cells, based on dendritic tree morphology, but this requires further study. Giant-cell axons join those of the pyramidal cells in making up the dorsal acoustic striae (DAS), which projects to the contralateral IC (Fernandez and Karapas, 1967).

Vertical cells (V) are found primarily in layer 3 (Lorente de Nó, 1981; Zhang and Oertel, 1993c); their cell bodies lie at the same level as the basal dendritic trees of pyramidal cells and their dendrites extend into layers 2 and 4. Their smooth dendritic trees are oriented vertically within the isofrequency sheets, hence their name. Vertical-cell axons ramify within the DCN in a fashion mainly parallel to their own isofrequency sheet and also give a collateral that projects to the VCN, where it ends tonotopically (Wickesberg and Oertel, 1988). Vertical cells stain prominently for glycine (Wenthold et al., 1987; Saint Marie et al., 1991) and are important inhibitory interneurons in the DCN, as is discussed below. They also inhibit VCN cells, and that inhibition is blocked by strychnine (Wickesberg and Oertel, 1990).

The basal dendrites of pyramidal cells and the vertical cell dendrites are flattened in the plane of the isofrequency sheet, so that the dendritic trees in Fig. 4.5 are shown at their maximal extent (Osen, 1983; Blackstad et al., 1984). As a result of this flattening, ANF's run approximately parallel to the dendritic trees of pyramidal and vertical cells, which constrains the BF range of the ANFs that can contact one cell.

Granule cells give rise to parallel fibers, which are the main source of excitatory synapses in the DCN's superficial layer. Granule cells are located in the DCN, as shown in Fig. 4.5 (gr), but they are also found in concentrations surrounding the principal cell areas of the VCN (Fig. 4.2). In the DCN, granule cells are concentrated in layer 2, but they are also found scattered through the other layers. Layer 1 of the DCN receives parallel fibers from granule cells in all these domains (Mugnaini et al., 1980b) and in fact, the superficial layer of the DCN seems to be the target of granule-cell axons, no matter where in the cochlear nucleus the cells are located. The granule-cell axons run perpendicularly to the isofrequency sheets and so run approximately perpendicular to the view in Fig. 4.5. Thus the major afferent systems of the DCN define a two-dimensional array of cells, with the tonotopic axis as one dimension and some, currently unknown, feature of granule cell responses defining the other dimension.

Granule cells receive inputs at specialized *glomerular synapses* in which a large synaptic terminal (mossy fiber) is partially surrounded by claw-like granule-cell dendrites, which in turn receive inhibitory synapses from other cells (Mugnaini et al., 1980a). One source of inhibitory input to similar glomerular synapses in the cerebellum are Golgi cells, and a similar Golgi system has been described in the DCN. Golgi cells are not shown in Fig. 4.5; there is still some uncertainty about the exact arrangement of cochlear-nucleus Golgi cells.

Granule cells receive a diverse set of inputs, including type II (Brown et al., 1988) and probably also type I ANFs (Liberman, 1993), efferents of the central auditory system (Kane, 1977; Caicedo and Herbert, 1993; Feliciano et al., 1995; Weedman and Ryugo, 1996), and nonauditory inputs from the somatosensory (Itoh et al., 1987; Weinberg and Rustioni, 1987; Wright and Ryugo, 1996) and vestibular systems (Burian and Gestoettner, 1988; Kevetter and Perachio, 1989). Thus the information carried to the pyramidal cells through the circuitry of the superficial DCN is quite different from that carried in the deep DCN.

Cartwheel (Ca) and *stellate* (St) cells are inhibitory interneurons in layer 1 of DCN (Mugnaini et al., 1980b; Wouterlood and Mugniani, 1984; Wouterlood et al., 1984). These cells stain for both glycine and GABA/GAD, with stellate cells showing strong GABAergic labeling and cartwheel cells showing stronger glycinergic labeling (reviewed by Osen et al., 1990). Stellate cells are small interneurons in the superficial layer; they appear to form an electrically coupled network through gap junctions between their dendrites. The destination of their axons is not known, but it appears to be other cells in the superficial DCN (Lorente de Nó, 1981). Cartwheel dendrites, like those of pyramidal cells, are densely covered with spines on which parallel fiber synapses are made. Cartwheel cells' axons distribute in layers 2 and 3 of the DCN and show a tendency to project parallel to the isofrequency sheets (Berrebi and Mugnaini, 1991; Manis et al., 1994). Cartwheel cells are similar to Purkinje cells of the cerebellum in several ways, including a similar embryological origin, similar expression of molecular markers, similarities in structure, and a similar fate in mutant mouse strains involving cerebellar degeneration (Berrebi et al., 1990). These similarities and the similarity of the cochlear-nucleus granule cells to those in the cerebellum suggests that there is an analogy between the cerebellum and the superficial DCN, with the pyramidal cells taking the role of deep-cerebellar neurons (see Chap. 7). There are many differences between the two structures, of course, including the lack of a climbing fiber in the DCN, but the analogy may be useful in considering the role of the DCN in the auditory system.

Two additional interneurons, the *unipolar brush cell* (UBC) and the *chestnut cell*, have been described in the granule-cell areas (Floris et al., 1994; Weedman et al., 1996). These cells receive mossy-fiber inputs, like granule cells, but do so with different patterns. Granule-cell dendrites form claws which partially cover mossy-fiber terminals and each granule cell contacts several mossy fibers, one on each of its several dendrites. By contrast, UBCs have a single large dendrite that envelopes a single mossy-fiber terminal and chestnut cells receive a dense termination of many mossy fibers that covers their somata and their single, stubby dendrite. These different patterns of synaptic convergence suggest three different computational roles (Weedman et al., 1996): granule cells could respond selectively to temporally coincident activity in subsets of their mossy-fiber inputs; UBCs in the cerebellum have been shown to serve as signal amplifiers, giving a prolonged response to their single mossy-fiber input (Rossi et al.,

1995); and chestnut cells could serve as a convergence point of several mossy-fiber inputs, forming their sum.

NUMBERS OF CELL TYPES AND CONVERGENCE

In cat, there are about 3000 IHCs and 50,000 type I ANFs (Ryugo, 1992). The total population of cells in the cochlear nucleus is similar in number to the ANFs. Most numerous are the bushy cells, with 36,600 SBCs and 6300 GBCs (Osen, 1970b). These numbers are consistent with the innervation ratios described above for SBCs (1–3 ANFs per cell) and GBCs ($\approx$35 LS terminals per cell), given that each ANF contacts, on average, 1 SBC soma and 3–6 GBC somas (Liberman, 1991). There are some 35,000 multipolar cells (Osen, 1970b), most of which are T-multipolars; the ratio of T- and D-multipolars is about 15:1 (Doucet et al., 1996). In the DCN, there are about 4350 pyramidal cells, and 1280 giant cells (Osen, 1970b; Adams, 1976). There is not a sufficient basis for accurately computing the convergence ratios onto these cell types, mainly because most ANF terminals are made on the dendrites of multipolar cells and DCN cells. However, assuming that all the synapse-like swellings in the neuropil (i.e., the nonsomatic swellings) in the VCN and DCN are synapses on multipolar cells or pyramidal/giant cells yields a convergence ratio of about 30–100 fibers per cell in both areas (Liberman, 1991, 1993). There are about 1500 octopus cells (Osen, 1970b) and each ANF contacts about 2 somas in the octopus-cell area (Liberman, 1993), yielding a convergence ratio of about 67 ANFs per octopus cell.

BASIC CIRCUIT

The intrinsic organization of neuronal elements and synaptic connections within the cochlear nucleus is summarized in the basic circuit diagram of Fig. 4.6. All the principal cells of the nucleus are shown, except for octopus cells. There is one set of circuits associated with the auditory inputs to the nucleus: auditory-nerve fibers (a.n.f) innervate all principal cell types as well as the vertical-cell (V) interneurons. As discussed above, the vertical cells are glycinergic; physiological evidence suggests that they inhibit DCN principal cells (Voigt and Young, 1980) as well as bushy and multipolar cells of the VCN (Wickesberg and Oertel, 1990). The projection pattern of the vertical-cell axons is tonotopic in both the DCN and VCN; that is, the axons of vertical cells distribute terminals in the same isofrequency sheets as the ANFs that innervate the vertical cell itself (Wickesberg and Oertel, 1988; Zhang and Oertel, 1993c). These anatomical observations are supported by physiological properties of inhibition in principal cells: as is discussed later, the inhibitory input to DCN principal cells that most likely comes from vertical cells has a BF equal to or slightly lower than the BF of the principal cell (Voigt and Young, 1990; Spirou and Young, 1991); similarly, in the VCN the inhibition that is blocked by strychnine is maximal near a neuron's BF and is weaker at adjacent frequencies (Caspary et al., 1994).

Although interneuronal circuits in the VCN have not been described, multipolar cells serve the role of interneurons through their axon collaterals, which terminate locally within the VCN as well as project to the DCN (Smith and Rhode, 1989; Oertel et al., 1990). A similar role has been ascribed to the axon collaterals of medium spiny neurons in the striatum (Chap. 9). Both T- and D- multipolars (T-M and D-M in Fig. 4.6)

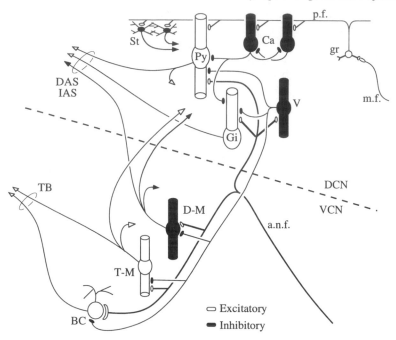

Fig. 4.6. Schematic drawing of the basic circuit of the cochlear nucleus. Excitatory neurons and terminals are shown unfilled; inhibitory elements are filled. Inputs to the cochlear nucleus come from auditory-nerve fibers (a.n.f.) and mossy fibers (m.f.); additional inputs that are not shown are efferents from the central auditory system as well as other parts of the brain. Output axons of the nucleus come from the principal cells: spherical and globular bushy cells (BC); T- and D-multipolars (T-M, D-M); giant cells (Gi); pyramidal cells (Py). Octopus cells are not shown. Vertical cells (V) form one major intrinsic circuit by projecting to all principal cell types except the octopus cell. A second circuit is formed by multipolar cell collaterals, which terminate in the VCN and the DCN. The axons of multipolar and vertical cells which travel between the DCN and AVCN make up a large part of the prominent bundle of fibers labeled *i.f.* in Fig. 4.2B. Granule cell axons form parallel fibers (p.f.) in superficial DCN; these terminate on pyramidal, cartwheel (Ca) and stellate cells (St). The exact termination patterns within the nucleus of terminals shown as arrows are not known. DAS, dorsal acoustic stria; IAS, intermediate acoustic stria; TB, trapezoid body.

have such collaterals. Based on the vesicle shapes in their terminals, it is likely that T-multipolars produce excitatory terminals and D-multipolars produce inhibitory terminals (Smith and Rhode, 1989). The targets of multipolar axons in the DCN have not been identified. However, the projection patterns of the collaterals place them in regions where they could contact pyramidal, vertical, and giant neurons. The properties of D-multipolar cells' responses to sound correspond to the properties predicted for an inhibitory input to DCN vertical and principal cells, based on their response properties (Nelken and Young, 1994; Winter and Palmer, 1995). The potential role of D-multipolars in generating the responses of DCN neurons is discussed below.

A few large multipolar cells project from the cochlear nucleus on one side of the brain to the contralateral cochlear nucleus (Cant and Gaston, 1982). These and other connections outside the cochlear nucleus are not shown in Fig. 4.6.

The second excitatory input to the cochlear nucleus is the mossy fibers (m.f.) and other inputs to the granule-cell domains. The diagram in Fig. 4.6 shows the destinations of the granule-cell axons (p.f.), which terminate directly on the apical dendrites of pyramidal cells and on the cartwheel (Ca) and stellate (St) cell inhibitory interneurons. The axons of cartwheel cells end in layers 2 and 3 where they produce inhibitory postsynaptic potentials (IPSPs) in pyramidal and giant cells (Zhang and Oertel, 1993b; Zhang and Oertel, 1994; Golding and Oertel, 1995). In addition, cartwheel cells interact with one another in a network (Wouterlood and Mugnaini, 1984; Berrebi and Mugnaini, 1991; Golding and Oertel, 1996); although cartwheel cells produce IPSPs in principal cells, the reversal potential of the cartwheel-to-cartwheel cell synapse is such that its effect is slightly depolarizing for the cell at rest, but slightly hyperpolarizing when the cell has been depolarized by other inputs (Golding and Oertel, 1996). Thus the effects of the cartwheel cell network are likely to be context dependent — excitatory when the cells are at rest, but stabilizing when the cells are excited. The cartwheel cells are the most numerous neuron in the DCN, excepting the granule cells (Wouterlood and Mugnaini, 1984); by virtue of their numbers, their network of interconnections, and their profuse terminal distribution, cartwheel cells represent a substantial computational resource for the DCN.

The final intrinsic circuit shown in Fig. 4.6 is formed by collaterals of pyramidal-cell axons, which terminate locally in the DCN (Smith and Rhode, 1985). These form SS-type terminals and terminals resembling the pyramidal-cell collaterals are seen on the somata and proximal dendrites of pyramidal cells.

MEMBRANE PROPERTIES AND INTEGRATION OF INPUTS

The differences in synaptic organization described in the previous sections are correlated with differences in the postsynaptic membrane properties of the cells. Figure 4.7 shows responses to sound and electrophysiological properties typical of two VCN cell types to illustrate these differences. Responses to short bursts of sound recorded in vivo using extracellular electrodes are shown in the left column; responses in vitro to intracellular injections of hyperpolarizing and depolarizing currents are shown in the right column. The sounds in this case were tones at the BF of the neuron at a loudness significantly above threshold, where the neurons' responses are stable and assume their typical form (Pfeiffer, 1966a; Godfrey et al., 1975a,b; Bourk, 1976). The responses of ANFs to this stimulus resemble those shown in Fig. 4.7C1. Following stimulus onset there is a rapid increase in discharge rate to a maximum, followed by a slower decline to a fairly steady discharge. An important aspect of auditory-nerve responses that is not shown is their irregularity. In this context, irregularity means a lack of repetitive firing behavior; the spikes of an ANF occur randomly in time, so the intervals between spikes are highly variable and the pattern of action potentials is different for each stimulus repetition.

T-MULTIPOLAR CELLS

Figure 4.7A and B show responses that are characteristic of T-multipolar cells (Rhode et al., 1983a; Wu and Oertel, 1984; Smith and Rhode, 1989; Feng et al., 1994). By contrast to ANFs, these cells show regular responses, meaning that they respond to

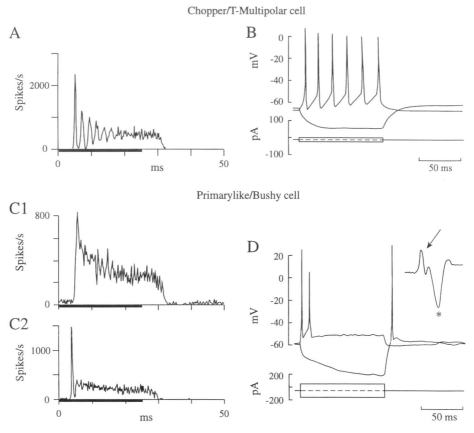

Fig. 4.7. Basic response characteristics of VCN bushy and T-multipolar cells to tones and electrical stimuli. The left column shows poststimulus time histograms (PSTHs) of responses to BF
tone bursts from extracellular recordings. The PSTH plots discharge rate versus time averaged
over several stimulus repetitions. The stimulus is on during the first half of the abscissa, as shown
by the heavy lines on the abscissae. The right column shows responses to intracellular injection
of depolarizing and hyperpolarizing currents. The top waveforms are the membrane potential
and the bottom waveforms are the current injected. Response types and the cells from which
they are typically recorded are as follows: **A,B:** Chopper responses from T-multipolar cells; **C:**
primarylike (**C1**) responses from SBC and primarylike-with-notch (**C2**) from GBC. **D:** Bushy
cell membrane currents. The inset shows a complex action potential with a prepotential (arrow),
probably from an SBC. (A and C redrawn from Blackburn and Sachs, 1989; Band D from Mavis
and Marx, 1991, with permission.)

stimuli with a highly reproducible pattern of spike trains in which the interspike intervals are all about the same length. Figure 4.7B shows an example of a regular spiking pattern in response to electrical depolarization that is typical of multipolar cells.
The responses to acoustic stimuli are similar, and the result is a poststimulus time histogram (PSTH) like the one shown in Fig. 4.7A. The pattern of peaks and valleys in
this PSTH is called *chopping*. Each peak in the histogram shows where a spike occurs
in response to the stimulus; because of the regularity of the response, a spike will occur in each peak on every repetition of the stimulus. The peaks are large at the onset

of the response because the latency to the first spike is quite reproducible in chopper neurons; the peaks fade away over the first 20 ms of the response as small variations in interspike interval accumulate and spike times in successive stimulus repetitions diverge.

BUSHY CELLS

Figure 4.7C and D show responses typical of bushy cells (Rhode et al., 1983a; Rouiller and Ryugo, 1984; Wu and Oertel, 1984; Smith and Rhode, 1987). The simplest case is the SBC which receives large axosomatic terminals from a small number of ANFs (Fig. 4.4F). Because these endbulb terminals are so large, it is reasonable to expect that the excitatory postsynaptic potentials (EPSPs) they produce should be large, with a high probability of generating a postsynaptic spike. In fact, large EPSPs are observed in bushy cells (Oertel, 1983) and the responses to sound of SBCs resemble those of ANFs (Smith et al., 1993; Feng et al., 1994). SBC responses are called *primarylike* (Fig. 4.7C1) because of their resemblance to ANFs. As expected, primarylike neurons fire as irregularly as ANFs (Rothman et al., 1993).

Evidence that primarylike responses reflect a one-spike-in, one-spike-out mode of processing is provided by their action potential shapes in extracellular recordings. Frequently, primarylike neurons show action potentials like the one in the inset of Fig. 4.7D with a *prepotential* (arrow) followed by a normal bipolar extracellular action potential (asterisk, Pfeiffer, 1966b). Prepotentials of this kind are seen in the SBC region of the AVCN and in the MnTB, where there are similar endbulb synapses on the bushy-cell-like principal cells (Guinan and Li, 1990). Using independent electrical stimulation of the presynaptic and postsynaptic cells, Guinan and Li (1990) showed that the prepotential is the spike discharge of the presynaptic endbulb. With this interpretation, the prepotential makes it possible to observe the action potentials of both components of the SBC synapse. In the AVCN, prepotentials are almost always followed by the postsynaptic component of the spike, demonstrating that this is a very secure synapse (Goldberg and Brownell, 1973; Bourk, 1976).

GBCs give a similar response, called *primarylike-with-notch* (pri-N) (Fig. 4.7C2). Pri-N responses differ from primarylike (and ANF) responses mainly in their behavior at the beginning of the response. The PSTH shows a large peak, followed by a short pause in firing (the notch), followed by a fairly steady discharge. The onset peak occurs because pri-N neurons have a very repeatable latency, so a spike occurs at the time of the peak in all repetitions of the stimulus; the neuron is refractory immediately following the peak, which produces the brief (<2 ms) notch. Following the notch, pri-N neurons fire irregularly like ANFs and primarylike neurons (Rothman et al., 1993). GBCs differ from SBCs in that many ANFs converge with smaller terminals on a GBC (Fig. 4.4H). The precisely timed onset spike of pri-N neurons can be explained by this convergence, by assuming that the postsynaptic cell will fire in response to the first input spike it receives from any of its inputs. Clearly, the more inputs that converge on the cell, the less time it will take for the first input spike to occur and the sharper will be the onset peak in the PSTH (Young et al., 1988).

The electrical characteristics of bushy cells are shown in Fig. 4.7D (Wu and Oertel, 1984; Manis and Marx, 1991). When depolarized, these cells fire only 1 to 3 spikes at stimulus onset and then their membrane potential settles to a slightly depolarized value.

This behavior is produced by a potassium conductance which is partly activated at rest and is strongly activated by depolarization (Manis and Marx, 1991; Reyes et al., 1994). When the cell is hyperpolarized, deactivation of this conductance can be seen in the slow hyperpolarizing drift in membrane potential in Fig. 4.7D; the anodal break spike at the termination of the hyperpolarizing current step reflects, in part, the reduced potassium conductance of the cell at this time. The effect of this low-threshold potassium conductance is to give the bushy cell a very short membrane time constant (2–4 ms at rest) and thereby block temporal integration of synaptic inputs (Oertel, 1983). Figure 4.8 shows postsynaptic potentials produced in a multipolar cell (A) and a bushy cell (B) by trains of electrical stimuli delivered to the auditory nerve. Temporal summation is clear in the multipolar cell but is minimal in the bushy cell. The difference between the two cells is mainly the time constant of the decay phase of the potential, which is noticeably faster in the bushy cell. We will see below that rapid temporal processing permits bushy cells to preserve stimulus waveform information that is necessary for sound localization computations done in the MSO (Irvine, 1986).

Bushy cells have an additional membrane specialization for rapid temporal processing. In the avian homologue of the bushy cell (nucleus magnocellularis), the postsynaptic glutamate receptor associated with the auditory-nerve terminals shows unusually rapid desensitization during sustained application of glutamate (Raman and Trussell, 1992). The desensitization plays two roles: the first is to minimize the possibility of temporal summation by making the EPSPs brief (because of the short bushy-cell-membrane time constant, the EPSP closely follows the synaptic conductance change); and second, the refractory period for action-potential generation after an EPSP is made shorter, because the cell repolarizes quickly, allowing the cell to respond to afferent inputs at higher rates (Raman et al., 1994).

OCTOPUS CELLS AND D-MULTIPOLAR CELLS

Octopus and D-multipolar cells give responses to sound that are called *onset* (Godfrey et al., 1975a; Smith and Rhode, 1989; Ostapoff et al., 1994). Onset responses have a prominent and reliable spike immediately at the beginning of a BF-tone stimulus, followed by little or no activity. Octopus cells give a pure onset response, wheras D-multipolars give a short burst of spikes followed by a varying level of steady-state discharge, called an *onset-C* response. The electrophysiological properties of these cells have not been characterized as well as those of bushy and multipolar cells; however, the existing work suggests that these cell types share with bushy cells a short membrane time constant generated by a low input resistance (Oertel et al., 1990; Golding et al., 1995). The source of the low input resistance appears to be different from that in bushy cells, however, at least in octopus cells, where an inward-rectifier potassium channel seems to be involved (Golding et al., 1995). Octopus and D-multipolar cells also share anatomical characteristics, the most important of which are a dense innervation of their somata by auditory-nerve boutons and the orientation of their dendrites across the tonotopic map (Kane, 1973; Smith and Rhode, 1989). Responses to sound in both the octopus-cell region and in onset-C neurons are characterized by broad tuning and somewhat elevated thresholds, which are consistent with cells that receive inputs across a broad range of BFs (Godfrey et al., 1975a; Rhode and Smith, 1986; Winter and Palmer, 1995). In fact, onset-C neurons seem to require coincident firing of inputs across a range of BFs in order to produce a strong response (Palmer et al., 1996).

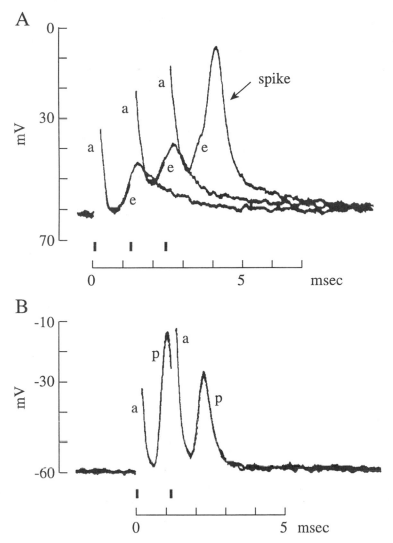

Fig. 4.8. Postsynaptic potentials in a likely multipolar (**A**) and a likely bushy (**B**) cell produced by electrical stimulation of the auditory nerve (heavy vertical bars on the time axis). **A:** Responses to one, two, and three stimuli are shown, a, stimulus artifact; e, EPSPs. Temporal summation leads to a spike after three stimuli. **B:** Large postsynaptic potentials (p) show rapid recovery time constants and no temporal summation. (Redrawn from Oertel, 1983 with permission.)

This characteristic has been used to explain why onset-C neurons respond weakly to stimuli containing a narrow range of frequencies, such as a tone, but vigorously to stimuli containing a broad range of frequencies, such as noise.

PYRAMIDAL AND CARTWHEEL CELLS

Classical studies indicated that pyramidal neurons in the DCN show the type of response to sound referred to as *pauser* or *buildup*. The PSTHs in Fig. 4.9A are typical of the responses of pyramidal cells in anesthetized animals, where the inhibitory circuits of the DCN are weakened. The response shows a poorly timed, long-latency onset spike followed by a prominent pause (Fig. 4.9A1) or a slow buildup in response with a long latency (Fig. 4.9A2). The membrane properties of pyramidal cells are complex and include the full complement of potassium, calcium, and sodium channels found in neurons elsewhere in the brain (Hirsch and Oertel, 1988; Manis, 1990). Despite this complexity and despite the inhibitory inputs that pyramidal cells receive, their basic pauser and buildup characteristics seem to derive from an A-type potassium conductance. Figure 4.9B shows intracellular responses to depolarizing currents that support this point (Manis, 1990). The cells were held hyperpolarized in between the depolarizing current pulses, as shown by the current waveforms; the dotted lines show the holding current necessary to place the cell at its resting potential. Depolarization in this case produced a pauser response (Fig. 4.9B1) or a buildup response (Fig. 4.9B2), depending on the strength of the depolarizing current. The pausing behavior was replaced by a multipolar-cell-like regular discharge when the cell was held at its resting potential. The simplest explanation for the pauser/buildup behavior is that an A-type potassium channel, which is inactivated at rest, is de-inactivated by hyperpolarization (Connor and Stevens, 1971). Thus hyperpolarizing–depolarizing current protocols like the ones in Fig. 4.9B should produce a significant transient outward potassium current through the A channel, resulting in the pause (Kim et al., 1994). In vivo, a hyperpolarization that is sufficient to de-inactivate the conductance is observed as an after-effect of a strong response to an acoustic stimulus (Rhode et al., 1983b). Properties of the A current are reviewed in Chap. 2.

Figure 4.9C shows responses to sound of cartwheel cells in the superficial DCN. Cartwheel cells are characterized by complex action potentials (Fig. 4.9D; Zhang and Oertel, 1993a; Manis et al., 1994) which presumably reflect a combined calcium and sodium spike. They are the only cells in the cochlear nucleus that have been shown to give such complex spikes. Many cartwheel cells respond weakly to sound (Fig. 4.9C1), whereas others give robust responses more like those of other cochlear nucleus cells (Fig. 4.9C2; Parham and Kim, 1995). No particular pattern of response is consistently observed in PSTHs of cartwheel-cell responses. The major excitatory inputs to cartwheel cells are from the granule cells (see Fig. 4.6); as discussed above, type I ANFs do not project into the granule-cell domains, although they probably do contact the granule cells that are scattered in the principal cell regions. The differences between weak and strong responses of cartwheel cells probably reflect differences in the relative amount of auditory-nerve input received by the granule cells connected to a particular cartwheel cell.

SOMATIC AND DENDRITIC PROPERTIES

Analysis of membrane properties has provided the basis for computational simulations that not only reproduce the properties of a given cell but also give insight into the mechanisms by which different features of the auditory input are encoded by different neuronal types and their synaptic connections.

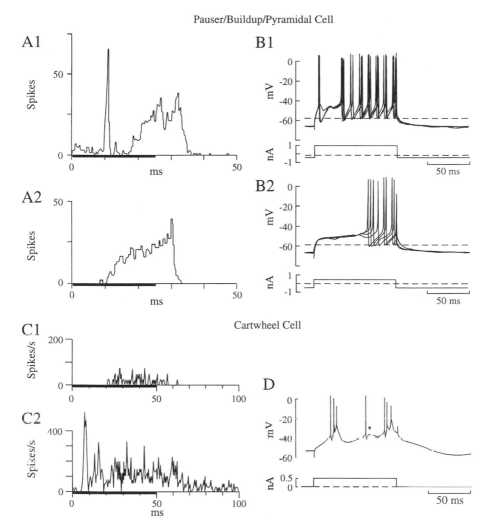

Fig. 4.9. Poststimulus time histograms (PSTHs) of BF-tone responses (left column) and responses to intracellular injection of depolarizing currents (right column) for two DCN cell types. Response types and the cells from which they are typically recorded are as follows: **A:** Pauser **(A1)** and build-up **(A2)** responses from pyramidal cells (Godfrey et al., 1975b). Note that the ordinates of these PSTHs are scaled as spike counts and not as discharge rate. **B:** Responses to current of a pyramidal cell; hyperpolarizing current was used to hold the cell below its resting potential (dashed line) to de-inactivate A-type K channels (Manis, 1990). **C:** Examples of weak **(C1)** and strong **(C2)** acoustic responses of cartwheel cells (Parham and Kim, 1995). **D:** Mixed complex and simple (triangle) spikes from a cartwheel cell (Manis et al., 1994). (Redrawn from the sources indicated, with permission; reprinted permission of Wiley-Liss)

CHOPPER NEURONS

The transformation in spike activity pattern that is observed between ANFs and chopper neurons can be explained through the use of straightforward computational models (Banks and Sachs, 1991; Arle and Kim, 1991; Hewitt and Meddis, 1993). The main component of the transformation is conversion of the irregular activity of ANFs to a regular spike train. Three features of models have been found to be important in producing a regular response: (*1*) the spike generators in the soma and axon tend to fire regularly, e.g., in response to a steady depolarization; (*2*) the larger the number of independent, subthreshold inputs to the cell, the more regular is the response; and (*3*) the farther away from the soma along the dendrites that inputs are applied, the more regular is the response.

The transformation has been studied systematically using the model shown in Fig. 4.10A (Banks and Sachs, 1991); the model consists of a soma and an axon containing voltage-gated sodium and potassium channels, with characteristics like those in the squid axon, connected to a simplified dendritic tree model. This model does not contain all the channels that are probably present in multipolar cells; nevertheless, it captures the basic input–output properties of these cells. Auditory-nerve inputs are applied to the model through the excitatory conductances g_E. The spike trains used to model auditory-nerve inputs are irregular and accurately duplicate the statistical features of real auditory-nerve spike trains. The responses of the model are regular, like those of choppers. Figure 4.10B shows an example of a model spike train and the conductance input that generated it. Note that there is little correspondence between the time of arrival of auditory-nerve spikes, as judged by the EPSPs, and the postsynaptic spikes. There is, of course, an EPSP preceding each output spike, but the basic pattern of the output is determined by the tendency of the neuron to fire regularly, as opposed to the time of occurrence of input spikes. Figure 4.10C is a PSTH of the model's output, showing the chopper pattern. Note the correspondence of spike times in Fig. 4.10B and peaks in the PSTH in Fig. 4.10C.

As discussed above, three features of the model are important in controlling its regularity. Of these, the properties of the somatic spike generator are most important (Hewitt et al., 1992; Wang and Sachs, 1995) and the number of independent inputs is more important than position in the dendrites. The effect of the number of inputs can be understood intuitively by considering that when the number of inputs is increased, the conductance change produced by each individual input is reduced to keep the overall average input to the cell fixed. The result of summing a small number of large inputs is more noisy than the result of summing a large number of small inputs, so regularity increases with the number of inputs (Molnar and Pfeiffer, 1968). The effect of input location on the dendritic tree can be understood from the properties of current flow in dendritic trees, which have the effect of smoothing out temporal fluctuations in the input (White et al., 1994); the smoothing effect is large when the inputs are further from the soma.

PRIMARYLIKE NEURONS

The membrane properties of bushy cells shown in Fig. 4.7D can be accurately reproduced by the model shown in Fig. 4.10D (Rothman et al., 1993). As discussed above, most of the synaptic input to bushy cells is on the soma, so the model consists of only one somatic compartment, containing the same channels as in the multipolar cell model

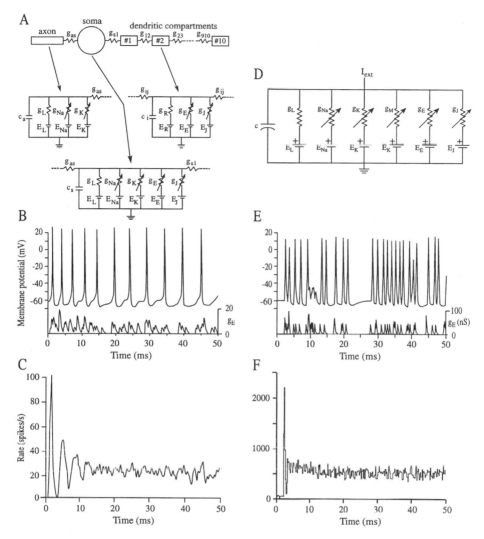

Fig. 4.10. Computational models used to study the input–output transformations in multipolar and bushy neurons. **A:** The multipolar neuron is broken into 12 compartments (Banks and Sachs, 1991). The axon and soma are each one compartment, containing a capacitance c_a, c_s, a leak conductance g_L, and voltage-dependent sodium g_{Na} and potassium g_K channels. The dendritic tree is collapsed into a single equivalent cylinder of 10 compartments, each containing a capacitance c_i, a resting conductance g_R, and excitatory g_E and inhibitory g_J synaptic conductances. The soma also contains excitatory and inhibitory synaptic conductances. **B:** Somatic membrane potential (above) and synaptic conductance (below) for the multipolar-cell model with 8 independent subthreshold excitatory inputs to the second dendritic compartment. **C:** PSTH of the model responses for the same input as in B. **D:** The bushy cell is modeled as a single somatic compartment containing capacitance c, leak conductance g_L, voltage-gated sodium g_{Na} and potassium g_K, g_M channels, and inhibitory g_J and excitatory g_E synaptic channels (Rothman et al., 1993). **E,F:** Membrane potential and PSTH for the bushy-cell model with 5 independent suprathreshold excitatory inputs. In both models, ANF-like spike trains drive the excitatory conductances; each spike arrival produces a transient alpha-wave conductance change $A(t/t_p)$ $\exp[(t_p - t)/t_p]$, where $t_p = 0.1$ (bushy) or 0.25 (multipolar) ms. (A–C redrawn from Banks and Sachs, 1991; D–F from Rothman et al., 1993, with permission.)

plus a voltage-dependent potassium conductance g_M. g_M models the potassium conductance which is activated at rest in these cells and gives the model electrophysiological characteristics similar to those of real bushy cells shown in Fig. 4.7D. The behavior of this model was studied as the number and strength of independent
auditory-nerve inputs was varied. The model accurately duplicates bushy-cell PSTHs,
producing primarylike responses if supplied with only one or two large (suprathreshold) auditory-nerve inputs and pri-N responses if supplied with more inputs (e.g., Fig.
4.10F with 5 suprathreshold inputs). The model's spike trains are as irregular as those
of ANFs and real bushy cells, if supplied with suprathreshold inputs, but tend to be
too regular with subthreshold inputs. Figure 4.10E shows a model spike train and the
underlying conductance waveform; in contrast with the multipolar model of Fig. 4.10B,
there is good temporal register of EPSPs and postsynaptic spikes. This correspondence
results in part from the lack of temporal summation of inputs and is traceable to the
effects of the low-threshold potassium conductance.

The model in Fig. 4.10D accounts well for the properties of SBCs and for some
properties of GBCs. However, there are problems in trying to account for all the properties of GBCs; one issue is that GBCs receive a large number of ANF inputs, up to
50 (Liberman, 1991; Ostapoff and Morest, 1991). Most of these inputs probably come
from ANFs with significant spontaneous discharge. Because the inputs have to be
suprathreshold in order to produce an irregular output, the result of applying a large
number of spontaneously active inputs to the bushy cell model is to give the model
substantial spontaneous activity. However, pri-N neurons frequently have low or zero
spontaneous activity (Blackburn and Sachs, 1989; Spirou et al., 1990). In addition,
there are problems accounting for the phase-locking behavior of pri-N neurons (phase-
locking is explained later in Fig. 4.11). The details of this issue are beyond the scope

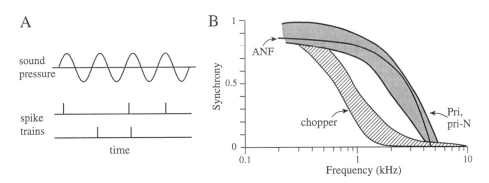

Fig. 4.11. Phase-locking in ANFs and VCN units. **A:** Top line shows the waveform of a tone
as the sound pressure at the eardrum. The next two lines show spike trains in two neurons responding to the tone. Phase-locking is the tendency of spikes to occur at a particular point during the stimulus cycle, in this case, near the positive peak. Note that each neuron does not necessarily produce a spike in every stimulus cycle. **B:** Plot of the strength of phase-locking versus
frequency for ANFs (line), primarylike and pri-N neurons (shaded region) and choppers (hatched
region). Phase-locking is measured as synchrony (Johnson, 1980), which varies from 0 (random
spike patterns with no phase locking) to 1 (perfect locking, spikes all occur at the same point in
the cycle). The line is the average of ANF data from Johnson (1980). Shaded and hatched regions surround most of the cochlear-nucleus data from Blackburn and Sachs (1989).

of this chapter and are discussed elsewhere (Joris et al., 1994; Rothman and Young, 1996).

One hypothesis that is suggested by attempts to model GBCs is that some of the inhibitory inputs known to be present on bushy cells (Altschuler et al., 1986; Adams and Mugnaini, 1987; Wenthold et al., 1988; Saint Marie et al., 1989) provide a continuous inhibition that is adjusted to maintain the cells at a stable, low-spontaneous operating point. The plausibility of this idea is supported by the fact, noted above, that inhibitory inputs to VCN neurons are centered on the cells' BFs and concentrated near BF (Caspary et al., 1994), so that the inhibition does not seem designed for the role of contrast enhancement through lateral suppression that is usually offered in sensory systems.

CIRCUIT FUNCTIONS

We have seen that each neuron type of the cochlear nucleus has specific structural and functional properties which, together with its distinctive synaptic connections, enable it to respond in a specific way to the auditory stimulus. We are now in a position to assess how the multiple features of the auditory stimulus are encoded by the parallel processing lines of the cochlear nucleus. It is the extraction of these multiple features that permit the auditory system to be adapted for a wide range of auditory signals, from the alerting signals of prey or predator to the discrimination of communication signals, and, in humans, the critical abilities of language and the emotional and cognitive appreciation of song and instrumental music.

PHASE-LOCKING IN BUSHY CELLS AND SOUND LOCALIZATION

An essential aspect of auditory processing is computing the location of the source of a sound. This computation begins in the superior olivary nuclei (Fig. 4.3B) where neurons compare the time of arrival (MSO; Goldberg and Brown, 1969) and the sound level (LSO; Boudreau and Tsuchitani, 1970) of the stimuli in the two ears. Such comparisons are useful because a sound originating, say, on the left will reach the left ear before it reaches the right ear and will be louder in the left ear (Irvine, 1986). These binaural differences in stimulus arrival time and loudness are cues to the location of the sound source. The inputs to the MSO and LSO are from the bushy cells of the VCN and, in the following paragraphs, the anatomical and membrane specializations of bushy cells are interpreted as necessary to support interaural time difference analysis in the MSO.

The means by which temporal information about the stimulus is encoded is shown in Fig. 4.11A. This figure shows the spike trains of two neurons responding to a tone; the responses are *phase locked* to the stimulus, in that spikes occur near a particular preferred portion of the stimulus waveform. Figure 4.11B shows that phase-locking occurs in cat ANFs (line) for frequencies up to about 5 kHz (Johnson, 1980). The shaded region shows that the phase-locking ability of primarylike and pri-N neurons (bushy cells) is similar to that of ANFs (Blackburn and Sachs, 1989). Although it is not well shown in Fig. 4.11B, bushy cells actually display enhanced phase-locking at low frequencies, below 1 kHz, where they may be entrained precisely to the stimulus waveform (Joris et al., 1994). By contrast, the phase-locking of chopper neurons (T-multipolars) is much weaker, essentially disappearing by 2 kHz (hatched region).

The differences between primarylike and chopper neurons derive from their membrane properties. Because of membrane capacitance, the postsynaptic processing of all neurons tends to be low-pass, i.e., fast fluctuations in the synaptic inputs are filtered out. In T-multipolars, where the inputs are on the dendritic tree, there is an additional component of low-pass filtering due to the dendrites (White et al., 1994). As a result, frequencies in the input above a few hundred Hz are severely attenuated. By contrast, in bushy cells, postsynaptic filtering effects are minimized by placing the synapses on the soma, by making the postsynaptic currents large so as to quickly charge the membrane capacitance, and by minimizing temporal integration of inputs, as described in Fig. 4.8. The tendency of bushy cells to follow the temporal patterns of their inputs, as opposed to T-multipolar cells which do not, was demonstrated by the model results in Figs. 4.10B and 4.10E.

A particular strong cue for sound localization is the interaural delay in the *waveform* of the stimulus. In fact, perceptual experiments show that the strongest cue for localization of sound in azimuth is the interaural delay of the stimulus waveform for frequency components below 1 kHz (Wightman and Kistler, 1992). Clearly, if the waveform of a stimulus like the tone in Fig. 4.11A is delayed in one ear, the ANF spikes that are phase locked to the tone will be delayed by the same amount. Thus MSO neurons can compare the time of arrival of the stimulus waveforms in the two ears by comparing the time of arrival of phase-locked spike trains from the two cochlear nuclei. MSO neurons accomplish this comparison by functioning as coincidence detectors (Goldberg and Brown, 1960), meaning that they respond when they receive coincident spikes from their bushy-cell inputs on the two sides. Coincidence detection is possible in MSO cells only because they share the short membrane time constant and the low-threshold potassium channel described above for bushy cells (Smith, 1995; Brughera et al., 1996). Thus the membrane specializations of both bushy and MSO cells can be understood as allowing the high-precision temporal responses that are necessary for binaural comparison of interaural time difference.

STIMULUS SPECTRUM REPRESENTATION IN CHOPPER NEURONS

In addition to localizing a sound, it is important to identify it, meaning to identify the source that produced the sound. The auditory system identifies sounds on the basis of their frequency content and their temporal fluctuations. A good illustration of the importance of frequency content is provided by the vowels of human speech. Figure 4.12A shows the frequency content of the vowel EH, as in "met", when spoken by a male voice. There are prominent peaks of energy at 512, 1792, and 2432 Hz (arrows); these peaks are called *formants* and correspond to the resonant frequencies of the vocal tract. Each vowel is characterized by a different combination of formant frequencies (Peterson and Barney, 1952) and our perceptual recognition of different vowels is closely tied to the frequencies of their first three formants.

Because of the importance of the frequency content of sounds for their perception, it is natural to consider the neural representation of sounds in terms of a plot of neural response versus BF (Pfeiffer and Kim, 1975; Sachs and Young, 1979). That is, we are considering the representation of a sound in terms of the tonotopic map established in the cochlea (Fig. 4.1), where each ANF represents the energy in the stimulus at frequencies near its BF. Figure 4.12B–E compare the tonotopic representation of the fre-

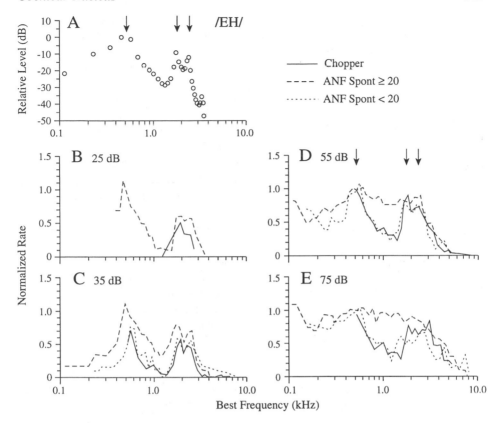

Fig. 4.12. Frequency content of a vowel-like stimulus and its neural representation in populations of auditory nerve fibers and chopper units. **A:** Distribution of energy across frequency for a synthetic version of the vowel EH, as in "met"; the points show the levels of a series of tones of different frequencies that are added together to make the vowel. The energy peaks (arrows) are the formants. **B–E:** Responses of populations of ANFs and chopper units to the vowel at four sound levels, ranging from very soft (25 dB, B) to conversational levels (75 dB, E). Response is plotted as normalized rate which varies from 0 (spontaneous rate) to 1 (maximal or saturated rate). The abscissa shows the BF of the neurons. Data from individual neurons are not shown; instead, the lines are averages of the responses of neurons computed with triangular weighting over a range of BFs of 0.25 octave. The three line types correspond to three neural populations, as given in the legend. ANFs are separated into two groups as described in the text. Lines are plotted only over the frequency range where significant numbers of neurons of each type were studied. The chopper data are from a subgroup of the chopper population, called *chop-T* (Young et al, 1988), but are typical of all choppers. (Redrawn from Blackburn and Sachs, 1990, with permission.)

quency spectrum of the EH for two subpopulations of ANFs and for chopper neurons (Blackburn and Sachs, 1990); the chopper neurons appear to derive a stable representation of the stimulus spectrum from the more variable ANF representation.

The plots in Fig. 4.12B–E show discharge rate versus BF; these plots were constructed by recording the responses of several hundred neurons to the vowel, plotting each neuron's discharge rate at an abscissa position equal to its BF, and then averaging the data using a moving window filter. The lines show the average values, which can be considered to be the vowel's neural representation at the input to the central auditory system. Response profiles are shown for three populations of neurons: (*1*) ANFs with spontaneous rates less than 20/s, (*2*) fibers with spontaneous rates above 20/s, and (*3*) cochlear-nucleus choppers. The two populations of ANFs are differentiated because their dynamic ranges are different. High spontaneous rate fibers have low thresholds, but have limited dynamic ranges, so that these fibers provide rate information at low sound levels. This is illustrated in Fig. 4.12 by the dashed lines for spont $\geq$20. At the lowest sound level (25 dB, Fig. 4.12B), the dashed-line rate profile provides a good representation of the vowel in that there are peaks of discharge rate among fibers with BFs equal to the formant frequencies. As the sound level increases this clear representation is lost as high spontaneous rate fibers of all BFs approach their maximal discharge rates (Fig. 4.12E), meaning normalized rates of 1. Note that this loss of rate representation occurs at conversational sound levels, i.e., at 75 dB, a level at which we comfortably communicate using speech.

Low spontaneous rate fibers, by contrast, have higher thresholds and wider dynamic ranges. This is illustrated in Fig. 4.12 by the dotted lines; at the lowest level (Fig. 4.12B) there is no response from the low-spontaneous rate fibers, because the stimulus is below threshold. As stimulus level increases, a good rate representation is observed, which is maintained to the highest level shown; that is, there are clearly defined peaks of response near the first and the second/third formant peaks (arrows) with a minimum of response in between.

The solid lines in Fig. 4.12 show responses of chopper neurons to the same stimulus. Note that the choppers maintain a representation that is at least as good as that of the better ANF group; there is a clear peak at BFs equal to the formants at all sound levels. This behavior can be easily explained if T-multipolar cells receive inputs predominantly from low spontaneous rate ANFs. However, two observations argue that choppers also receive significant input from high spontaneous rate fibers: (*1*) chopper neurons have thresholds as low as those of high spontaneous rate ANFs (Bourk, 1976); and (*2*) direct demonstration of functional connections between chopper neurons and ANFs has been done with cross-correlation analysis (Sachs et al., 1993). In this method, simultaneous recordings of an ANF and a cochlear-nucleus cell are done and the spike trains are analyzed to show that the probability of spiking is enhanced in the chopper immediately following spikes in the ANF. When such an enhancement is seen, it is evidence that the two neurons are connected by a monosynaptic, excitatory synapse (Moore et al., 1970). Such connections were frequently found for choppers and high spontaneous rate ANFs, but were rarely found for low spontaneous rate fibers; this result cannot be used to rule out a connection of low spontaneous rate fibers to choppers, but it does mean that high spontaneous rate fibers are connected. Finally, note that Fig. 4.12B shows a substantial rate response of choppers to the vowel at the lowest sound level, where low spontaneous rate ANFs give little or no response (choppers with BFs near F1 presumably respond to the vowel at 25 dB, but were not studied in sufficient numbers to be plotted in the figure).

The evidence thus suggests that chopper neurons receive both low and high spontaneous rate auditory-nerve inputs. This raises the question of how choppers avoid the saturation of their discharge rate which is inherent in the responses of their high spontaneous rate inputs (Figs. 4.12D and E). One way would be to turn off the high spontaneous rate inputs at sound levels where there is substantial low spontaneous rate activity and respond to low spontaneous rate inputs instead. That is, choppers could respond to their high spontaneous rate inputs at low sound levels and then switch to their low spontaneous rate inputs at moderate or high levels. A means by which T-multipolar cells could perform this switching has been demonstrated (Lai et al., 1994). Computational modeling shows that inhibitory terminals activating conductances that are sufficiently large can cancel the effects of excitatory inputs located at more distal sites on the dendritic tree; at the same time, excitatory inputs that are proximal to the inhibitory inputs are not affected (Koch et al., 1983; see Chap. 1). Thus, by placing high spontaneous rate terminals in the distal portion of the dendritic tree and intermingling them with strong inhibitory inputs, the effect of the high spontaneous rate inputs can be canceled by activation of the inhibitory inputs. If low spontaneous rate inputs are placed on the proximal dendritic tree, their effect on the cell would not be affected by the inhibitory inputs. Thus the cell can be induced to switch from its high spontaneous to its low spontaneous inputs by an inhibitory input driven by, for example, low spontaneous rate fibers averaged over a broad range of BFs. Although direct evidence for this idea is lacking, it provides a possible explanation for the behavior of chopper neurons shown in Fig. 4.12.

Thus chopper neurons, or T-multipolar cells, provide a representation of the shape of the stimulus frequency spectrum which is stable as sound level changes. This representation provides information about the identity of the sound, one speech sound versus another for example, which complements the information about sound source location provided in parallel through the bushy-cell/superior-olive pathway. Thus we begin to see how aspects of the acoustic environment are separated out at the brainstem level and selectively represented. It is important to point out, however, that the separation is not complete. Information about the stimulus frequency spectrum is also encoded in the bushy-cell pathway, although in a different form which depends on phase-locking. For a description of this temporal representation, see Sachs (1984) and Blackburn and Sachs (1990).

ENHANCEMENT OF MODULATION RESPONSES

Important real-world acoustic signals such as speech or music are dynamic, meaning that their amplitude and frequency contents fluctuate in time. An example of *amplitude modulation* of a signal is shown in Fig. 4.13A. This signal is basically a tone whose amplitude fluctuates with a period of 8 ms; three cycles are shown. The amplitude modulation in Fig. 4.13A is modeled after the modulation normally seen in vowels; the rate of amplitude fluctuation (in this case 125 Hz, or once per 8 ms) corresponds to the pitch of the voice and it is this rate of fluctuation which is varied to sing different musical notes. The *envelope* of the stimulus is the time-varying amplitude of the signal, which can be approximated by connecting the positive peaks of the waveform. The envelope of speech or music is a complex signal in itself. Envelopes vary from the relatively fast fluctuations associated with vowels (as in Fig. 4.13A) to slower fluctuations corresponding to the sequence of speech sounds and syllables or the sequence of musical notes. In the case of speech, substantial information can be obtained from only the envelope of the signal (Van Tasell et al., 1987); this can be demonstrated

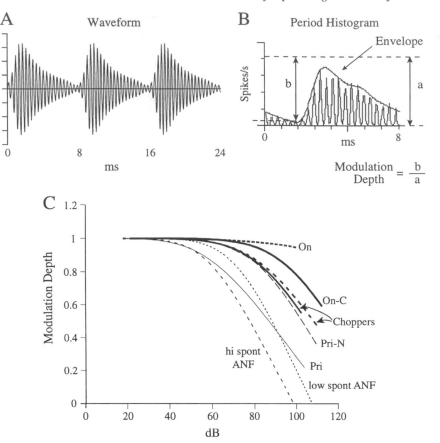

Fig. 4.13. **A:** Stimulus used to investigate modulation responses. The signal is narrowband with a bandwidth comparable to the formant resonances of speech; it is centered at the BF of the neuron under study and approximates a BF tone modulated by an envelope typical of a vowel. **B:** Period histogram of a neuron's response to the stimulus in A, showing rate versus time through one cycle of the envelope (8 ms), averaged over the whole response. Note the modulation of the histogram indicated by the line marked *Envelope*. A measure of envelope response is the *modulation depth b/a*. **C:** Average modulation depth for populations of neurons plotted versus stimulus level. Data are shown separately for 8 neuron types, as indicated by the labels. Two lines are shown for choppers, corresponding to choppers of low and high degrees of regularity (chop-T and chop-S, Young et al., 1988); the behaviors of these two groups are essentially identical. Note the enhanced modulation response in cochlear-nucleus neurons, especially onset neurons (Redrawn with permission from Wang and Sachs, 1994.)

by extracting the envelope of the signal and using it to modulate the amplitude of a noise, so that all cues related to the frequency content of the stimulus are lost (i.e., the formant peaks in Fig. 4.12A). Listeners are able to make many basic speech discriminations based on this impoverished signal; indeed, the cochlear implant, an auditory prostheses for the deaf, provides much of its information through the signal envelope (see Shannon et al., 1995 for a discussion of this issue). Thus, the representation of the envelope of complex signals is an important aspect of auditory analysis.

A feature seen in almost all the cell types in the cochlear nucleus is enhancement of the response to the envelope of the acoustic signal (Frisina et al., 1990; Rhode and Greenberg, 1994; Wang and Sachs, 1994). Fig. 4.13B shows the response of an ANF to a signal like that in Fig. 4.13A (Wang and Sachs, 1993, 1994). In this case, the fiber responds to both the waveform of the tone which underlies the signal and the envelope of the tone's amplitude modulation. Phase-locking to the tone waveform is reflected in the series of peaks making up the histogram and the response to the envelope is reflected by the variation in the amplitude of those peaks. A line shows the envelope of the histogram, which is a neural representation of the envelope of the signal. A measure of the strength of the envelope representation is the *modulation depth* = b/a. As the sound level increases, the modulation of neural responses is lost because of the neurons' limited dynamic ranges; essentially, as the stimulus level increases, the amplitude of the signal at all points in the envelope eventually reaches the upper end of the neuron's dynamic range. When this happens, the neuron responds at its maximal rate to all portions of the envelope and the modulation of the response disappears.

The average modulation depth of responses like Fig. 4.13B is plotted against stimulus level in Fig. 4.13C for ANFs and for VCN neurons (Wang and Sachs, 1994). As described above, modulation depth decreases as the signal level is increased for all neuron types. The decrease occurs at the lowest level for ANFs and primarylike neurons (mostly SBCs). Because low spontaneous rate ANFs have wider dynamic ranges than high spontaneous rate fibers, the modulation response survives to higher levels in the low spontaneous rate population. It is not surprising that primarylike neurons behave like ANFs, given the model for SBCs described above. Pri-N and chopper neurons show a substantially amplified response to modulation at high sound levels, but the best modulation responses are observed in onset neurons (Frisina et al., 1990; Rhode and Greenberg, 1994). The range of sound levels over which modulation responses are amplified in the cochlear nucleus relative to the auditory nerve (above 60 dB on the abscissa of Fig. 4.13C) includes the range of loudness commonly encountered in conversational speech and extends upward into the range of loud backgrounds, like a crowded room, where our auditory systems frequently function.

The means by which modulation responses are amplified in the cochlear nucleus have been investigated using the chopper model described in Fig. 4.10A (Wang and Sachs, 1995). A cochlear-nucleus neuron can only show modulation response if there is some modulation of its inputs. Modulated inputs are maintained over a wide range of levels in the model by combining activity across high and low spontaneous rate fibers, as in the previous section, and by adding inputs from ANFs over a range of different BFs. It turns out that, for the narrowband stimulus of Fig. 4.13A, ANFs give enhanced modulation responses when their BFs are different from the center frequency of the stimulus; the responses are strongest when the energy in the stimulus is at the edge of the neurons' frequency response areas (Wang and Sachs, 1993). This may explain why onset neurons give the strongest modulation responses, because they receive auditory-nerve inputs over the widest range of BFs and therefore take best advantage of the enhanced off-BF modulation responses. In addition, it is possible in the model to amplify the modulation in the inputs by making the inputs subthreshold, so that coincident firing of several inputs is required to exceed threshold. This has the effect of amplifying peaks of the input envelope. Finally, saturation of the model was avoided by applying inhibitory inputs to maintain the model near the center of its dynamic range.

Amplification of the envelope of the signal occurs in all of the cochlear nucleus' output pathways, except the SBCs. In this sense, the cochlear nucleus begins the processing of information encoded in the temporal fluctuations of the stimulus; in more central auditory nuclei, like the IC and the auditory cortex, responses to stimulus modulation are further elaborated (see Langner, 1992 for a review).

DORSAL COCHLEAR NUCLEUS

The discussion of VCN neurons has focused on the effects of their auditory-nerve inputs and their membrane properties. In the DCN, by contrast, the neurons' acoustic response properties are dependent on the synaptic circuitry of the nucleus. The components of the DCN circuit were discussed in connection with Figs. 4.5 and 4.6. The deep layers receive inputs from the auditory nerve and VCN and the superficial layer receives inputs from granule cells, which carry both auditory and nonauditory information. The acoustic response properties of DCN principal cells are complex but can be accounted for largely by the synaptic circuits of the deep DCN.

The response properties typical of DCN vertical cells and principal cells are shown in Fig. 4.14A and B. These plots are response maps which show the neurons' responses to tones at various frequencies and sound levels. Response-map shapes of cochlear-nucleus neurons are classified into five types on the basis of the distribution of the excitatory and inhibitory areas within them (Evans and Nelson, 1973; Young and Brownell, 1976). Figure 4.14A shows the response map of a type II neuron; this type has been associated with vertical cells, because type II neurons can be antidromically activated from the VCN (Young, 1980) and vertical cells are the only known projection from the DCN to VCN (Lorente de Nó, 1981). Type II neurons have a frequency selectivity that is similar to most neurons in the peripheral auditory system. There is a central V-shaped excitatory area (black) with surrounding inhibitory sidebands (shaded). Type II neurons are characterized by two features in addition to this response map shape: they are not spontaneously active and they respond weakly or not at all to broadband noise (Young and Voigt, 1982). The weak noise response is a distinguishing characteristic of type II responses; no other neuron in the cochlear nucleus behaves this way, including other neurons with prominent inhibitory sidebands. Presumably, broadband noise activates inhibitory inputs that are strong enough to prevent the cell from firing; one explanation for the weak noise response is to assume that the inhibitory inputs to type IIs are from neurons that respond strongly to noise, but weakly to tones. A likely candidate are the onset-C neurons (D-multipolar cells) of the VCN (Winter and Palmer, 1995). Onset-C neurons give weak responses to tones and strong responses to broadband noise, as required, and D-multipolar neurons have been shown to project inhibitory-type terminals into the DCN (Smith and Rhode, 1989; Oertel et al., 1990).

Figure 4.14B shows the response map of a type IV neuron; this response type has been associated with DCN principal cells (pyramidal and giant cells) because type IV neurons can be antidromically activated from the efferent-fiber pathway of the DCN (Young, 1980). Type IV response maps are complex and vary in shape from neuron to neuron (Spirou and Young, 1991); however, in unanesthetized (decerebrate) cats

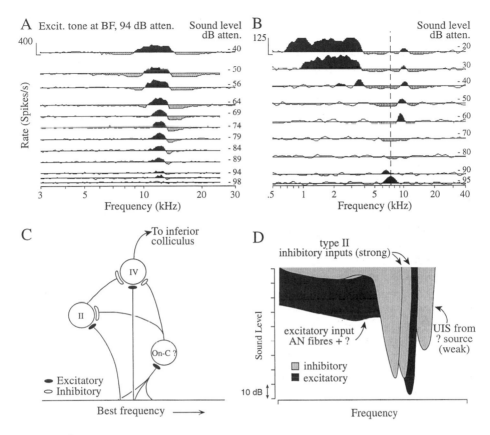

Fig. 4.14. Response maps of type II and type IV neurons in the DCN. A: Type II response map showing excitatory and inhibitory areas as a function of frequency and sound level of a tone stimulus. Each trace shows discharge rate of the neuron versus tone frequency at a fixed sound level, given at right. Sound levels become louder from bottom to top. Because the type II neuron had no spontaneous activity, a BF tone slightly above threshold was presented along with the test tone bursts to generate the background activity necessary to demonstrate inhibition. The straight horizontal lines are the background rate, i.e., the rate in response to the background tone alone. The rate scale is given at top left. Excitatory responses are increases in rate above background (colored black); inhibitory regions are decreases in rate below background (shaded areas). B: The same for a type IV neuron, except no background tone was presented and the horizontal lines are the neuron's spontaneous discharge rate. The dashed line marks the neuron's BF. C: Model of the excitatory and inhibitory interactions believed to underlie principal cell responses in the DCN. Principal cell responses are type IV; they receive excitatory input from ANFs and perhaps T-multipolar cells (the tonotopic array of excitatory inputs to the DCN is represented by the horizontal line at bottom) and inhibitory inputs from two interneurons: type II neurons (vertical cells) and On-C neurons (D-multipolar cells). The strengths of synaptic connections are indicated schematically by their size. On-C neurons respond strongly to broadband stimuli, but weakly to tones; type Ii neurons do the opposite because of the strong inhibitory input from On-C neurons. Type IV neurons are inhibited strongly by type II neurons and weakly by On-C neurons. D: Schematic to explain the response map shape of type IV neurons in terms of excitatory ANF (black) and inhibitory type II (shaded) response maps. The upper inhibitory sideband (UIS) is not accounted for by these two inputs (see text). (Reproduced with permission from Spirou and Young, 1991.)

153

they are characterized by a strong inhibitory area which is centered near, usually just below, the BF of the neuron (called the *central inhibitory area*, CIA). In Fig. 4.14B, the BF is 7.4 kHz, shown by the dashed line. The CIA is the inhibitory area between 4 and 9 kHz. Type IV neurons give excitatory responses to low-level BF tones, but inhibitory responses to BF tones at levels 10–30 dB above threshold, within the CIA (follow the dashed line vertically in Fig. 4.14B). Other features in Fig. 4.14B that are typical of most type IV response maps are a thin excitatory area along the upper frequency edge of the CIA (near ≈ 10 kHz), a broad excitatory area at frequencies below the CIA (<4 kHz in this case), and an inhibitory sideband at high frequencies (>10 kHz in this case).

A variety of evidence suggests that the CIA in type IV response maps is produced by monosynaptic inhibitory input from vertical cells. The most direct evidence comes from cross-correlation studies in which the spike trains of a type II and a type IV neuron are studied simultaneously (Voigt and Young, 1980, 1990). Figure 4.15 shows an example of cross-correlation analysis applied to a type II–type IV pair. Simplified response maps of the neurons are shown in Fig. 4.15A and B; these maps show excitatory (black) and inhibitory (unfilled) areas only, rather than discharge rates as in Fig. 4.14. Note the correspondence of the excitatory area of the type II neuron and the CIA of the type IV neuron; the arrows above the response maps point to the BFs of the two neurons for orientation. Figure 4.15D shows a cross-correlogram of the spike trains of the two neurons; the correlogram can be thought of as the average discharge rate in the presumed postsynaptic neuron (type IV) as a function of time relative to spikes in the presumed presynaptic neuron (type II). Note the prominent dip in the cross-correlogram just to the right of the origin. The dip called an *inhibitory trough*, corresponds to a decrease in the probability of response of the type IV neuron immediately following spikes in the type II neuron. This is the feature expected in the cross-correlogram of a pair of neurons connected by a monosynaptic inhibitory synapse (Moore et al., 1970). The plots in Fig. 4.15C show the discharge rates of these two neurons in response to a tone at various sound levels; the tone is at the BF of the type II neuron, which is slightly below the type IV BF. The decrease in discharge rate of the type IV neuron below its spontaneous rate (dashed line) marks the lower boundary of the CIA. These data are typical of type II–type IV pairs with an inhibitory trough in their cross-correlograms in that the decrease in discharge rate in the type IV neuron occurs at the threshold of the type II neuron (Young and Voigt, 1981).

Type II inhibitory input to type IV neurons accounts for many of the features of type IV response maps. Figure 4.14D shows a schematic to illustrate this point. Shown is the response map of an excitatory input (black area) with the excitatory portions of the response maps of two type II inhibitory inputs superimposed (shaded area). The shape of the excitatory input's response map is typical of the behavior of ANFs and T-multipolar cells, the known excitatory inputs to the deep DCN. The type II response maps show higher thresholds and lower BFs, as is consistent with experimental results (Young and Brownell, 1976; Voigt and Young, 1990), e.g., Fig. 4.15A and B. The excitatory input has a *low-frequency tail* in its response map, meaning a region of roughly constant threshold, which is about 40–60 dB above its BF threshold. The type II neurons also have tails, but at very high levels (Young and Voigt, 1982). If the type II inhibitory input is very strong, then the type IV response map will look about like the model

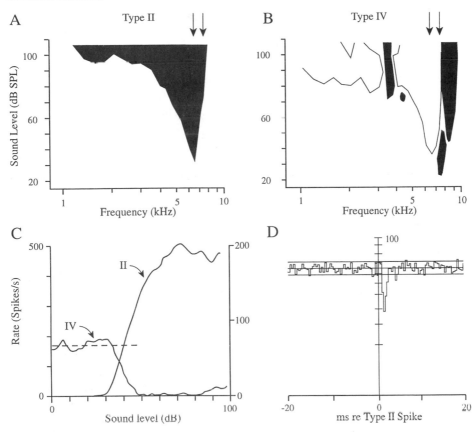

Fig. 4.15. Cross-correlation analysis of a simultaneously recorded type II–type IV pair showing evidence for a monosynaptic inhibitory connection. A,B: Simplified response maps for a type II (**A**) and type IV (**B**) neuron; excitatory regions are shown filled and inhibitory regions are shown unfilled. Inhibitory regions of the type II neuron were not determined. The arrows at the top point to the BFs of the two neurons (6.5 kHz for the type II and 7.4 kHz for the type IV neuron). The two neurons were recorded simultaneously in the same DCN with two microelectrodes. **C:** Rate versus sound level for the same two neurons. The stimulus was a 6.5 kHz tone, at the BF of the type II neuron. The type II rate is on the left ordinate and the type IV rate is at right. Note that when the type II rate begins to increase, the type IV rate begins to decrease (horizontal dashed line is the type IV spontaneous rate). **D:** A cross-correlogram of the spike trains of these two neurons. Note the inhibitory trough (see text). The horizontal lines show the expected value of the correlogram if the two neurons were independent with ±2 S.D. confidence limits. (Redrawn from Young and Voigt, 1981, with permission.)

shown in this figure. The most common features of type IV response maps are accounted for by this simple model (compare with Fig. 4.14B; Reed and Blum, 1995). One feature not accounted for is the upper inhibitory sideband (UIS) which frequently occurs; one possibility is that the UIS is produced by the additional inhibitory input described below.

The type II–type IV circuit accounts for some additional unusual features of type IV responses to sound (Young and Brownell, 1976; Spirou and Young, 1991; Nelken and

Young, 1994). Most prominent among these is that type IV neurons usually respond strongly to broadband stimuli like noise, even though their responses to tones may be predominantly inhibitory. Because type II neurons do not respond to noise, the model allows type IV neurons to respond to noise as strongly as do their excitatory inputs. However, the model does not account for the responses of type IV neurons to a noise-notch stimulus, meaning a broadband noise with the energy removed over some range of frequencies, forming a notch. If the notch is placed at frequencies surrounding the BF of a type IV neuron, then the neuron is inhibited (Spirou and Young, 1991; Nelken and Young, 1994). This inhibition is unexpected from the tone-response map of the neuron (Fig. 4.14B), because over most of the range of levels, the frequencies near BF (dashed line) are inhibitory, so their removal should produce a net excitation. It turns out that the inhibitory response to notched noise requires a second inhibitory input to type IV neurons that responds strongly to broadband stimuli; it has been proposed that the onset-C (D-multipolar) cell provides the needed inhibition (Nelken and Young, 1994). With the addition of this second inhibitory source, the known response properties of type IV neurons can be accounted for, at least qualitatively. The circuit model in Fig. 4.14C summarizes the connections among type II (vertical cell), type IV (principal cell), and onset-C (D-multipolar) neurons that are sufficient to explain currently known response properties of type IV neurons.

As shown in Fig. 4.6, the circuitry of the superficial DCN provides both excitatory inputs to principal cells through direct granule-cell terminals as well as inhibitory inputs through the cartwheel and stellate interneurons. The nature of the information carried in the superficial layer depends on the sources of the mossy-fiber inputs to the granule cells. Among several known sources, only one has been studied in detail; this is the somatosensory projection from the dorsal column and spinal trigeminal nuclei (Itoh et al., 1987) which terminates as mossy fibers in the granule-cell areas (Wright and Ryugo, 1996). DCN principal cells are inhibited by manual movement of the pinna; the neurons are not responsive to light touch or movement of hairs on the pinna, but rather to back-and-forth movements of the whole auricle (Young et al., 1995). This inhibition is carried to the principal cells through the granule-cell system and the cartwheel cells (Davis et al., 1996). The cat, of course, has a mobile pinna; when the pinna moves, as happens frequently in an awake cat that is exploring its environment, the acoustics of the ear change significantly; one important consequence is that the cues for sound localization move with the pinna (Young et al., 1996). Thus, information on pinna movement is necessary to the processing of sound localization; such information is apparently provided to the auditory system, through the DCN, at an early stage.

The role of the DCN in the auditory system has been difficult to establish because lesions of the DCN or DAS do not produce dramatic auditory deficits, whereas lesions of the trapezoid body produce a state of deafness (Masterton and Granger, 1988; Masterton et al., 1994). From the descriptions above, it is apparent that DCN output neurons are inhibited by sharp spectral features, such as peaks or notches in the frequency content of the stimulus, or by movement of the pinna. All of these are important events to the auditory system. Sharp spectral features convey information; for example, spectral peaks identify vowels and other speech sounds, and spectral notches convey information about sound localization to augment the binaural cues described earlier in the chapter (Middlebrooks and Green, 1991). Movements of the pinna are important events to the auditory system, because of the acoustic effects mentioned above. Thus the DCN may serve a role of detecting and signaling, by inhibition of its output cells, important auditory events.

The components of the cochlear nucleus provide examples of a wide range of modes of neural integration. The different cell types in the cochlear nucleus form the beginnings of at least four parallel systems in the brainstem auditory system. The role in audition of these parallel systems can be inferred to some extent from the nature of the representation of sound that each system conveys at the output of the cochlear nucleus. A sound grasp of the mechanisms in the cochlear nucleus is the necessary starting point for understanding the nature of auditory processing at subsequent levels of the auditory pathway.

5

OLFACTORY BULB

GORDON M. SHEPHERD and CHARLES A. GREER

The olfactory bulb is an outgrowth of the forebrain, specialized for processing the molecular signals that give rise to the sense of smell. It receives all of the input from the olfactory sensory neurons (see Fig. 5.1), and sends its output directly to the olfactory cortex (see Chap. 10). This basic relationship is seen in the most primitive fish, and has endured throughout the evolution of nearly all vertebrates.

As a region for experimental analysis, the olfactory bulb is attractive for several reasons. In its position in front of the brain, it is easily accessible. The sensory nerves to the bulb are completely separated from its output fibers to the brain. This enables input and output to be manipulated individually, whether by electrical stimulation or tracer injection, similar to the situation in the spinal cord (Chap. 4). Within, the bulb is a distinctly laminated structure, containing sharply differentiated cell types, particularly in terrestrial animals. All of these features facilitate the application of different experimental techniques and the precise interpretation of results.

Historically, these advantages have been put to good use. Work on the olfactory bulb by Ramon y Cajal and the classical histologists in the nineteenth century contributed to the evidence that led to acceptance of the neuron doctrine (reviewed in Shepherd, 1991b). Studies by modern workers have contributed to emerging principles of synaptic organization, as outlined in Chap. 1. It has been realized that many aspects of the synaptic organization of the bulb reflect general principles shared with other sensory regions, especially the retina (Chap. 6) and thalamus (Chap. 8).

Until recently, a disadvantage of working on the olfactory bulb has been the limited knowledge available concerning the sensory mechanisms in the olfactory pathway—in particular, the nature of odor-receptor interactions and the modes of processing of these molecular signals. However, advances on both these fronts have led to an emerging consensus on at least the outlines of the mechanisms whereby information carried in odor molecules is first transduced by the sensory neurons and then processed by the olfactory bulb. A full discussion of olfactory transduction lies outside the bounds of this chapter (see Ache, 1994; Breer, 1994; Hildebrand and Shepherd, 1997, for reviews). Studies of the olfactory bulb itself have also become too extensive to review completely here (see Nickell and Shipley, 1993; Trombley and Shepherd, 1994; Mori and Yoshihara, 1995). Our focus will therefore be on the principles of synaptic orga-

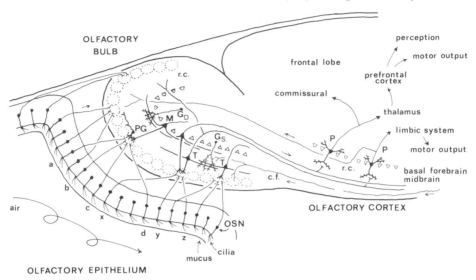

Fig. 5.1. Overview of the olfactory pathway. The olfactory bulb receives input from the receptor neurons in the olfactory epithelium and projects to the olfactory cortex. The diagram indicates some essential aspects of the projection patterns between the regions, as well as the main neural elements within the olfactory bulb. Note that the olfactory epithelium is arranged in overlapping populations of receptor neurons (a–d, x–z) which project to individual glomeruli. Some of the central olfactory connections to limbic brain structures are also indicated. Abbreviations: OSN, olfactory sensory neuron; PG, periglomerular cell; M, mitral cell; T, tufted cell; G_S, superficial granule cell; G_D deep granule cell; r.c., recurrent axon collateral; c.f., centrifugal fiber; P, pyramidal cell.

nization underlying a critical function of the olfactory system: the ability to discriminate between different odor molecules.

NEURONAL ELEMENTS

As in other brain regions, the neuronal elements fall into three categories: input, output, and intrinsic. In describing these elements, we will also relate them to their histological layers (see Fig. 5.2). The classical descriptions were based on Golgi-impregnated neurons (cf. Cajal, 1911); they have been confirmed and amplified by more recent studies employing Golgi methods and intracellular staining (see below).

INPUTS

Afferents. The sensory input consists of the parallel array of axons from the olfactory sensory neurons in the nasal cavity (Fig. 5.2A). A detailed consideration of the sen-

Fig. 5.2. Neural elements of the mammalian olfactory bulb, grouped according to subdivision into inputs (afferent fibers), principal neurons, and intrinsic neurons (local interneurons). Diagrams based on various studies using the Golgi method and HRP (see text). Abbreviations for layers: ONL, olfactory nerve layer; GL, glomerular layer; EPL, external plexiform layer; MCL, mitral cell layer; IPL, internal plexiform layer; GRL, granule cell layer. **A:** ONm and ONl in-

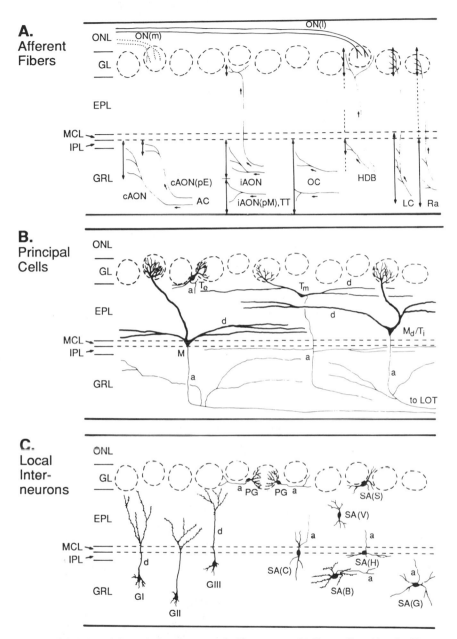

A.
Afferent Fibers

B.
Principal Cells

C.
Local Interneurons

dicate medial (m) and lateral (l) subtypes of olfactory nerve fibers. Centrifugal afferents are from the contralateral anterior olfactory nucleus (cAON), ipsilateral anterior olfactory nucleus (iAON), tenia tecta (TT), olfactory cortex (OC), horizontal limb of the diagonal band (HDB), locus coeruleus (LC), and rapine nucleus (Ra). pE, pars externa of the AON; pM, pars medialis of the AON. **B:** The dendrites and axon collaterals of a mitral cell (M), an internal tufted cell (Ti, or a displaced mitral cell, Md), a middle tufted cell (Tm), and an external tufted cell (Te), a, axon, d dendrite; LOT, lateral olfactory tract. **C:** Three types of granule cells (GI, GII, GIII); PG, periglomerular cell; SA(B) Blanes' cell; SA(C), Clandins' cell; SA(G), Golgi cell; SA(H), Hensen's cell; SA(S) Schwann cell; SA(V) van Gehuchten cell. [Modified from Mori, 1987, with permission.]

161

sory neuron is not possible here (see Farbman, 1994, for review), but several facts are relevant. Traditionally, it has been believed that the sensory neurons are morphologically homogeneous. However, there is evidence for at least one small population of a morphologically distinct subtype (cf. Jourdan, 1975; Moran et al., 1982), and plentiful evidence for molecular subtypes (see below). The sensory axons are all unmyelinated; their diameters form a unimodal spectrum with a mean of approximately 0.2 μm and a range of 0.1–0.4 mm.

This morphological uniformity appears to stand in contrast to the variety of input fibers that characterize many regions of the brain. There is nonetheless a heterogeneity of physiological specificities of the sensory neurons for different odor molecules. Insight into this heterogeneity has been provided by evidence for a large multigene family that may encode for up to 1,000 different olfactory receptors (Buck and Axel, 1991). It is currently believed that a given neuron expresses one or a few types of these putative receptors. Subsets of receptor neurons expressing mRNA for a given type of receptor are distributed within four zones within the olfactory epithelium (Strotman et al., 1992; Ressler et al., 1993; Vassar et al., 1993). Within a zone the subsets appear to be distributed randomly, although physiological studies indicate regions of neurons most sensitive to a given odor (MacKay-Sim and Kesteven, 1994; Youngentob et al., 1995; Ezeh et al., 1995); this issue continues to be under investigation.

As the axons of the sensory neurons pass through the basal lamina of the olfactory epithelium they fasciculate into mesaxons that are surrounded by a specialized ensheathing glial cell (see below). The tight packing of many axons within a single Schwann cell mesaxon provides the opportunity for ephaptic interactions between neighboring axons in which K^+ extruded during impulse activity may play a role (Bliss and Rosenberg, 1979; Gesteland, 1986; Eng and Kocsis, 1987); there is a close similarity in this respect with parallel fibers in the cerebellum.

The olfactory axons are grouped in bundles, which enter the bulb surface where the bundles splay out and interweave. Recent studies suggest that the axons reorganize into functionally related subsets (Treloar et al., 1996; Mombaerts et al., 1996). Following refasciculation, the axons terminate in spherical regions of neuropil called *gomeruli*. In situ hybridization studies have shown that the mRNA for a given olfactory receptor hybridizes to one or a few glomeruli (Vassar et al., 1994; Ressler et al., 1994; Mombaerts et al., 1996). While this does not rule out the possibility of inputs to the same glomerulus from subsets expressing other receptor types (Treloar et al., 1996), it does indicate that molecular subsets of sensory neuron axons fasciculate and the fascicles converge on specific glomerular targets.

In fish and amphibians, the glomeruli are small (20–40 μm in diameter) and not distinctly demarcated; in mammals, they are spherical with sharp borders, and range in size from 30–50 μm in diameter in small mammals (e.g., mice) to 100–200 μm in rabbits or cats (cf. Allison, 1953). The olfactory glomeruli are among the clearest examples in the brain of the principle of grouping neural elements and synapses into anatomically defined modules. They are analogous to the multineuronal "barrels" and "columns" in cerebral cortex (Chap. 12), and represent a higher level of organization than the synaptic glomeruli of the cerebellum (Chap. 7) and thalamus (Chap. 8).

The olfactory axons do not branch on their way to the glomeruli, but once inside, they ramify to varying extents prior to terminating. The arborization of the axons within the glomerulus is spatially limited, involving an average of 7 bifurcations and 8 terminal boutons and *en passant* varicosities (Halasz and Greer, 1993). During early development in rats, some axons terminate transiently in deeper layers (Monti-Graziadei et al., 1980; Farbman, 1994), but these are pruned back, and in the adult all sensory terminals are within the glomeruli.

A notable feature of the sensory neurons is that they are continuously replaced from stem cells in the epithelium throughout adult life (Graziadei and Monti-Graziadei, 1979; Caggiano et al., 1994). Thus, the specificity of synaptic connections in the glomeruli is maintained despite a constant remodeling due to turnover of the sensory terminals (Shepherd, 1994a; Singer et al., 1995b). This degree of plasticity is unique among the regions of the brain considered in this book.

Central Inputs. There are several types of inputs from the brain, each of which has a distinctive laminar pattern of termination (reviewed in Macrides and Davis, 1983; Mori, 1987; Scott and Harrison, 1987; Nickell and Shipley, 1993). One type consists of axon collaterals from pyramidal neurons in the *olfactory cortex* (Chap. 10); these end mostly in the granule cell layer (see OC, Fig. 5.2A). Extensive connections are made by fibers from different parts of the *anterior olfactory nucleus* (AON); their different laminar projections possibly relate to different populations of granule cells (see below). The nucleus of the *horizontal limb of the diagonal band* (HDB) is one of the basal forebrain cholinergic centers; it sends fibers to both the granule layer and the periglomerular parts of the glomerular layer. From the brainstem, the *locus coeruleus* (LC) and the *raphe nucleus* (Ra) send fibers diffusely to the granule layer and specifically to the interiors of the glomeruli (see Fig. 5.2A).

These central inputs are also referred to as *centrifugal* inputs, to indicate their outward orientation from the brain. It is obvious that the olfactory bulb is under extensive and highly differentiated control by the brain. This is true of many other sensory regions in the brain; the retina, by contrast, receives few centrifugal fibers (Chap. 6).

PRINCIPAL NEURONS

The output from the olfactory bulb is carried by the axons of mitral and tufted cells (Fig. 5.2B). The morphology of these cells has been the subject of several studies (Mori et al., 1981a, 1983; Macrides and Schneider, 1982; Kishi et al., 1984; Orona et al., 1984).

Mitral Cells. In fish and amphibia, the principal neurons are relatively undifferentiated. In reptiles, birds, and mammals, however, distinctive mitral cell bodies lie in a thin sheet 200–400 μm deep to the glomerular layer (see Fig. 5.2B). The cell bodies are 15–30 μm in diameter, a medium size for a principal neuron in the brain.

In mammals, each mitral cell tends to give rise to a single *primary* dendrite, which traverses the external plexiform layer (EPL) and terminates within a glomerulus in a tuft of branches. The tuft has a diameter of 50–150 μm, extending throughout most of its glomerulus. The diameter of the dendrite ranges from 2 to 12 μm (depending on the size of the cell body from which it arises); the length is 200–800 μm, depending on how much it angles across the EPL. Each mitral cell also gives rise to several *secondary* (basal) dendrites; laterally directed, they branch sparingly and terminate in the EPL. They are 1–8 μm in diameter, and in mammals extend 500–800 μm. In turtles, HRP-injected mitral cells commonly display two thin (1–2 μm) primary dendrites up to 700 μm in length, and several thin secondary dendrites which extend over 1 mm, and may reach up to halfway around the circumference of the EPL (Mori et al., 1981a). In mammals, subtypes of mitral cells have been identified on the basis of the branching pattern of their secondary dendrites (Macrides and Schneider, 1982; Mori et al., 1983; Orona et al., 1984). As shown in the HRP-stained cells in Fig. 5.2B, type I mitral cells send their secondary dendrites into the deepest region of the EPL, whereas type II (displaced) mitral cells send their secondary dendrites into the middle region of the EPL. These two types form synaptic microcircuits with corresponding subtypes of interneurons (see below). The field of the secondary dendrites may be "dislike" (Mori, 1987) or oriented in the anterior–posterior axis (Shepherd, 1972a).

The primary and secondary dendrites of mitral cells have generally smooth surfaces. Thus they are *aspiny* neurons, like motoneurons, but unlike *spiny* principal neurons, such as cortical pyramidal cells. The highly differentiated terminal tuft, which segregates primary sensory afferents and their associated microcircuits from the rest of the bulb, is virtually unique among principal neurons, and exemplifies the attractiveness of the olfactory bulb as an experimental model.

The mitral cell axons proceed to the depths of the bulb and then pass caudally to gather at the posterolateral surface to form the lateral olfactory tract (LOT). Within the bulb the axons give off *recurrent collaterals*. According to the classical studies (Cajal, 1911), some collaterals recur to terminate in the EPL, and some remain in the deep granule layer. However, studies of cells visualized by intracellular (Kishi et al., 1984) or extracellular (Orona et al., 1984) injections of HRP show that the collaterals remain within the granule layer (GRL) and internal plexiform layer (IPL) (Kishi et al., 1984; Orona et al., 1984). Age or species differences may account for some of this discrepancy. The collaterals distribute diffusely within the deep layers.

The output axons in the LOT give off numerous collateral branches, which terminate in the olfactory cortex, as described in Chap. 10. The distances traveled are relatively short, up to 10–15 mm. This is similar to the projection distances of some other principal neurons, such as cerebellar Purkinje cells or dentate granule cells, but contrasts with the extremely long axons of motoneurons and cortical pyramidal cells.

Tufted Cells. Output cells similar to mitral cells but located more superficially in the EPL are called *tufted cells* (Fig. 5.2B). The subgroups and their nomenclature have become rather complex, but for present purposes we can identify three main groups according to their laminar position. The main population, *middle tufted cells* (T_m), lies near the middle of the EPL. These have a cell body diameter of 15–20 μm, several thin basal dendrites (300–600 μm), and a primary dendrite (200–300 μm) ending in a relatively confined tuft of branches in a glomerulus. The axons gives off collaterals that are mostly confined within the IPL and then joins the LOT. Its projection sites in olfactory cortex differ from those of mitral cells (see Chap. 10).

There are also several varieties of *external tufted cells* (T_e), whose dendrites have distinctive branching patterns (see contrasting examples in Fig. 5.2B). All of these give

off collaterals in the IPL or adjacent GRL, where they constitute a topographically ordered intrabulbar association system (Schoenfeld et al., 1985). Some send an axon into
the LOT, whereas others do not and thus should be classified as intrinsic neurons (see
below). Finally, some *internal tufted cells* (T$_i$) overlap in distribution and morphology
with outwardly displaced type II mitral cells.

Traditionally, tufted cells were considered to be smaller versions of mitral cells (Allison, 1953). However, Cajal (1911) noted that their axon collateral patterns are different, and it was suggested that this could provide for distinctive types of modulation
of granule cells (Shepherd, 1972a). Subsequent research has established that the two
types differ genetically (Greer and Shepherd, 1982); in the mouse mutant *pcd* (i.e.,
Purkinje cell degeneration), there is selective degeneration of mitral cells without affecting the tufted cells. The careful studies of Macrides et al. (1985), Orona et al.
(1984), and Mori (1987) have documented the detailed morphology of the different
subtypes of mitral and tufted cells. Transmitter differences will be noted below. It thus
appears that, as in many other regions of the brain, the principal neurons are differentiated into multiple subgroups, on the basis of genetics, position, dendritic morphology, intrabulbar axonal connections, extrabulbar projection sites, and neurotransmitters and modulators.

INTRINSIC NEURONS

There are two main types of intrinsic neuron in the olfactory bulb: periglomerular cells
(PG) and granule cells (GC) (see Fig. 5.2C).

Periglomerular Cells. Surrounding the glomeruli are the cell bodies of PG cells. The cell
body is only 6–8 μm in diameter, among the smallest of neurons in the brain. As shown
by Cajal (1911) and confirmed by modern studies (see Pinching and Powell, 1971a,b;
Schneider and Macrides, 1978), each PG cell has a short bushy dendrite that arborizes
to an extent of 50–100 μm within a glomerulus; bitufted PG cells, to two glomeruli,
are infrequently seen. The dendritic branches intermingle with the terminals of olfactory axons and the branches of mitral and tufted cells. The PG axon distributes laterally within extraglomerular regions, extending as far as 5 glomeruli away (Pinching
and Powell, 1971a,b). Because the axon remains within the olfactory bulb, the PG cell
falls within the category of *short-axon cell.* Morphologically, the PG cells appear to
be a homogeneous population, but biochemical subtypes containing different transmitters have been identified (see below).

Whereas mitral and tufted cells are differentiated prenatally, PG cells are generated
far into the postnatal period and perhaps the adult (Frazier-Cierpial and Brunjes, 1989;
Luskin, 1993; Ono et al., 1994; Rousselot et al., 1995; Lois et al., 1996). Interestingly,
this late migration appears to occur within a spatially defined tube, the rostral migratory stream, leading from the anterior horn of the lateral ventricle to the ependymal
core of the bulb. The tangential migration within the tube depends on the presence of
embryonic polysialic acid (PSA) nerve-cell adhesion molecules (N-CAM) and may include a unique mechanism of interaction between the migrating cells (Hu et al., 1996).
Within the bulb, the subsequent radial migration has not yet been elucidated, although
it is of interest to note that the distribution of radial glia in the bulb declines rapidly
during the early postnatal period (Chiu and Greer, 1996).

Granule Cells. Deep to the layer of mitral cell bodies is a thick layer containing the cell bodies of granule cells (GRL in Fig. 5.2). These cell bodies are also very small (6–8 μm in diameter); they appeared as grains (hence the term *granule*) to the early microscopists, who applied this term to many types of small cells in the brain. The cell bodies are grouped in clusters in the granule layer.

Each granule cell gives rise to a superficial process which extends radially toward the surface and ramifies and terminates in the EPL, the branching field extending laterally some 50–200 μm. There is also a deep process which branches sparingly in the granule layer. It was early noted that granule cells located at different depths would have different functional roles to play in intrabulbar circuits (Shepherd, 1972a). This notion has been greatly amplified by recent studies. Both intra- and extracellular HRP injections have shown that there are three main cell types in rodents (see Fig. 5.2C). *Superficial* granule cells (Orona et al., 1983; type G_{III} of Mori et al., 1983) have peripheral dendrites that ramify mainly in the superficial EPL, among the dendrites of tufted cells. *Deep* granule cells (G_{II}) send their dendrites mainly to the deep EPL, among the dendrites of mitral cells. *Intermediate* granule cells (G_I) have dendrites that ramify at all levels of the EPL. It thus appears that mitral and tufted cells have both segregated and overlapping microcircuits through granule cells, as discussed below (see also Macrides et al., 1985). Other subtypes of granule cells have been reported on the basis of light and dark staining of the cell bodies by toluidine blue (Struble and Walters, 1982), and localization of neuropeptides (see below).

Granule cells, like PG cells, continue to be generated late into the postnatal period, arriving in the bulb via tangential migration within the rostral migratory stream (Kishi, 1987). The continuing genesis and migration of these neurons suggests that remodeling occurs continually within the local synaptic circuits of the bulb, parallel to the remodeling of sensory neuron synapses within the glomeruli.

The granule cell dendrites are notable for bearing numerous spines (also called *gemmules*). In general, the spines are larger but less numerous than spines of dendrites of pyramidal cells in the cerebral cortex. In a developmental study, Greer (1984) found that the density of spines increased from 1 per 10 μm of dendritic branch length at birth to a peak of 2–3 at 12 days, settling to an adult value of approximately 2. This is much lower than the spine densities of striatal cells (see Chap. 9), and of pyramidal neurons in the hippocampus (Chap. 11) and neocortex (Chap. 12).

The most notable feature of the granule cell is that it lacks an axon. This was evident in the first studies by Golgi (1886), and has been repeatedly confirmed by use of Golgi methods, HRP, and electron microscopy. The resemblance to amacrine cells in the retina was early recognized. Electron microscopic studies have clearly shown that the granule cell processes are dendrites on the basis of their fine structural features and their close resemblance to cortical dendrites (Price and Powell, 1970a,b). The lack of an axon meant that these cells always stood out as exceptions to the classical "law of dynamic polarization" (Cajal, 1911). This problem was solved by the discovery of the output functions of the dendritic spines of these cells (see Chap. 1 and below).

It remains to note that a third type of intrinsic neuron, *short-axon cell*, is represented sparingly in the glomerular layer and more frequently in the granule layer. The latter consist of several subtypes (Pinching and Powell, 1971a,b; Schneider and Macrides,

1978), with dendritic trees of variable extent, and axons that ramify in the EPL or granule layer (see Fig. 5.2C).

CELL POPULATIONS

Olfactory sensory neurons in one side of the nose number approximately 50×10^6 in the rabbit, giving rise to as many axons entering each olfactory bulb. This is a relatively large array of sensory input channels, exceeded only by the photoreceptors in the retina (Chap. 6). This array converges onto approximately 2,000 glomeruli, to which are connected approximately 50,000 mitral cells and 100,000 tufted cells (see Allison, 1953). Thus, the convergence ratios are very high: onto glomeruli, 25,000:1; onto mitral cells, 1,000:1; and onto tufted cells, 500:1. The data remain incomplete for most species but it appears that many have fewer numbers of receptor cells and therefore somewhat less convergence onto glomeruli. For example, in the rat the number of olfactory receptor neurons has been estimated at 20×10^6 while the number of glomeruli is estimated at about 1,700 (J. Schwob, personal communication). This yields a convergence ratio of about 12,000 axons:glomerulus, or half of that previously estimated in the rabbit. Although more complete data are necessary, it is still evident that the convergence of receptor cell axons onto glomeruli and projection neurons is very high.

The ratios of intrinsic neurons to principal neurons are also high. Some order-of-magnitude estimates for these ratios are: PG to mitral, 20:1; granule to mitral, 50–100:1; short-axon to mitral, 1:1 (Shepherd, 1972a). Better data are needed for different species. However, even these rough estimates suggest an extensive array of intrinsic circuits for information-processing in the bulb.

SYNAPTIC CONNECTIONS

The distinct laminae and cell types of the olfactory bulb have greatly simplified the electron microscopic analysis of synaptic connections. In many cases, identification of processes has been further confirmed by serial reconstructions. Because of these advantages, the olfactory bulb was among the first brain regions in which identification of the main patterns of synaptic connection was on a secure basis. These patterns are found in the four main layers of synaptic neuropil in the bulb, which we will describe in sequence.

GLOMERULAR LAYER

Intraglomerular Connections. As noted above, all sensory neuron axons terminate in the glomeruli. This means that, by definition, a glomerulus defines a subset of the olfactory neuron population that projects exclusively to it. Early anatomical studies suggested that a subset does not ramify randomly throughout a glomerulus, but rather, there are intraglomerular compartments of axonal projections (Land et al., 1970; Land and Shepherd, 1974). This is supported by recent studies using molecular markers (Treloar et al. (1996). Using an olfactory marker protein (OMP)-driven LacZ reporter that marked subsets of receptors, they found some glomeruli that were only partially labeled, suggesting that the input to some glomeruli may be heterogeneous. Similar observations have been made using DiI staining of subsets of axons (Dembner and Greer, 1994).

Within the glomeruli the olfactory sensory terminals make axodendritic synapses onto the dendritic tufts of both the relay neurons (mitral and tufted cells) and the intrinsic neurons (PG cells) (Pinching and Powell, 1971a,b). As shown in Fig. 5.3A, the axon terminals are relatively large, especially compared with the thin axons from which they arise. The terminals are filled with small round vesicles. The contacts are type 1 chemical synapses. In at least one strain of mouse (BALB/c), the sensory connection onto the PG cell dendrites is absent. This finding has been documented by White (1972), using serial reconstructions. This strain may lack a PG cell subpopulation that receives the olfactory input, or a receptor cell subpopulation that normally terminates on the PG cells. An interesting question is whether this genetic difference in synaptic connectivity is associated with specific behaviors expressed by this strain.

The dendrites within the glomerulus not only receive the sensory input but are themselves presynaptic in position. The most common pattern is dendrodendritic contacts from mitral/tufted cells to PG cells; these are type 1 synapses. The presynaptic dendrites contain only a few synaptic vesicles at the synaptic sites, in contrast to the sensory axon terminals (see above). Another common pattern is dendrodendritic contacts in the opposite direction, from PG cells to mitral/tufted cells; these are type 2 synapses. As indicated in Fig. 5.3, the two types of synapse may be arranged in reciprocal, side-by-side pairs (approximately 25% of the total), or in more widely spaced serial sequences. The type 2 dendrite may in turn receive a type 2 synapse from another, presumably also PG, dendrite. No dendrite has been observed to be presynaptic to an axon terminal (in contrast to dorsal horn [Gobel et al., 1980] and retina [Dowling and Boycott, 1966]). Patterns of connections form complex microcircuits involving groups of axons and dendrites, sometimes set apart by an incomplete glial wrapping (see below). Finally, there are terminals of certain types of centrifugal fibers.

Interglomerular Connections. In addition to the PG cell bodies there is an extraglomerular neuropil between the glomeruli. Several types of synaptic connections occur here (Pinching and Powell, 1971a,b). First, the axons of PG cells make type 2 synapses onto the somata and dendrites of other PG cells, and onto the primary dendrites of mitral and tufted cells as they emerge from the glomeruli. Second, there are type 1 synapses

Fig. 5.3. Synaptic connections in the mammalian olfactory bulb. **A:** Axodendritic and dendrodendritic connections in the olfactory glomerulus. ON, olfactory nerve; Md, mitral dendrite; PGd, periglomerular cell dendrite; PGa, periglomerular cell axon. Note the serial and reciprocal synaptic sequences. **B** (Top): Dendrodendritic connections in the external plexiform layer between a mitral secondary dendrite (Md) and a granule cell dendritic spine (Grs); note also the centrifugal axodendritic connection onto the spine. Grd, granule dendrite. Bottom: Axodendritic connections in the granule layer. **C:** Electron micrograph of a dendrite (M) and a granule cell spine (S) in the mouse. Note that M → S synapse has round presynaptic vesicles and thick postsynaptic densities, indicative of type 1, whereas S → M synapse has flattened presynaptic vesicles and more symmetrical membrane densities, indicative of type 2. **D:** Computer reconstruction of serial EM sections through a granule spine, showing long, thin neck and larger head which bears a reciprocal synapse (asterisk). [A after Andres, 1965; Reese and Brightman, 1970; Pinching and Powell, 1971a,b; White, 1972; B after Rall et al., 1966; Price and Powell, 1970a; C,D from Greer et al., 1989, with permission.]

A. Glomerular Layer

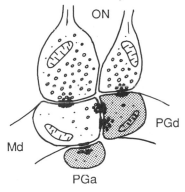

ON

Md

PGd

PGa

B. Granule Layer

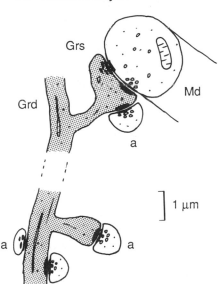

Grs

Grd

Md

a

a

a

] 1 μm

C. Reciprocal Synapse

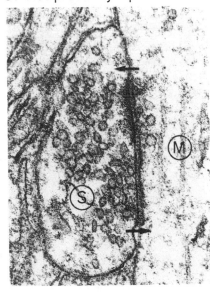

M

S

D. Granule Spine

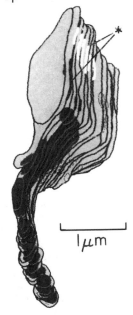

*

|1μm

from tufted cell axon collaterals onto tufted cell dendrites. Third, there are synaptic terminals of various types of centrifugal fibers.

EXTERNAL PLEXIFORM LAYER

In the EPL, the dominant type of synaptic connection is a pair of reciprocal contacts (Hirata, 1964; Andres, 1965; Rall et al., 1966). Serial reconstructions (Rall et al., 1966) established that these contacts occur, as indicated in Fig. 5.3B, between the secondary dendrite (Md) of a mitral/tufted cell and the spine (gemmule) of a granule cell dendrite (Grs). These were the first dendrodendritic synapses identified in the nervous system. An electron micrograph (EM) of a typical reciprocal synapse is shown in Fig. 5.3C. A recent reconstruction of a granule cell spine, bearing reciprocal synapses as indicated by (*), is shown in Fig. 5.3D. In the reciprocal pair, the mitral-to-granule synapse is type 1, whereas the granule-to-mitral synapse is type 2 (Price and Powell, 1970b). Over 80% of all synapses in the EPL are involved in such reciprocal pairs. Electron micrographs show the EPL to be a neuropil composed almost entirely of mitral/tufted and granule cell dendrites and their synaptic interconnections (see Reese and Shepherd, 1972). If we consider that there are up to 100 granule cells for each mitral cell, and that each granule cell has 50–100 spines in the EPL (Greer, 1987; Mori, 1987), it is obvious that these dendrodendritic microcircuits provide for extremely powerful and specific interactions with the mitral cells. Because the basal dendritic fields of most mitral and tufted cells occupy separate zones in the EPL, their microcircuits through granule dendrites are correspondingly separated.

In single EM sections the granule-to-mitral/tufted synapse sometimes appears indistinct or missing. Ramón-Moliner (1977) suggested that the inhibitory action of granule cells might therefore be mediated by a nonsynaptic mechanism. However, Lieberman and colleagues carefully reinvestigated the question (Jackowski et al., 1978) using several EM techniques, and confirmed that the granule-to-mitral synapses are approximately equal partners in the reciprocal pairs, as originally described. This of course does not rule out the possibility of additional nonsynaptic interactions between the cells.

In addition to synapses made by dendrites, the EPL also contains axon terminals from several sources: intrinsic short-axon cells, and centrifugal fibers (as noted above, recurrent mitral collaterals, thought by Cajal to terminate in the EPL, are now believed to be restricted to the IPL). These axon terminals make type 1 synapses predominantly on the presynaptic granule spines (Price and Powell, 1970b); no contacts have been seen on mitral dendrites.

Development and Plasticity. How is the dendrodendritic microcircuit assembled during development? The mechanism in fact appears to be relatively simple. According to Hinds (1970), the mitral- (or tufted)-to-granule synapse appears first, at about E17 in the mouse, followed a day later by the granule-to-mitral (or tufted) synapse. Whether each neuron has its own genetic timetable of synapse expression, or the earlier mitral synapse induces the granule synapse, requires further study. The later expression of granule synapses is consistent with the general rule that intrinsic neurons develop later than projection neurons (Jacobson, 1978). In the retina, more complex microcircuits also appear to be assembled according to a similar genetic algorithm consisting of sequential expression of individual synaptic types (Nishimura and Rakic, 1987).

Recent studies have revealed a great deal of plasticity in these microcircuits. In the mutant mouse strain *pcd*, the specific degeneration of mitral, but not tufted, cells occurs at about 3 months of age (Greer and Shepherd, 1982). The number of reciprocal synapses between granule spines and tufted cell dendrites increases in compensation, suggesting that many denervated granule-to-mitral spines survive and establish new efferent and afferent synapses with tufted-cell dendrites (Greer and Halasz, 1987). By contrast, olfactory deprivation causes a reduction in incidence of dendrodendritic synapses, which is more severe in the granule-to-mitral contacts (Benson et al., 1984). It has been suggested that "the reciprocal pair of synapses exists in a dynamic equilibrium in which each sustains the other through trophic or feedback mechanisms" (Shepherd and Greer, 1988).

Odor deprivation has been effectively used to demonstrate the role of afferent input during bulb development (Brunjes, 1994). Unilateral deprivation leads to down-regulation of global metabolic indices such as 2-deoxyglucose as well as a loss of dopamine in subsets of periglomerular cells (Baker et al., 1983). Deprivation also causes changes in the membrane properties of mitral and tufted cells through a down-regulation of Na^+ channel subunits (Sashihara et al., 1996). By contrast, pairing of specific odors with arousal during early development may lead to structural changes within the bulb, including the appearance of supernumerary glomeruli (Woo et al., 1987). Odor deprivation also causes a reduction in the incidence of dendrodendritic synapses, which is most severe in the granule-to-mitral contacts (Benson et al., 1984). This is consistent with the suggestion of Hinds (1970) that the mitral-to-granule contacts form first, followed by the granule-to-mitral contacts.

GRANULE LAYER

In the granule layer, axon terminals are found on the shafts and spines of the granule-cell dendrites (see Fig. 5.3B). The studies of Price and Powell (1970b) showed that these axon terminals derive from both intrinsic and extrinsic (central) inputs. The *intrinsic* sources include the axon collaterals of mitral and tufted cells, and the axons of the deep short-axon cells. There is evidence that the synapses of these terminals are types 1 and 2, respectively. The *extrinsic* sources make connections at different levels of the granule dendritic tree (see Fig. 5.2A). The anterior commissure (AC) distributes mainly to the deep processes. The AON distributes over the middle part of the dendrites, including the spines in the EPL. The HDB axons distribute mainly to the spines in the EPL; some terminals are also found at the borders of the glomeruli. The synapses made by these inputs from the brain appear to be type 1.

It should be noted that all of the synaptic connections in which the granule cell takes part are oriented toward the granule cell, with the sole exception of the dendrodendritic synapses from the granule spines onto the mitral dendrites in the EPL. The latter are therefore the only output avenue from the granule cells.

Gap junctions are also found between adjacent perikarya in the granule cell layer (Reyher et al., 1991; Paternostro et al., 1995). Freeze-fracture replicas show particle aggregates in the perikaryon membrane, while immunocytochemical analyses revealed punctate staining for gap-junction protein. Lucifer yellow injections into single granule cells result in the staining of small subsets of adjacent cells. These findings suggest that granule cells may be organized into syncytial subsets (Paternostro et al., 1995).

GLIA

As noted above, olfactory receptor axons are organized into bundles of 100–200 axons surrounded by the ensheathing glia cell of the olfactory nerve (Valverde and Lopez-Mascaraque, 1991; Doucette, 1993; Ramon-Cueto and Valverde, 1995). These specialized glia have several interesting properties, including the expression of CNS glial fibrillary acidic protein (GFAP), which distinguishes them from the PNS Schwann cell (Barber and Lindsay, 1982). In addition, ensheathing cells express laminin throughout life, as well as the low-affinity nerve growth factor receptor, both of which may be associated with the continued turnover of the olfactory receptor-cell axons (Leisi, 1985; Turner and Perez-Polo, 1993; Kafitz and Greer, 1997). At the juncture of the olfactory nerve layer and the glomerulus the glial phenotype changes abruptly (Gonzalez et al., 1993). Conventional CNS astrocytes surround the glomerulus, and intraglomerular synaptic complexes (i.e., Fig. 5.3A) are often surrounded by one or more loose folds of glial membrane. This is similar to, though not nearly as distinct as, the synaptic glomeruli of the cerebellum and thalamus (Pinching and Powell, 1971a,b). Glial folds are also sometimes seen around the reciprocal dendrodendritic synapses in the EPL. This appears to be generally consistent with the role of glial in isolating synaptic complexes elsewhere in the CNS.

Within the EPL, in most vertebrate species, several loose folds of glial membrane surround the primary dendrites of mitral and tufted cells near the glomerular boundary. In mice and primates, typical myelin has been found at this site, which may surround not only the primary dendrite but even extend to the cell body in the case of tufted cells (Pinching, 1971; Burd, 1980). This shows that a dendrite may be myelinated and that myelin is not exclusively associated with axons. The function of the myelin may be associated with generation of fast prepotentials and impulses in the primary dendrite (Mori et al, 1983; Shen et al, 1997; see below).

BASIC CIRCUIT

The synaptic organization of the olfactory bulb is summarized in the basic circuit diagram of Fig. 5.4. The output cells (mitral and tufted cells) receive the sensory input in their glomerular tufts and give rise to the bulbar output from their cell bodies. The two main functions, *input processing* and *output control*, that characterize all local regions of the brain (Chap. 1) are therefore separated into two distinct levels in relation to the output cells. We will summarize the organization at these two levels.

INPUT PROCESSING

Intraglomerular Microcircuits. The olfactory glomeruli are the most characteristic feature of the olfactory bulb in all vertebrates. Within the glomeruli, the basic elements of the synaptic triad (see Chap. 1) come together: input (olfactory-axon terminals), output (mitral/tufted-cell dendrites), and intrinsic (PG-cell dendrites). As discussed in Chap. 1, the synapses between the input and principal elements provide the necessary basis for input–output transmission, whereas synapses between the principal and intrinsic elements provide for elaboration and control of the input–output transfer.

The synaptic triad in the glomerulus involves input synapses onto both the principal and (in most species) the intrinsic elements. This is a common pattern in the brain;

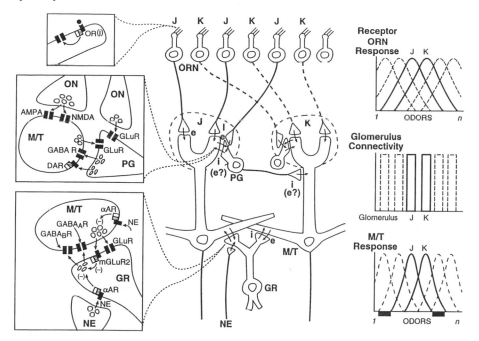

Fig. 5.4. Basic circuit of the mammalian olfactory bulb. Abbreviations (left, molecular components): OR, olfactory receptor; ON, olfactory nerve; AMPA, 2-amino-5-phosphonovaleric acid;
NMDA, N-methyl-D-aspartate; M/T, mitral/tufted cell; PG, periglomerular cell; GluR, ionotropic
glutamate receptor; GABA R, GABA receptor; DAR, dopamine receptor; NE, norepinephrine;
αAR, α adrenoreceptor; mGluR2, metabotropic glutamate receptor; GR, granule cell. Middle
(synaptic circuit): ORN, olfactory receptor neuron; J,K, ORN subsets; e, excitatory; i, inhibitory.
Right (structure–function relations) top: overlapping response spectra of ORNs to a range of
odors (1–n); middle: connectivity of subsets to individual glomeruli; bottom: response spectra
of M/T cells show less overlap because of lateral inhibition (black bars below abscissa).

the same type of arrangement is found, for example, in the retina, cerebellum, and thalamus (Shepherd, 1979). In the latter regions, the synapses onto the principal and intrinsic elements arise from a single large input terminal, whereas in the olfactory
glomeruli, the synapses are made by separate terminals (see Chaps. 1, 6–8). The
arrangement of separate terminals appears to permit considerable combinatorial complexity in processing odor information. Do the separate terminals arise from separate
olfactory axons; if so, do some olfactory sensory cells project only to the principal neuron, others only to the intrinsic neuron? These questions are under investigation.

After the initial input to the principal and intrinsic elements, further processing takes
place within the glomerulus through the dendrodendritic microcircuits. There is increasing evidence that a glomerulus may act to some extent as a functional unit. This
has been long suspected on anatomical grounds (see Clark, 1957). Tract-tracing studies gave the first clear evidence of this (Land et al., 1970), and further indicated that
there may be several levels of organization within a single olfactory glomerulus (Land
and Shepherd, 1974). There is physiological evidence for glomerular specificity for

different olfactory stimuli (Leveteau and MacLeod, 1966). The strongest evidence thus far has come from activity mapping with the 2-deoxyglucose (2DG) technique, which revealed individual glomeruli as well as groups of glomeruli responsive to a given odor (Sharp et al., 1977; see further below). High-resolution 2DG methods show a relatively homogeneous distribution of activity throughout a glomerulus during odor stimulation (Benson et al., 1985). Monoclonal antibody staining for several cell-surface glycoproteins shows sharply defined glomerular borders (reviewed in Schwob, 1992; Mori and Yoshihara, 1995). Finally, as noted above, olfactory receptor-cell axons containing the mRNA for a putative odor-ligand receptor converge and terminate in 1 to 3 glomeruli (Vassar et al., 1994; Ressler et al., 1994; Mombaerts et al., 1996).

If glomeruli have this functional specificity, then the group of mitral, tufted, and PG cells with dendrites connected to a particular glomerulus will all share this specificity. There is growing evidence to support this suggestion (Wilson and Leon, 1987a; Buonviso and Chaput, 1990; Mori et al., 1992; Mori and Yoshihara, 1995). Mitral cells near each other and innervating the same glomerulus tend to have much more similar responses to odor stimuli than mitral cells that are distant from each other. Radial arrays of active glomeruli and deeper cells have in fact been visualized, using both 2DG (Stewart et al., 1979) and voltage-sensitive dyes (Kauer and Cinelli, 1993). This implies a horizontal constraint on the organization of functionally related neurons in the bulb, which may be analogous to the functional columns of the cerebral cortex (Shepherd, 1972a).

Interglomerular Microcircuits. Activity in one glomerulus can affect other glomeruli through interglomerular connections. The main route is PG-cell axons, which through their terminals can affect the transmission of information out of neighboring glomeruli (see Fig. 5.4). There is evidence that these interglomerular actions may be excitatory (Shepherd, 1963; Freeman, 1974) or inhibitory (Getchell and Shepherd, 1975a,b). If glomeruli function as units, then one function of the interglomerular microcircuits could be to enhance the contrast between glomeruli of different specificities, which parallels intercolumnar interactions in the neocortex (see Chap. 12). Conversely, the connections might function to recruit neighboring glomeruli as the concentration of an odor increases. It is a measure of our ignorance that we cannot yet distinguish experimentally between these alternatives.

OUTPUT CONTROL

The connection between the levels of input processing in the glomeruli and output control from the mitral and tufted cell bodies is made by the primary dendrites of the mitral and tufted cells. Thus, in species such as most mammals in which there are single primary dendrites, a glomerulus defines a translaminar glomerular unit formed of all the mitral and tufted (and PG) cells connected to it. This anatomical unit has also been shown to be a functional unit in the processing of odor stimuli. This was first seen in 2DG studies as translaminar densities (cf. Stewart et al, 1979); it has also been seen in in situ hybridization for early immediate genes (Sallaz and Jourdan, 1993; Guthrie et al., 1993), and in salamanders, using voltage-sensitive dyes (VSDs) (cf. Kauer and Cinelli, 1993; Cinelli and Kauer, 1994). An example in which VSDs are used is shown in Fig. 5.5. One may refer to these as *odor columns*, in analogy with ocular dominance

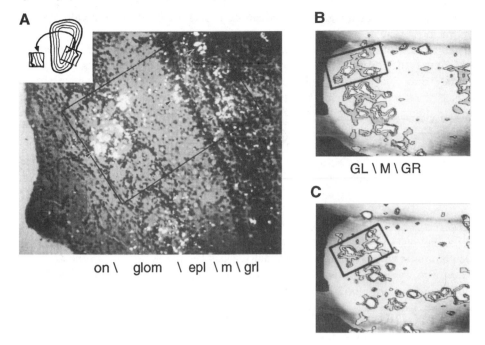

Fig. 5.5. Columnar arrangement of functional glomerular units. **A:** Dark-field view of 2-deoxyglucose (2DG) autoradiography in the olfactory bulb of a rat exposed to odor, showing localization over a glomerulus and small clusters of periglomerular, mitral, and granule cell bodies (arrowheads). Inset shows site of histological section. Olfactory bulb layers indicated at bottom. **B:** Functional glomerular units in the salamander olfactory bulb revealed by voltage sensitive dye fluorescence, in response to stimulation with amyl acetate. **C:** The same animal, after simulation with ethyl-n-butyrate, which activates a glomerular unit that is shifted by overlaps with the unit in B. Olfactory bulb layers indicated at bottom. [From Kaucr and Cinelli, 1993, with permission.]

columns and orientation columns in the visual cortex (see Chap. 12). These columns thus define the units that are the basis for control of the output from the olfactory bulb.

At the level of output control, the main type of microcircuit is the reciprocal dendrodendritic synapse between mitral/tufted cells and granule cells. At this level, the mitral/tufted primary dendrite functions as the afferent element of the synaptic triad, conveying the input directly to the soma and secondary dendrites, which function as the principal neuron component. The triad is completed by the intrinsic element, the granule cell spine.

As we shall soon see, there is strong evidence that in the reciprocal synaptic microcircuit, the mitral-to-granule synapse is excitatory and the granule-to-mitral synapse is inhibitory. Because the granule-to-mitral/tufted synapse is the sole output of the granule cell, the inhibition it delivers is very powerful, and it is the main means for mediating control of output from the olfactory bulb. Although the reciprocal synaptic microcircuit seems to be a simple and inflexible arrangement, in fact it can generate several types of functions. The most obvious functions are self- and lateral inhibition of the mitral/tufted cells, but this microcircuit is also involved in temporal patterning and memory storage, as will be discussed below.

The spatial constraints on these circuits controlling output obviously contrast with those involved in processing the input. As we have seen, input processing is organized according to glomerular modules, each presumably limited to processing a specific subset of sensory inputs. By contrast, output control is mediated through the long mitral/tufted secondary dendrites, whose fields are extensive and overlapping. A given output neuron is modulated according to a graded summation of effects from a wide range of other output cells, thus reflecting the context of information being processed in neighboring parallel channels. This modulation is important in determining not only the patterns of excitation and inhibition in space but also sequences of excitation and inhibition in time.

Parallel Output Pathways. The organization of the olfactory bulb contains several types of parallel pathways for processing olfactory input. The most obvious are the hundreds of glomerular units. Although traditionally it has been believed that in the vertebrate these ordinary glomeruli and their columns are all similar, anatomically identifiable glomeruli have begun to be recognized. The first and most clearly demarcated type is a *modified glomerular complex* (MGC) that forms a separate "labeled line" within the main olfactory bulb (Teicher et al, 1980; Greer et al, 1982). It is believed to mediate information concerning odor cues related to suckling in young animals (Pedersen et al., 1986). The possible analogy between this MGC and the macroglomerular complex involved in pheromone signaling in insects is intriguing (reviewed in Hildebrand and Shepherd, 1997). Allied with the MGC in vertebrates are *necklace glomeruli* at the border of the main olfactory bulb facing the accessory olfactory bulb (AOB) (Zheng and Jourdan, 1988). The accessory olfactory bulb will be discussed below.

In addition to these parallel pathways related to the glomeruli, there are also parallel pathways through the mitral and tufted cell populations (see Fig. 5.4). It is not known whether, at the level of input processing within the glomeruli, the dendritic tufts of the two types receive input from different receptor cell axons, or if they interact with common (as shown) or different PG cell dendrites. However, at the level of output control in the EPL, each type is dominated by different subpopulations of granule cells: superficial granule cells (G_S) control superficial and middle tufted cells (T_M), and deep granule cells (G_D) control mitral cells (M_1); granule cells forming a third subpopulation appear to interact with both tufted and mitral cells. These cell types can be identified in the drawings of Fig. 5.2.

When differing projection sites of mitral and tufted cells in olfactory cortical areas were first recognized, it was suggested by Skeen and Hall (1977) that there might be an analogy in this regard to the different classes of retinal ganglion cells. The differing morphologies of the dendritic trees of these cells further support that analogy (Macrides and Schneider, 1982). As noted by Orona et al. (1984), in the retina, the particular sublamina of dendritic ramification of a ganglion cell has been found to be the main morphological feature correlated with the physiological type of its response (see Chap. 6). The fact that both mitral and tufted cells are further divided into subclasses on the basis of dendritic morphology indicates that multiple parallel pathways exist; this may be important in the mediation of different types of information about molecular stimuli. A point of interest is that tufted cells are more readily excited by orthodromic stimulation than mitral cells. This may be a reflection of the size principle (Henneman et al., 1965), that small cells tend to be more excitable due to their higher input impedance. Other differences, such as in primary afferent input, local circuit connectivity, or intrinsic properties, could also be involved.

Accessory Olfactory Bulb. Odor information is processed via the AOB in parallel with the main olfactory system; the AOB appears to be receptive to both volatile and non-volatile ligands. The sensory neuron is found in a tube-like structure, the vomeronasal organ (VNO), located at the base of the nasal septum. Similar to the sensory neurons found in the main epithelium, the vomeronasal receptor cells express different mRNAs for putative odorant receptors (Dulac and Axel, 1995). The axons of the vomeronasal cells run in several distinct fascicles along the medial aspect of the main olfactory bulb toward its dorsal–caudal aspects where the AOB is located. The cytoarchitecture and synaptic organization of the AOB is similar to that of the main olfactory bulb although the laminar organization is less distinct. The receptor cell axons terminate in glomerular regions on the dendrites of the primary projection neuron, the mitral cells. Periglomerular cells are few in number and are also likely to receive direct afferent input. Intraglomerular circuits appear similar to those described for the main bulb. Modulation of mitral cell output occurs in the external plexiform layer where reciprocal dendrodendritic synapses are formed with granule cells. Despite these similarities, there are also differences. The glomeruli are small and fewer in number. Although the projection neurons are called mitral cells, they are generally smaller and more polymorphic than their counterparts in the main bulb. There are also differences in some neurotransmitters (see below).

The output of the AOB is exclusively to the medial anterior, medial posterior, and posterior cortical nuclei of the amygdala and to the bed nucleus of the stria terminalis From these regions multiple paths carry AOB information to the hypothalamus. The accessory pathway is believed to be involved in processing contact signals involved in mating in many mammals, as well as hormonally regulated odor-stimulated behaviors (see Keverne, 1995, for review). In fact, the AOB provides one of the clearest examples of a correlation between a synaptic circuit and a specific learned behavior in the nervous system (see below).

CENTRIFUGAL MODULATION

In addition to processing sensory information, the bulbar microcircuits are also involved in gating and modulating that information by the brain. A key site for this control is the dendritic spine of the granule cell. As can be seen in Fig. 5.4, a synaptic triad is formed by the centrifugal fiber terminal, the granule spine, and the mitral/tufted dendrite. Through this connection, the centrifugal fiber can exert direct and exquisite control over the function of the reciprocal microcircuit. The nature of that control will be discussed later.

From these considerations it appears that mitral and granule cell synapses are concerned both with olfactory processing and with integration of information passing forward from the brain through the granule cell. Some of the information from the brain may be in the form of feedback through long loops from the olfactory projection areas. Some of it, however, may be in the form of nonolfactory signals from hypothalamic and limbic structures. The granule-to-mitral synapse is therefore of interest as a specific site at which there is an overlap of functions. One may characterize it in this regard as a *multifunctional*, or *multiplex*, synapse. It is a good example of the spine as a multifunctional integrative unit (see Chap. 1).

A second level of centrifugal control occurs in the glomerular layer. Most of the centrifugal fibers that reach this layer have connections restricted to the interglomerular neuropil. However, the serotonergic fibers from the dorsal raphe enjoy a special privilege of being allowed to enter and ramify within the glomeruli. This presumably enables these fibers to modulate in a very specific way the initial processing of the olfactory input to the bulb.

SYNAPTIC ACTIONS

Synaptic circuits in the vertebrate olfactory bulb have been analyzed in several types of preparations. First were anaesthetized animals, particularly rabbit, rat, and salamander. The separation of input and output pathways, in the olfactory nerves and lateral olfactory tract, respectively, enabled these studies to identify the basic types of synaptic actions and synaptic circuits, as well as permit analysis of these circuits during odor stimulation. The next step was the introduction of isolated preparations. The first of these was the isolated olfactory bulb of the turtle, which enabled exhaustive studies to be carried out of synaptic excitation by olfactory axons and synaptic inhibition by the dendrodendritic synapses. Most recently, a mammalian slice preparation is being developed that provides for adequate preservation of the olfactory bulb microcircuits. Finally, cell cultures have been introduced as a means of analyzing the pharmacology of specific types of excitatory and inhibitory synapses.

GLOMERULAR SYNAPTIC ACTIONS

In the isolated turtle olfactory bulb, a single shock stimulus of the olfactory nerves gives rise to a series of potentials in the mitral cell. As shown in Fig. 5.6A(a), this consists of an initial excitatory–inhibitory sequence (E_1–I_1), followed by a second E_2–I_2 sequence. These potentials are graded in amplitude with stimulus strength, and represent synaptic potentials. E_1 and E_2 reflect the excitatory synaptic response in the glomerulus. I_1 and I_2 are associated with an increased conductance, have reversal potentials near resting potentials (Mori et al., 1981b), and thus appear to be inhibitory synaptic responses.

When sufficiently strong, E_1 gives rise to an action potential (Fig. 5.6A,b). The action potential at the cell body is generated by both Na^+ and Ca^{2+} currents (Mori et al., 1981a; Jahr and Nicoll, 1982a). As described in Chap. 2, voltage-gated Ca^{2+} influx is an important means of activating K^+ conductances involved in regulating impulse frequency. In the mitral cell, it has a further significance in view of the role of Ca^{2+} in controlling neurotransmitter release from the presynaptic soma and dendrites (cf. Chap. 1; see below).

In order to identify the components of this complex response that are due to glomerular synapses, we can make a comparison with the response to antidromic activation. A single shock stimulus to the lateral olfactory tract sets up an impulse volley that in-

A. Fast Orthodromic Response **B.** Fast Antidromic Response

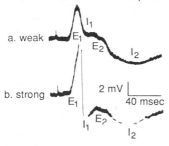 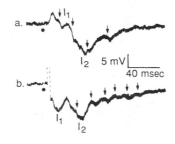

C. Slow Inhibitory Response

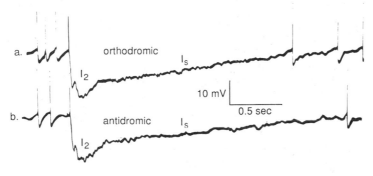

D. Slow Excitatory Response (Orthodromic)

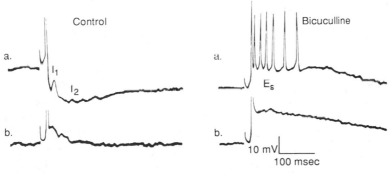

Fig. 5.6. The main types of synaptic actions in mitral cells. Intracellular recordings from the in vitro turtle olfactory bulb show responses to a single volley in the olfactory nerves (orthodromic activation) or lateral olfactory tract (LOT) (antidromic activation). **A:** The fast orthodromic response, just below (a) and above (b) threshold for impulse generation. The synaptic potentials consist of excitatory (E_1 and E_2) and inhibitory (I_1 and I_2) components. **B:** The fast antidromic response, similarly just below (a) and above (b) threshold for impulse generation in the LOT axon. Arrows indicate small, unitary hyperpolarizing potentials. **C:** The slow inhibitory response (I_S), elicited by orthodromic (a) and antidromic (b) stimulation. **D:** A slow excitatory response (E_S) to orthodromic input is revealed by adding bicuculline, a $GABA_A$ blocker, to the medium. The control shows the response at the normal resting potential (a) and during hyperpolarizing current injection (b), which reversed the I_1 and I_2 components and reduced but did not reverse I_S. The bicuculline traces show the hyperpolarizing current injection, which increased the amplitude of E_S. [A,B from Mori et al., 1981b; C from Mori et al., 1981c; D from Nowycky et al., 1981b, with permission.]

vades the mitral cells antidromically. Responses just below and just above threshold for the axon of the cell from which one is recording are shown in Fig. 5.6B. This antidromic response lacks the excitatory synaptic potentials E_1 and E_2, but shows a sequence of inhibitory synaptic potentials I_1 and I_2 that are similar to those in the orthodromic response. This is to be expected if these inhibitory potentials are generated in the secondary dendrites of the mitral cells by the actions of granule cells (see below). In favorable recordings, small hyperpolarizing potentials are seen (arrows in Fig. 5.6B), which may represent unitary inhibitory potentials.

Following these early synaptic events, there is a long-lasting hyperpolarization, referred to as I_S. As shown in Fig. 5.6C, it is elicited by both antidromic and orthodromic stimulation. It may last up to 10 sec or more, and the effects of the inhibition may be seen for up to 1 min. The later part of this potential is not associated with an increased membrane conductance, and a reversal potential cannot be obtained (Mori et al., 1981c). This potential appears also to be generated in mitral-cell secondary dendrites by granule cells, though by a separate transmitter mechanism (see Transmitters, below).

Further analysis of the glomerular components of the orthodromic synaptic responses has had to rely on soma recordings, because intracellular recordings from the glomerular tuft have not yet been possible. When inhibitory potentials are blocked by either bicuculline or low Cl^-, a prolonged EPSP (E_s) is revealed (Fig. 5.6D). This response is not seen when the cell is activated antidromically, and has therefore been ascribed to a large EPSP generated in the glomerular tuft of the mitral cell. When unopposed by inhibition, this EPSP renders the mitral cell hyperexcitable so that it responds with a burst of impulses (Fig. 5.6D,a). This is similar to findings in many other regions, and demonstrates how important inhibition is in controlling and shaping the responses of a neuron.

Studies of this kind have suggested several types of synaptic actions within the glomeruli. These include (*1*) the large EPSP (E_s) set up by the olfactory nerve synapses onto mitral/tufted cells; (*2*) prolongation of the excitatory response, possibly by autoreceptors; (*3*) inhibition of the glomerular tuft, by serial and reciprocal microcircuits through synapses from inhibitory PG cell dendrites; and (*4*) additional prolongation of the excitatory response, possibly by intrinsic axon terminals on mitral/tufted dendrites. It can be seen that all of these actions are correlated with the synaptic connections identified in anatomical studies (see above). They remain to be verified by combined anatomical and physiological studies in the same animal. The neurotransmitters at these synapses are discussed below.

An important general point is the wealth of synaptic integration, involving both excitation and inhibition, that takes place in the most distal part of the mitral/tufted dendritic tree. This is the level of input processing as defined earlier. There is currently great interest in the functions of distal dendrites in cells such as pyramidal neurons in the cortex (see Chaps. 10–12). The olfactory bulb provides one of the clearest examples in the nervous system that inhibition is important in distal dendrites as well as at the cell body, and that a significant amount of synaptic integration and sensory processing occurs locally in distal dendritic branches before transmission to the site of impulse output in the cell body. The role of active properties in dendritic function is considered in Chap. 1 and further below.

DENDRODENDRITIC INHIBITION BY GRANULE CELLS

We turn next to consider synaptic actions at the level of the cell body and secondary dendrites of mitral/tufted cells—that is, at the level of output control. The predominant property is inhibition, mediated by the reciprocal synapses between mitral/tufted and granule cells.

The evidence for the reciprocal microcircuit and its physiological actions came in several steps. First, intracellular and extracellular unit recordings showed that antidromic invasion of mitral cells is followed by long-lasting inhibition (Phillips et al., 1963). Recordings from granule cells suggested that the inhibition could be mediated by the granule cell dendrites operating in an output mode (Shepherd, 1963). A computational model was then constructed of the intracellular potentials and the associated extracellular field potentials in order to identify precisely the timing and placement of the synaptic actions (Rall et al., 1966; Rall and Shepherd, 1968). This indicated that the backward spreading impulse in the mitral secondary dendrites is appropriately timed and placed to make these dendrites the presynaptic elements for synaptic excitation of the granule cell spines. The EPSP in the granule cell spines in turn is appropriately timed and placed to mediate the long-lasting inhibition of the mitral cells. The final step was an electron microscopic study, using serial reconstructions, which showed that the mitral secondary dendrites and granule spines are interconnected by reciprocal synapses appropriately located and oriented for mediating the interactions predicted by the model (Rall et al., 1966). The excitatory mitral-to-granule synapse was shown to be type 1 and the inhibitory granule-to-mitral synapse, type 2 by Price and Powell (1970b) (see Fig. 5.3 above).

The functioning of the reciprocal synapses as a microcircuit module was previously described in Chap. 1, and is illustrated in greater detail in Fig. 5.7. In A (diagram 1), depolarization (D) of the mitral cell dendrite, by spread of an antidromic or orthodromic impulse from the cell body, activates the excitatory (E) synapse onto the granule spine (shaded area). The EPSP in the spine activates the inhibitory (I) synapse back onto the mitral dendrite (diagram 2). This causes a hyperpolarizing (H) IPSP in the mitral dendrite (diagram 3), which suppresses the excitability of the mitral cell until the inhibitory action has worn off. The long-lasting nature of this inhibitory action, in the absence of impulse activity in the interneuron, was early recognized (Phillips et al., 1963; Rall and Shepherd, 1968).

The generation of the impulse at the soma-axon hillock, with backspread into the dendrites during both orthodromic and antidromic activation, was in accord with the classical model of the functional organization of the neuron. Both actively and passively spreading impulses were tested and found to be adequate for extensively invading the mitral secondary dendrites (Rall and Shepherd, 1968). Since most of the reciprocal synapses are located on the secondary dendrites, it was concluded that they can be activated by the spread of either antidromic or orthodromic impulses from the cell body, as shown in Fig. 5.7. The mitral cell thus provided examples of specific functions (feedback and lateral inhibition) mediated by a backpropagating or backspreading impulse (cf. Chap. 1 and below). As we describe below, these functions in turn underlie several specific operations in the processing of sensory input, including the tuning of response spectra, oscillatory behavior, and memory storage.

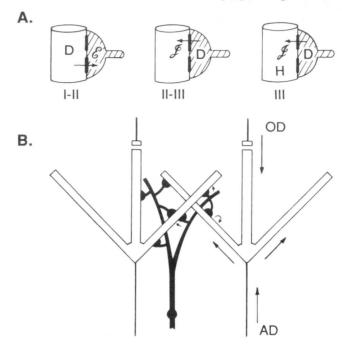

Fig. 5.7. **A:** Postulated mechanisms of action of the dendrodendritic synaptic pathway between mitral (open) and granule (shaded) cells, during successive time periods I, II, and III following an antidromic volley. D, depolarization; H, hyperpolarization; *E*, excitation; *I*, inhibition. **B:** Diagram of the pathways for self- and lateral-inhibition through dendrodendritic connections. OD, orthodromic (normal) activation; AD, antidromic activation. [From Rall and Shepherd, 1968, with permission.]

Physiological Testing of the Model. The isolated turtle brain preparation, with its preservation of intrinsic circuits, has permitted direct physiological testing of the model. Jahr and Nicoll (1982a) carried out a particularly elegant experiment to verify the presynaptic role of mitral cell dendrites. As shown in Fig. 5.8A, in a normal mitral cell, injected depolarizing current elicited a fast spike (Fig. 8A, top), which was followed by a slow IPSP (Fig. 8A, bottom). When tetrodotoxin (TTX) was added to the bath to block Na^+ conductance (Fig. 5.8B), the cell responded with a smaller, slower spike (top), presumably because of Ca^{2+} ions. This spike was still followed by the slow IPSP (bottom). (Tetraethylammonium [TEA] was also added to block K^+ conductance, which otherwise shunts out the depolarizing Ca^{2+} conductance.) When bicuculline (a $GABA_A$ blocker) was added to the bath, the mitral cell still responded with an impulse, but the IPSP was eliminated (Fig. 5.8C). Because the only active mitral cell was the one injected, this experiment shows several critical features: that the mitral-cell soma-dendrites act as a presynaptic terminal to the granule cell; that the circuit is recurrent onto the injected cell; and that the inhibitory transmitter is GABA.

As we have seen, regenerative calcium conductances are important properties of dendritic membranes. In many neurons they play key roles in promoting intradendritic transmission and synaptic integration (see Chap. 2). The experiments of Figs. 5.6 and

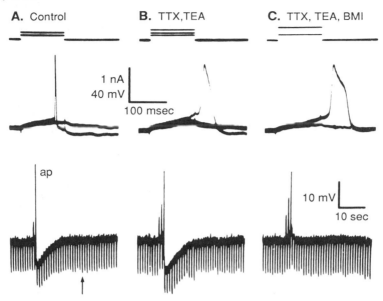

A. Control   **B.** TTX,TEA   **C.** TTX, TEA, BMI

1 nA
40 mV

100 msec

ap

10 mV

10 sec

Fig. 5.8. An electrophysiological test of the reciprocal dendrodendritic microcircuit between mitral and granule cells. These tracings are intracellular recordings from a mitral cell in the in vitro turtle olfactory bulb. The top trace is a monitor of the depolarizing pulses injected into the cell. The middle trace is the intracellular recording of the response of the cell on a fast sweep. The bottom trace is a slow trace, showing the intracellular impulse response (ap) and the hyperpolarizing pulses used to monitor input resistance (arrow). A: Control responses, showing rapid spike (middle) followed by inhibition (bottom). B: In TTX (to block Na$^+$ conductances) and TEA (to block K$^+$ conductances, which would shunt Ca^{2+} currents), the spike is broader, but is still followed by inhibition. C: Addition of bicuculline (BMI), a GABA$_A$ blocker, removes the inhibition, presumably by blocking granule to mitral inhibition. See text. [Modified from Jahr and Nicoll, 1982a, with permission.]

5.8 show that they may also control Ca^{2+} entry and synaptic transmitter release in presynaptic cell bodies and dendrites. In fact, a number of types of Ca^{2+} currents have been identified in acutely isolated mitral cells of the rat, including I_T, I_L, and I_N (Wang et al., 1996).

In its presynaptic role, the mitral cell soma dendrites can be considered analogous to the large terminal arborization at the neuromuscular junction (NMJ). The NMJ has multiple active zones that are activated by an impulse to release acetylcholine (ACh) into the postsynaptic muscle endplate membrane (cf. Chap. 1). Similarly, the mitral soma dendrites have multiple synapses that are activated by an impulse to release their neurotransmitter onto postsynaptic granule cell spines. The mitral cell is therefore an attractive model for analysis of presynaptic release mechanisms at central synapses.

Oscillatory Activity. The sequence of dendrodendritic interactions described above provides one possible basis for the generation of rhythmic activity in the neuronal populations of the bulb (Rall and Shepherd, 1968; Freeman, 1975). As illustrated in Fig. 5.9, the sequence begins with a long-lasting EPSP in the mitral dendritic tufts (MT) in

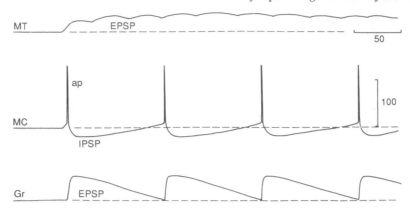

Fig. 5.9. Postulated mechanism whereby the dendrodendritic pathway may provide for rhythmic activity in the olfactory bulb. Postulated intracellular potentials are shown for the mitral dendritic tuft in the glomerulus (MT), mitral cell body (MC), and granule cell (Gr). See text. [From Shepherd, 1979, with permission.]

the glomeruli, due to the olfactory nerve input or the intrinsic activity at the glomerular level. The first mitral cell impulse generated by the EPSP (MC) synchronously activates all the granule cells with which that mitral cell has synaptic connections (Gr). These deliver feedback inhibition of the activated mitral cell and feedforward inhibition of neighboring inactive mitral cells in the way already described above for Fig. 5.7. As the mitral IPSP subsides, a point is reached at which the EPSP is again at threshold; an impulse is again initiated, and the cycle repeats itself. Through the extensive interconnections between the mitral and granule cells, a steady input in the glomeruli is converted into a rhythmic impulse output in the mitral cell population, locked to a rhythmic activation of the granule cell population. Also contributing to the rhythmic activation are the voltage-gated membrane conductances of the cells.

The activity in these populations generates electric current, which spreads through the cells according to the electrotonic properties described below (see also Johnston and Wu, 1995; Segev, 1995; Shepherd, 1998). The current paths of the individual neurons summate in the extracellular spaces in and around the olfactory bulb and thereby give rise to summed extracellular potentials, which are recorded by an electroencephalograph (EEG). Such rhythmic EEG potentials are a prominent characteristic of the olfactory bulb in the resting state as well as during olfactory-induced activity (Adrian, 1950). Explicit models have been developed for the role of these oscillations in processing sensory input (Freeman, 1983; Laurent et al., 1996).

NEUROTRANSMITTERS

One might suppose that the olfactory bulb, with its relatively stereotyped architecture, would have a simple set of neurotransmitters to mediate its synaptic interactions. In fact, the opposite is true: the bulb is enormously rich in neuroactive substances, rivaling any other brain region in this respect. Why this should be so is not fully understood, but it is likely related to the fact that the bulb mediates information about crucial behaviors such as feeding, social organization, and reproduction, which are dependent on a number of behavioral state variables.

A summary of the putative neurotransmitter and neuromodulator substances of the main type of neurons is shown in Fig. 5.10. We will discuss briefly the evidence as it relates to the main types of synaptic connections within the basic circuit (reviewed in Halasz and Shepherd, 1983; Trombley and Shepherd, 1994; Nickell and Shipley, 1994; Shipley and Ennis, 1996).

OLFACTORY SENSORY NEURONS

As noted earlier, the olfactory sensory neurons turn over from stem cells in the neuroepithelium throughout adult life. The sensory neurons contain a special peptide (olfactory marker protein; OMP) and have a high concentration of the dipeptide carnosine (reviewed in Margolis et al., 1986). Electrophysiological experiments show that the olfactory axons are excitatory (see above), but neither OMP nor carnosine has been shown to be neuroactive at this synapse.

Several recent studies have indicated that glutamate is a transmitter at the olfactory nerve synapse onto the mitral, tufted, and PG cell dendrites in the glomeruli. Intracellular recordings from mitral cells in the isolated turtle olfactory bulb (Berkowicz et al., 1994) and extracellular unit recordings in the rat olfactory bulb slice (Ennis et al., 1996) have shown that the EPSP in response to an olfactory nerve shock has both AMPA and NMDA components (Fig. 5.11). Glutamate is colocalized with carnosine in axon terminals in the glomeruli (Sassoè-Pognetto et al., 1993). Several glutamate receptor ionic and metabotropic subtypes are found in the glomerular layer, but it has not yet been determined whether they are related to postsynaptic targets of the olfactory nerves or of the presynaptic dendrites in the glomeruli (see Shipley and Ennis, 1996, for review).

PERIGLOMERULAR CELLS

The first definitive study of glomerular transmitters showed, by histofluorescence and EM autoradiography, that some periglomerular (PG) cells are positive for dopamine (DA)-synthesizing enzymes (Halasz et al., 1977). The dopamine is transneuronally regulated; degeneration and regeneration of olfactory nerves following olfactory nerve transection are paralleled by a decrease and increase of DA and dihydroxyphenylacetic acid (DOPAC) levels in the olfactory bulb (Baker et al., 1983; Baker, 1988).

Some PG cells and their dendrites contain glutamic acid decarboxylase (GAD), the GABA-synthesizing enzyme, as well as take up GABA (Ribak et al., 1977). In rabbit olfactory bulb slice preparations, GABA-activated whole-cell currents and single-channel currents recorded from PG cells show $GABA_A$ receptor properties (block by bicuculline, etc.; Bufler et al., 1992). GABA also acts on $GABA_A$ receptors to elicit inhibitory currents in cultured rat olfactory bulb cells (Trombley and Shepherd, 1994). Evidence for inhibitory actions of glycine on PG and other bulbar neurons has also been obtained (see below).

DA and GABA may be colocalized in the same PG cell in some species and restricted to separate PG cell subpopulations in others (Mugnaini et al., 1984; Baker, 1988; see Fig. 5.10). This demonstrates two principles: (*1*) a single morphological cell type may be fractionated into more than one neurotransmitter subtype, and (*2*) the mix

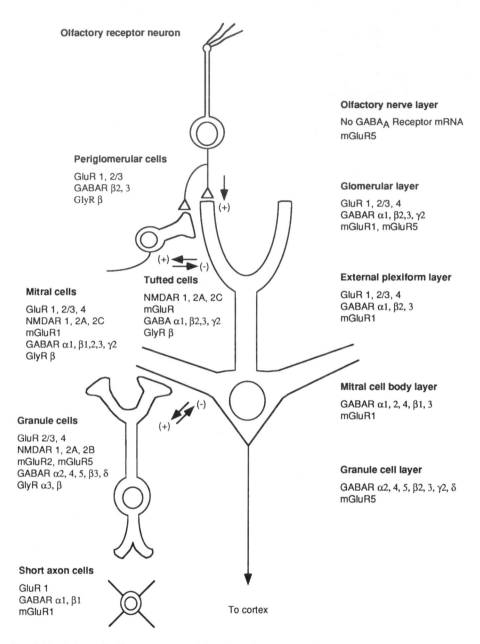

Olfactory receptor neuron

Olfactory nerve layer

No GABA$_A$ Receptor mRNA
mGluR5

Periglomerular cells

GluR 1, 2/3
GABAR β2, 3
GlyR β

Glomerular layer

GluR 1, 2/3, 4
GABAR α1, β2,3, γ2
mGluR1, mGluR5

(+)

(+) ◄► (-)

Tufted cells

NMDAR 1, 2A, 2C
mGluR
GABA α1, β2,3, γ2
GlyR β

External plexiform layer

GluR 1, 2/3, 4
GABAR α1, β2, 3
mGluR1

Mitral cells

GluR 1, 2/3, 4
NMDAR 1, 2A, 2C
mGluR1
GABAR α1, β1,2,3, γ2
GlyR β

(-)

(+)

Mitral cell body layer

GABAR α1, 2, 4, β1, 3
mGluR1

Granule cells

GluR 2/3, 4
NMDAR 1, 2A, 2B
mGluR2, mGluR5
GABAR α2, 4, 5, β3, δ
GlyR α3, β

Granule cell layer

GABAR α2, 4, 5, β2, 3, γ2, δ
mGluR5

Short axon cells

GluR 1
GABAR α1, β1
mGluR1

To cortex

Fig. 5.10. Schematic diagram summarizing the cellular and laminar distribution of receptor subunits for amino acid transmitters in the olfactory bulb. Glutamate AMPA receptor subunits: GluR1, 2/3, 4. Glutamate NMDA receptor subunits: NMDA R1, 2A, 2B, 2C. Metabotropic glutamate receptors: mGluR1, 2, 5. GABA$_A$ receptor subunits: α1, 2, 3, 4, 5; β1, 2, 3; γ2. Glycine receptor subunits: α3, β. [From Trombley and Shepherd, 1997, with permission.]

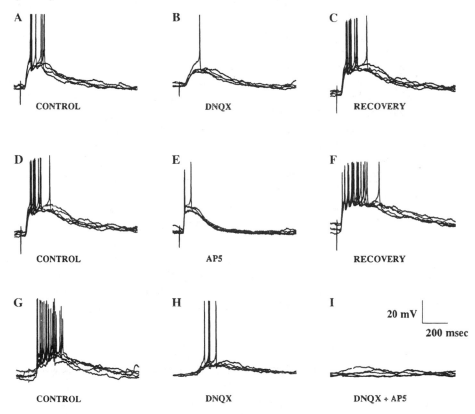

Fig. 5.11. Evidence for glutamate as the transmitter from olfactory nerve terminals. Intracellular recordings from mitral cells in the isolated turtle olfactory bulb. A–C: DNQX in the bath blocks the early rapid AMPA phase of the EPSP response to an olfactory nerve volley. D–F: AP5 blocks the slow NMDA phase of the EPSP response. G–I: DNQX plus AP5 eliminates the EPSP entirely. [From Berkowicz et al., 1994, with permission.]

of neurotransmitters in a single morphological cell type is phylogenetically flexible. Dopaminergic and GABAergic subpopulations of intrinsic neurons are also seen in other parts of the nervous system (cf. retina, Chap. 6). As pointed out by Oertel et al. (1982), such dual subtypes may reflect an important principle of synaptic circuits.

PG cells have been postulated to have either excitatory or inhibitory synaptic actions at their dendrites and axons (see above). It is tempting to presume that both dopamine and GABA (as well as glycine) have inhibitory actions. However, the issue may not be that simple. For example, there is still controversy about whether DA has excitatory or inhibitory actions in the basal ganglia (see Chap. 9). Excitatory actions of GABA mediated by GABA$_A$ receptors are well known during early development and at distal dendritic sites (cf. Chap. 2). In the olfactory glomerulus, there is electrophysiological evidence that GABA may have excitatory actions (Rhoades and Freeman, 1990), as well as electron spectroscopic evidence for accumulations of Cl$^-$ in intraglomerular dendrites, which could reflect reversed chloride gradients underlying excitatory GABAergic actions (Siklos et al., 1995).

MITRAL CELLS

Studies of the mitral-to-granule excitatory synapse have emphasized the importance of knowledge of synaptic organization in interpreting neuropharmacological results. For example, microionophoresis of amino acids, particularly aspartate and DL-homocysteate, tends to inhibit mitral cell activity. At first, this appeared to be confusing, in view of the usual excitatory effects of these amino acids on other neurons. However, closer consideration suggested that these substances, when released from the micropipette, act to excite the granule cell spines, which then inhibit the mitral cells (McLennan, 1971; Nicoll, 1971). This serves as a model for the local interactions that must be taken into account in interpreting microionophoresis studies.

The evidence for glutamate, acting at both AMPA and NMDA receptors on mitral/tufted and PG cell dendrites, has been mentioned above. The candidacy of glutamate as the transmitter of the output synapses from the presynaptic mitral cell soma-dendrites has been strengthened by the finding of NMDA receptors in the EPL of the olfactory bulb (Cotman et al., 1987). The AMPA receptors in olfactory bulb cells have a low permeability to Ca^{2+}. Glutamate also appears to be the transmitter of the mitral axon terminals in the olfactory cortex (see Chap. 10). Because the mitral cell has synaptic output from both its dendrites and axon, it provides a model for testing whether the same transmitter is released from all synapses of a neuron, a possibility known as *Dale's law* (Dale, 1935).

TUFTED CELLS

It is generally believed that tufted cells share the same neurotransmitters at their dendritic and axonal output synapses with mitral cells. However, some tufted cells appear to be dopaminergic, which makes them more similar to PG cells (Halasz et al., 1977). This may be correlated with other differences between mitral and tufted cells, as noted above.

GRANULE CELLS

Numerous studies point to GABA as the neurotransmitter released by the dendrodendritic synapses of the granule spine onto the mitral/tufted cell dendrites. Granule cells take up GABA (Halasz et al., 1978). The GABA-synthesizing enzyme GAD has been localized to the granule cells and their dendritic spines by EM immunohistochemistry (Ribak et al., 1977).

In the in vitro preparation of the turtle olfactory bulb, the early hyperpolarizing components of the IPSP in a mitral cell have several GABAergic properties: they are blocked by bicuculline and low Cl^- in the bathing medium, reversed by Cl^- filled electrodes, associated with an increased conductance, and have clear reversal potentials (Mori et al., 1981b; Nowycky et al., 1981a,b; Jahr and Nicoll, 1982a). These reflect properties of $GABA_A$ receptors. Similar evidence has been obtained in the salamander (Wellis and Kauer, 1993). The later, slow, inhibitory potential (I_S) does not have a reversal potential, suggesting that it may be mediated by a different synaptic receptor (possibly $GABA_B$ receptors) or at a more distant locus on the mitral cell dendrites (Mori et al., 1981c).

Evidence for glycine as a transmitter in the olfactory bulb has recently been obtained. Glycine was found to evoke chloride-mediated membrane currents in rabbit olfactory bulb slices (Bufler et al., 1992) and to have powerful inhibitory effects on both mitral/tufted cells and granule cells in culture (Trombley and Shepherd, 1994). Immunoreactivity for monoclonal antibodies against glycine and glycine receptors is found in the EPL and around mitral cell bodies (van den Pol and Gorcs, 1988). In situ hybridization experiments have shown that the $\alpha3$ glycine receptor subunit, the ligand-binding subunit of the strychnine-sensitive glycine receptor, is present in the olfactory bulb (Malioso ct al., 1991). The olfactory bulb thus has emerged as one of the best examples that glycine is a neurotransmitter in the brain as well as the spinal cord (cf. Kuhse et al., 1991).

PEPTIDES

The olfactory bulb offers a smorgasbord of delectable peptides. Besides carnosine and OMP, it is especially rich in taurine, thyroid hormone–releasing hormone (TRH), insulin, and cholecystokinin (CCK). However, absolute levels are not the only measure of the significance of a neuroactive substance. Location at a critical site in a synaptic circuit is even more significant. Examples of this are substance P, present in tufted cells, and enkephalins, present in both PG cells and granule cells. Nicoll et al. (1980a,b) studied the effect of a stable enkephalin analogue D-Ala-Mets-enkephalin (DALA) in the in vitro turtle olfactory bulb. DALA in the bathing medium reduced the IPSPs induced in mitral cells, especially the recurrent inhibition elicited by intracellular activation of a mitral cell. They suggested that the primary action of enkephalins is to suppress inhibitory interneurons, thereby producing indirectly an increase in excitability of the principal neurons. This would be an example of disinhibition within a synaptic circuit (see Chap. 1), and illustrates again how an understanding of synaptic organization is essential for interpreting pharmacological actions.

Peptides are colocalized with neurotransmitters at most synapses in the olfactory bulb, but the significance is not yet understood. There is evidence that some enkephalin is contained in granule cells, suggesting that it may be coreleased with GABA and have a direct action on mitral cells (Bogan et al., 1982; Davis et al., 1982). One possibility is that it produces the slow inhibitory potential (see above). There are, however, many types of interactions between transmitters and peptides, as discussed in Chap. 2.

GASEOUS MESSENGERS

Histochemical staining for nitric oxide synthase (NOS) and NADPH diaphorase has shown that the highest densities of NOS occur in the cerebellum and olfactory bulb, a finding supported by in situ mRNA hybridization for NOS (Bredt et al., 1991). The stained elements include mainly fibers within the glomeruli, subpopulations of PG cells, and fibers around the granule cells. Neighboring glomeruli characteristically show distinct levels of staining (Zhao et al., 1994). Mitral, tufted, and granule cells are not stained. It has been hypothesized (Breer and Shepherd, 1993) that the NO released from PG cell dendrites may act on neighboring dendrites, a new form of local, diffuse, dendrodendritic interaction to supplement the specific synaptic interactions between PG dendrites and the dendrites of mitral/tufted cells (see above). A likely target of NO is soluble guanylate cyclase (sGC). Recent in situ hybridization studies indicate localization of sGC mRNA in mitral/tufted cells as well as mRNA for subunits of the cyclic nucleotide gated (CNG) channel (Kingston et al., 1996). It can therefore be hypothesized that activation of subsets of PG cells may lead to modulation of CNG channels in mitral/tufted cells, which could alter the excitability of those cells and the processing of odor output from the glomeruli.

An interesting point regarding the NO released from subsets of fibers and from PG cell dendrites within a glomerulus is that their action would likely be confined to that glomerulus because of the short acting nature of NO (Breer and Shepherd, 1993). NO thus appears to be well adapted to contribute to the functioning of the glomerulus as a unit. Neighboring glomeruli could function relatively independently because of the confinement of NO in the glomerulus within which it is released.

CENTRIFUGAL FIBERS

As noted previously, there are three main types of centrifugal fiber, each associated with a specific classical neurotransmitter.

Noradrenaline (NA)-containing fibers arrive from the locus coeruleus, and distribute mostly within the granule layer and IPL, as well as the glomerular layer (see Fig. 5.2 above). The actions of NA on mitral cells are complex. One action suggested by the ionophoretic studies of Jahr and Nicoll (1982b) is that NA acts on granule cells to reduce their release of GABA. In primary cultures of bulb cells, it has been found that NA acts on an α_2 receptor to suppress inhibition of mitral cells (Trombley and Shepherd, 1993). The mechanism appears to involve reduction of a Ca^{2+} conductance in the presynaptic terminal (Trombley, 1992).

Serotonin-containing fibers arrive from the dorsal raphe. They distribute preferentially to different laminae in different species (Takeuchi et al., 1982). Of special interest are the fibers that terminate within the glomeruli, thus permitting a brainstem system direct access to the initial level of input processing of olfactory signals. These could be significant in mediating behavioral-state variables set by brainstem systems involved in hunger, satiety, arousal, and sleep. Judging from ionophoresis experiments, the action of serotonin on mitral cells is inhibitory (Bloom et al., 1971).

Cholinergic fibers arrive from the basal forebrain and distribute relatively evenly through the laminae. According to Rotter et al. (1977), the external plexiform layer "has the highest concentration of muscarinic receptors in the brain . . . and high levels occur in the glomerular layer, mitral cell layer, and the granule cell layer" as well. Because these fibers terminate mainly on granule cell spines, they are well placed to modulate the dendrodendritic inhibition of mitral cells at the level of output control. Ionophoresis of ACh in vivo has mostly depressant effects on mitral cell firing (Bloom et al., 1971), but ACh action has not yet been studied in vitro nor interpreted in relation to the specific details of synaptic organization.

DENDRITIC PROPERTIES

We have considered the anatomy of the neurons, the physiology of their synaptic actions, and the neurotransmitters mediating those actions, and we are now in a position to consider how these properties are involved in the processing of information within the synaptic circuits of the olfactory bulb. Processing can be divided into two parts: synaptic integration that occurs within neurons, and synaptic interactions that occur between neurons. Synaptic integration involves intraneuronal transmission within dendrites, which will be considered first; we then take up interneuronal synaptic interactions in the final section. Each of the three main cell types of the bulb provides a model for illustrating important principles of dendritic signal processing.

MITRAL CELL

In studying the mitral cell, it soon becomes apparent that its dendritic tree is not one homogeneous unit. Rather, it is divided into several distinct anatomical entities, each with its own distinct function. The *glomerular dendritic* tuft is concerned primarily with reception and processing of the olfactory input; it is analogous in this respect to the entire dendritic tree of a thalamic relay neuron. The *primary dendritic shift* has as its distinct function the transfer of information from the glomerular tuft to the cell body; in this radial transfer function it is analogous to a retinal bipolar cell. The *secondary dendritic branches* are exclusively concerned with controlling bulbar output through interactions with the granule cells. These divisions are so distinct that one can regard the mitral cell as not one but three cells, transfer between them taking place through intraneuronal continuity rather than interneuronal synapses. This means that we must assess dendritic properties in relation to the different functions of each of these entities.

Glomerular Tuft. We have seen that the glomerular tuft forms a small dendritic tree within an olfactory glomerulus. The trunks of the tuft have relatively small diameters of 1–3 μm. As a first approximation, assume that each dendritic trunk divides in such a way as to conform to the 3/2 power constraint on the diameter (see Johnston and Wu, 1995; Segev, 1995; Shepherd, 1998). Each trunk will thus give rise to a small equivalent cylinder; taken together, they will form an equivalent cylinder for the entire tuft. Assuming a range of values for electrical parameters that is typical of neurons, we can obtain an estimate of a characteristic length of 150–600 μm for the case of 1-μm diameter trunks and 300–1,000 μm for 3-μm diameter trunks.

These estimates are considerably higher than the actual extent of the tufts, which range from 150 to 200 μm. The electrotonic length ($L = x/A$) of an equivalent cylinder for the tuft might therefore be estimated at <1, and possibly <0.5 μm. Thus, the smaller branches of the tuft are counterbalanced by their shorter lengths, an expression of the scaling principle (see Shepherd, 1998). Because of the short electrotonic length of the tuft, current flow through the tuft must be relatively effective by passive means alone, and synaptic responses to sensory inputs can spread effectively to the primary dendrite. However, recent patch recordings from the primary dendrite near the glomerular tuft indicate that synaptic responses may also be boosted by active properties of the tuft dendritic branches (Chen et al., 1997a,b).

Primary Dendrite. This is a single unbranched process, and therefore it is easy to make a model for it. For the mammal, likely estimates for the characteristic length of a typical primary dendrite of 6-μm diameter fall in the range of 300–1500 μm. Since a primary dendrite has a length of some 400 μm, it appears that the electrotonic length of this example is less than 1, and perhaps even less than 0.5. Electrotonic spread should, therefore, be relatively effective through such a process (Rall and Shepherd, 1968). In the turtle, primary dendrites are thinner (2–3 μm) and longer (500–700 μm), but this is offset by a higher specific membrane resistance (in the range of 50,000 ohm cm^2), promoting better signal spread (Mori et al., 1981a).

Earlier computational (Rall and Shepherd, 1968) and experimental (Mori et al., 1982) studies indicated that some primary dendrites might have active properties, and this has been borne out by recent patch recordings in the rat olfactory bulb slice. As already illustrated (Fig. 1.9), double patch recordings from soma and distal primary dendrite (Chen et al., 1997a,b) have shown that, with weak synaptic excitation from the olfactory nerves, the site of impulse initiation is in the soma-axon hillock region, with back propagation into the distal primary dendrite. This is fully in accord with the electrotonic properties we have discussed, which should provide for effective coupling between the EPSP and the axon hillock by passive means (see below). With stronger EPSPs, the site of impulse initiation shifts to the distal site, as shown previously in Fig. 1.9. IPSPs elicited in the secondary dendrites can also cause a shift to the distal site (see below). It is hypothesized that this provides a means for the mitral cell to provide for coupling between glomerular tuft and axonal output even in the face of strong lateral inhibition. We have noted above that myelin has been observed wrapped around the distal primary dendrites of some species. Possibly the myelin is associated with active properties of the dendrites; alternatively, it may serve to enhance passive spread. More work on the function of myelin here is needed.

Secondary Dendrites. The key question with regard to this compartment of the mitral dendritic tree has been the extent to which an impulse at the cell body would invade the secondary dendrites and activate the mitral-to-granule synapses. In the course of investigating the extracellular potential fields in the olfactory bulb, a compartmental model was developed for the mitral cell dendrites that is relevant to just this problem. This investigation provided the basis for postulating dendrodendritic synaptic interactions in the bulb (Rall et al., 1966; Rall and Shepherd, 1968).

The steps for modeling the dendrites follow those already outlined. An equivalent cylinder for the tree of dendrites is illustrated in Fig. 5.12. Individual secondary dendrites are 2–6 μm in diameter and 400–600 μm in length. Their electrotonic lengths, as well as the values for the equivalent cylinder for the entire tree, have been estimated to lie in the range of 0.5–1.0.

In the investigation of the properties of the dendrites, a model for the action potential was also developed, so that it was possible to simulate an experiment in which an impulse propagates into the cell body and spreads into the dendrites (Rall and Shepherd, 1968). Computational experiments were carried out in which different assumptions were made about the electrotonic lengths of the dendrites and their active and passive properties. The use of compartmental models to perform experiments that simulate situations, often inaccessible in the biological preparation itself, is a powerful approach that was introduced by Rall (1964); the widespread use of such compartmental simulations is evident in most of the chapters in this book.

The main result obtained from the model was that impulse spread into both primary and secondary dendrites is very effective by passive means alone. This is illustrated schematically in the diagram of Fig. 5.12. Passive spread is in fact so effective that in

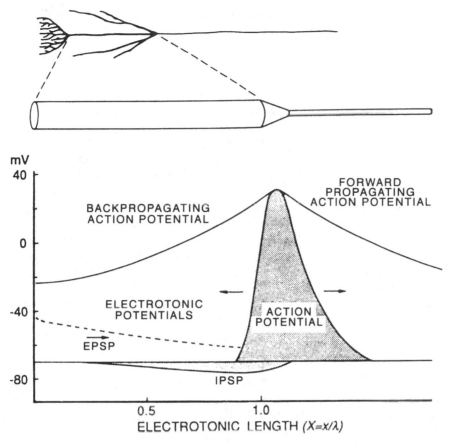

Fig. 5.12. Electrotonic model of the mitral cell, illustrating the spread of potentials in the primary and secondary dendrites. Top: Schematic diagram of a mitral cell. Middle: Equivalent cylinder for the 1° to 2° dendrites, together with the soma, axon hillock, and axon. Bottom: Theoretical spatial distributions of the excitatory synaptic potential (EPSP: dashed line) and action potential and their associated electrotonic potentials for the case of a relatively weak EPSP that causes action potential initiation in the soma-axon hillock-initial axon segment region. The diagram illustrates the moment of action potential initiation; this is followed by active backpropagation into the dendrites. (Stronger excitation causes impulse initiation in the distal primary dendrite, with forward propagation to the axon). Also shown is the early distribution of a recurrent IPSP in the secondary dendrites. See text. [Modified from Shepherd and Greer (1990), with permission; based on Rall and Shepherd (1968), Bhalla and Bower (1993), and Chen et al. (1997)].

some cases it was difficult in the computations to distinguish a passively spreading impulse from an actively propagating one; this was also true for the primary dendrites. The recent patch recordings (Chen et al., 1997) provide evidence that at least some mitral secondary dendrites appear to support active impulses. Fig. 5.12 indicates that, like the primary dendrite, the impulse would be likely to invade quite effectively the long secondary dendrites by either active or passive means. Thus, the IPSP produced by feedback from the granule cells would be expected to be distributed throughout the dendritic tree, as indicated in Fig. 5.12. Simulations of impulse spread in the mitral cell dendrites support these interpretations (Bhalla and Bower, 1993).

GRANULE CELL

Because the granule cell lacks an axon, study of its dendritic properties is obviously crucial to understanding all of its input-output functions.

In the investigation of the recurrent dendrodendritic pathway by Rall and Shepherd (1968), a model for the granule cell was developed and explored. The branching tree within the EPL was represented by an equivalent cylinder; branch diameters of 0.2–0.8 μm were assumed, and an electrotonic length of about 0.4 was estimated. The shaft diameter of the granule cell is on the order of 1 μm; for an average shaft length of 600 μm, an electrotonic length of 1.7 was estimated for the model of the combined tree and shaft. The model was used to simulate synaptic depolarization of the granule spines in the EPL. The model demonstrated that this synaptic depolarization gives rise to the extracellular potentials generated just after an antidromic impulse invades the mitral cell dendrites (Phillips et al., 1963). When the mitral cell model and the granule cell model were joined in sequence, it could be postulated that the EPSP in the granule dendritic spines results from a dendrodendritic input from the mitral secondary dendrites. As described in the previous section, the localization and timing indicated that the spine EPSP activates inhibitory synapses onto the same secondary dendrites, to produce the long-lasting IPSP recorded in the physiological experiments (Phillips et al., 1963).

Dendritic Spines. The properties of the granule dendritic spines must be critical in controlling the relative effectiveness of recurrent inhibition from a single spine and lateral inhibition mediated by spread of activity to neighboring spines (see Fig. 5.7, above). This question has been addressed directly by making precise measurements of dendrites and spines in reconstructions from serial electron micrographs (Woolf et al., 1991a) and in material observed in the high-voltage electron microscope (Greer, 1988). Computational models of these measured structures have then been constructed to explore the spread of activity.

An example of two common arrangements of spines is shown in Fig. 5.13. In the top panel, spines (A–D) are arranged in a linear fashion along the dendritic branch (E). Excitatory input (from a mitral/tufted cell dendrite) to spine C produces a large EPSP in C, which undergoes electrotonic decrement in spreading into the branch E. However, there is very little decrement in spreading in the other direction, from the branch into the other spines (A,B,D), because of the impedance mismatch between dendrite and spines. A different arrangement is shown in the bottom panel, where several spines (B–D) arise from a common stem, a so-called complex spine. Spread of activity from C to the neighboring spines now occurs in distinct steps. These considerations have been discussed in terms of spread of electrical potential, but they also apply to the diffusion of Ca^{2+} and other ions and metabolites between spine head and dendritic branch (Woolf and Greer, 1994).

These results confirm that, although the stems of the spines may be narrow (0.2 i.e., μm), reasonable assumptions about the electrical properties of the membranes lead to the conclusion that electrotonic spread from spine to spine is considerable over the

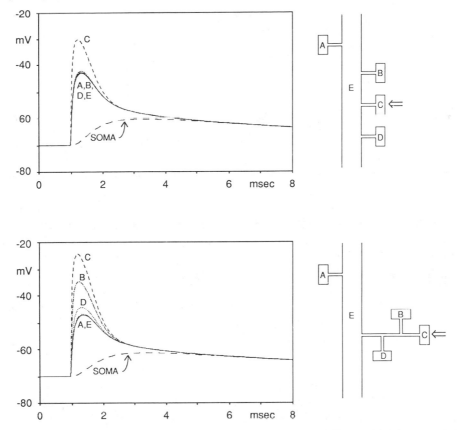

Fig. 5.13. Electrotonic models of granule cell dendrites and spines. The models, shown at right, are based on reconstructions of serial electron micrographs. An excitatory synaptic conductance change was simulated in spine C, and the synaptic potentials were measured in each spine (A–D) and in the dendritic branch. Upper panels: Linear arrangement of spines. Lower panels: A single and a complex spine. For these simulations, Rm = 4000 ohm cm^2. [From Greer, 1988, with permission; Woolf, T.B., Greer, C.A., Shepherd, G.M., unpublished observations.]

short distances involved. It appears therefore that lateral inhibition can be mediated by passive spread alone through the dendritic tree in the EPL. The inhibition is spatially graded according to the electrotonic decrement of the potentials in the tree. Depending on the spatial arrangements, individual spines may act as subunits in the manner discussed in Chap. 1. A computational study has shown how groups of spines may function together as a complex input–output population (Woolf et al, 1991b), dependent on the underlying membrane electrotonic properties, in much the same way that such units arise in the dendrites of amacrine cells (Koch et al, 1982).

These considerations do not rule out the possibility of active properties of the granule dendritic membrane in addition to electrotonic properties. Might the spines themselves have active properties, so that spread into the branches is more effective? And might the branches have active properties? The original model of the granule cell did not rule out active spine properties, but it indicated that active properties must be limited and not lead to propagation from the branches in the EPL into the main dendritic shaft (Rall and Shepherd, 1968). Subsequently, Jahr and Nicoll (1982a) found that recurrent inhibition persists despite the presence of TTX (see Fig. 5.8 above), implying that voltage-gated sodium channels do not contribute to the potentials in granule dendritic spines.

PERIGLOMERULAR CELL

The PG cell has already been discussed as an example of a short-axon cell, a type found in many parts of the brain. Being small, the PG cell has been relatively inaccessible to experimental studies, and there is as yet no biophysical model as in the cases of the mitral and granule cells. For a first approximation to its overall electrotonic properties, the dendritic tuft may be regarded as a smaller version of the mitral dendritic tuft described above. Taking into account both the smaller diameters and the shorter lengths of the branches, it seems reasonable to conclude that an equivalent cylinder for the PG cell tuft would be similar to that for the mitral tuft, that is, $L = 0.5–1.0$. This is, again, an expression of the scaling principle for dendritic trees of different size.

PG cell functions appear to be exquisitely dependent on levels of input activity. Electrophysiological studies have suggested that at threshold there is mainly straight-through excitation of mitral cells by receptor axons; long-lasting facilitation is sometimes detectable (Getchell and Shepherd, 1975a,b). As input activity increases, the activation of PG cells, both by direct olfactory axon input and by indirect dendrodendritic synapses, begins to bring about inhibitory feedback from the PG cell dendrites. Small EPSPs probably mediate only local input–output paths through the dendrites; moderate EPSPs will lead to more extensive inhibitory actions within a glomerulus; large EPSPs, by spreading to the axon hillock, set up impulses that mediate inhibition of dendrites arising from neighboring glomeruli.

Studies of responses to natural stimulation with odors have demonstrated even more complex interactions, including the presence of an initial brief hyperpolarization at weak levels of stimulation (see next section). It thus appears that several levels of interaction can be identified within the glomerular layer, governed by the amplitudes of EPSPs and their electrotonic spread within the PG cell dendrites. Functionally, these interactions enhance transmission at detection thresholds and provide the lateral inhibition necessary for discrimination between odors at higher odor concentrations. The PG cell dendritic tree thus provides for *multiple state-dependent input–output functions*. Similar properties have been postulated for thalamic short-axon cells and may apply to other types of cells.

FUNCTIONAL CIRCUITS

We have described the basic circuit of the olfactory bulb and the excitatory and inhibitory potentials that arise through interactions between the mitral/tufted cells and their two sets of intrinsic neurons: PG and granule cells. How do these interactions provide the neural basis for the ability to discriminate between odor stimuli? We will summarize briefly how these interactions are organized to generate odor maps, how they are involved in contrast enhancement underlying odor discrimination, and how they provide mechanisms for odor memory.

GLOMERULAR MODULES FORM AN ODOR IMAGE

In order to analyse synaptic circuits during normal function, one must know where one is in the neural map representing the sensory space. Odor stimuli do not carry information about external space as do visual or somatosensory stimuli, and the olfactory pathway can therefore use its "neural space" to represent the intrinsic properties of the odor molecules. The 2-deoxyglucose method first showed how these properties are mapped into spatial patterns (see Fig. 5.14): the patterns tend to be bilaterally symmetrical; they differ with different odors; the patterns for a given odor occur in the same glomerular domain in different animals; the weakest odor concentrations elicit activity in one or a few glomeruli, reflecting input from the olfactory cells with the highest-affinity receptors for that odor; and stronger stimuli elicit activity more widely within a domain, reflecting input from cells with lower-affinity receptors (Sharp et al.,

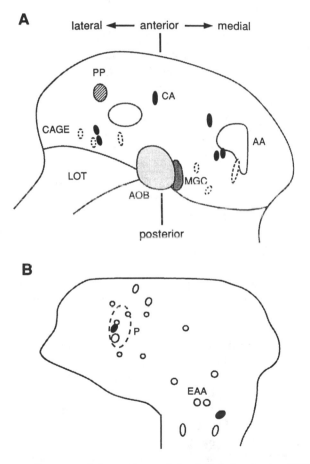

Fig. 5.14. Summary diagrams of the patterns of focal 2-deoxyglucose (2DG) uptake in the glomerular layer of the rat olfactory bulb elicited by odor stimulation. Flat map of the glomerular layer, opened out from a cut along the ventral anterior–posterior meridian. Abbreviations: PP, peppermint; CA, camphor; AA, amyl acetate; CAGE, cage air; MGC, modified glomerular complex; AOB, accessory olfactory bulb; LOT, lateral olfactory tract. [A. From Shepherd and Firestein, 1991, B. From Jourdan, 1982, with permission.]

1975; 1977; Stewart et al., 1979; Jourdan et al., 1982). These properties have been confirmed and extended by studies of the patterns shown by in situ hybridization for c-fos mRNA (Sallasz and Jourdan, 1993; Guthrie et al., 1993; Guthrie and Gall, 1995), and by voltage-sensitive dyes (Kauer and Cinelli, 1993; Cinelli and Kauer, 1994). A recent study using Ca^{2+} sensitive dyes in the zebrafish has demonstrated particularly clearly the different patterns of glomerular activation related to different amino acid stimuli; the properties of these patterns are virtually identical to those from the 2DG studies in mammals (Friedrich and Korsching, 1996).

The principles obtained from these functional studies are receiving support from the more recent analysis of the localization of olfactory receptor mRNA in the olfactory axon terminals within the glomeruli. Thus, these studies are showing that receptor-specific glomeruli are bilaterally symmetrical and reproducible from animal to animal (Vassar et al., 1994; Ressler et al., 1994), which is fully consistent with the functional results.

Taken together, all of these studies suggest that odors are represented as "odor images" or "odotopic maps" in the glomerular sheet. Activation of individual identified glomeruli (Teicher et al., 1980; Lancet et al., 1982) has supported a variety of anatomical and molecular evidence that the glomerulus is a functional unit in the processing of odor stimuli (reviewed in Shepherd, 1994a; Hildebrand and Shepherd, 1997).

For the analysis of synaptic circuits, these findings mean, first, that it is essential to know where in the glomerular sheet one is when stimulating with a given odor. Second, they mean that analysis is focussing on the role of circuits in relation to the glomerular functional units as they process the input from a given odor relative to others.

Following these guidelines, Mori and colleagues have carried out electrophysiological recordings to analyze the responses of mitral cells in the rabbit to stimulation with homologous series of odor compounds (Mori et al., 1992; summarized in Mori and Yoshihara, 1995). Their recordings were made from functionally identified regions of the glomerular sheet, which allowed them to explore systematically the responses to a wide range of chemically related odor compounds. The spectrum of odor molecules that can activate a given cell was called its *molecular receptive range* (MRR), by analogy to the spatial receptive field of a cell in the visual pathway. A key finding was that the mitral cells all showed narrow MRRs, with responses to only two or three neighbors in a given series of compounds from C2 to C12. Compounds of the same or similar carbon lengths were often activated in different but related series. These results provided the first direct physiological evidence that "conformational features (odotopes) of odor molecules are mapped spatially in the olfactory bulb" (Mori and Yoshihara, 1995). The fact that these recordings were from mitral cells implies that the olfactory sensory neurons providing direct input to the mitral cells encode the odotopes (determinants, epitopes) of the odor molecules as postulated by receptor modeling studies (Singer and Shepherd, 1994; Singer et al., 1995a). The olfactory sensory neurons in fact show similar properties to mitral cells in response to odors in a homologous series (Sato et al., 1994). The role of inhibition in processing this information in the bulb will be discussed below.

In summary, we now have a consistent outline for the initial encoding of odor information in the mammal as a basis for odor discrimination, which may be summarized by referring back to the basic circuit diagram of Fig. 5.4. First, odor molecule functional groups interact with receptor molecule subsites. Next, second-messenger pathways lead to differential impulse discharges. Third, the axons of a given subset converge on a few target glomeruli in the olfactory bulb. An olfactory glomerulus is thus a functional unit reflecting the molecular receptive range (MRR) of the subset(s) projecting to it. Finally, the map of olfactory glomeruli encodes odor space; given odor stimuli thus elicit "odor images" within the neural space of the glomeruli sheet. It is these "images" that are the basis for further processing by the synaptic circuits of the olfactory bulb.

EXCITATORY–INHIBITORY INTERACTIONS ARE INVOLVED IN ODOR PROCESSING

In analyzing synaptic mechanisms underlying odor processing it is critical to have precise control over the stimulus so that very brief step-pulses of odor can be used as stimuli, in the same manner as brief flashes of light or sound tones might be used in respective analyses. Mitral cell responses to such stimuli show three main response patterns (Kauer, 1974; Kauer and Shepherd, 1977). First, the neuron may be suppressed at all odor concentrations, the S (suppression) type. Second, a slow spike discharge at low odor concentrations may change to an early brief spike burst followed by suppression at higher concentrations, the E (excitatory) type. Finally, there may be no detectable response to a given odor, the N (no response) type. These types have many minor variations; they are seen in their simplest form in fish and salamander, and in more complex forms in mammals (cf. Wellis and Scott, 1987).

Intracellular recordings in vertebrates (Hamilton and Kauer, 1985; Wellis and Scott, 1987) and invertebrates (Christensen and Hildebrand, 1987; Christensen et al., 1996) have revealed the synaptic potentials underlying these response types. Similarities across phyla are emphasized in the intracellular recordings from mitral cells and antennal lobe projection neurons shown in Fig. 5.15. In salamanders (A, left), an odor pulse produces an initial brief hyperpolarization of the mitral cell, followed by an EPSP generating a burst of impulses, followed by a long-lasting IPSP; a similar sequence of potentials is seen in the odor response of a projection neuron in the moth (A, right). This similarity extends to the responses to an electric shock to the olfactory nerves (B). In the salamander (B, left), a subthreshold nerve volley elicits an EPSP–IPSP sequence (trace marked by open circle); when above threshold, the mitral cell generates a brief EPSP and one or two spikes, followed by a long-lasting IPSP; a similar sequence is seen in the moth projection neuron (B, right).

It has been concluded (see also Hildebrand, 1995, 1996) that a common mechanism is invoked by an odor pulse. In the mitral cell, with weak input levels the EPSP spreads through the primary dendrite to elicit the impulse at the soma-axon hillock with subsequent forward and backpropagation (Figs. 1.6, 5.13). The large amplitude of the IPSP suggests that it is generated at or near the recording site in the soma, where granule cell inhibition predominates. An interesting point is that the initial brief hyperpolarization is common across phyla in response to odor stimulation but not electric shocks. The route of this IPSP is not yet clear, because the main inhibitory pathway in the olfactory bulb, through granule cells, requires initial excitation of the mitral cells. One possibility is that the granule cells may be activated initially by tufted cells, which have lower thresholds for activation than the larger mitral cells (Schneider and Scott, 1983),

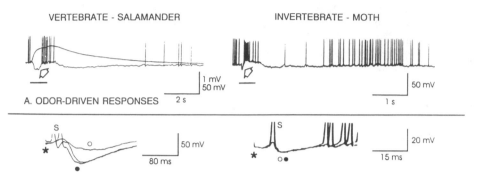

POSTSYNAPTIC RESPONSES OF OUTPUT NEURONS
IN THE OLFACTORY BULB AND THE ANTENNAL LOBE

VERTEBRATE - SALAMANDER   INVERTEBRATE - MOTH

A. ODOR-DRIVEN RESPONSES   2 s   1 s

B. ORTHODROMIC ELECTRICAL STIMULATION

Fig. 5.15. Intracellular responses of vertebrate mitral cells and invertebrate antennal lobe output cells, showing close similarity of response properties across phyla. **A:** Odor stimulation (horizontal bar) produces a sequence of potentials in the salamandar mitral cell consisting of a brief hyperpolarization (open arrowhead) followed by an EPSP giving rise to a burst of action potentials, followed by a long-lasting IPSP. A similar sequence is produced in the moth output neuron. **B:** An electrical shock (*) to the olfactory nerves in the salamandar produces if it is below impulse threshold and EPSP–IPSP sequence (○); above threshold the larger EPSP elicits spikes, followed by a larger IPSP (●). On the right, these is a similar EPSP–IPSP sequence in the moth output neuron. [Salamander recordings adapted from Hamilton and Kauer, 1988, 1989; moth recordings adapted from Christensen and Hildebrand, 1987 and Christensen et al., 1993; in Christensen et al., 1996.]

an expression of the size principle (see Chap. 4). Another possibility is that the hyperpolarization is due to a large IPSP in the glomerular tuft mediated by dendrodendritic connections through PG cells. This would require sensory input to PG cell dendrites.

Analysis of odor responses in principal neurons of the antennal lobe of the insect has thus yielded excitatory–inhibitory sequences similar to those described above in vertebrates (cf. Christensen et al, 1996). The similarity extends even to the brief hyperpolarization that precedes the initial EPSP and impulse burst. This suggests that despite differences in the morphological types of neurons, the synaptic circuits provide for common principles of odor-processing across phyla (reviewed in Hildebrand, 1995, 1996; Hildebrand and Shepherd, 1997).

LATERAL INHIBITION MEDIATES ODOR CONTRAST ENHANCEMENT

With the evidence that the fundamental units of odor information are sets of odor determinants processed by individual glomeruli, Mori and collaborators have tested for the role of the dendrodendritic microcircuits in processing that information (Yokoi et al., 1995). As noted above, the response of a mitral cell to a homologous series is limited to 2–3 neighboring members of a homologous series. A characteristic finding was that the members immediately flanking these compounds in a series elicited inhibition of the mitral cell (Fig. 5.16). This appears to be directly analogous to the contrast enhancement that characterizes the receptive field properties of cells in other systems,

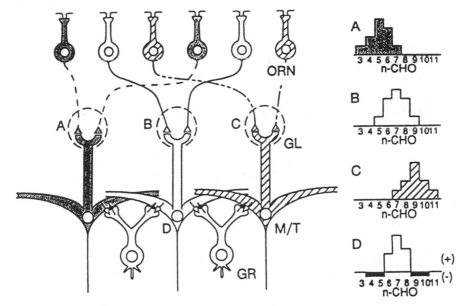

Fig. 5.16. Summary of the physiological evidence for contrast enhancement between responses of mitral cells connected to neighboring glomeruli. Diagram illustrates response spectra of olfactory receptor neuron (ORN) subsets that project to three neighboring glomeruli (GL), and the role of dendrodendritic lateral inhibition in sharpening the contrast. M/T, mitral/tufted cell; GR, granule cell; open arrowhead, excitatory mitral-to-granule synapse; closed arrowhead, inhibitory granule-to-mitral synapse. **A–C:** Different glomeruli receiving inputs from different ORN subsets, with different response spectra (A–C at right) to a series (3–11) of aliphatic aldehydes (n-CHO); **D:** mitral cell receiving input from glomerulus B has narrower response range because of lateral inhibition of neighbors, shown by horizontal black bars below abscissa in D on right. [From Yokoi et al., 1995, with permission.]

except that here it involves not spatial contrast to enhance edge detection between light and dark fields but rather molecular determinant contrast to enhance detection between differing odotopes (functional groups) in related compounds. Application of bicuculline abolished the inhibition, indicating that it is mediated by $GABA_A$ receptors; further evidence suggested that this GABAergic inhibition is mediated by the interactions of granule cells with the mitral/tufted cells.

These experiments thus provide the most direct evidence to date that a critical role of the dendrodendritic lateral inhibition of mitral cells by granule cells is to enhance contrast between the activity of mitral cells transmitting information about different odor stimuli. In view of the evidence for the action of the glomerulus as a functional unit, it is reasonable to hypothesize that the contrast enhancement occurs between mitral cells relaying information from different glomeruli (Fig. 5.4, 5.16). These mechanisms are likely to play a critical role in the ability to carry out odor discrimination, whether between single-odor compounds or between complex odors.

The combinations of excitatory and inhibitory MRRs have further suggested that "odor-opponent" interactions exist between mitral cells belonging to different glomerular units, which is analogous to color-opponent interactions in the retina (Shepherd,

1992; Mori et al., 1992; Mori and Shepherd, 1994; Mori and Yoshihara, 1995). This is a useful hypothesis to be tested.

MODULATION OF RECURRENT INHIBITION MEDIATES ODOR MEMORY

The dendrodendritic synaptic microcircuit has emerged as an attractive model for examining the factors underlying plasticity at single synapses. Olfactory learning can be demonstrated early in development; rat pups, for example, use odors present in utero to identify the location and behavioral meaning of their mother's nipple after birth. Olfactory learning is not restricted to early development and can be demonstrated at all ages. Adult female mice, for example, learn the odor of an impregnating male. However, if she later is exposed to the odor of a strange male, the pregnancy is blocked because the fertilized egg is rejected. This blockade, known as the *Bruce effect* (Bruce, 1959), is believed to enhance outbreeding by the female mice.

Many of the morphological, metabolic, and physiologic changes that result from olfactory learning occur in the olfactory bulb. Early studies demonstrated the involvement of glutamate receptors and GABAergic transmission in olfactory learning. Several types of olfactory learning are also dependent on the presence of norepinephrine,

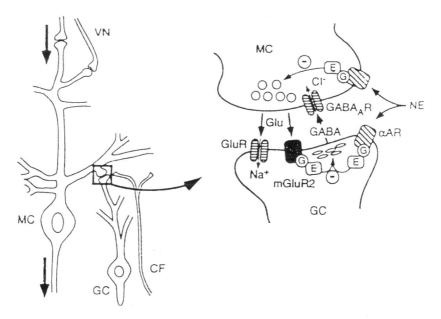

Fig. 5.17. Synaptic mechanism proposed to underly memory storage in the mouse accessory olfactory bulb. Left: Schematic diagram of basic circuit, showing axons from vomeronasal (VN) organ making synapses on mitral cell. Right: Diagram of synaptic receptors and second-messenger actions at the dendrodendritic reciprocal synapses between mitral cell (MC) dendrite and granule cell (GC) dendritic spine. Activated mitral cell releases glutamate, acting on GluR to generate EPSP but also activating mGluR, which produces long-term depression of recurrent GABAergic inhibition of the activated mitral cell. See text. Abbreviations: CF, centrifugal (noradrenergic) fibers; G, G protein; E, intracellular effector; for other abbreviations, see Fig. 5.4. [From Kaba et al., 1995, with permission.]

and noradrenergic modulation of dendrodendritic inhibition has been proposed as its site of action.

Recent studies suggest that changes in the efficacy of dendrodendritic reciprocal excitatory–inhibitory synapses between mitral and granule cells in the accessory olfactory bulb mediate the olfactory learning represented by the Bruce effect. The mGluR2 subtype of the metabotropic glutamate receptor family, found predominantly on granule cell dendrites, may play a critical role in this learning. The evidence for this role is summarized as follows (see Fig. 5.17). Release of glutamate from a mitral cell activates the mGluR2 receptor on the granule cells it contacts and reduces reciprocal inhibitory transmission from those granule cells, thereby enhancing the mitral cell's output to the cortex. Infusions of a specific mGluR2 agonist, DCG-IV, into the accessory olfactory bulb of a female mouse, coupled with exposure to the odor of a male mouse, induces the formation of a memory of that pheromone which ordinarily would occur only during mating to this male. If the female now mates with a second male, she forms a memory for the second male's odor in the usual manner. However, the memory for the first odor, formed by mGluR2 activation but without mating, prevents the pregnancy block that ordinarily would occur on re-exposure to the first male after the female has mated with the second male. Thus, a reduction of reciprocal inhibition from granule cells to mitral cells, through mGluR2 activation, mimicks the memory formation that occurs during mating.

It has been suggested (Marty and Llano, 1995) that these data constitute the best evidence in a mammalian system of a link between a specific learned behavior and changes in the efficacy of an identified synapse.

6

RETINA

PETER STERLING

The retina is a thin sheet of neural tissue lining the posterior hemisphere of the eye ball. It is actually part of the brain itself ($\sim$0.5%), evaginating from the lateral wall of the neural tube during embryonic development. The optic stalk grows out from the brain toward the ectoderm, inducing it to form an optical system (cornea, pupil, lens), which projects a physical image of the world onto the retina. The retina's task is to convert this optical image into a "neural image" for transmission down the optic nerve to a multitude of centers for further analysis. The task is complex—which is reflected in the synaptic organization.

The transformation from optical to neural image involves three stages: (*1*) transduction of the image by *photoreceptors*; (*2*) transmission of these signals by excitatory chemical synapses to *bipolar neurons*; and (*3*) further transmission by excitatory chemical synapses to *ganglion cells*. Axons from the latter collect in the optic nerve and project forward to the brain. At each synaptic stage there are specialized laterally connecting neurons called, respectively, *horizontal* and *amacrine* cells. These modify (largely by inhibitory chemical synapses) forward transmission across the synaptic layers. These elements are shown schematically in Fig. 6.1.

A closer look at this apparently simple design (three interconnected layers and five broad classes of neuron) reveals additional complexity (Figs. 6.2, 6.3). Each neuron class is represented by several or many specific *types*. Each cell type is distinguished from others in its class by its characteristic morphology, connections, neurochemistry, and function (Rodieck and Brening, 1983; Sterling, 1983). This diversity, amounting to some 80 cellular types (Kolb et al., 1981; Sterling, 1983; Vaney, 1990), was puzzling at first, but a broad explanation has gradually emerged: it is impossible to encode all the information in an optical image using a single neural image. Therefore, the retina uses different cell types to create parallel circuits for simultaneous transmission of *multiple neural images* to the brain. The retina also creates separate circuits for different light levels—daylight, twilight, and starlight—but these share certain circuit components and use the same final pathways to the brain (Smith et al., 1986).

This chapter describes key cell types and their interconnection in parallel circuits. It also discusses how the functional architecture of a circuit depends on the functional architecture of its synapses. Finally, it suggests how the flow of visual information shifts between circuits that are specialized for different light levels and how the cir-

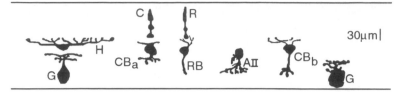

Fig. 6.1. Neuronal elements of the mammalian retina (same scale as diagrams for other regions). Symbols are defined in Fig. 6.2 legend.

cuits are switched. The chapter focuses on mammalian retina because that is where the combined knowledge of circuitry and cell physiology is best known. Early efforts centered on cat, so specific measurements, counts, etc. cited here refer to cat central retina. But recent efforts have broadened to include rabbit, rat, monkey, and human. These demonstrate strongly conserved patterns in the circuitry, as well as special adaptations, and some of both will be mentioned.

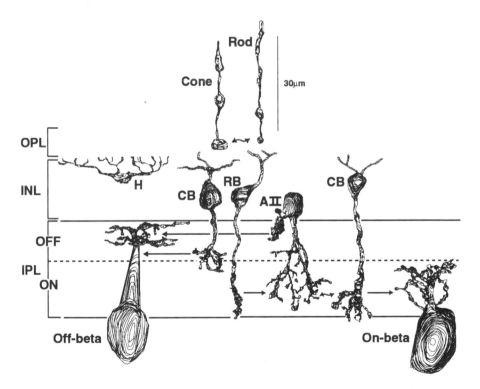

Fig. 6.2. Neuronal elements, scale enlarged in the vertical axis, to show more clearly the cell morphology and layers. Inputs: rod and cone photoreceptors. **Principal neurons:** ON and OFF ganglion cells. **Intrinsic neurons:** rod bipolar (RB) and cone bipolar (CB) neurons; horizontal (H), and amacrine neurons (A). OPL, outer plexiform layer; INL, inner nuclear layer; IPL, inner plexiform layer. AII designates a specific type of amacrine cell that serves the starlight circuit (see text).

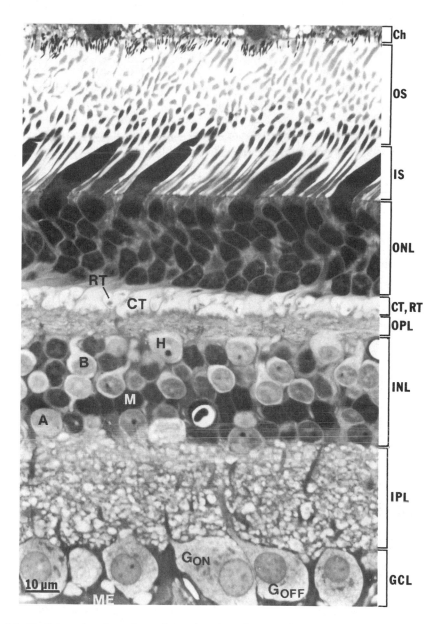

Fig. 6.3. Radial section through monkey retina about 5 mm (~25 degrees) from the fovea. Here cone and rod inner segments are easily distinguished from each other, as are their terminals in the outer plexiform layer. Pigmented cells of the choroid layer (Ch) attach the active form of vitamin A (aldehyde) to opsin and return it to the outer segments. Pigment cells also phagocytose membrane discs shed daily from the outer segment tips. OS, outer segments; IS, inner segments; ONL, outer nuclear layer; CT, cone terminal; RT, rod terminal; OPL, outer plexiform layer; INL, inner nuclear layer; IPL, inner plexiform layer; GCL, ganglion cell layer; B, bipolar cell; M, Müller cells; H, horizontal cells; A, amacrine cells; ME, Müller end feet; G_{ON}, ON ganglion cell; G_{OFF}, OFF ganglion cell. [Light micrograph from N. Vardi.]

NEURONAL ELEMENTS

INPUT ELEMENTS: RECEPTORS

Photoreceptors are elongated (Fig. 6.4). The distal tip points toward the back of the eye, away from the light, and is embedded in folds of melanotic epithelium. The outer segment contains about 900 membranous discs, stacked perpendicular to the cell's long axis (Fig. 6.4B). The disc surface is densely packed with molecules of the photopigment rhodopsin at nearly 60,000 per disc (reviewed in Pugh and Lamb, 1993). The inner segment is filled with mitochondria. These fuel the ion pumps essential for transduction and raise the refractive index, thereby creating a wave-guide that traps photons and funnels them to the outer segment (Enoch, 1981).

The photoreceptor between the mitochondrial segment and the soma contains the usual machinery for protein synthesis and packaging. Because the soma is stouter than

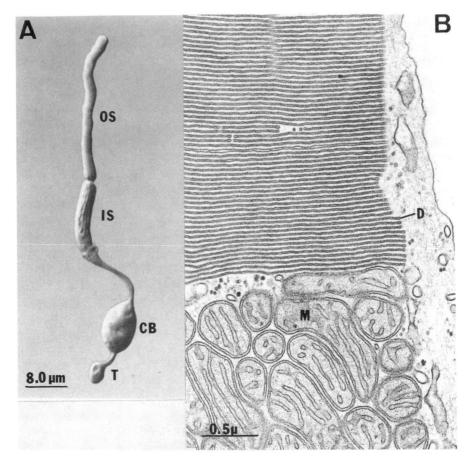

Fig. 6.4. **A:** Isolated rod photoreceptor (rabbit) showing the cell's distinct regions. Light micrograph. **B:** Radial section through rod outer/inner segment junction (salamander) showing regularly spaced membranous discs (D) and densely packed mitochondria (M). [Electron micrographs from Townes-Anderson et al., 1985; 1988, with permission.]

the inner segment (which packs densely with its neighbors), the somas pile up in tiers (outer nuclear layer; Fig. 6.3). The photoreceptor axon is generally short, 50 microns or less, except those in the fovea, where extremely dense packing of cones leaves no room for connections to the second- and third-order neurons. Then receptor axons can be as long as 500 microns (Polyak, 1941; Schein, 1988; Hsu et al., 1997). The photoreceptor axon ends without branching, in a single, highly specialized synapse that contains one or more synaptic "ribbons" (see Figs. 6.4, 6.13).

Intensity Range. Light intensity in the natural environment varies over a range of about 10^{10}, and we can see over this entire range. Two types of receptor divide the range: rods for night and cones for day. In mammals both have a narrow outer segment; which is 1–2 μm diameter for the rod and 3–5 μm diameter for the cone. This ensures a small cytoplasmic volume, which is essential to a rapid response time, and this in turn matches our rapid movements. By comparison, the rods of sluggish amphibians have a 5-fold greater diameter (25-fold greater volume) and partly as a consequence are 10-fold slower (Pugh and Lamb, 1993). So, if our photoreceptors were large, sports such as baseball or tennis would be out of the question.

This design feature (of narrow diameter) limits the number of photons that a receptor can collect within an "integration time." A rod integrates photon signals over about 300 msec (Yau, 1994); yet starlight presents it with only 1 photon per 10 minutes! So even when the light is 2000 times brighter, there is still only 1 photon per rod per integration time. Thus from dusk to dimmest starlight the rod detects single photons and needs to transmit only a *binary signal:* 0 photons or 1. The task of transmitting this irreducibly simple message shapes the circuit design at all stages proximal to the outer segment. For example, the rod axon is extremely thin (0.25 μm), and the synaptic terminal is small, with a single ribbon synapse (see Figs. 6.4, 6.13).

A cone integrates photon signals over about 50 msec. During this interval, bright sun delivers about 10^5 photons per cone, and twilight, with color just barely discernible, delivers about 100 photons per cone (Schnapf et al., 1990). Thus, a cone integrates many photons to give a *graded signal* with good temporal resolution. The cone, having much more information to transmit than a rod, employs a thicker axon (1.6 μm) and a larger terminal with many ribbon synapses (see Fig. 6.13). At dusk, as light intensity drops below cone threshold (marked by loss of color perception), the rod is collecting up to 100 photons per integration time. Thus, over a modest range (2 log units of intensity) the rod produces a graded signal that fills in for the failing cone. This graded rod signal for twilight is routed differently from the binary signal for starlight (see Circuits, below).

Spectral Sensitivity. Mammals have a single type of rod (peak spectral sensitivity at 500 nm). This makes sense because at night photons are too sparse to be worth segregating by wavelength. But in daylight there are plenty of photons, so most mammals gain extra information by using two cone types with different spectral sensitivity (Barlow, 1982). Most cones (at least 90%) are tuned to middle wavelengths (~550 nm), termed "M" or "green" (reviewed by Jacobs, 1993). A few are tuned to short wavelengths (~450 nm), termed "S" or "blue." Because S cones can be distinguished by morphology, by staining with Procion dye, and by antibody to the photopigment, we know that they form a sparse, but regular mosaic (de Monasterio et al., 1981; Szél et al., 1988; Ahnelt et al., 1990; Curcio et al., 1991). These anatomical methods confirm psychophysical maps of punctate sensitivity to S cone stimuli (Williams et al., 1981). S cones connect via a selective circuit to a special type of ganglion cell (see Circuits, below).

Old World primates (including humans) are special in being "trichromatic," meaning that there is an additional cone type tuned to long wavelengths (peak ~570 nm), termed "L" or "red." The M and L cone pigments are nearly identical except for a few critical amino acids in the transmembrane region, so antibodies have not yet distinguished them (Neitz et al., 1991). Spectral sensitivity mapped for cone populations in situ shows M and L cones in monkey to be equally numerous and to distribute in small, apparently random clusters (Mollon and Bowmaker, 1992; Packer et al., 1996). How these cones connect to ganglion cells is naturally of great interest and is presently controversial (Dacey, 1996; Calkins and Sterling, 1997a).

Some animals using three cone pigments, such as fish, turtles, and birds, may express up to seven types of cone! This trick is accomplished by fitting the inner segment with an oil droplet of specific color/absorbance (red, yellow/ultraviolet). These serve as filters to limit the spectral composition of the light entering the outer segment (e.g., Ohtsuka, 1985). Also, evolution tunes cone pigments to match the environment's spectral content. For example, Lake Baikal is very clear and deep, but longer wavelengths fail to penetrate at greater depths. Consequently, fish species at greater depths shift their cone pigments down the spectrum (Bowmaker et al., 1994). Equally wonderful in its vision capability is the kestrel (a falcon), which has a cone type tuned to ultraviolet (~350 nm). Soaring high with this receptor, it can identify the urine trails of its prey (meadow vole), which in sunlight fluoresce UV (Viitala et al., 1995).

INTRINSIC ELEMENTS FOR FORWARD TRANSMISSION: BIPOLAR AND AII CELLS

Bipolar Cells. Bipolar somas occupy the middle region of the inner nuclear layer (Fig. 6.3). Their dendrites ascend to collect synapses from photoreceptors. In amphibia a given bipolar cell collects from both rods and cones, probably because both give graded signals. But in mammals one bipolar type collects only from rods, and other types collect only from cones. Bipolar axons descend to the inner plexiform layer where they provide ribbon synapses, each directed at a pair of postsynaptic processes, termed a "dyad" (see below; Dowling and Boycott, 1966).

The rod bipolar soma (7 μm) is located high in the outer nuclear layer (Fig. 6.5). The narrow, candelabra-like, dendritic arbor penetrates the stratum of cone terminals to reach the overlying rod terminals where it collects signals from 20 rods in cat and up to 80 rods or more in rabbit (Dacheux and Raviola, 1986; Young and Vaney, 1991). The rod bipolar axon descends without branching to the deepest stratum of the inner plexiform layer where it contacts, not ganglion cells, but a third-order, intrinsic neuron, termed the "AII" amacrine cell (Fig. 6.2; Kolb and Famiglietti, 1974; McGuire et al., 1984; Freed et al., 1987; Strettoi et al., 1990; Wässle et al., 1991). The rod bipolar terminal employs 30 ribbon synapses, with little variation within or between animals (McGuire et al., 1984; Rao and Sterling, 1991).

The cone bipolar somas are also small (~8 μm), and the dendritic fields are narrow (~15 μm; Fig. 6.6). The dendritic arbor typically collects from 5 to 10 overlying cone

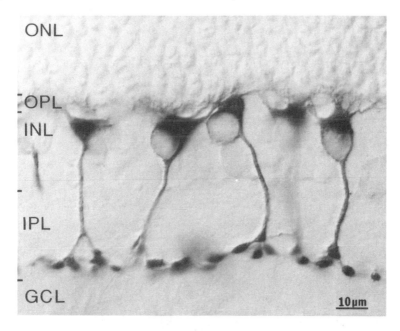

Fig. 6.5. Rod bipolar array (rabbit) immunostained for protein kinase C. Dendrites of adjacent cells overlap modestly in OPL, but axon terminals simply "tile" the deepest level of the IPL without overlap. [Light micrograph from Young and Vaney, 1991, with permission.]

terminals without skipping any (Cohen and Sterling, 1990a,b; Boycott and Wässle, 1991; Calkins and Sterling, 1996). An exception is the S cone bipolar cell which *does* skip overlying M and L cones to contact S cones exclusively (Mariani, 1984; Kouyama and Marshak, 1992). The S cone bipolar cell has been defined clearly in monkey and probably corresponds to the wide-field cone bipolar in cat and other mammals that also skips certain cones (e.g., type **b₅**, Fig. 6.6). Cone bipolar axons descend to the IPL where each type selects a particular stratum and contacts both amacrine and ganglion cells (Fig. 6.6). Cone bipolar terminals employ 30–100 ribbon synapses, depending on cell type (Cohen and Sterling, 1990a; Calkins et al., 1994).

ON vs. OFF Bipolar Types. It was discovered early that some bipolar cells are excited (i.e., depolarized) by light onset whereas others are excited by light offset (Werblin and Dowling, 1969; Kaneko, 1970). How the cone synapse manages to drive these cells in opposite directions is explained later (see Fig. 6.15). But here we note that the two categories of axon terminate at different levels: OFF axons end in the upper half of the inner plexiform layer, and ON axons arborize in the lower half (Fig. 6.2). Within these OFF and ON laminae, multiple types segregate in different strata (Fig. 6.6; Kolb et al., 1981; Cohen and Sterling, 1990a; Boycott and Wässle, 1991; Euler et al., 1996). It was unexpected that ON and OFF bipolar cells would comprise so many types (~4–5 types of each category). Since all types (except for the S cone bipolar cell) collect from the same cones, their spatial and spectral inputs are identical. Therefore, one surmises that they carry different *temporal* components of the cone signal. Indeed, two types of ON

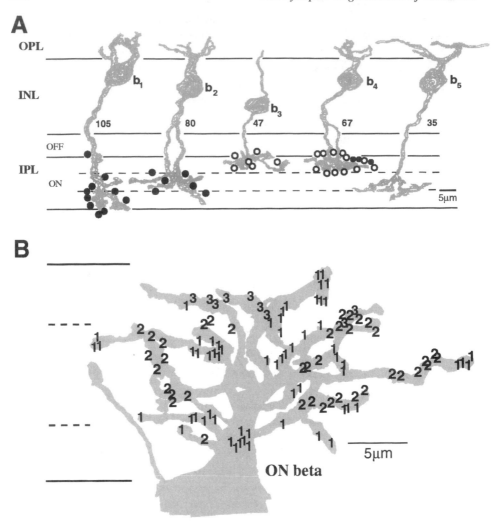

Fig. 6.6. **A:** Multiple types of ON cone bipolar cell with axons in the ON sublayer of the IPL. Each type expresses a different number of ribbon outputs (noted at the right of each axon) and a different pattern of gap junctions (filled, open circles). Types b_1–b_4 collect signals from all the overlying cones without skipping any; type b_5 ignores the immediately overlying cones and reaches widely to collect signals from outlying cones. [Reconstructions from Cohen and Sterling, 1990a,b, with permission.] **B:** ON-beta ganglion cell arborizes among all types of ON cone bipolar axon, but collects ribbon synapses from only three types (b_1, b_2, b_3) in the proportion 80:40:20. [From Cohen and Sterling, 1992, with permission.]

bipolar cell in carp do differ temporally, one depolarizing sustainedly to steady illumination, the other depolarizing transiently (Saito et al., 1985).

All Cell. The AII soma in the amacrine cell layer sends a thick stalk to the ON level of the inner plexiform layer where it arborizes richly to collect chemical synapses from rod bipolar terminals (Fig. 6.2; Kolb and Famiglietti, 1974; Vaney, 1985; Sterling et al., 1988; Strettoi et al., 1990). This arbor also forms numerous, large gap junctions with the axon terminals of ON cone bipolar cells. When these gap junctions are in a conducting state, depolarizing currents, resulting from rod bipolar excitation, spread from AII into the cone bipolar terminals, evoking their transmitter release onto ganglion cells (see Fig. 6.20). The AII also forms "lobular appendages" at the OFF level of the inner plexiform layer. These structures, jammed with mitochondria and synaptic vesicles, provide inhibitory chemical synapses to OFF bipolar terminals and OFF ganglion cell dendrites (McGuire et al., 1984; Kolb and Nelson, 1993). This wiring explains how a single type of rod bipolar cell can simultaneously excite the ON and inhibit the OFF ganglion cells (Sterling, 1983; Mastronarde, 1983).

OUTPUT ELEMENTS: GANGLION CELLS

Ganglion cell bodies form the innermost cellular layer of the retina (Figs. 6.2, 6.3). Their dendrites penetrate the inner plexiform layer to collect excitatory synapses from bipolar axons and both excitatory and inhibitory synapses from amacrine cells. Ganglion cell axons enter the optic nerve and extend to the brain. The domestic cat optic nerve contains about 160,000 axons (260,000 for its wild progenitor; Williams et al., 1993a); the human nerve contains about 1.2 million axons and the macaque optic nerve contains about 1.8 million axons (Potts et al., 1972). Since the number of fibers in the optic nerve can vary 10-fold, it does not seem to be a physical "bottleneck" for information outflow as was commonly thought. Thus many cones converge onto a single ganglion cell—not to reduce the number of transmission channels in the nerve, but for deeper reasons, to which we shall return.

Ganglion cell somas look pretty much alike (Fig. 6.3), but Golgi impregnations revealed the dendritic arbors to be remarkably diverse—twenty types or more (e.g., Polyak, 1941; Boycott and Dowling, 1969; Cajal, 1972; Boycott and Wässle, 1974; Kolb et al., 1981). Now that one can record data from a ganglion cell in vitro and render its dendritic arbor visible by injecting dye, we realize that each morphological type has a distinctive physiology. For example, the ganglion cell with a planar, "loopy" dendritic arbor responds selectively to stimuli moving in a particular direction (see Fig. 6.12; Amthor et al., 1989). This structure–function correspondence was first shown in rabbit, but holds also for cat (Berson et al., 1996, 1997; Isayama et al., 1997) and probably also for primate. Thus, a ganglion cell type carrying a particular sort of information can (like a gene) be conserved across species.

Each type of ganglion cell distributes to a particular brain region, which uses the special information carried by that cell. Thus, the nucleus of the optic tract, which controls optokinetic eye movements, collects from the directionally selective ganglion cell (Pu and Amthor, 1990; Pu et al., 1997). And the suprachiasmatic nucleus, which uses light to reset circadian rhythms, collects from other types branching over extremely wide areas. Still other types of motion-selective ganglion cell project to the superior colliculus, which uses the information to orient the head and eyes (Rodieck and Watanabe, 1993; Berson et al., 1996, 1997; Isayama et al., 1997). Such subcortical "housekeeping" centers use about 40% of the cat's ganglion cells. But these cells have small somas ($\sim$10 μm) and fine axons (0.3 μm in diameter), so they occupy less than 5% of the optic nerve cross section. Similar numbers of housekeeping ganglion cells are required in primates, but obviously their proportion of all ganglion cells is much smaller (Rodieck et al., 1993).

The key region for mammalian visual processing is the striate cortex, which receives its main thalamic input from the dorsal lateral geniculate nucleus. Thus, it is to this nucleus that most ganglion cells project (60% in cat; 90% in monkey). Two major classes of ganglion cell in cat are geniculate-bound: "beta" and "alpha" cells (Fig. 6.7; Boycott and Wässle, 1974; Wässle et al., 1981a,b). The beta cell has a narrow, bushy dendritic tree and a sustained (tonic) discharge of action potentials to a maintained stimulus (Figs. 6.2, 6.7). The alpha cell has a wider, sparser dendritic tree and a transient (phasic) discharge (Cleland and Levick, 1974; Stone and Fukuda, 1974; Saito, 1983). The beta and alpha cells are each of two types, one with dendrites in the ON strata of the inner plexiform layer, the other with dendrites in the OFF strata (Fig. 6.7; Famiglietti and Kolb, 1976). The former are excited by light onset; the latter are excited by light offset (Fig. 6.7; Nelson et al., 1978). Thus they are termed ON beta, OFF beta, ON alpha, and OFF alpha.

The primate retina expresses a similar division into ON and OFF versions of narrow-field, tonic cells and wider-field, phasic cells (e.g., de Monasterio, 1978). The narrow-field types are termed *midget cells* because in central retina the dendritic arbor collects from a midget bipolar cell with input from a single cone (Polyak, 1941; Kolb and Dekorver, 1991; Calkins et al., 1994), but more peripherally the arbor broadens to collect from many midget bipolar axons (Watanabe and Rodieck, 1989; Dacey, 1993; Goodchild et al., 1996b). Midget cells are also termed "P" cells because they project to the lateral geniculate's **p**arvocellular layers. The wider-field cells are of at least two types: *parasol*, with flat dendritic arbors, and *garland*, with gnarly, 3-D arbors (Polyak, 1941; Boycott and Dowling, 1969). The two types are commonly lumped together as

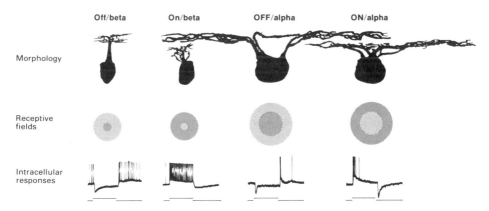

Fig. 6.7. Form and function of cat ganglion cells. Beta cells have a narrow dendritic field, and alpha cells a broad one (top row, vertical views). Cells are maximally excited by stimuli covering the whole dendritic field, corresponding to the *receptive* field "center" and maximally suppressed by stimuli filling the outer annulus, termed the receptive field "surround" (middle row, tangential views). ON cells, excited by *in*creased intensity on the center, arborize deep in the inner plexiform layer; OFF cells, excited by *de*creased intensity on the center, arborize superficially. Beta cells give a transient plus sustained response; alpha cells give mainly a transient response. [Intracellular recordings from Saito, 1983.]

"M" cells because they project to the geniculate's magnocellular layers (Perry et al., 1984; reviewed by Kaplan et al., 1990). Two physiological types of M cell, linear and nonlinear (Kaplan and Shapley, 1982; Shapley and Perry, 1986), may correspond, respectively, to the parasol and garland morphologies (Sterling et al., 1994).

Over a decade of intense description, physiologists divided ganglion cells into different functional categories: Y (brisk-transient), X (brisk-sustained), and W (other, including edge-detector, directionally sensitive, etc.). Simultaneously morphologists categorized ganglion cells by dendritic branching patterns: alpha (planar-radiate), beta (3-D-bushy), gamma (other, including planar-sparse, planar-loopy, etc.). It was quickly appreciated that functional categories might map onto the morphological ones, but to prove this directly by recording, followed by tracer injection, required almost another decade (e.g., Saito, 1983). This correspondence of structure to function in ganglion cells is now firmly established as a principle of retinal organization, and consequently a type can be named for its function (e.g., directionally sensitive; see Fig. 6.12C) or its morphology (alpha, beta; Fig. 6.7) without any confusion. However, when a category is named for its central projection, such as M or P, one must remember that several types can project to the same locus. Thus one expects multiple types of M and P cell.

INTRINSIC ELEMENTS FOR LATERAL TRANSMISSION: HORIZONTAL AND AMACRINE CELLS

Horizontal Cells. Horizontal cell somas form the upper tier of the inner nuclear layer (Fig. 6.3), and the processes connect exclusively within the outer plexiform layer. Collecting widely from receptors, their main task is to average the signals and feed negatively back onto receptor terminals and forward onto bipolar dendrites. Horizontal cells couple to each other electrically. The strength of this coupling changes with adaptive state and is modulated by dopamine secreted by certain cells in the amacrine layer (reviewed by Murakami et al., 1995). In fish these are "interplexiform" cells which are contacted in turn by centrifugal axons from the brain (Dowling, 1986). Catfish horizontal cells send axons to the inner plexiform layer (Sakai and Naka, 1985), but this is not the general plan.

Two types of horizontal cell in diurnal mammals connect with cones (Fig. 6.8). One has thick dendrites, a wide field, and couples strongly to its neighbors; the other has slender dendrites, a narrow field, and couples weakly (reviewed by Vaney, 1994a; Mills and Massey, 1994; Sandmann et al., 1996). Generally each type connects to all the cone terminals in its dendritic field. However, in primate the large-field cell avoids S cones, and the narrow-field cell connects especially strongly to them (Dacey, et al., 1996; Goodchild et al., 1996a; see also Sandmann et al., 1996). Within this general framework there are some quite spectacular morphological variations whose functions remain mysterious (see, e.g., Müller and Peichl, 1993).

One type of horizontal cell connects with rods. It does so by emitting a fine axon that in cat meanders for several millimeters and then breaks into an elaborate arbor that contacts several thousand rods (Fig. 6.8). This axon also couples to its neighbors and thus pools signals from tens of thousands of rods (Vaney, 1993). This is not the usual sort of axon for it lacks action potentials; further, cone input to the dendrites does not reach the rod axon arbor, so it must be electrically isolated from the soma (Nelson, 1977). On the other hand, the horizontal cell soma *does* receive strong rod sig-

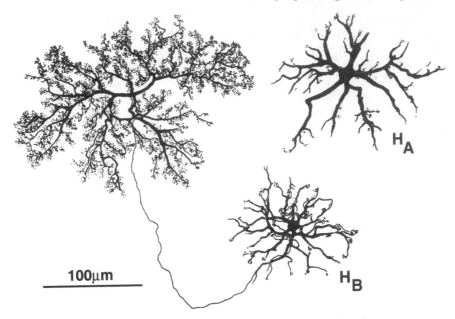

Fig. 6.8. Two types of horizontal cell from cat retina as seen in tangential view following Golgi impregnation. Dendrites of types A and B both connect with cones; axon arbor of type B connects with about 3000 rods. [From Fisher and Boycott, 1974, with permission.]

nals (e.g., Steinberg, 1969; Nelson, 1977; Lankeet et al., 1996), which must therefore come via rod-to-cone gap junctions (Raviola and Gilula, 1973; Kolb, 1977; Smith et al., 1986). Thus the soma serves metabolically two processes with utterly different connections. It doesn't seem to matter which type of horizontal cell produces the axon, since in cat and rabbit it is the wide-field cell, and in primate it is the narrow-field cell (reviewed by Sandmann et al., 1996).

Amacrine Cells. Amacrine somas form the lower tier of the inner nuclear layer and are also numerous in the ganglion cell layer, here they are called *displaced.* Amacrine cells connect exclusively within the inner plexiform layer (plus some synapses in the ganglion cell fiber layer) and are diverse in the extreme; there are 40 types or more (Kolb et al., 1981; Vaney, 1990). Given such diversity, attempts to generalize are likely to be inadequate, but consider the following: (*1*) The AII amacrine, being narrow field (Fig. 6.2), distributes densely and thus constitutes about 20% of the amacrine layer cells. As noted, the AII collects purely from rod bipolars and serves a feedforward link in the rod's starlight pathway. (*2*) Certain narrow-field amacrines collect purely from cone bipolar terminals. These amacrines feed back reciprocally onto the bipolar terminal and forward onto the ganglion cell (see Fig. 6.14). These types, which exist as both ON and OFF forms, must distribute densely to tile the plane (Polyak, 1941; Kolb et al., 1981). This pattern of connection may reflect lateral inhibition across a small spatial scale covering tens of microns rather than hundreds as for the horizontal cells. (*3*) Certain medium-field amacrines collect from cone bipolars and arborize intimately with dendrites of certain ganglion cell types. For example, the *starburst* amacrine cell associates with other members of its own type (Fig. 6.9A; Tauchi and Masland, 1984) to form a loopy pattern that in rabbit associates with dendrites of the direction-selective ganglion cells (Vaney et al., 1989a; Famiglietti, 1992b), and in cat the alpha ganglion cell (Vardi et al., 1989). The starburst cell is also present in primate (Rodieck, 1989), where it probably associates with the co–planar arbors of parasol ganglion cells. There are separate starburst populations for the ON and OFF levels of the inner plexiform layer. The starburst cell responds phasically to glutamatergic bipolar input (kainate receptors; Linn et al., 1991) and releases a pulse of acetylcholine onto the ganglion cells (Masland et al., 1984; Massey and Redburn, 1985). The acetylcholine, binding to nicotinic receptors, excites ganglion cells (e.g., Schmidt et al., 1987; Kaneda et al., 1995). Thus, the starburst circuit probably boosts ganglion cell transient responses, enhancing sensitivity to motion. Several studies suggest that the starburst cell fires action potentials (Bloomfield, 1992; Jensen, 1995), but recent studies with whole cell recording report purely passive responses (Taylor and Wässle, 1995; Peters and Masland, 1996). (*4*) Certain types of wide-field amacrine collect exclusively rod bipolar input (A17; Nelson and Kolb, 1985), but other wide-field types arborize in strata supplied only by cone bipolar terminals. The "dendritic" fields reach about 500 to 1000 μm, which is probably near the electrotonic limit for fine, passive cables (Fig. 6.9C; Dacey, 1989a, 1990; Famiglietti, 1992a). However, the proximal region of each dendrite sprouts a fine axon that travels centripetally for at least 3 mm (Fig. 6.9B). Such a cell resembles a wagon wheel, with the dendritic field for a hub and the axons as radiating spokes (Fig. 6.9C). These axons conduct full action potentials (Dacheux and Raviola, 1995; Freed et al., 1996; Stafford and Dacey, 1996) which appear to travel centrifugally (Cook and Werblin, 1994). These long-range amacrine cells are obvious candidates to mediate the strong excitation of certain ganglion cells evoked by stimuli millimeters beyond the conventional receptive field (e.g., McIlwain, 1966; Derrington et al., 1979).

Interplexiform Cells. These cells have somas in the amacrine layer but send processes to both outer and inner plexiform layers (Cajal, 1972). The interplexiform cell receives synapses on its inner processes and provides synaptic outputs in both the inner and outer plexiform layers. In cat it forms chemical synapses upon both rod bipolar and cone bipolar dendrites (Kolb and West, 1977; Nakamura et al., 1980; McGuire et al., 1984; Cohen and Sterling, 1990a), and in fish it contacts horizontal cells (Dowling, 1986). Some authors refer to the interplexiform as a "sixth cell class", but it seems equally reasonable to consider it as one more extraordinary type of amacrine cell.

The interplexiform cell in New World monkey and fish contains dopamine (Dowling, 1986). In cat, the dopaminergic amacrine cell sends sporadic processes to the outer plexiform (Oyster et al., 1985). Since dopamine regulates horizontal cell coupling (Teranishi et al., 1984; Piccolino et al., 1984; Hampson et al., 1992; reviewed by Murakami et al., 1995) which shapes the inhibitory surround of cones and bipolar cells (see Fig. 6.17), the dopamine cells may adjust the surround's depth and extent to ambient image statistics.

Cat and rabbit interplexiform cells use GABA and contact bipolar dendrites, so they probably have a different function. Bipolar cells, being only 30–50 μm long, are isopo-

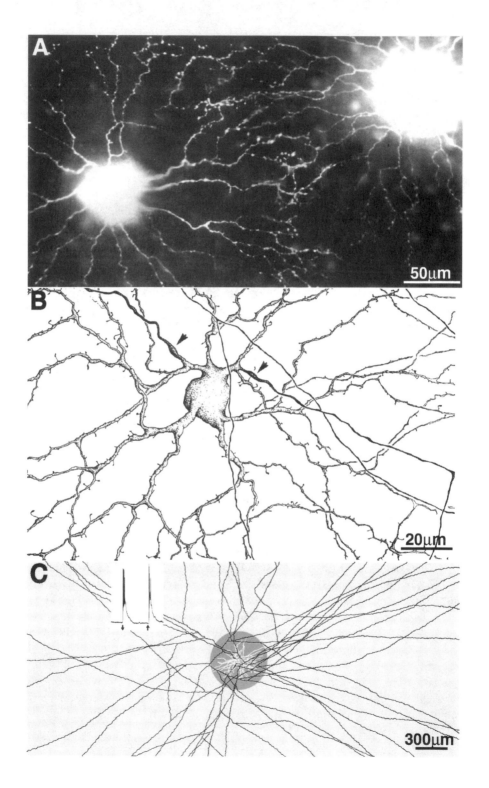

tential. Thus, if receptors postsynaptic to the interplexiform cell coupled directly to an ion channel (as do GABA$_A$ or GABA$_C$ receptors), there would be no advantage to placing the synapse distally on the bipolar dendrite versus placing it in the usual locus for an amacrine synapse, on the bipolar axon terminal. However, the concentration of a diffusible substance decays over extremely short distances (<1 μm; Berg, 1993), so placing the interplexiform synapse distally might imply a receptor coupled to a second messenger.

Centrifugal Fibers. Specific brain regions in certain vertebrates, including fish, amphibia, reptiles, and birds, produce efferent axons that travel in the optic nerve to terminate in the inner retina. In birds the "isthmo-optic nucleus", a substantial structure with a definite retino-topic organization, projects about 10,000 fibers centrifugally to the inner retina to terminate on a special type of amacrine cell (Dowling and Cowan, 1966; Uchiyama and Ito, 1993). In fish the olfactory bulb sends fibers containing a peptide (LHRH) to contact interplexiform cells (Zucker and Dowling, 1987). Thus, the idea is not entirely far fetched that an odor, a memory, or a feeling could modify the construction of a visual image in the retina—that beauty could be literally in the eye of the beholder. However, little is known regarding the function of these centrifugal pathways (Uchiyama and Barlow, 1994).

CELL POPULATIONS

Spatial Density of Receptors. Cones and rods pack densely, occupying 90% of the two-dimensional receptor sheet, with a residual extracellular space of about 10% (Fig. 6.10; Packer et al., 1989). Animals active in both day and night, such as human, macaque, cat, and rabbit, assign about 5% of their receptors to cones and the rest to rods. If this seems counterintuitive, simply recall that the photon flux in daytime is many orders of magnitude greater than at night. So in daytime the retina can operate effectively on a fraction of the photons striking the receptor sheet, whereas from dusk to dawn, every photon counts.

Cone density always peaks in central retina. Species whose lifestyle requires high spatial acuity, e.g., raptors scanning for prey from great heights, or primates foraging for fine morsels at close range, pack cones so densely at the center (*fovea*) that rods are completely excluded (Fig. 6.10). Then, through the connecting of each cone to a private (midget) bipolar cell followed by a midget ganglion cell, a neural image can be established at the output as fine as the *grain* of the cone array. In human fovea, cone density reaches nearly 200,000/mm^2 (Fig. 6.10), providing 120 cones/degree,

Fig. 6.9. Two types of amacrine cell in tangential view. **A:** Medium-field, "starburst" amacrine cells. Processes from adjacent cells associate to form a planar network with input from cone bipolar ribbon synapses and output to motion-sensitive ganglion cells, including the alpha and directionally selective ganglion cells. **B:** Wide-field amacrine cell whose proximal dendrites (spiny) emit multiple axons (arrowheads). **C:** Same cell at lower magnification. Cell fires transient burst of action potentials (inset) to ON and OFF of a stimulus to receptive field center (black disc) which corresponds to the dendritic field; action potentials travel centrifugally from the cell in all directions. [A from Tauchi and Masland, 1984; B and C from Stafford and Dacey, 1997, with permission.]

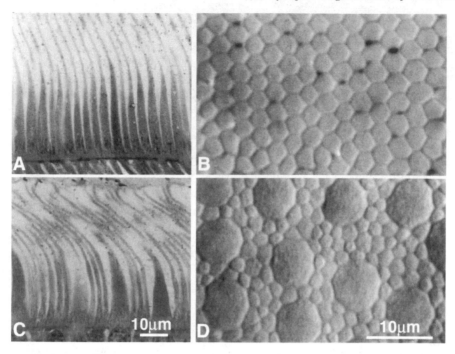

Fig. 6.10. Mosaic of photoreceptors (human). **A:** Fovea: vertical section shows cone inner segments to be narrow and gently tapered, the outer segments to be long and fine. **B:** Fovea: tangential section through base of inner segments shows hexagonal packing. Thus fovea provides fine spatial sampling in daylight, but absence of rods renders it useless in twilight. **C:** Periphery: vertical section shows cone inner segments to be squatter but still tapered and surrounded by rod inner segments that are much finer and untapered. **D:** Periphery: tangential view shows about 10 rods per cone, which can boost the cone signal in twilight (see text). Although cones comprise only 10% of the mosaic, their apertures occupy about 40% of the available collecting area. Yet at night, cones collect disproportionately few photons. As the pupil dilates, photons reach the retina over a wide range of angles, but the cone's wave-guide mechanism rejects all but the few arriving nearly perpendicular to the retina. Thus the wave-guide mechanism, which in daylight efficiently captures photons arriving from a narrow locus in space, in starlight is relatively transparent. [Light micrographs from Curcio et al., 1990, with permission.]

which is adequate to create a neural image of a grating as fine as 60 cycles/degree (Curcio et al., 1990; Williams, 1992, Smallman et al., 1996). In the eagle's fovea cone density and spatial acuity are about double this, apparently reaching a biophysical limit. Higher cone densities would require still finer inner segment, with a wave-guide mechanism that could no longer prevent photons from escaping to neighboring cones (Reymond, 1985).

Naturally, once light intensity falls below cone threshold, the fovea, lacking rods, becomes a blind spot. It is easy to convince yourself of this. At dusk, just as your perception of color fades completely, note that you have also lost the ability to read fine print (as in the *New York Times*). Now hold your thumb at arm's length and, as your gaze steadies upon it, it will disappear. At this distance, the thumb subtends about 1° on the retina, corresponding to the fovea's rod-free region. Thus, while your eyes are free to move, vision seems entirely normal and you do not suspect that 10^6 cones (and consequently about half of your striate cortex) have been silenced. So species that can accept somewhat coarser vision in daylight, but need to preserve it at night, reduce cone density at the center to accommodate rods. Thus, cat cone density is almost 10-fold lower than that of human in the central area ($30,000/mm^2$), yet allows for rods at $200,000/mm^2$ (Williams et al., 1993a). Rod density commonly peaks at about 15–25° from the center (Young and Vaney, 1991; Williams et al., 1993a; Curcio et al., 1990; Packer et al., 1989).

Receptor density declines toward the periphery. Conversely, receptor diameter generally increases, for example, in macaque by about 4-fold for cones and 2-fold for rods (Fig. 6.10D; Packer et al., 1989). This would make sense if the light-gathering efficiency of the optics declines toward the periphery, for then a larger receptor could still collect enough light to fill its dynamic range. Such factors must be considered in comparing densities. For example, peak rod density is about 2-fold greater in cat than in human ($400,000/mm^2$ vs. $175,000/mm^2$; see, e.g., Curcio et al., 1990; Williams, et al., 1993a), but the cat rod's collecting area is smaller by about the same factor. Thus, in terms of photon-collecting area these densities may be equivalent. One reason to make the cat rod finer is that the cat's eye collects more light (larger pupil, reflecting tapetum, etc.); therefore a finer cross section allows the rod to serve as a single photon detector over a wider intensity range.

Spatial density of different cone types also varies with retinal location. For example, the very center of human retina, termed *foveola*, includes M and L but not S cones (Williams et al., 1981; Curcio et al., 1990). This makes functional sense because when middle and long wavelengths are in sharp focus, short wavelengths are strongly blurred (Williams et al., 1993b). Therefore, to provide maximum spatial acuity, the foveola sacrifices trichromacy. S cones in mouse are sparse in superior retina but distribute densely to inferior retina, presumably because inferior retina views the sky (Szél et al., 1992).

That photoreceptor density is so finely sculpted across the retina implies an extremely efficient postreceptoral circuitry. Such local sculpting could evolve only if the small trades of rods for cones (or vice-versa) at each locus offered selective advantage. The improvement in signal quality would be proportional to the square root of the ratio in receptor density between two regions. For example, a 2-fold greater cone density would improve signal/noise for day vision by at most 1.4. If subsequent neural stages added noise by this factor or more, then any potential advantage to such a difference would be swamped. This alerts one to identify in the postreceptoral circuitry the key contributions to efficiency (see Functional Circuits, below).

Spatial Density of Postreceptoral Neurons. Postreceptoral cell types also distribute with characteristic spatial densities (Wässle and Riemann, 1978). These have been determined by standard histological methods, by reconstruction from electron micrographs (e.g., Sterling et al., 1988; Cohen and Sterling, 1990a; Klug et al., 1997), and also by immunostaining for a particular protein or epitope that fortuitously selects a particular type and stains the whole array. Thus, antibody to protein kinase C reveals the complete rod bipolar cell array (Fig. 6.5; Young and Vaney, 1991); anti-$G_{o\alpha}$ shows the ON cone bipolar cells (Vardi, 1997b); anti-recoverin shows OFF midget bipolar cells

(Fig. 6.11A; Milam et al., 1993; Wässle et al., 1994); anti-CCK shows S cone bipolars (Kouyama and Marshak, 1992); anti-calbindin shows the wide-field horizontal cells in cat and rabbit (Röhrenbeck et al., 1989); anti-calretinin shows the AII amacrine cells (Wässle et al., 1995), and so on. Also, because many cell types couple to their neigh-

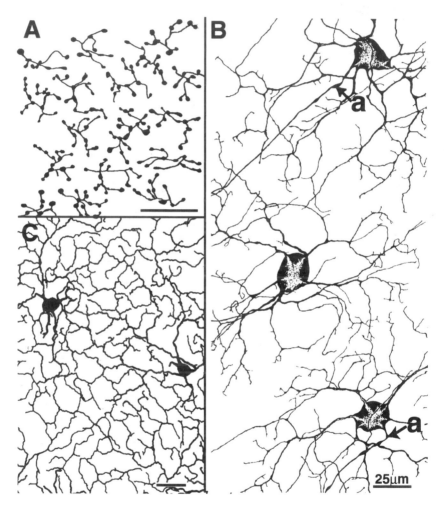

Fig. 6.11. **A:** Array of OFF midget bipolar terminals (macaque) in tangential view. Drawn from tissue immunostained for recoverin, about 10 mm beyond the fovea. The terminals "tile" the plane without overlap. **B:** Array of ON midget ganglion cells (human) in tangential view. Cells injected individually with neurobiotin, about 12 mm beyond fovea. The dendrites tile the plane without overlap and would collect input from many axons in the midget bipolar array shown in A. **C:** Array of directionally selective ganglion cells (only the OFF dendrites of the ON/OFF type are shown). One cell was injected with neurobiotin, which then spread to adjacent cells. Note the characteristic loopy dendrites that tile the plane without overlap. Such tiling behavior holds for all ganglion cells studied so far, with one exception discussed in the text. [A from Wässle et al., 1991; B from Dacey, 1993; C from D. Vaney after Vaney, 1994a, with permission.]

bors in the array, intracellular injection of a small tracer molecule (e.g., neurobiotin) has been used to establish the spatial densities (Figs. 6.11C, 6.12).

The spatial densities of postreceptoral neurons follow the photoreceptors in peaking centrally and declining toward the periphery. As spatial density falls, a cell type's arbor typically expands to compensate, so "tiling" or a specific degree of overlap (see below) is maintained (see, e.g., Wässle et al., 1978b, 1981a,b). However, the number of neurons converging upon a particular cell type may increase or remain constant. For example, rods converging onto the rod bipolar cell increase from about 15 in macaque central retina to about 60 in the periphery, whereas the number of cones converging upon a given type of cone bipolar cell remains constant at 5 to 10 (Grünert et al., 1994). Photoreceptors converging upon a ganglion cell increase linearly. For example, about 35 cones converge upon a central beta cell, but 180 cones converge on a peripheral beta cell (Tsukamoto et al., 1990).

Visual Acuity Set by the Finest Ganglion Cell Array. Spatial resolution is set by the finest sampling array at the retinal output. To discriminate the fine lines of a grating from a homogeneous field requires one ganglion cell for each dark or bright line (reviewed by Wässle and Boycott, 1991; Tsukamoto and Sterling, 1991). In the fovea, since a midget ganglion cell connects to only one cone, resolution corresponds to the cone sampling frequency. But outside the fovea, many cones converge on a midget ganglion cell (Fig. 6.11B), so resolution is set by the midget cell array. Similarly, in cat, resolution is set by the beta cell array. Since pairs of ON and OFF of the same cell class (e.g., midget, beta) sample the same territory (see Fig. 6.15), resolution is set by the density of one of these arrays, but not their sum (reviewed in Wässle and Boycott, 1991).

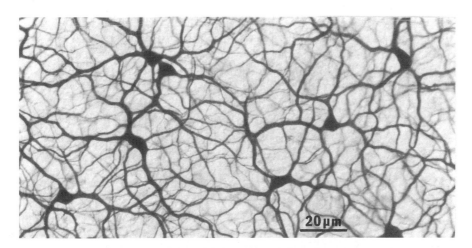

Fig. 6.12. Array of type A horizontal cells (rabbit) in tangential view. One cell was injected with neurobiotin, which then spread through gap junctions to reveal the whole array. Note the characteristics of this array: stout cables, strong coupling, and extensive overlap (cf. Fig. 6.11). [From S. Mills, after Mills and Massey, 1994, with permission.]

Tiling vs. Overlap of Neuronal Arbors. Along the *forward pathways from cones* the neural arbors of a given type do not overlap. Instead they show *mutual avoidance*, also termed *territoriality* (Wässle et al., 1981b). Consequently, their fields tend to "tile" the plane of the retina, forming a quasi-regular meshwork (Panico and Sterling, 1995). This rule holds for cone dendrites of each bipolar type and also for their axon terminals (Fig. 6.11A; Cohen and Sterling, 1990a,b; Boycott and Wässle, 1991.

Ganglion cell dendritic fields also tile. This has been shown for alpha cells and delta cells in cat (Dann et al., 1988; Dacey, 1989b), for ON-OFF directionally selective ganglion cells in rabbit (Fig. 6.11C; Vaney, 1994b), and for parasol and midget ganglion cells in primate (Fig. 6.11B; Dacey and Brace, 1992; Dacey, 1993). Although beta ganglion cell dendrites in cat central retina appear to overlap (Cohen and Sterling, 1992), their dendrites extend through several strata of the inner plexiform layer (IPL) (Fig. 6.6B) and may tile each stratum separately. Thus their apparent overlap may be an artifact of conventional light microscopy which collapses their 3-D dendritic fields. In short, tiling by ganglion cell dendritic arbors appears to be a general rule waiting for an exception. The lattice structures formed by presynaptic cone bipolar axon arbors and postsynaptic ganglion cell dendritic arbors are complementary (compare Fig. 6.11A with B). That is, the bipolar axon terminals just about fit the "holes" in the ganglion cell lattice. This connects the two arrays reliably while minimizing cost in materials and in the volume occupied by the lattices (Panico and Sterling, 1995).

Overall, a cone terminal, being narrower than the bipolar dendritic field, contributes most of its synapses to one member of each bipolar array and a few synapses to some neighbors (Sterling et al., 1988; Cohen and Sterling, 1990b). Similarly the cone bipolar axon arbor is narrower than the ganglion cell dendritic field (compare Fig. 6.6A with B; Fig. 6.11A with B) and contributes most of its synapses to one ganglion cell. Consequently, cone signals diverge very little on their course toward the retinal output, and a cone contributes most of its synapses to one member of a ganglion cell array (Sterling et al., 1988).

Along *forward pathways from rods*, certain neural arbors *do* overlap. Thus, rod bipolar dendrites overlap enough that every rod synapse, though approximating a point in the plane of the retina, contacts at least two bipolar cells (Fig. 6.5; Sterling et al., 1988; Young and Vaney, 1991). Similarly, the AII cell's collecting arbor in the inner plexiform layer overlaps more extensively, by 2- to 3-fold in central retina of cat, rabbit, and monkey and up to 10-fold in peripheral retina of rabbit (Vaney, 1985; Sterling et al., 1988; Vaney et al., 1991; Wässle et al., 1995). Thus, although the rod bipolar axon arbors tile without overlap (Fig. 6.5; Sterling et al., 1988; Young and Vaney, 1991), the circuit leading from one rod via amplifying chemical synapses diverges markedly (Sterling et al., 1988; Vardi and Smith, 1996).

Along *lateral pathways* a given cell type does not show simple territorial behavior; instead it overlaps with its neighbors, and sometimes they actually associate. Horizontal cell processes overlap enough that each retinal locus is "covered" by the arbors of 3–8 cells (Wässle et al., 1978a; Röhrenbeck et al., 1989). Furthermore, where horizontal cell processes of a given type cross each other, they form gap junctions and thus couple electrically. This holds for both the wide-field and narrow-field horizontal cells that connect with cones and also for the axon arbors that connects to rods; thus divergence in these systems, generated both by chemical and electrical synapses, is extensive. Experimentally this is convenient because a small tracer molecule injected into one neuron can reveal much of the network (Fig. 6.12; Mills and Massey, 1994; Vaney, 1994a).

Wide-field amacrine cells behave similarly: their processes cross each other extensively and couple. Thus, though their somas distribute sparsely, their processes and synapses distribute densely, forming a rather fine meshwork (Masland, 1986; Vaney, 1990; Dacey, 1989a). Certain narrow-field amacrine cells are labeled by neurobiotin injected into an alpha or a parasol ganglion cell (Vaney, 1994a; Dacey and Brace, 1992). Thus coupling in lateral pathways is not limited to wide-field types, nor invariably to members of the same type. The massive evidence of extensive cytoplasmic coupling between neurons is sobering in historical perspective. One hundred years ago, debate was fierce as to whether neurons were coupled (*reticularism*) or entirely separate (*neuronism*). The two schools, led respectively by Camillo Golgi and Santiago Ramon y Cajal, heaped scorn upon each other and refused to consider seriously each others' observations. For about 50 years it seemed that Cajal and the "neurone doctrine" had triumphed. But now it is clear that Cajal jumped to conclusions well beyond the resolution of the light microscope. Furthermore, the drawings by reticularists, such as Ehrlich, of apparently coupled ganglion cells may well have reflected spread of tracer (methylene blue) between coupled cells.

The cholinergic amacrine cells form a different and distinctive pattern. The spatial densities are intermediate and their arbors are medium-field, so each retinal locus is covered by about 80 arbors. Yet, the individual processes do not cross each other but instead associate in bundles, thus forming a coarse, quasi-regular meshwork (Fig. 6.9A).

Foveal Architecture Implies "Pursuit" Eye Movements. The foregoing aspects of retinal architecture reflect the broad CNS strategy for sensory surfaces: specialize one region to "sample" finely and assign a relatively large volume of brain to analyze the data. Concurrently, render the specialized surface mobile and evolve "attentional" mechanisms that allow the organism to select which region of the environment to analyze. In the present case, about half of the cones and ganglion cells in primate retina are concentrated in the fovea, and half of striate cortex is devoted to the fovea (reviewed by van Essen et al., 1992). Apparently the fovea occupies only its fair share of cortex, i.e., in proportion to the ganglion cells that it contributes (Schein, 1988; Wässle et al., 1989; Schein and de Monasterio, 1987). Although this is still disputed (Azzopardi and Cowey, 1993), it seems parsimonious to think that the brain allots computational space proportional to the information content of the input. Therefore, to devote more space than warranted purely by ganglion cell density would seem, prima facie, a poor investment.

The strategy of using the central retina for fine spatial sampling requires *smooth-pursuit* eye movements to stabilize regions of interest object upon the center. This minimizes motion in the image, reducing the need for central ganglion cells to code temporal information. But conversely this strategy maximizes image motion seen by peripheral ganglion cells (Eckert and Buchsbaum, 1993a,b). Thus, within a given cell type, response properties should vary with retinal location. A cat beta cell or primate midget cell that fires tonically to stabilized stimuli in central retina should fire more transiently in peripheral retina. This has been found experimentally (Cleland et al., 1971; de Monasterio, 1978) and may partly explain why peripheral ganglion cells collect from more cones (Tsukamoto et al., 1990)—the better to measure transient signals. This also predicts an increase in the proportion of amacrine synapses on a given cell type toward the periphery.

SYNAPTIC CONNECTIONS

OUTER PLEXIFORM LAYER

Ribbon Synapse. The chemical synapse of the photoreceptor terminal employs a synaptic ribbon. This is a flat, elongated organelle whose long axis anchors near the presynaptic membrane (Fig. 6.13). Synaptic vesicles tether to both faces of the ribbon via short filaments, so vesicles along the ribbon's basal edge touch the presynaptic membrane. Here they appear to "dock" ready for release. This occurs when the photoreceptor depolarizes, admitting calcium through channels in the presynaptic membrane all along the region where the ribbon anchors (reviewed by Matthews, 1996). The elongated active zone docks about five- to ten-fold more vesicles than at a conventional synapse, and since a vesicle need move only 30 nm on the ribbon to reach an emptied docking site, the ribbon has long suggested a mechanism for rapid "reloading" (Rao-Mirotznik et al., 1995).

This idea is now supported by capacitance measurements on isolated cells and terminals. A vesicle fusing to the presynaptic membrane increases the capacitance by about 26 attoFarads (von Gersdorff et al., 1996). When synchronous fusion of many vesicles is induced by a step depolarization, the increase in capacitance becomes measurable. Where the number of ribbon synapses is known, the peak fusion rate has been calculated at about 500 vesicles/ribbon/sec (Parsons et al., 1994; von Gersdorff et al., 1996). Furthermore, the capacitance jump corresponds to the total number of vesicles tethered on all the ribbons in a terminal (von Gersdorff et al., 1996). Thus vesicles must move rapidly on the ribbon, but whether this is via diffusion or by cytoplasmic "motor" is unknown. These maximum evoked rates appear to represent the peak of the operating range, so normal rates may be more like 50–100 vesicles/ribbon/sec (Rao et al., 1994a; Freed et al., 1997). Indeed, a milder stimulus, raising intracellular calcium by 2 μM, fuses 400 vesicles/sec in salamander rod, or about 50/sec/ribbon (Rieke and Schwartz, 1996; Townes-Anderson et al., 1985). Yet, even these lower rates are much higher than a conventional synapse can sustain (Borges et al., 1995; Stevens and Tsujimoto, 1995). Ribbon synapses appear to be present in all cases where transmitter release is modulated by graded potentials rather than by spikes, probably because they permit much higher rates of information transfer (de Ruyter and Laughlin, 1996).

The rod terminal employs a single active zone with one ribbon and one invagination (Fig. 6.13B). The latter houses two types of postsynaptic process: horizontal cell spines and bipolar dendritic tips. The paired spines from overlapping horizontal cell axons penetrate deeply to place their glutamate receptors near the vesicle release sites, within about 16 nm. The dendritic tips from two or more cells also penetrate but end quite far from the release sites, about 100–600 nm. In cross–section the invagination often seems to contain only three processes, so it was termed a *triad*, but now we know that the invagination contains at least four processes (i.e., it is at least a *tetrad*; Fig. 6.13B; Rao-Mirotznik et al., 1995). The crescent shape of the rod ribbon, its size (600

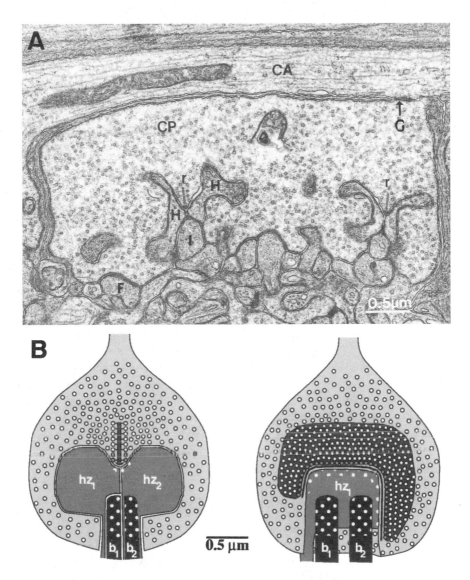

Fig. 6.13. **A:** Cone terminal in radial section (electron micrograph, macaque fovea). Two "triads" are present, each with a synaptic ribbon (r) pointing between two horizontal cell processes (H) toward an invaginating bipolar dendrite (IB). There are also "basal contacts" onto bipolar dendrites distant from the ribbon (B), and a gap junction (G) with the adjacent cone axon (CA) (CP, cone pedicle; F, flat bipolar). The complete terminal contains about 20 ribbon synapses. **B:** Rod terminal in orthogonal views (from 3-D reconstruction, cat central area). A single "tetrad" is present, with one ribbon pointing between two horizontal cell processes (hz) toward two rod bipolar dendrites (b). Note that bipolar dendrites are hundreds of nanometers distant from docked vesicles. [A from Tsukamoto et al., 1992; B from Rao-Mirotznik et al., 1995, with permission.]

tethered vesicles), and the length of the active zone (130 docked vesicles) are all conserved across mammalian species.

The cone terminal employs multiple active zones, each with a ribbon and an invagination (Fig. 6.13A). There are about 20 active zones per terminal in the fovea and 40 or more per terminal in the periphery (Ahnelt et al., 1990; Calkins and Sterling, 1996; Chun et al., 1996). Each invagination houses paired horizontal cell processes— one from a wide-field, the other from a narrow-field cell, and these penetrate deeply to end near the release sites (Fig. 6.13A; Kolb, 1970; Boycott and Kolb, 1973). One or two bipolar dendrites also invaginate at each active zone, but less deeply, terminating 100–200 nm from the release sites (Fig. 6.13A; Kolb, 1970; Calkins and Sterling, 1996; Chun et al., 1996). The external, basal surface of the cone terminal forms symmetrical junctions termed *flat* or *basal* contacts with the tips of bipolar dendrites (Kolb, 1970; Calkins and Sterling, 1996). All the invaginating positions are occupied by ON bipolar dendrites, and many of the basal positions are occupied by OFF bipolar dendrites. The cone terminal membrane at the basal contacts bears neither a ribbon nor a conventional cluster of docked vesicles. So it is widely thought that ribbon synapses serve the ON dendrites by exocytosis and that basal synapses serve the OFF dendrites by some transmitter release mechanism yet to be identified (e.g., Kolb, 1994).

However, this simple rule does not hold. Many ON bipolar dendrites also receive basal contacts (Calkins and Sterling, 1996; Chun et al., 1996), and it has become apparent that the key functional difference between OFF and ON dendrites depends not on the junctional morphology but on which type of glutamate receptor they express: GluR for OFF cells and mGluR6 for ON cells. Also, despite the relatively huge distance from vesicle release sites to invaginating and flat bipolar dendrites (hundreds of nanometers), a single vesicle can still deliver pulses of transmitter in the 10 μM range (Rao-Mirotznik et al., 1997). This concentration, which would be sustained for several milliseconds, corresponds to the effective concentrations for ON and OFF bipolar dendritic tips (de la Villa et al., 1995; Sasaki and Kaneko, 1996). Thus vesicles released at the ribbon synapse may actually serve both invaginating and basal dendrites.

Nonribbon Synapses. Horizontal cell processes contain synaptic vesicles and in one case (primate rod) clearly form conventional synapses onto the photoreceptor (Linberg and Fisher, 1988). But this is the only case, so it is uncertain whether GABA is released from horizontal cells via conventional vesicular mechanism or by a calcium-independent mechanism, such as a GABA transporter (Schwartz, 1987). In cold-blooded species the photoreceptor terminal is sensitive to GABA (e.g., Tachibana and Kaneko, 1984; reviewed by Piccolino, 1995), so one expects this as well in mammals. However, this has yet to be confirmed by physiology or immunocytochemistry, since antibodies to various subunits of GABA$_A$ and GABA$_C$ receptors do not stain the terminals. Cone bipolar dendrites do stain strongly for GABA$_A$ receptor just outside the invagination (Vardi and Sterling, 1994), and rod bipolar dendrites stain for GABA$_C$ receptor (Enz et al., 1996). So horizontal cells may release transmitter diffusely along the interface between bipolar dendrites and photoreceptor terminals.

A few conventional synapses are present in the outer plexiform layer (OPL). Mostly these are from GABAergic interplexiform processes onto bipolar dendrites (McGuire et al., 1984; Cohen and Sterling, 1990a). However, other transmitters may affect the

OPL without benefit of conventional synapses. For example, the dopamine-containing processes ascending from the amacrine cell layer meander through the OPL without making conventional contacts. D_1 receptors are present in OPL (Veruki and Wässle, 1996), and dopamine potently uncouples horizontal cell gap junctions (Hampson et al., 1994; reviewed by Murakami et al., 1995). In short, there is ample evidence here for "paracrine" effects of a transmitter (Witkovsky et al., 1993).

Electrical synapses (gap junctions) are present at three critical sites in the OPL. First, each cone terminal couples to its immediate neighbors via relatively small junctions (Fig. 6.13A). For example, each terminal in primate fovea could have at most 170 connexons (the multimeric channel that forms the junction) with its neighbors (Raviola and Gilula, 1973; Tsukamoto et al., 1990). Second, each rod terminal forms a gap junction with each of two neighboring cone terminals (Kolb, 1977; Smith et al., 1986). Since there are about 20 rods for every cone, a cone must couple to about 40 rods (Sterling et al., 1988). These junctions feed rod signals into the cone terminal (Nelson, 1977; Schneeweis and Schnapf, 1995). Third, there are numerous, extensive gap junctions between horizontal cells. Wide-field cells couple and narrow-field cells couple, but the two types do not cross-couple (Vaney, 1994b; Mills and Massey, 1994).

INNER PLEXIFORM LAYER

The sole input to this layer derives from bipolar axon terminals. These, like receptor terminals, form ribbon synapses, but the ribbons are generally smaller and more numerous. For example, a ribbon in a rod bipolar terminal tethers only 100 synaptic vesicles and docks only about 20 vesicles (Rao and Sterling, 1991). The rod bipolar terminal (cat) contains about 30 ribbons, whereas a cone bipolar terminal can contain more than 100 ribbons. The number of ribbons is distinctive for a given cell type at a given eccentricity and is highly regular, varying at most by 5–10% (McGuire et al., 1984; Cohen and Sterling, 1990a; Calkins et al., 1994).

The bipolar terminal does not invaginate, so one ribbon synapse cannot accommodate many postsynaptic processes. Instead, two postsynaptic processes align on either side of the linear active zone, forming a dyad (Fig. 6.14; Dowling and Boycott, 1966). The postsynaptic elements at a dyad can be two ganglion cell dendrites, two amacrine processes, or one of each. Often, the amacrine process feeds back a conventional synapse onto the bipolar axon, in which case it is called a *reciprocal synapse* (e.g., Calkins and Sterling, 1996). Each bipolar type expresses a specific pattern. For example, the rod bipolar dyad always includes one process from an AII amacrine and another from a small subset of different amacrine types. The AII *never* gives a reciprocal synapse at the rod bipolar dyad, but the other amacrine types *always* do. Beta ganglion cell dendrites are *never* found at the rod bipolar dyad, but alpha cell dendrites are present at about 1 dyad out of 30 (McGuire et al., 1984; Freed et al., 1987; Freed and Sterling, 1988).

Lateral connections in the IPL use conventional chemical synapses and gap junctions. Amacrine cells are the sole source of conventional synapses (Dowling and Boycott, 1966). Synaptic vesicle morphology is invariant (no round vs. pleomorphic vesicles); nor is Gray's scheme (type I vs. type II synapses) applicable (see Chaps. 1, 2). Commonly in cold-blooded (small-brained) animals conventional synapses are arranged such that adjacent processes contact each other serially in long sequences (Dubin, 1976).

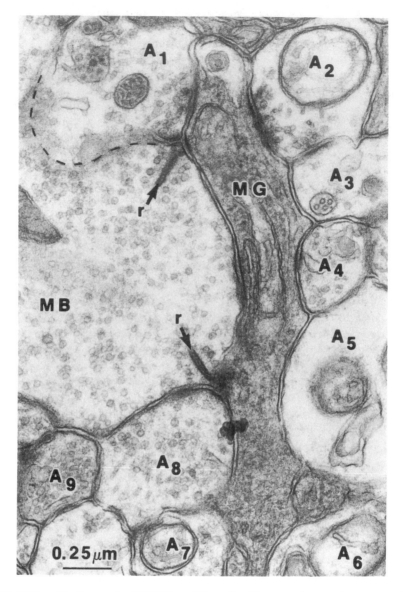

Fig. 6.14. Midget bipolar terminal (MB) in radial section (electron micrograph, macaque fovea). Two dyads are present, each with a presynaptic ribbon. The ribbon points between two postsynaptic processes, the dendrite of a midget ganglion cell (MG) and an amacrine process (A_1, A_8) that feeds back onto the bipolar terminal and forward onto the ganglion cell (A_8). Many other amacrine processes also contact the ganglion cell. [From Calkins and Sterling, 1996, with permission.]

These sequences might perform complex, local computations. However, the underlying circuits have not yet been worked out, and their actual function is unknown.

Electrical synapses are present at five classes of connections in the IPL. First, they interconnect certain types of cone bipolar cell, both homotypically (b_4-b_4) and heterotypically (b_3-b_4; Cohen and Sterling, 1990a). Second, they couple particular types of amacrine cell homotypically, such as the AII and wide-field types (Vaney, 1994a). Third, they couple particular amacrine types to bipolar cells. For example, the largest electrical synapses in the IPL couple AII amacrine dendrites to ON cone bipolar axon terminals (Kolb and Famiglietti, 1974; Sterling et al., 1988; Strettoi et al., 1990). This connection is apparently critical for vision under starlight, as will be discussed. Fourth, certain narrow-field amacrine cells couple to particular types of ganglion cell (alpha, parasol; Vaney, 1994a; Dacey and Brace, 1992). Finally, certain types of ganglion cell couple homotypically without amacrine participation, e.g., the directionally sensitive ganglion cell (Fig. 6.11C; Vaney, 1994b).

The ganglion cell differs from output cells in other brain regions. The cell is relatively small, with 10–25 μm soma, compared to 50–80 μm for the motoneuron and Purkinje cell. And ganglion cell dendrites extend for only 20–200 μm, compared to 1000 μm for the motoneuron. Correspondingly, the ganglion cell collects relatively few synapses: 60–100 for a central midget cell; 200 for a central beta cell; 3000 for a peripheral beta and a central alpha cell (Freed and Sterling, 1988; Cohen and Sterling, 1992; Kier et al., 1995; Calkins et al., 1996). In contrast, a spinal alpha motoneuron collects about 10,000 synapses, and cerebellar Purkinje cell collects more than 100,000 synapses! Another difference is that a ganglion cell collects synapses exclusively on dendrites and not the soma. By contrast, the motoneuron is encrusted with synapses over its entire surface (Chap. 3), and the very design of the Purkinje cell seems to hinge on an antagonism between excitatory inputs to the dendritic tree and inhibitory inputs to the soma (Chap. 7).

DEVELOPMENT

The understanding of how retinal circuits develop is rather fragmentary at present, so rather than attempt a synthesis, we note some current lines of investigation. A key effort is to identify mechanisms that generate the plethora of retinal cell types. This seems to involve specific transcription factors. For example, the *Brn-3* family of POU domain transcription factors are expressed in subsets of retinal ganglion cells. These proteins first appear in ganglion cell precursors migrating from the zone of dividing neuroblasts to the future ganglion cell layer. Targeted disruption of the *Brn-3b* gene causes selective loss of 70% of ganglion cells but not other types (Gan et al., 1996); also, transgene expression of *Brn-3* members labels various types of amacrine and ganglion cells but not other types (Xiang et al., 1996). Still another POU-domain protein, RPF-1, is expressed in neuroblasts destined to become ganglion and amacrine cells (Zhou et al., 1996).

Another effort concerns the mechanisms that regulate cell number (Williams and Herrup, 1988). As is generally the case, excess cells are produced and then "pruned" by cell death (*apoptosis*). Thus, in cat by embryonic day 39, about 700,000 ganglion cells send axons into the optic nerve. They connect centrally and fire action potentials that drive geniculate neurons (Katz and Shatz, 1996). Nevertheless, by birth only 270,000 axons remain and by 6 weeks postnatal the adult number (~180,000) is reached (Williams et al., 1986). Why certain ganglion cells live while others die remains to be established, but the current best guess is that the process involves competition for a specific neurotrophin (reviewed by Katz and Shatz, 1996).

Prenatal firing of optic axons shapes geniculate development since blocking the action potentials by intraocular tetrodotoxin prevents segregation of eye-specific geniculate layers. The activity may also help establish the orderly 2-D maps of retina in central structures (Katz and Shatz, 1996). This ganglion cell firing is not random but rather sweeps across the retina in waves, so that adjacent cells fire together (Meister et al., 1991). The waves of firing are also associated with waves of intracellular calcium fluctuation in amacrine and ganglion cells that may be triggered by cholinergic amacrine cells (Wong et al., 1995; Feller et al., 1996). The waves may also be coordinated via electrical coupling and shared levels of extracellular potassium (Penn et al., 1994; Burgi and Grzywacz, 1994). Since "neurons that fire together, wire together," these waves of correlated activity may contribute to the orderly relationships at the far end of the optic nerve. The need to generate these early waves of activity may explain why the earliest synaptic connections in retina involve lateral rather than forward elements (Maslim and Stone, 1986).

At birth, the main ganglion cells in cat (alpha, beta, etc.) are easily recognized (Ramoa et al., 1988; Dann et al., 1988). But they are not yet connected to their intraretinal circuits because the photoreceptors are still proliferating, and the bipolar axons are just descending toward the IPL. As the eyes open (6–10 days postnatal), synaptogenesis enters high gear and is nearly complete by 4 weeks (Vogel, 1978; Maslim and Stone, 1986). Each cell type probably has its own programmed period and rate of synaptogenesis, and there is no simple way to characterize the sequence. Thus, it proceeds neither strictly centrifugally (ganglion cell → bipolar → receptor) nor vice-versa (McArdle et al., 1977; cf. Nishimura and Rakic, 1987b). Furthermore, the genesis of retinal wiring, despite its coincidence with eye opening, appears to follow a genetic program and to be little affected by light or patterned stimulation. Thus, neither dark rearing nor occlusion by lid-suture (which prevents patterned stimulation) affects adult retinal morphology or physiology, even though such procedures profoundly alter the structure and function of the visual cortex (Hubel and Wiesel, 1977).

Perinatal alpha and beta ganglion cells display immature dendritic arbors with excessive branches and spines, and their ON/OFF dendritic stratification is incomplete (Dann et al., 1988; Ramoa et al., 1988). Pruning of the ganglion dendritic arbors proceeds almost normally in the presence of tetrodotoxin (TTX). Therefore, action potentials, which crucially shape the axon arbor, hardly affect the dendritic arbor (Wong et al., 1991). On the other hand, bipolar input (insensitive to TTX) apparently does shape the dendritic arbors. Thus, tonically hyperpolarizing ON bipolar cells during eye opening (by intraocular application of the mGluR6 agonist APB) arrests the normal progress of stratification (Bodnarenko et al., 1995).

The synaptic connections in adult mammalian retina appear not to be "plastic". But in lower vertebrates (such as fish and amphibia) the retina continues to grow throughout life, adding nerve cells in concentric rings at the periphery to all three layers. The optic tectum, the main target of the fish and amphibian optic nerve, also continues to add neurons, but in concentric crescents rather than in complete rings. This creates a topological mismatch between the retina and its map on the tectum. Consequently, the map requires continuous readjustment. This is accomplished by the continuous retraction of old retino-tectal synapses, growth of the optic axons across the tectum, and the formation of new synapses (Easter and Stuermer, 1984; Reh and Constantine-Paton, 1984). If the neural retina is totally removed from the eye of a fish or amphibian, cells from the pigment epithelium de-differentiate, divide, and regenerate a whole new neural retina whose ganglion cell axons find their way to the brain and reconnect properly.

Another fascinating developmental plasticity is the shift in retinal wiring that in certain organisms accompanies changes in lifestyle. For example, the adult frog eats flies and has a type of ganglion cell tuned by specific "circuits" (patterns of connection between specific cell types) to "fly-like" stimuli (Barlow, 1953; Maturana et al., 1960). But the tadpole eats algae and lacks this cell type. The fly-detecting ganglion cell and its neural circuitry develop as part of the many complex changes that accompany metamorphosis (Frank and Hollyfield, 1987). However, it seems fairly certain that its emergence is directed by a genetic program that operates regardless of whether the frog is ever confronted with a fly.

VISUAL TRANSDUCTION

Rods and cones share the same transduction mechanism (Fig. 6.15). The outer segment bears numerous cation channels permeable to Na^+ and Ca^{2+}. A channel flickers open upon binding two molecules of cGMP, and in the dark the intracellular concentration of cGMP is high. Therefore, at any instant about 10^4 channels are open. The result in darkness is a continuous inward sodium current at the outer segment which is balanced by an outward potassium current at the inner segment. This circulating dark current depolarizes the receptor to about -40 mV. The cell's ionic balance is maintained by an active sodium/potassium exchanger operating continuously at the inner segment, which explains the large energy demand at this site and thus its need for densely packed mitochondria (Fig. 6.4; reviewed by Yau, 1994; Pugh and Lamb, 1993).

The optical image focuses at the level of the *inner* segments (Figs. 6.4; 6.10). A photon contributing to this image penetrates the plasma membrane to enter the inner segment. Entering a rod, the photon may simply pass through, continuing on until it is finally trapped in a neighboring receptor. It doesn't matter which rod captures a given photon because at night the optical image is poor and subsequent pooling of rod signals is great. But if a photon enters a *cone* inner segment, it is trapped because of the densely packed mitochondria that raise the refractive index. Thus the cone inner segment's "wave guide" funneling photons toward the outer segment preserves the correspondence between the optical image and the transduced image (Enoch, 1981).

A photon reaching the outer segment penetrates the stacked membrane discs (Fig. 6.4) until it encounters a molecule of photopigment (rhodopsin) and transfers its energy. This isomerizes the vitamin A group attached to the opsin protein, activating the molecule and causing it to activate several hundred molecules of the G protein transducin. This in turn activates hundreds of phosphodiesterase molecules that rapidly hydrolyze cGMP, lowering its concentration, closing the cation channels, and reducing the Na^+ influx (*dark current*). The outer segment hyperpolarizes, and signal descends

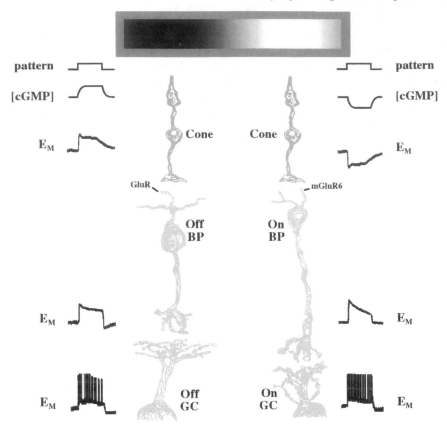

Fig. 6.15. Basics of cone transduction and forward signal transfer. One cycle of a dark/bright grating flashes briefly on a steady background. Light *decrement* for the left cone allows guanyl cyclase to raise [cGMP], thus opening cation channels in the outer segment and depolarizing the cone membrane potential (E_M). The cone terminal increases its discharge of glutamate onto ionotropic receptors (GluR), depolarizing the OFF bipolar cell, thus releasing glutamate onto the OFF ganglion cell and causing it to spike. Light *increment* for the right cone isomerizes rhodopsin, triggering the G protein cascade that lowers [cGMP], thus closing cation channels in the outer segment and hyperpolarizing the cone membrane potential. The cone terminal ceases its tonic release of glutamate onto metabotropic (mGluR6) receptors, depolarizing the ON bipolar cell, thus releasing glutamate onto the ON ganglion cell and causing it to spike. This key step at the cone terminal, use of paired neurons to separately encode light decrement and increment, carries forward to the ganglion cells that feed the geniculostriate pathway, doubling their dynamic range.

through the inner segment where voltage-gated channels shape it temporally and boost its amplitude (reviewed by Pugh and Lamb, 1993; Yau, 1994).

The rod achieves the ultimate sensitivity: one photon isomerizing one rhodopsin molecule (Rh*) lowers the cGMP concentration enough to suppress about 4% of the dark current. This gives a ~0.7 pA signal with a signal/noise ratio (~5) adequate for transmission forward (Baylor et al., 1984; Smith et al., 1986). Although the rhodopsin molecule is quite stable, it can be isomerized in the absence of light by thermal agitation, producing ~0.006 Rh*/rod/sec. Since subsequent stages cannot distinguish a photic isomerization from a thermal one, this rate of "dark light" sets the lower limit of visual sensitivity (reviewed by Barlow, 1982). The rod sums linearly up to about 20 Rh* delivered as a flash, saturating completely to 100 Rh*/flash (Baylor et al., 1984). But to a background that steadily evokes 100 Rh* per integration time (corresponding to twilight), the rod can reduce its sensitivity and thus avoid saturation when the cone signal is declining toward its threshold (Tamura et al., 1991).

The cone is less sensitive by nearly 70-fold: one Rh* suppresses only about 0.06% of the dark current. But this response is buried in the random fluctuations of the membrane current and so is undetectable. The cone signal rises above the noise when about 100 Rh* arrive within its integration time; thus its threshold for signaling uses about the same fraction of the dark current as the rod (Schnapf et al., 1990). The cone signal turns on at the same rate as the rod, but turns off much faster, which is key to its shorter integration time (Pugh and Lamb, 1993). Several mechanisms turn down its sensitivity as intensity rises to retain its linear response, and even in the brightest light the response does not saturate completely. The mechanisms that arrest transduction and turn down its sensitivity involve feedback control by calcium at many levels of the cascade but are as yet incompletely understood (reviewed by Yau, 1994).

DENDRITIC AND AXONAL PROPERTIES

PATTERNS OF FUNCTIONAL POLARIZATION

Classically, "dendritic" has implied passive, centripetal current flow toward the soma and axon hillock. "Axonal" has implied active centrifugal propagation away from the soma toward the presynaptic terminal. But in retina as elsewhere (Chaps. 1, 2), these simple definitions tend to dissolve. It is true that the forward relay neurons do display typical polarity. Indeed, the sequence photoreceptor → bipolar cell → ganglion cell was Cajal's primary exemplar (together with the olfactory bulb mitral cell; see Chap. 5) for his "law" of polarized conduction. But photoreceptor and bipolar axons do not normally spike; rather, they are passive, releasing transmitter upon graded depolarization (von Gersdorff and Matthews, 1994; Rieke and Schwartz, 1996). Also, these axon terminals *receive* modulatory inputs. Both points violate classical theory.

The lateral elements break *all* the classical rules (Piccolino, 1986). In fact their designs seem almost ad hoc, each suited to accomplish a particular task. Thus, a horizontal cell collects input all along its processes and gives output at the same sites. Furthermore, because they are strongly coupled, horizontal cells present essentially a continuous sheet, passively integrating inputs and modulating outputs rather widely in space and time (R.G. Smith, 1995). Narrow-field and medium-field amacrine cells are also nonpolarized since their inputs and outputs tend to be near each other (Famiglietti, 1991; Calkins and Sterling, 1996). But these amacrine processes are quite fine caliber, are not coupled, and may be passive. Consequently, the output of such a cell, e.g., the starburst cell, is modulated by local inputs. This is evident because its excitatory influence on a ganglion cell extends no further than the ganglion cell dendritic arbor even though starburst cells with input to the ganglion cell extend considerably beyond it (Yang and Masland, 1992).

The wide-field amacrine cells present a bizarre twist to the theme of polarized conduction. As noted above, these cells collect input conventionally via a dendritic tree that funnels postsynaptic potentials (PSPs) toward the soma. Action potentials arise, also conventionally, at an axon hillock and propagate for millimeters across the retina (Fig. 6.9). But unconventionally, each primary dendrite emits its own axon; thus although the cell segregates its passive dendrites and spiking axons, the latter broadcast spikes radially in two dimensions.

The AII amacrine cell represents still another twist to the theme of functional polarity and active vs. passive membrane. The cell collects its key inputs from rod bipolar synapses on its main arbor in the ON layer of the IPL and uses its gap junctions with cone bipolar axon terminals as a local excitatory output. Since the AII collecting arbor is narrow-field, it should not require active membrane to propagate its signal. Yet the cell produces large, fast depolarizations that are sensitive to TTX (Nelson, 1982; Boos, et al., 1993). Here a voltage-sensitive membrane, rather than spreading signals beyond where passive conduction could take them, seems to provide a "thresholding" mechanism that amplifies small signals nonlinearly to protect them from noise (Freed et al., 1987; Smith and Vardi, 1995). Only a few of the 40 amacrine types have been studied, so further surprises are to be expected.

INDIVIDUAL RETINAL NEURONS ARE ELECTROTONICALLY COMPACT

The axons and main dendrites of feedforward neurons are relatively short and thick. Thus rod and cone axons, respectively, 0.5 and 1.6 μm in diameter, range from 20 to 400 μm long (Hsu et al., 1997). Bipolar dendrites and axons are about the same thickness as photoreceptor axons, but even shorter. Ganglion cell dendrites (beta and alpha) are also about 0.5–1.5 μm in diameter, and the arbors range from about 30 to 250 μm across. Consequently, all synapses onto these cells are calculated to be well within one space constant of the soma. Electrotonic considerations indicate that photovoltages transmitted to rod and cone terminals and EPSPs transmitted from distal dendrites to the ganglion cell soma are little attenuated (Koch et al., 1982; Freed et al., 1992; Kier et al., 1995; Hsu et al., 1997).

NEUROTRANSMITTERS AND POSTSYNAPTIC RECEPTORS

Essentially all of the transmitters identified elsewhere in the brain exist also in the retina. A transmitter can be assigned to a cell type upon immunocytochemical detection of (*1*) the endogenous transmitter; (*2*) its synthetic enzyme; and (*3*) transmitter receptors on postsynaptic cells. When no antibody is available, in situ hybridization for mRNA of the appropriate molecule also provides a clue, but the conclusion remains tentative because the mRNA may not be expressed. Commonly, a neuron that uses a particular transmitter also expresses a transporter molecule on its surface that binds the transmitter in the extracellular space and actively pumps it back into the cell. Glia cells do not release transmitters, but they do express receptors for transmitters and also GABA and glutamate transporters (reviewed by Newman and Reichenbach, 1996).

PHOTORECEPTORS TO HORIZONTAL AND BIPOLAR CELLS

Photoreceptors contain the excitatory amino acid glutamate, and they release it when depolarized. Two experimental *tours de force* seem conclusive. First, a turtle rod was sucked by its outer segment into a micropipette through which it could be electrically stimulated. The tip of a second pipette, bearing a patch of neuronal membrane ripped from a cultured hippocampal neuron, was moved close to the rod axon terminal. The membrane patch, which was "outside out" (see Chap. 2), contained the N-methyl-D-aspartate (NMDA) type of glutamate receptor. The electrically depolarized rod released a transmitter that opened ion channels gated by the NMDA receptors on the "sniffer" patch (Copenhagen and Jahr, 1989). Second, the rod axon terminal was sucked into a pipette containing glutamate dehydrogenase plus NAD; release of glutamate was then measured directly by an increase in fluorescence resulting from the formation of $NADH_2$ (Ayoub et al., 1989).

Neurons postsynaptic to photoreceptors all express ionotropic receptors for glutamate. Horizontal cells express the GluR (AMPA/kainate) and NMDA types of glutamate receptor that open a cation channel with a reversal potential near zero (reviewed by Massey and Maguire, 1995). Thus, as the photoreceptor depolarizes to dark stimuli, releasing glutamate (see above), the horizontal cells depolarize. The OFF bipolar cell dendrites also express a GluR receptor and thus also depolarize to dark stimuli. Although horizontal and OFF bipolar cells express the same broad class of receptor (GluR), the particular combinations of subunits probably differ. This would explain how the effective concentration for a half-maximal response (EC_{50}) could be 0.5 mM for the horizontal cell and 10 μM for the bipolar cell (Sasaki and Kaneko, 1996). This difference seems key to assembling multiple postsynaptic processes into a complex where they can all be activated by the same point source of glutamate (Fig. 6.13; Rao-Mirotznik et al., 1997).

The ON bipolar dendrites express a *metabotropic* glutamate receptor, mGluR6 (Fig. 6.15A). This receptor, which is highly localized to the tips of rod bipolar and ON cone bipolar dendrites (Nomura et al., 1994; Vardi and Morigiwa, 1997), couples to a second messenger system requiring cGMP and phosphodiesterase (Nawy and Jahr, 1990; Shiells and Falk, 1990). Dark stimuli, releasing glutamate onto this receptor, close an ion channel with a reversal potential near zero and thus hyperpolarize the cell. Bright stimuli, suppressing the photoreceptor's glutamate release, open this cation channel and depolarize the cell. This synapse has been termed *sign-reversing* and *inhibitory* because glutamate's action is to hyperpolarize, but the reversal potential is positive (i.e., excitatory). Therefore, it may be simplest to consider the ON bipolar cell as excited by bright stimuli and the OFF bipolar cell as excited by dark stimuli (both referred to the local mean intensity level).

By this molecular trick of employing two different receptors for the same transmitter, cone bipolar cells double the dynamic range for encoding intensity differences across a natural scene (see below). Half of the bipolar cells carry signals greater than the local mean, and half carry signals less than the local mean. Their ganglion cells and corresponding cells in the lateral geniculate nucleus follow suit. Finally, at the level of simple cells in striate cortex, these signals recombine so that the parallel, elongated subregions antagonize each other with equal strength (Palmer and Davis, 1981; Ferster 1988). An important lesson here is that to understand the reason for a particular encoding procedure at one synapse, one may need to look ahead another 4 to 5 stages!

Since ON bipolar cells require cGMP and phosphodiesterase, it was natural to think that they use the same transduction mechanism as the photoreceptor: glutamate bound to mGluR6 would activate transducin and then phosphodiesterase (PDE) lowering cGMP and closing a cGMP-gated cation channel (Nawy and Jahr, 1990; Shiells and Falk, 1990). However, the molecules key to the phototransduction cascade are not found by immunocytochemistry (Vardi et al., 1993). Instead, a different G-protein, G_o, co-localizes with the mGluR6 receptor, so quite a different second messenger cascade may be involved (Vardi, 1997).

HORIZONTAL TO PHOTORECEPTOR AND BIPOLAR CELLS

Horizontal cells use GABA. Although mammalian horizontal cells do not demonstrably accumulate exogenous GABA, they do contain it (Chun and Wässle, 1989). They also express the GABA-synthetic enzyme glutamic acid decarboxylase (GAD) in one of two isoforms, GAD_{65} or GAD_{67}, (Vardi et al., 1994). Furthermore, $GABA_A$ and $GABA_C$ receptors are expressed by cone bipolar and rod bipolar dendrites, respectively, which implies a local source of GABA, presumably horizontal cells (Vardi et al., 1992; Vardi and Sterling, 1994; Enz et al., 1996). The cone axon terminal in lower vertebrates hyperpolarizes to ionophoresis of GABA, suggesting GABA feedback onto it (e.g., Tachibana and Kaneko, 1984; Wu, 1992), so one expects this also in mammals.

BIPOLAR TO GANGLION AND AMACRINE CELLS

Bipolar neurons use glutamate as a transmitter. Here the evidence rests mainly on the responsiveness of ganglion and amacrine cells to ionophoresed glutamate and its various agonists and antagonists. GluR and NMDA receptors are both expressed by ganglion cells and specific amacrine types (Cohen et al., 1994; reviewed by Massey and Maguire, 1995). Many different subunits of each receptor type are present (Hamassaki-Britto et al., 1993; Peng et al., 1995; Vardi and Morigiwa, 1997). Furthermore, various processes in the inner plexiform layer, including bipolar terminals, express metabotropic glutamate receptors (Brandstätter et al., 1996).

Certain bipolar neurons accumulate exogenous glycine and contain endogenous glycine (Cohen and Sterling, 1986; Pourcho and Goebel, 1987). Also, some ganglion cells bear glycine receptors (Koulen et al., 1996) and respond to ionophoretic glycine with an increased Cl^- conductance that is blocked specifically by strychnine (Bolz et al., 1985). So one might think that some bipolar neurons are glycinergic. Yet, many amacrine-to-ganglion cell synapses accumulate glycine (Freed and Sterling, 1988), and glycine receptors localize postsynaptically to amacrine rather than to bipolar synapses (Pourcho and Owczarzak, 1991; Sassoè-Pognetto et al., 1994). Thus current evidence favors glycine as a transmitter for narrow-field amacrine cells and not for bipolar cells.

One striking complication is that certain bipolar cells contain endogenous GABA and express GAD (Wässle and Chun, 1989; Vardi and Auerbach, 1995). These cells represent a distinct type with axon in the OFF layer of the IPL (Vardi and Shi, 1996). It will be interesting to learn whether this type releases only one transmitter or both. If it releases both, a differential arrangement of postsynaptic receptors would permit this synapse to excite one member of its postsynaptic dyad (ganglion cell) while simultaneously inhibiting the other (AII amacrine cell).

AMACRINE CELLS

About half of all amacrine somas contain glycine and half contain GABA + GAD (Vardi and Auerbach, 1995). But GABA occurs in many amacrine types that also express other transmitters. For example, the starburst amacrine cells that synthesize acetylcholine also synthesize GABA using both isoforms of GAD (Brecha et al., 1988; Kosaka et al., 1988; Vaney and Young, 1988; Vardi and Auerbach, 1995).

Other GABA amacrine cells contain dopamine, indoleamines (reviewed by Vaney, 1990), neuropeptides such as somatostatin (Sagar, 1987; White et al., 1990), vasoactive intestinal polypeptide (Casini and Brecha, 1992), and substance P (Vaney et al., 1989b). Still others contain NADPH diaphorase, which synthesizes nitric oxide (Sandell, 1985; Sagar, 1987), so conceivably, GABA in amacrine cells is never the sole transmitter. In no case is it yet clear whether a cell coreleases GABA with its other transmitter/modulator, or whether they are released at different spatial loci or in response to different electrical or chemical signals (O'Malley et al., 1994).

Processes postsynaptic at amacrine synapses bear the standard receptor molecules. Thus, where glycine is presynaptic, there are postsynaptic glycine receptors (Pourcho and Owczarzak, 1991; Sassoè-Pognetto et al., 1994); where GABA is presynaptic, there are postsynaptic $GABA_A$ or $GABA_C$ receptors (Vardi and Sterling, 1994; Enz et al., 1996). However, since dopamine can also act in paracrine fashion, tens of microns beyond its site of release (Witkovsky et al., 1993), the D_1 receptors distribute much more widely than the conventional dopaminergic synapses (Veruki and Wässle, 1997). Neuropeptide receptors tend to have many subtypes. For example, for somatostatin there are five types (Reisine and Bell, 1995), one of which, SSRT2a, has been localized in retina to the rod bipolar terminal (Vasilaki et al., 1996).

Matters already seem complicated by multiple presynaptic transmitters and multiple subtypes of postsynaptic receptor. But they are profoundly more so because many postsynaptic receptors, including those for glutamate, GABA, dopamine, indoleamines, and peptides, couple to various G proteins, and these trigger a variety of second messenger systems. For example, G_{olf} is expressed by wide-field horizontal cells, and ganglion cells in the IPL; G_o is expressed by ON bipolar cells and by certain amacrine processes in the IPL (Vardi, 1997a,b). Since a given G protein can couple to more than one type of downstream effector, the possible signaling pathways must be very large. Thus one senses an underlying neurochemical network at least as complex as the network of anatomical connections.

FUNCTIONAL CIRCUITS

HOW EFFICIENT IS THE RETINA?

Having described the main types of retinal neuron, their connections and transmitters, we are nearly ready to consider how the anatomical wiring serves function. But first we should ask, how well does the retina perform? The first steps of phototransduction are inefficient: only about one-third of the photons striking the retina are absorbed by a rhodopsin molecule, and only half of these cause isomerization (reviewed by Sterling et al., 1987). Yet once activated, a rhodopsin molecule (Rh*) projects this information through subsequent stages with remarkable reliability. Thus a single Rh* activates several hundred transducin (G protein) molecules, leading reliably to 2–3 spikes in several ON ganglion cells and to suppression of 2–3 spikes in several OFF ganglion cells (Barlow et al., 1971; Matronarde, 1983; Vardi and Smith, 1996).

Once a single photon signal reaches a ganglion cell, to be useful it must sum efficiently with other such signals. If noise were added along the way, e.g., from random release of synaptic vesicles; or if the signal were to saturate some stage along the transmission pathway, information would be lost and the image would be degraded. Yet we discriminate stimuli near threshold with very little information loss along neural circuits. The evidence stems from "ideal observer" computer models that perform any specified discrimination based on the number of photons counted. The models take account of losses due to optics, photoreceptor sampling, and transduction. But thereafter, they operate ideally, i.e., with no further information loss owing to neural mechanisms (Geisler, 1989). It turns out that for suitable stimulation we approach the sensitivity of an ideal observer to within a factor of 2–3 in both dim and bright light (Crowell and Banks, 1988; Savage and Banks, 1992). Therefore, the sum of all stages—from transduction to the ultimate site of discrimination—must not lose any more information than this. Thus retinal circuits must be extremely efficient—as implied by the fine sculpting of the receptor mosaic (described earlier). This alerts us to circuit mechanisms that prevent noise and saturation.

CIRCUITS FOR GANGLION CELL RECEPTIVE FIELD

Center. The center circuit turns out to be fairly simple: the cones co-spatial with the ganglion cell dendritic field modulate glutamate release onto dendrites of cone bipolar cells whose axons contact the ganglion cell dendritic tree. Brightening these cones depolarizes the ON bipolar cells and delivers glutamate to ON ganglion cell dendrites; dimming these cones depolarizes the OFF bipolar cells and delivers glutamate to OFF ganglion cell dendrites (Fig. 6.15A). Thus, the center circuit is purely excitatory.

How many cones connect directly to a ganglion cell dendritic arbor depends on species, retinal location, and ganglion cell type. For example, in cat about 35 cones overlie a central beta cell dendritic field and employ about 15 bipolar cells to contact it with nearly 200 synapses (Fig. 6.16; Cohen and Sterling, 1992). About 625 cones overlie a central alpha cell and employ about 150 bipolar cells with nearly 450 synapses (Fig. 6.16; Freed and Sterling, 1988). In these respects a peripheral beta cell resembles a central alpha cell (Kolb and Nelson, 1993; Kier et al., 1995; Freed et al., 1997).

In primates the receptive field centers are much smaller. For example, a single cone

Fig. 6.16. Circuits for the ganglion-cell receptive field center. **A:** Sensitivity profiles of central beta and alpha cell receptive fields. A beta cell is 8-fold more sensitive than an alpha cell to a small spot (just covering the beta center). Beta centers are narrow and closely spaced; alpha centers are broader and more coarsely spaced. **B:** Beta cell collects about 80 synapses from the b_1 bipolar array, whereas the alpha cell collects 450 b_1 synapses. **C:** Beta gaussian sensitivity profile is shaped mainly by the bipolar receptive field center, which is broad because of optical blur and cone coupling (see Fig. 6.17); the synapse distribution across the narrow beta dendritic tree

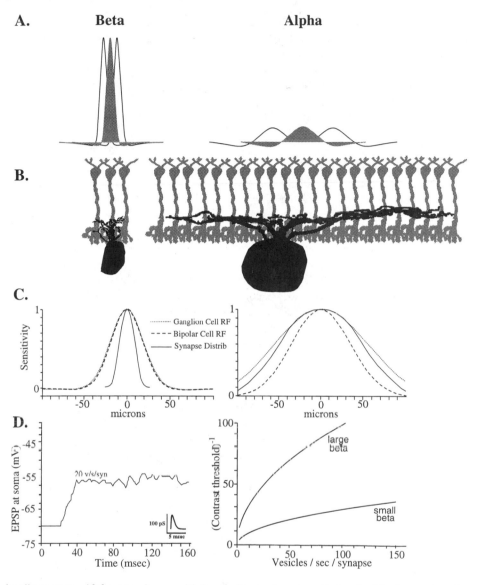

A. Beta   Alpha

B.

C.

Ganglion Cell RF
Bipolar Cell RF
Synapse Distrib

Sensitivity

-50   0   50
microns

-50   0   50
microns

D.

EPSP at soma (mV)

20 v/s/syn

100 pS

5 msec

Time (msec)

(Contrast threshold)$^{-1}$

large beta

small beta

Vesicles / sec / synapse

hardly matters. Alpha gaussian sensitivity profile is shaped partly by the bipolar centers, but more importantly by the dome-like distribution of synapses across the dendritic tree. The beta cell's greater peak sensitivity is due to its greater density of synapses/retinal area. **D:** Left, beta cell's response to simulated epscs (inset). Sustained depolarization of ~12 mV requires an average rate of 20 vesicles/sec/synapse, but random release causes the membrane potential to fluctuate. Right, higher mean rates of vesicle release improve the ratio of the sustained EPSP to its fluctuation. This ratio probably limits the smallest detectable intensity change within a receptive field center (contrast threshold). A peripheral beta cell with 10-fold more synapses than the central beta should achieve about 3-fold lower threshold for a given rate of random release, so for the small beta to achieve a contrast threshold comparable to the large one would require implausibly high sustained rates of vesicle release. [After Freed and Sterling, 1988; Freed et al., 1992, 1997, with permission.]

in the fovea contacts a pair of midget bipolar cells (ON and OFF) that in turn contact ON and OFF midget ganglion cells. This 1:1 bipolar-to-ganglion cell connection is accomplished with only 30–50 synapses. Peripherally, e.g., 20°, about 10 cones overlie the midget ganglion cell. Here, although each cone still contacts its own private midget bipolar cell, several of these converge onto a midget ganglion cell (Dacey, 1996; Goodchild et al., 1996b). The wider-field ganglion cells in primate, parasol and garland cells, collect on the order of 20 cones in the fovea (Calkins and Sterling, 1997b).

What explains the alpha cell's fast transient response to a steady center stimulus versus the beta cell's sustained response (Fig. 6.7)? Multiple mechanisms cooperate: (*1*) Only one type of bipolar cell contacts the alpha cell, and it has a large transient response, whereas three types of bipolar cell contact the beta cell and may carry sustained as well as transient responses (Fig. 6.6B; Nelson and Kolb, 1983; Freed and Sterling, 1988; Cohen and Sterling, 1992). (*2*) Starburst amacrine processes, which are coplanar with the alpha dendritic arbor, associate with it, whereas starburst processes have access to only a small fraction of the beta dendritic arbor (Vardi et al., 1989; Luo et al., 1996). (*3*) Bipolar input to the starburst cell uses fast kainate receptors (vs. slow NMDA receptors), transiently releasing acetylcholine onto ganglion cell dendrites (Linn et al., 1991; Famiglietti, 1991). (*4*) Nicotinic receptors activated in this way depolarize and rapidly desensitize (Kaneda et al., 1995). (*5*) Voltage-gated sodium channels for the alpha cell action potential inactivate rapidly (Kaneda and Kaneko, 1991). In short, this key physiological difference between the alpha and beta cell types arises partly from differences at the level of *inter*cellularly different wiring and partly from differences at the *intra*cellular level (different receptor and channel molecules).

Surround. The inhibitory surround arises first at the cone terminal (Fig. 6.17; see, e.g., Baylor et al., 1971; Smith and Sterling, 1990). Whereas a bright spot hyperpolarizes a central cone, a bright annulus hyperpolarizes surrounding cones. This suppresses their tonic excitation of horizontal cells, reducing GABA released onto the central cone and causing it to *de*polarize, in antagonism to its light response (Fig. 6.17D). Illuminating a small patch of cones corresponding to the ganglion cell center hardly affects horizontal cells because the patch constitutes at most a few percent of the horizontal cell input. But covering a wide field of cones (50–80 times as many cones as the center) is effective.

The bipolar cell, summing center–surround receptive fields of 5–10 converging cones, thus establishes its own center–surround receptive field at the OPL level (Werblin and Dowling, 1969; Kaneko, 1970). Then the response pattern carries forward via excitatory bipolar synapses onto the ganglion cell. Consequently when a beta cell sums 100 excitatory cone signals in its center, it also sums the antagonism of their surrounds; when an alpha cell sums 625 cone signals for its center, it likewise sums their antagonism. Because the alpha surround represents many more cone surrounds than a beta surround, it is noticeably stronger (Fig. 6.16; Freed and Sterling, 1988; Smith and Sterling, 1990). The efficacy of this lateral inhibitory circuit was demonstrated by injecting current into a horizontal cell and observing its suppression of light-evoked firing in ganglion cells (Mangel, 1991).

Lateral circuits of the IPL also contribute to the ganglion cell surround. Bipolar axons beyond the ganglion cell dendritic field excite amacrine arbors and spread signals

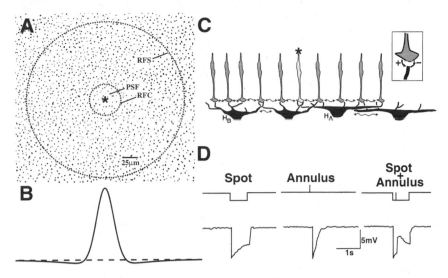

Fig. 6.17. **A:** Cone array in cat central area ($24,000/mm^2$). A point of light striking the cornea spreads, due to optical blur, to stimulate about 10 cones (PSF = point spread function). The signal spreads further, due to coupling at cone terminals, to create a receptive field center (RFC) for one cone (*) that encompasses about 50 cones. Inhibitory feedback via horizontal cells causes a receptive field surround (RFS) encompassing about 1200 cones. **B:** Sensitivity profile (difference-of-Gaussians) calculated for the cone receptive field. **C:** Neural circuit thought to shape the cone-sensitivity profile: center shaped by optics + coupling; surround shaped by inhibitory feedback (inset): its narrow, deep region set by narrow, weakly coupled H_B cell; its broad, shallow region set by broad, strongly coupled H_A cell. **D:** Intracellular recordings from turtle cone demonstrate its center–surround receptive field: a spot hyperpolarizes the center cone (*); an annulus causes a brief hyperpolarization by scattering light onto the center; the annulus plus the spot demonstrates the surround's depolarizing effect. [A–C from Smith, 1995; D from Gerschenfeld et al., 1980, with permission.]

toward the ganglion cell where they release glycine or GABA onto presynaptic bipolar terminals and ganglion cell dendrites (Pourcho and Owczarzak, 1989; Grünert and Wässle, 1990; Crooks and Kolb, 1992; Vardi and Sterling, 1994; Calkins and Sterling, 1996). Correspondingly, inhibitory conductances are recorded in the ganglion cell to broad stimuli but not to narrow ones (Freed and Nelson, 1994).

HOW RETINAL CIRCUITS SERVE VISION

NATURAL SCENES CONTAIN FINE DETAIL AT LOW CONTRAST

To appreciate how retinal circuitry serves visual performance, consider a scene from nature: a sheep among cottonwoods as viewed by a predator (wildcat) at 10 meters (Fig. 6.18A). At this distance the retinal image contains detail that is fine with respect to the grain of the ganglion cell mosaic. For example, the dark tip of the sheep's nose projected on the cat's retina fills a beta cell's receptive field center. But the detail in this scene is unlike that in an eye chart or a newspaper where the contrast is high (black/white = 1/10). In nature, the contrast tends to be low, more like 90/100 and

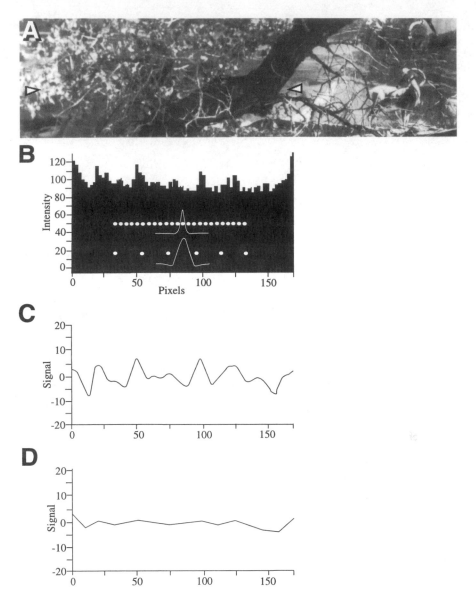

Fig. 6.18. How beta and alpha cell arrays "filter" the transduced image of a natural scene. **A:** Photograph of a bighorn sheep among the cottonwoods. Spatial detail is represented as peaks and troughs of intensity around some mean level. **B:** Photometer scan across the middle of the image (between the arrows). Much discernable structure, e.g., fine branches, differs from the mean by only a few percent. Were this scene viewed by a cat at 10 meters, one pixel would correspond roughly to one cone, and the intensity axis would correspond roughly to the signal amplitude across the cone array. Dimensions and spacings of the beta and alpha cell receptive fields are also indicated. **C:** Signal amplitude after filtering by beta cell array. Subtraction by the surrounds of the shared signal component has reset the mean to zero; pooling by the centers has reduced the noisy fluctuations. **D:** Signal amplitude after filtering by the alpha cell array. Again, a zero mean, but the broad pooling and sparse sampling has removed all but the coarsest spatial detail—thereby clearing the alpha cell dynamic range to efficiently encode motion. [Photograph by A. Pearlman; computations for B–D by R. Rao-Mirotznik and M. Eckert.]

even 99/100; this is apparent in the photometer reading across the scene (Fig. 6.18B; Srinivasan et al., 1982).

To create the optical image of a low contrast scene requires lots of light. One can verify this simply by viewing fine detail at a distance where it begins to blur. Decrease the intensity, either by dimming the light or by viewing through a dark glass, and the detail is utterly lost. Increase the intensity, and further detail emerges until the light is very bright. This can hardly be news, for who is unaware that visual acuity deteriorates after sunset? But why does this happen? Consider the explanation by Albert Rose, a pioneer in video engineering.

Rose (1973) likens the retina to a black canvas on which photons paint a scene in the pointillist style. To render one picture element (pixel) black and the others white (high contrast) requires at least $N - 1$ photons, where N = the number of pixels in the array. However, to render this pixel *gray*, say, an intensity 99% of the surrounding white pixels, requires the gray pixel to receive 99 photons while the others get 100. Thus the number of photons needed to render this scene is $100N - 1$; more generally, the lower the contrast in a scene, the more light is needed to represent it in an image.

There is an additional fact of physics to consider: photons arrive at a given point randomly in time. Their temporal fluctuation causes uncertainty regarding the true intensity at this point and is thus termed *photon noise*. As for all random processes that follow Poisson distribution, this noise is proportional to the square root of the mean. Consequently, to paint a pixel pale gray (1% dimmer than its neighbors) using random photons requires not 100 photons per pixel, as with the determinate dots of a pointillist, but the *square* of 100, i.e., 10,000 photons! To represent for an instant (~50 ms) in gray the finest detail that human optics can project on the retinal canvas would require a single cone to register about 10,000 photons—and that is about what is available in strong daylight. In short, to register fine detail at low contrast every possible photon must be transduced to minimize photon noise. This explains why baseball players tracking a white fly ball (subtending only a few cones) against a bright sky do not wear sunglasses (Sterling et al., 1992).

TO TRANSMIT A LOW CONTRAST NEURAL IMAGE REQUIRES MANY SIGNALING EVENTS

One problem in transmitting a low contrast image is that photon fluctuation in the optical image carries forward into the neural image at the level of the cones. Here, there are additional sources of noise because each step in transduction depends on random processes whose noise levels follow the same "square-root law" as photons. For example, cation channels in the cone outer segment flicker open and shut as they bind and release molecules of cGMP. The closing of a given channel at any instant does not represent a fall in the concentration of cGMP (any more than a single bump of a gas molecule on the wall of a container represents pressure) and therefore does not represent a transduction event. Only a fall in the average number of open channels signifies transduction, so again, the signal-to-noise ratio is $N/\sqrt{N}$. To represent at the first neural stage a 1% difference in the optical image requires 10,000 photosuppressible channels—and that is about what is available at any instant in one cone (Attwell, 1986; Yau, 1994).

The next problem is that a synapse can transmit only a limited number of intensity levels. This is determined by the number of synaptic vesicles that it can modulate over its modest integration time. For example, a cone terminal has been calculated to re-lease 100 vesicles/sec at each of 20 ribbon synapses (Rao et al., 1994b), but over its integration time of about 50 ms, this is only 100 vesicles. Assuming that vesicle re-lease is temporally random, the terminal could transmit at most 10 levels ($\sqrt{100}$). This may be somewhat fewer levels than a cone outer segment could encode, given that a threshold stimulus uses 6% of its photosuppressible conductance. So how can the cone terminal match the information content at its output to the number of vesicles avail-able for transmission? The question applies equally to the ganglion cell—which fires hundreds of spikes/sec (Kuffler, 1953), but over its 100 ms integration time, only 10–20 spikes. So the broad question is how to transfer a low contrast signal using noisy ele-ments of limited information capacity?

EFFICIENT CODING STRATEGIES

It is well known in the fields of information theory and image-processing that a chan-nel's capacity to transmit information increases as the logarithm of S/N ratio and lin-early with temporal bandwidth (Shannon and Weaver, 1949; reviewed by Laughlin, 1994; Attick and Redlich, 1992; van Hateren, 1992; Boahen, 1996). So given a neural channel's limited capacity, circuits should ensure that it is efficiently used by maxi-mizing the S/N ratio, removing redundancy, and subdividing the signal to segment the spatial, and especially the temporal, bandwidths.

Center Mechanisms Improve S/N. First, wherever possible, a circuit reduces accumulated noise *before* transmitting the signal forward. This prevents noise from occupying pre-cious channel capacity needed for the signal; it also prevents noise from being ampli-fied, which would make its removal at a later stage more difficult. To reduce photon noise and transduction noise, adjacent cone terminals pool their signals by electrical coupling. This hardly reduces their amplitudes because signals in adjacent cones are similar (correlated). However, the noise is strongly attenuated because random fluctu-ations in adjacent cones are *un*correlated. Consequently, the ratio of signal to noise (S/N) improves (Lamb and Simon, 1976). Pooling has some cost: loss of the very finest detail in the optical image (compare Fig. 6.18B with C). However, some of what seems to be "fine detail" in this static image is simply photon fluctuation captured over the brief integration of the photographic exposure. The improvement of S/N achieved by coupling human foveal cones is calculated for middle spatial frequencies to be about 2-fold (Hsu et al., 1997). Given an overall postreceptoral sensitivity loss of only 2- or 3-fold, this is highly significant.

Further pooling of cone signals occurs through convergence of cones onto bipolar cells and bipolar cells onto the ganglion cell (Fig. 6.16). Thus the final weighting of cone signals across the ganglion cell center is the combination of many factors: opti-cal blur, cone–coupling, cone–to–bipolar–to–ganglion cell convergence, and the domed distribution of bipolar synapses across the ganglion cell dendritic field (Fig. 6.16C; Kier et al., 1995; Freed et al., 1997). The net effect is a Gaussian weighting (Rodieck, 1965; Enroth-Cugell and Robson, 1966; Linsenmeier et al., 1982). This seems to be no accident but rather to express another computational strategy. Such a dome-like weighting for summing partially correlated signals optimally improves the beta gan-glion cell S/N ratio compared with that of a single cone by about 5-fold (Tsukamoto et al., 1990). Thus ganglion cells can achieve contrast thresholds of a few percent or less, matching what is needed to transmit the low contrast features in a natural scene.

Surround *Mechanism Reduces Redundancy.* The second image-processing strategy is to strip the signal in each cone of nonessential information. This permits what is truly essential to occupy more of the channel capacity. Since the *mean* intensity across the scene (Fig. 6.18B) is shared by neighboring cones, it is redundant. Therefore, it can be removed without loss of the essential news that a given cone (or patch of cones) is dimmer or brighter than the mean. This is the key contribution of horizontal cells: they average broadly to measure the local mean and then subtract it from the cone terminal. By stripping the redundant information at this stage, only the *difference* between the local signal and the mean need be transmitted forward along the excitatory pathway. This greatly expands the proportion of the dynamic range devoted to the differences and thus the fineness with which they can be transferred.

Note that the ganglion cell surround seems not to be concerned, as is commonly suggested, with edge detection or image sharpening. Rather, it simply reflects another standard image-processing strategy, termed *predictive coding* (Srinivasan et al., 1982). A signal averaged over some region predicts a value for the center; then only the difference between the predicted and the actual value is propagated. The best theoretical prediction weights the values near the center most strongly because they best predict the center value. The theory also suggests that in dim light the surround should become broader and shallower to get the best prediction, and indeed, the ganglion cell surround becomes broader and shallower (Derrington and Lennie, 1982).

The computational value of imparting a precise shape to the surround and of adjusting it for different intensities to get the optimal prediction may explain why there are two types of horizontal cell with different and variable coupling. When in a model only a wide-field horizontal cell feeds back onto the cone, the surround is too broad and shallow compared with its shape computed from the ganglion cell receptive field; and when only a narrow-field horizontal cell feeds back, the surround is too narrow and deep. But when both contribute, the cone surround has the proper shape (Smith, 1995). Increasing horizontal cell coupling broadens and flattens the modeled cone surround. This is one reason to suppress dopamine release in darkness—to increase horizontal cell coupling and thereby achieve the optimal predictive coding computation for the image's deteriorating S/N ratio.

Parallel Circuits Expand Dynamic Range and Divide Spatio-Temporal Bandwidth. The third image-processing strategy is to employ multiple, parallel circuits, each specialized for a different aspect of the image. This permits a given circuit to devote its full channel capacity to a small component of the original signal and transmit that component efficiently. The ON and OFF cone bipolar cells provide a good example: predictive coding at the cone terminals (see above) increases the signal fluctuations about the mean from a few percent about a mean of 100 to 10-fold about the mean zero (Fig. 6.18C). Furthermore, circuits that excite ON bipolar cells carry signals above the mean and circuits that excite OFF bipolar cells carry signals below the mean, allowing each bipolar group to encode only half of the total deviation, with a consequent doubling of the dynamic range. This also permits the corresponding ganglion cells to use high spike rates to signal decrements as well as increments, which improves their transfer. As would be expected, blocking the ON bipolar circuits with an mGluR6 agonist reduces behavioral sensitivity to light increments but not to decrements (Schiller et al., 1986).

Beta and alpha cells represent another key example of parallel processing strategy to achieve efficient coding. The beta cell's narrow center and fine sampling array render it sensitive to fine spatial detail at low contrast but *in*sensitive to coarser structure; thus, the beta cell's contrast sensitivity declines at low spatial frequencies (Derrington and Lennie, 1982). The alpha cell fills this gap. Although its broad center and sparse sampling array render it insensitive to fine stationary detail, these same properties improve its sensitivity to lower spatial frequencies. It is as though the two arrays view the world through screens of a different mesh.

And there is another advantage to parallel processing: the alpha cell can do for fine temporal correlations in the visual scene what the beta cell does for fine spatial correlations. A low contrast spot moving rapidly across the cone mosaic adds to each cone only modest numbers of extra photons. It would be impossible, by examining the output of any single cone, to distinguish this signal from photon fluctuation. However, the S/N ratio could be improved by summing the temporally correlated signals from a sequence of cones. In this case the most valuable information in the signal is that which is most sharply demarcated in time, that is, the transient. Furthermore, the larger the region that can be devoted to temporal averaging, the greater the sensitivity to high velocity. Thus, both major features of the alpha cell—its large receptive field center and its transient response—suit it to extend the range of motion detection beyond what the beta cell can do.

Since a channel's information capacity depends linearly on temporal bandwidth and only on the log of the S/N ratio, retinal circuits could transmit more information by segmenting the temporal bandwidth than by incrementally improving the S/N ratio. This might explain why ON and OFF classes of cone bipolar cell both comprise *four* different types. Since each type collects from the same set of cones, they are bombarded by synaptic vesicles at the same rate and should have similar S/N ratios. However, by expressing differention channels, different glutamate receptors, etc., they might carry different temporal bandwidths from the cone (Cohen and Sterling, 1990a,b). Some observations from fish support this (Saito et al., 1985), but the corresponding work on mammalian bipolar cells remains to be done.

Ribbon Synapses Transfer Information at High Rates. When noise has been reduced by spatial pooling, when redundant information has been stripped by predictive coding, and when different temporal bandwidths have been assigned to different bipolar types, there remains the final problem: how to transfer the signal to the ganglion cell? Assuming vesicle release to be temporally random (reviewed by Korn and Faber, 1991; Frerking and Wilson, 1996), a ganglion cell would require many vesicles to signal a small change within the receptive field center. Beta and alpha cells respond to gratings optimized to stimulate the receptive field center at contrasts as low as a few percent. A 1% contrast would require at least 10,000 vesicles over the ganglion cell's integration time (100 ms). For a ganglion cell bearing about 1000 bipolar (ribbon) synapses, this would require 100 vesicles/sec/synapse. Smaller beta cells in cat central retina and midget ganglion cells in primate fovea, which collect 10- to 40-fold fewer synapses, are far noisier and do not achieve such low contrast thresholds (Fig. 6.16).

Additional Strategies and Circuits Needed to Optimize Signal Transfer. The retina needs many additional strategies (and circuits) to optimize information transfer. For example, one expects an efficient computational strategy and a corresponding circuit for color (Buchsbaum and Gottschalk, 1983; reviewed by Calkins and Sterling, 1997b). Also, there may be mechanisms to reduce randomness in timing of transmitter release (Laughlin and de Ruyter, 1996) and mechanisms to generate strong temporal correlations in firing by adjacent ganglion cells (Meister, 1996)—both of which could improve coding efficiency.

To prevent saturation, which as noted would reduce efficiency (i.e., lose information), there need to be many mechanisms to adjust local sensitivity, i.e., mechanisms for adaptation/gain control. For example, an ON ganglion cell's sensitivity to a steady, bright stimulus to its center resets downward within about 100 ms (Cleland and Freeman, 1988). This adaptation occurs in small subunits across the center. It cannot be due to horizontal cells, whose fields are broader than the ganglion cell center, so the best candidate is some type of narrow-field amacrine cell that responds to focal stimuli and feeds back negatively onto the bipolar axon terminal (Fig. 6.14; Calkins and Sterling, 1996). In addition to adaptive mechanisms for such first order image properties as wavelength and intensity, there are also adaptive mechanisms for second-order image statistics, such as contrast and motion (Smirnakis et al., 1997). In short, although there are scores of circuits yet to be identified anatomically, there are also numerous functional problems for them to solve.

CIRCUITS FOR DAYLIGHT, TWILIGHT, AND STARLIGHT

Ambient intensity across a natural scene can vary by 100-fold. Over this range a ganglion cell responds quasi-linearly, although its range for maximum gain is limited to about 10-fold (Sakmann and Creutzfeldt, 1969), and this is why local gain control mechanisms are needed (Laughlin et al., 1987). But over the course of the day, intensity shifts by *ten billion-fold*, and no single circuit can cover the whole range. Two fundamentally different circuits are required, a *cone bipolar circuit* for graded photoreceptor signals (Fig. 6.15), and a *rod bipolar circuit* for binary signals (Fig. 6.19). By using gap junctions as neural "switches", the two circuits share key components (Fig. 6.20).

Daylight, of course, activates the cone bipolar circuit, whose key features for efficiently transferring graded signals include coupling of cone terminals (reduce noise), negative feedback (reduce redundancy), and multiple ribbon synapses at both synaptic stages (high vesicle rates to encode finely graded signals). At twilight, when ambient light intensity falls below cone threshold (100 photons/cone/integration time), this circuit fails (see above). However, rods are now desaturating. Since there are 20 rods per cone, and since a rod integrates for about 6-fold longer, signals are available from 12,000 photons transduced by rods. The 40 rod terminals immediately surrounding each cone terminal couple to it via gap junctions and thus inject this graded signal to be carried forward by the cone bipolar circuit (Kolb, 1977; Nelson, 1977; Smith et al., 1986; Sterling et al., 1988; Schneeweis and Schnapf, 1995).

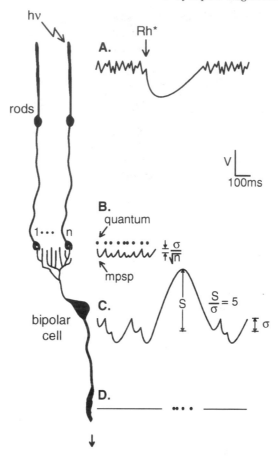

Fig. 6.19. Transmission of a binary signal. **A:** *0* (no photon) is represented at outer segment by tonic depolarization; *1* (a photon, hv) is represented by one rhodopsin isomerizing (Rh*) caus-ing a hyperpolarization. **B:** *0* is represented at the rod terminal by tonic, random release of trans-mitter quanta causing miniature hyperpolarizing PSPS at the bipolar dendrite; *1* is represented by supression of transmitter release. **C:** *0* is represented at the soma by tonic, hyperpolarization due to integrated PSPS from *n* rods (n = 20–60); *1* is represented by depolarization due to sup-pression of transmitter release at one rod terminal. **D:** *1* is represented at the bipolar terminal as a pulse of transmitter quanta. A false positive (spurious *1*) would occur if an extra-long interval between quanta at the rod terminal (due to random release) were read at the bipolar as the pause in release due to a photon. But when tonic release is at least 40 quanta/sec, the probability of a false positive is calculated to be extremely low. [From Rao et al., 1994a, with permission.]

When ambient intensity falls to one photon/rod/integration time, photons are spread too thinly to provide a graded signal. Thus the cone bipolar circuit is not needed, and worse, the coupling of many receptors that lack photons to one rod that captures a pho-ton would inject "dark noise" from the transduction cascade. Noise in the single rod would increase by the square root of the number of noisy rods coupled to it (i.e., ~6-fold), and this would obliterate its single Rh* response. To protect the Rh* response

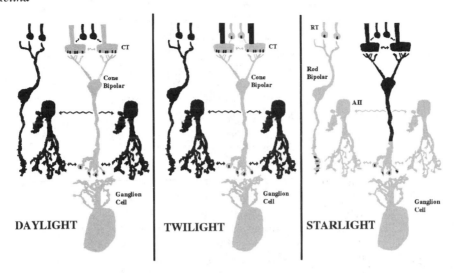

Fig. 6.20. To convey the full range of environmental intensities efficiently (i.e., minimizing neural noise and retinal thickness), requires three different circuits that partially overlap, plus three sets of gap junctions ($<\!\!\sim\!\sim\!>$) to switch between them. In *daylight* cone signals are graded and thus require many ribbon synapses for transfer (both at the OPL and IPL). In *twilight* rod signals are graded and thus also require many ribbon synapses. Rods obtain access to these by turning on their gap junctions to cone terminals, in effect, parasitizing the multiple ribbon synapses available at both stages of the cone bipolar circuit. In *starlight* rod signals are binary and thus require only a one-ribbon synapse (Fig. 6.19). The single photon response cannot transfer via coupling to the cone terminal because the many rods lacking a photon add too much noise. Therefore, the rod-cone junction turns off, and the binary signal transfers via the rod's single-ribbon synapse to the rod bipolar cell. The latter's response will be coarsely graded over some part of the intensity range (due to rod convergence) and will thus require multiple ribbon synapses—which are present in the rod bipolar terminal. The AII cell's response will be more finely graded (because of rod bipolar convergence) and will thus require yet more ribbon synapses. The AII cell obtains access to these by turning on its gap junctions with cone bipolar terminals. Coupling the AII cells, indirectly via the cone bipolar terminals and also directly via AII–AII junctions, spreads current widely enough to enlarge the ganglion cell's summation area well beyond its dendritic tree. This improves the signal/noise ratio in very dim light, but would degrade acuity in brighter light. Therefore, both sets of junction are regulated and presumably uncouple in twilight and daylight. See text.

from noise and to preserve its amplitude, the rod-cone gap junctions should uncouple at very low intensities, switching over to the rod bipolar circuit (Smith et al., 1986). Although rod–cone uncoupling has not been demonstrated directly, two rod pathways have been demonstrated psychophysically: a fast one for middle intensities (twilight) and a slower one for lowest intensities (starlight). Since their intensity ranges overlap somewhat, for certain rates of a flickering stimulus, they can be made to cancel (Stockman et al., 1995). Presumably these pathways correspond, respectively, to the rod-driven cone bipolar circuit and to the rod bipolar circuit (Fig. 6.20; reviewed by Sterling et al., 1995).

The starlight circuit's first task is to transfer a binary signal: 0 or 1 Rh*. *0* is represented by tonic vesicle release from the rod's single ribbon synapse, and *1* is represented by a pause in release (Fig. 6.19). But assuming release is temporally random, some extra-long intervals between quanta will occur that might be "mistaken" by the bipolar cell for a pause. Therefore the release rate should be high enough to prevent this source of spurious single photon signals. A model of the circuit suggests that 50–100 vesicles/sec might be enough (Rao et al., 1994a). This fits measured rates for ribbon synapses (as noted above) and suggests why the rod bipolar circuit requires only one ribbon synapse at the first stage.

However, at the next stage the rod bipolar cell collects from 20 to 60 rods, so except at the very lowest intensities, it needs to transfer a coarsely graded signal. This requires greater vesicle release than for a binary signal. Consistent with this, instead of using one ribbon synapse (as at the rod output), the rod bipolar axon uses 30 ribbon synapses at its output (Sterling et al., 1988). The AII cell collecting from about 30 rod bipolar cells needs to transfer a more finely graded signal, and for this it couples electrically to cone bipolar terminals that contribute 150–2000 synapses to a ganglion cell. Thus the overall pattern of the rod bipolar circuit is a stepwise expansion in number of ribbon synapses to match the stepwise increase in signal pooling. The rod bipolar circuit's "parasitic" use of the cone bipolar terminals as final input to ganglion cells saves space which, in the retina constrained to be thin (≤ 250 μm), is at a premium.

Tuning the Circuits. The rod circuits, like the cone circuit, are "tuned" for efficiency at different intensities by modulated coupling (reviewed in Sterling, 1995). In twilight, to preserve spatial acuity, ganglion cell receptive field centers should be narrow. But if cone bipolar axons were coupled to AII cells, cone signals would spread laterally in the AII network and degrade spatial acuity (Sterling, 1983). Therefore the cone bipolar–AII junctions should remain uncoupled until starlight, when the noisy optical image can be transmitted most efficiently by expanding the ganglion cell center (Barlow et al., 1957). Indeed, AII-cone bipolar junctions *do* uncouple when cGMP rises within the bipolar cell in response to nitric oxide production (Mills and Massey, 1995), and this mechanism may serve the transition to starlight intensities. Also in starlight, as noted, rods should uncouple from cones, and apparently do, but the mechanism is unidentified.

Finally, in starlight the AII–AII junctions should couple, but to a variable degree. This coupling reduces noise by signal averaging, and also interacts with the AII cell's voltage-sensitive mechanism (Nelson, 1982; Boos et al., 1993). This mechanism, by *thresholding*, may remove noise that would otherwise swamp the Rh* signals when 30 rod bipolar cells converge on an AII cell (Freed et al., 1987; Smith and Vardi, 1995). But it could also spread spurious spikes through the AII network. A computational model suggests that by matching coupling to the noise level (which shifts with intensity), the circuit can maximize thresholding and minimize spurious spiking (Smith and Vardi, 1995). Dopamine synapses on the AII soma (Pourcho, 1982; Voight and Wässle, 1987) uncouple AII–AII junctions (Hampson et al., 1992), and since retinal dopamine declines in darkness, AII coupling should rise progressively. Of course, once neuromodulators of coupling are identified, such as NO and dopamine, the question arises: what signals and effectors modulate the modulators? Here, at present, the trail grows cold.

CONCLUDING REMARKS

We have noted that once photons are transduced, most of their information reaches the brain. Retinal circuits achieve this astonishing efficiency in part by finely dividing responsibility. Thus we have distinguished circuits that (*1*) divide the dynamic range around the local mean intensity (ON and OFF); (*2*) divide the spatio-temporal bandwidth (beta vs. alpha, P vs. M); (*3*) divide the color spectrum (blue-yellow; red–green); and (*4*) divide vast diurnal shifts in intensity (cone bipolar vs. rod bipolar). Also key to efficient forward transfer are the ribbon synapses that can fuse vesicles and reload at very high rates. Also contributing are various linear mechanisms that reduce noise at each stage of summation by spatial averaging and optimal weighting.

One *non*linear mechanism was noted, thresholding for the Rh* signal, but there are many more. For example, the alpha cell displays nonlinear subunits that extend far beyond the conventional receptive field of (see, e.g., Hochstein and Shapley, 1976; Cox and Rowe, 1996; Derrington et al., 1979); there are also nonlinear mechanisms for rapid and slower contrast gain control (reviewed by Kaplan et al., 1990; Smirnakis et al., 1997). Intuitively, the amacrine cells should be involved, with their many different types and their rich possibilities for chemical signaling. So far we know little about amacrine *inter*cellular, synaptic circuitry, and little about their *intra*cellular, second messenger circuitry. These are puzzles for the future. However, rapid technical advances in unraveling the retina's synaptic organization, new methods for in vitro recording, and advances in molecular biology lead one to think that the future is near.

7

CEREBELLUM

RODOLFO R. LLINÁS AND KERRY D. WALTON

The cerebellum, a very distinct region of the brain, derives its name as a diminutive of the word *cerebrum*. To the ancient anatomists this was a second, smaller brain in its own right. This is particularly explicit in the German language, where *Kleinhirn* ("cerebellum") translates literally to "small brain." It occupies, in all vertebrates, a position immediately behind the tectal plate and straddles the midline as a bridge over the fourth ventricle. In addition, it is the only region of the nervous system to span the midline without interruption.

The cerebellum has undergone an enormous elaboration throughout evolution, in fact, more so than any other region of the central nervous system (CNS), including the cerebrum. Indeed, in *Homo sapiens* the cerebellum has increased in size fourfold in the past ten million years, as opposed to the entire brain, which has increased in mass threefold (Jansen, 1969; Romer, 1969). On the other hand, the cerebellum has maintained its initial neuronal structure, almost invariant, throughout vertebrate evolution. Thus, its size but not its wiring has changed in evolution. As an example, the cerebellar cortex in a frog has an area approximately 12 mm^2—that is, 4 mm wide (in the mediolateral direction) and 3 mm long (in the rostrocaudal direction). In humans, the cerebellar cortex is a single continuous sheet having an area of 50,000 cm^2 (1,000 mm wide and an average of 50 mm long). This is 4×10^3 times more extensive than that of a frog (Braitenberg and Atwood, 1958). This cortex folds into very deep folia (Fig. 7.1), allowing this enormous surface to be packed into a 6 cm $\times$ 5 cm $\times$ 10 cm volume. Because the cerebellar cortex is very long in the rostrocaudal direction, most of the foldings occur in that direction.

The basic functional design of the cerebellum is that of an interaction between two sets of quite different neuronal elements, those of the *cortex* and those in the centrally located *cerebellar nuclei*. The cerebellar cortex receives two types of afferents, the climbing and the mossy fibers, and generates a single output system, the axons of Purkinje cells (Cajal, 1904). The cerebellar nuclei receive collaterals from the climbing and mossy fibers (Bloedel and Courville, 1981) and are the main targets for the Purkinje cell axons. The cerebellum as a whole is connected to the rest of the central nervous system by three large fiber bundles, the cerebellar peduncles.

The function of the cerebellum must be considered within the context of the rest of the nervous system since it is not a primary way station for sensory or motor function;

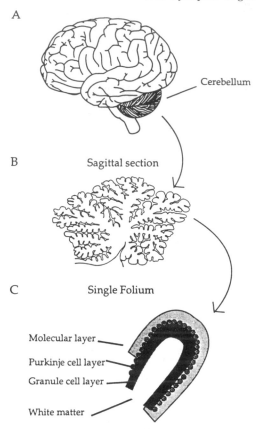

A

Cerebellum

B   Sagittal section

C   Single Folium

Molecular layer
Purkinje cell layer
Granule cell layer

White matter

Fig. 7.1. **A:** Drawing of the lateral view of the human brain showing the cerebellum. **B:** Mid-sagittal section of the cerebellum. **C:** Drawing of a single folium, showing the three layers of cerebellar cortex and the white matter.

that is, its destruction does not produce sensory deficits or paralysis. Nevertheless, lesions of the cerebellum are accompanied by well-defined and often devastating changes in the ability of the rest of the nervous system to generate even the simplest motor sequences used to attain motor goals. Indeed, the cerebellum is essential to the execution of specific movements as well as to placing motor sequences in the context of the total motor state of the individual at a given instant. Such a function is called *motor coordination* and relates to many different levels of brain function. It is not surprising then that the cerebellum should have a complex neuronal organization and that it should be vigorously connected with the rest of the brain. The enormous Purkinje cells are the sole link between the cerebellar cortex and the cerebellar nuclei. These neurons are the largest neuronal elements in the brain, with respect to the number of synapses they receive, and probably also with regard to the complexity of their integrative properties. In this chapter we will show how the role of the cerebellum in motor coordination arises from the interplay between the intrinsic excitability of the Purkinje cell and of the cerebellar nuclear cell membrane, and from the crystal-like organization of the synaptic connectivity in the cerebellar cortex (see Fig. 7.2).

NEURONAL ELEMENTS

The cerebellar cortex is one of the least variable of CNS structures with respect to its neuronal elements (Cajal, 1904; Palay and Chan-Palay, 1974). In fact, a basic circuit present in all vertebrates is now well recognized as being composed of the Purkinje cell, the single output system of the cortex, and two inputs: (*1*) a monosynaptic input to the Purkinje cell, the climbing fiber; and (*2*) a disynaptic input, the mossy fiber–granule cell–Purkinje cell system.

Because the Purkinje cell bodies are arranged in a single sheet, the Purkinje cell layer, the cerebellar cortex is divided into two main strata: (*1*) the level peripheral to the Purkinje cell layer known as the *molecular layer;* and (*2*) the layer deep to the Purkinje cells (i.e., toward the white matter), the *granular layer*. Central to the granular layer is the white matter formed by the input and output nerve-fiber systems of this cortex (Fig. 7.1B,C).

INPUT ELEMENTS

Climbing Fibers. The two types of cerebellar afferents, the climbing fibers and the mossy fibers, represent opposite extremes among the afferents in the central nervous system. The climbing fibers originate from only one brainstem nucleus, the inferior olive. The main inputs to the olive originate in the spinal cord, the brainstem, the cerebellar nuclei, and the motor cortex. Olivary axons are long, fine (1–3 μm), and myelinated. They cross the brainstem at the level of the inferior olive, after which they course rostrally to enter the cerebellum via the inferior cerebellar peduncle. Upon entering the cerebellar mass, they give off collaterals to the cerebellar nuclei and proceed toward the cerebellar cortex after branching into several fine fibers. The fibers lose their myelin as they penetrate through the granular layer before meeting with the Purkinje cell dendrites in the molecular layer (Fig. 7.3,CF). Each fiber branches repeatedly to "climb" along the entire Purkinje cell dendritic tree, thus they were named *climbing fibers* by Ramón y Cajal. Each Purkinje cell receives only one climbing fiber. However, a given inferior olivary cell axon branches to form several climbing fibers. There may be as many as ten climbing fibers generated by a single inferior olivary cell.

Mossy Fiber–Parallel Fiber Pathway. The other cerebellar afferents, the mossy fibers, originate from many CNS regions. Chief among them are the vestibular nerve and nuclei, the spinal cord, the reticular formation, the cerebellar nuclei, and the cortex via the pontocerebellar pathway, perhaps one of the most massive pathways in the brain. These fibers enter through the middle and rostral cerebellar peduncles and send collaterals to the deep cerebellar nuclei before branching in the white matter and synapsing on the granule cells (Chan-Palay, 1977). Thus, unlike the climbing fibers, mossy fibers do not synapse directly on Purkinje cells, but on the small granule cells lying directly below them (Fig. 7.3B). This connectivity increases the number of Purkinje cells ultimately stimulated by one mossy fiber axon. Also, because mossy fibers branch

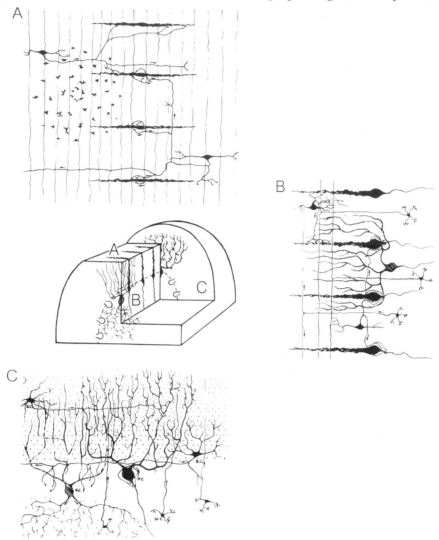

Fig. 7.2. Geometric organization of the neuronal elements of the cerebellar cortex. Three planes of section through a cerebellar folium: **A:** tangential plane (looking down on the cortical surface); **B:** transverse (medial to lateral) plane; and **C:** sagittal (anterior to posterior) plane.

profusely in the white matter, a given mossy fiber innervates several folia. The synapses between mossy fibers and granule cells occur as the fine branches of the mossy fibers twine through the granule layer axons. The contacts are made as the mossy fiber enlarges and generates tight knottings along its length. These portions of contact are called *mossy fiber rosettes.* One mossy fiber may have 20–30 rosettes (See Fig. 7.5B).

An integral part of the mossy-fiber input pathway is the granule cell axon, which completes the disynaptic input connection to the Purkinje cells. The axon of the granule cell, usually nonmyelinated, projects upward, past the Purkinje cell layer, into the molecular layer. On its way, it may form synapses with the dendritic trunk of Purkinje cells. In the molecular layer, the axon splits into two branches which take diametrically opposite directions, forming the shape of an uppercase T (Fig. 7.3B). Fibers forming the horizontal part of the T are found in all depths of the molecular layer. Because these fibers are precisely arrayed parallel to each other along the length of a folia, they have been named *parallel fibers*. These are perpendicular to the plane of the Purkinje cell dendrites (Fig. 7.3B), so that each Purkinje cell dendritic tree in humans may be intersected by as many as 200,000 parallel fibers (Braitenberg and Atwood, 1958).

OUTPUT ELEMENTS

Purkinje Cells. As stated above, the Purkinje cell is the only output element of the cerebellar cortex. These cells, which reach numbers as high as 15×10^6 in humans, were among the first neurons recognized in the nervous system (Purkinje, 1837) (Fig. 7.4A). Each cell has a large and extensive dendritic arborization, a single primary dendrite, a sphere-like soma (20–40 μm), and a long, slender axon that is myelinated when it leaves the granule cell layer. The dendrites of a typical human Purkinje cell may form as many as 200,000 synapses with afferent fibers—more than any other cell in the CNS.

The Purkinje cell dendrites extend densely above the Purkinje cell layer through the molecular layer toward the boundary of the cortex. The unusual arrangement of the Purkinje cell dendrites makes them at once the most conspicuous structural element in the cerebellar cortex and provides an important clue to its functional organization. The entire mass of tangled, repeatedly bifurcating branches is confined to a single plane, very much like a pressed leaf. Moreover, the planes of all the Purkinje cell dendrites in a given region are parallel, so that the dendritic arrays of the cells stack up in neat ranks; adjacent cells in a single plane form equally neat, but overlapping files (Fig. 7.2A). To a large extent, this orderly array determines the nature and number of contacts made with other kinds of cells. Thus, parallel fibers running perpendicular to the plane of the dendrites intersect a great many Purkinje cells, by the very manner in which these elements are organized.

The Purkinje cell is not merely a transmitter or repeater of information originating elsewhere. As we shall see, its output is determined by its synaptic interactions with other neurons, by their interactions with one another, and by its quite complex intrinsic membrane properties.

INTRINSIC ELEMENTS

The basic circuit common to all cerebella contains only one excitatory intrinsic neuron, the granule cell. This basic circuit is augmented by three types of inhibitory interneurons: the Golgi cells of the granule cell layer (Fig. 7.3C, GrC), and the basket (Fig. 7.3C, BC) and stellate cells of the molecular layer which are elaborated progressively in evolution. We will begin with the granule cells.

Granule Cells. These are the smallest cells in the cerebellum, with an oval or round soma 5–8 μm in diameter. They are densely packed in the granule cell layer, which occupies about one-third of the cerebellar mass. In fact, these cells are the most numerous in the CNS; there are about 5×10^{10} cerebellar granule cells in the human

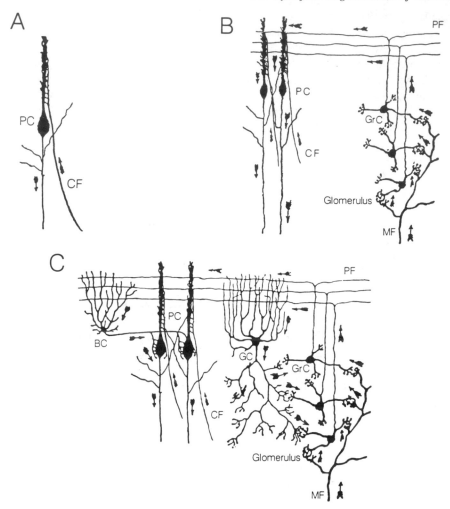

Fig. 7.3. Drawing of the cerebellar afferent circuits and intrinsic neurons. **A:** The climbing fiber–Purkinje cell circuit. A fine branch of an axon from the inferior olivary nucleus (CF) climbs over the extensive arborization of the Purkinje cell (PC) dendritic tree; note the axon collaterals of the Purkinje cell axon. The Purkinje cell is viewed in profile here since it is drawn from a coronal section of the cerebellar cortex. **B:** in the glomeruli, activity in the mossy fibers (MF) excites granule cells (GrC), whose axons project toward the surface of the cortex where they bifurcate to form parallel fibers (PF); these in turn pass through many Purkinje cell dendrites with which they form excitatory synapses. **C:** In this drawing, the two afferent systems shown in A and B are combined and the two main types of intrinsic neurons are depicted: (*1*) the Golgi cells (GC), with cell bodies just below the Purkinje cell layer; and (*2*) the basket cells (BC), with cell bodies in the molecular layer. [Modified from Cajal, 1904, with permission.]

brain. Each cell has four or five short dendrites (each less than 30 μm long) that end in an expansion (Fig. 7.4C). Their thin (0.1–0.2 μm in diameter), ascending axon has varicosities where synapses are formed, before it bifurcates to form the parallel fibers (see above). After bifurcating, the parallel fiber may run for 6 mm (3 mm on each side) before coming to an end (Fig. 7.3C).

Golgi Cells. There are two sizes of Golgi cells: (*1*) large ones (somata 9–16 μm in diameter), which are found mainly in the upper part of the granular cell layer; and (*2*) smaller ones (somata 6–11 μm in diameter), which are found in the lower half of the granular layer. They have extensive radial dendritic trees (Fig. 7.2A) that extend through all layers of the cortex (Fig. 7.3C). They receive input from the parallel fibers in the molecular layer and from climbing and mossy fiber collaterals in the granular layer. Their axons branch repeatedly in the granular layer, where they terminate on granular cell dendrites in the cerebellar glomeruli (see below). There are approximately as many Golgi cells as Purkinje cells.

Basket and Stellate Cells. These are both found in the molecular layer, receive input from parallel fibers, and may be considered to be members of a single class. The processes of both cell types are oriented transversely to the long axis of the folia (see Fig. 7.3C, BC).

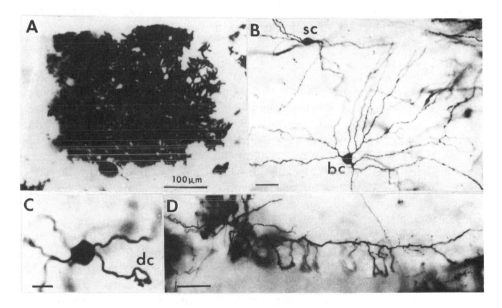

Fig. 7.4. Golgi preparations of cerebellar neurons. **A:** Purkinje cell soma, axonic initial segment and dendritic arbor in a sagittal plane of section. The extent of the dendritic tree is from the Purkinje cell layer and spreads rostrocaudally to reach the cerebellar surface. **B:** Molecular layer interneurons, stellate (sc) and basket cells (bc). The stellate cell is found in the upper 3/4 of the molecular layer. Their dendrites have few branching points and project in the same plane as the Purkinje cell dendrites. Basket cells are found deeper in the cortex, their dendrites project horizontally subtending over 180° of arc. The interneuron axons (not shown) project horizontally to the Purkinje cell layer where they contact Purkinje cell dendrites (see D below). **C:** Granule cell showing a soma with five emerging dendrites. Note that the dendrite ends in the form of a claw (dc) for contact with a mossy fiber and Golgi cell axons. **D:** Basket cell axon projects horizontally above and along the Purkinje cell layer in the same plane as Purkinje cell dendrites. Short projections of the basket axon descend about 30 μm into the Purkinje cell layer and each clasps a Purkinje cell soma. Scale: A = 100 μm; B = 20 μm; C = 5 μm; D = 50 μm. Micrographs courtesy of Dean Hillman.

The stellate cells are generally found in the outer two-thirds of the molecular layer. The smallest stellate cells, in the most superficial regions of the molecular layer, have 5- to 9-μm-diameter somata, a few radial dendrites, and a short axon (Fig. 7.4B, sc). Deeper stellate cells are larger, have more elaborate dendritic arborizations that radiate in all directions, and varicose axons that can extend parallel to the Purkinje cell dendritic plane as far as 450 μm. There are about 16 times as many small stellate cells as Purkinje cells.

Basket cells are found in the deep parts of the molecular layer, near the Purkinje cell layer. Their dendrites ascend into the molecular layer, in some instances as far as 300 μm (Fig. 7.4). Their axons extend along the Purkinje cell layer at right angles to the direction of the parallel fibers. They may spread over a distance equal to 20 Purkinje cell widths and 6 deep, and may contact as many as 150 Purkinje cell bodies. During its course, the horizontal segment of a basket cell axon sends off groups of collaterals that descend and embrace the Purkinje cell soma and initial segment (Figs. 7.3C and 7.4D; see also below). As many as 50 different basket cells are thought to wrap their axon terminals around each Purkinje cell soma, forming a basket-like meshwork resembling that on a Chianti bottle (Hámori and Szentágothai, 1966). Basket cell axons also ascend to contact the Purkinje cell dendritic tree. There are about six times as many basket cells as Purkinje cells.

CEREBELLAR NUCLEI

The Purkinje cell axons proceed through the granular cell layer, where they are myelinated, and course through the white matter to the cerebellar nuclei. Here they make inhibitory synapses on the projecting cells of the nuclei (Ito et al., 1964). There are three cerebellar nuclei on each side of the midline; each receives input from a region of the cortex directly above it and projects to specific brain regions. The most medial nuclei, the fastigial, receive input from the midline region of the cerebellar cortex, the vermis. They project caudally to the pons, medulla, vestibular nuclei, and spinal cord and rostrally to the ventral thalamic nuclei. Lateral to the vermis are the newer parts of the cerebellar cortex, the paravermis (projecting to the interposed nuclei) and the hemispheres (projecting to the convoluted dentate nuclei). These two deep cerebellar nuclei project rostrally to the red nucleus and ventral thalamic nuclei. Fibers also project to the pons, cervical spinal cord, reticular formation, and inferior olive. There is a pattern of innervation of the cerebellar nuclei within this broad radial organization whereby the rostrocaudal and mediolateral groups of Purkinje cell axons parcel each cerebellar nucleus into well-defined territories (Voogd and Bigaré, 1980).

These cells are not uniform in size: cells of small, medium, and even large diameter (≈ 35 μm) are found. The large cells have 10–12 long dendrites (about 400 μm long) that radiate to encompass a sphere. There are a few small cells with short axons, but the majority have long axons that leave the nuclei. The cerebellar nuclei are quite complex; there are two distinguishable cell populations in the fastigial and interpositus nuclei, and three populations in the dentate nucleus in cat (Palkovits et al., 1977).

The cerebellar nuclei are not simply "throughput" stations; rather, the synaptic integration that takes place here is a fulcrum for cerebellum function. Indeed, it is here that information from the cerebellar cortex is integrated with direct input from the mossy and climbing fibers. (This will be discussed in the section on Basic Circuits).

As in Purkinje cells, the intrinsic properties of the nuclear neurons are very important to their function (see Intrinsic Membrane Properties).

SYNAPTIC CONNECTIONS

Over 100 years ago, Ramón y Cajal (1888) published his description of the cerebellum. In this study of Golgi-stained material, the synaptic connections were already indicated, as shown in Fig. 7.2, as were the directions of flow of impulses in this cortex. Recent electron microscopic studies, which have provided additional information about the type of synaptic connections and their fine structure (cf. Palay and Chan-Palay, 1974), have confirmed Cajal's initial description. The synaptic connections among the elements in the cerebellum will be discussed by layer, not by cell type, in order to highlight the local circuits at each level of the cerebellum. We will begin with the granular cell layer.

GRANULAR CELL LAYER

Two cell types receive input here, the granule cells and the Golgi cells. The synapses onto granule cells take place in the cerebellar "glomeruli." The rosettes, which occur along the fine branches at the terminals of mossy fibers, form the core of each glomerulus. Excitatory synapses (Gray's type 1) are made between the rosettes and the interdigitating dendrites from as many as 20 granule cells. This can be seen in the electron micrograph in Fig. 7.5B, where a large mossy fiber presynaptic terminal (mf) is seen to be surrounded by several granular cell dendritic claws (dc). The presynaptic terminal contains spherical presynaptic vesicles about 450 Å in diameter. Golgi cell axon terminals surround the rosettes, where they make inhibitory (Gray's type 2) synapses onto the granule cell dendrites (Fig. 7.5B, ga). All are encapsulated by a glial lamella which marks the border of each glomerulus.

In the granular layer, Golgi cells receive excitatory (type 1) input from the mossy fibers. These synapses are formed on the Golgi cell dendrites and somata. Thus, mossy fiber volleys excite Golgi and granule cells. Climbing fibers also contact Golgi cells in the granular cell layer. Finally, Purkinje-cell recurrent axon-collateral varicosities and terminals make inhibitory (type 2) synapses on Golgi-cell dendritic trunks and primary branches.

PURKINJE CELL LAYER

The synapse formed in this region is between the basket-cell axon terminal and the Purkinje-cell soma and initial segment. As many as 50 basket-cell axon branches make intricate arborizations surrounding the somata, which form many axosomatic synapses, as shown in the electron micrograph in Fig. 7.5C, which illustrates basket cell axon (ba) contacts on the soma and initial segment of a Purkinje cell. Even though basket cell terminals cover both the soma and the axon hillock of the Purkinje cells, only a few synapses with the typical structure of Gray's type 2 (see Chap. 1) have been observed at the axon hillock level; however, a rather impressive morphological structure known as the *pinso terminale* may be found at this level (Cajal, 1888). This terminal portion is not a chemical synapse, but is similar to the electrical inhibitory synapse in Mauthner cells. These synapses very effectively shut down the output of the cortex.

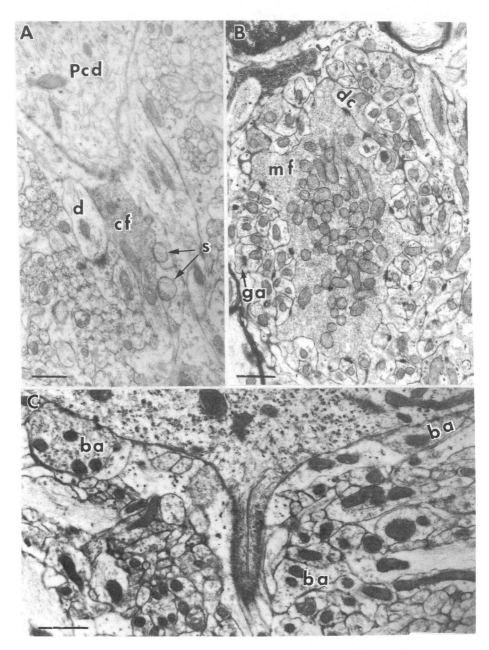

Fig. 7.5. Electron micrographs of parallel fiber and basket axon synaptic relationships. **A:** Climbing fiber (cf) synapse with spines from a large adjacent Purkinje cell dendrite (Pcd). The contact is made on Purkinje cell spines (s) as the climbing fiber follows the main Purkinje cell dendrite. Note that glial projections surround the dendrite and synaptic spines. A stellate cell or Golgi cell dendrite is adjacent to the climbing fiber and is contacted by a parallel fiber. **B:** A mossy fiber rosette (mf) filled with synaptic vesicles and mitochondria. Surrounding the mossy fiber axon are numerous profiles from dendritic claws (dc) making synaptic contacts. Golgi axon

MOLECULAR LAYER

Climbing Fiber–Purkinje Cell Connection. Among the afferent systems of central neurons, none is more remarkable in extent and power than the climbing fiber junction with Purkinje cells. This junction is unusual not only for its large coverage of a considerable portion of the Purkinje cell dendritic tree but also because, as we have seen, only one climbing fiber afferent contacts each Purkinje cell. The synapses are made between varicosities (2 μm across) on the climbing fiber and stubby spines on the soma and main dendrites of the Purkinje cell; as many as 200 contacts may be made between a climbing fiber and its Purkinje cell. Each contact synapses on 1 to 6 spines. A climbing fiber terminal (cf) contacting a Purkinje cell spine (s) near a dendrite (Pcd) is shown in Fig. 7.5A. A dendrite (d) from a Golgi or stellate cell is adjacent to the climbing fiber terminal. The presynaptic vesicles are round and 440–590 Å in diameter. Morphologicallay the presence of a climbing fiber synapse seems to exclude nearby parallel fiber–Purkinje cell contacts. The Purkinje cell dendrites can thus be divided into a central area covered by the climbing fibers and the more peripheral, spiny dendritic portion that is contacted by parallel fibers.

Parallel Fiber Connections. In contrast to the climbing fibers which contact mainly Purkinje cell dendrites, the parallel fibers terminate on the dendrites of all the neuronal elements in the cerebellar cortex, the only exception being the granule cells. Thus, parallel fibers contact the dendrites of Purkinje cells, basket cells, stellate cells, and Golgi cells. On the Purkinje cells, parallel fibers synapse with the spines on the terminal regions of the Purkinje cell dendrites, in regions called *spiny branchlets*. These are shown in Fig. 7.6A where an antibody against calbindin has been used to reveal the great density of spines on the dendritic trees of two Purkinje cells. The synaptic junction is formed between the head of a spine and a globular expansion of the parallel fiber; the spine penetrates the swollen part of the fiber. The electronmicrograph in Fig. 7.6B illustrates a Purkinje cell spiny branchlet (sb) with at least three spines (one is marked). A synapse with a parallel fiber is clearly seen on each of the three right-hand spines. The synaptic vesicles are spherical and 260–440 Å in diameter. A parallel fiber forms synapses with one out of the 3 to 5 Purkinje cells that it traverses. Thus, most of the parallel fibers passing a dendritic tree will not form synapses. There is such a large number of parallel fibers that as many as 200,000 synapses on one Purkinje cell dendrite may be formed in humans, by far the largest number of synaptic inputs to any central neuron. The ascending portion of the granule cell axon has varicosities that are presynaptic to spines on the lower dendrites of Purkinje cells. A Golgi cell dendrite (Gcd) with a spine (s) emerging from the dendritic shaft is shown in Fig. 7.6C. Parallel fiber boutons (b) synapse directly on the dendrite, the dendritic spine (s) head and the spine shaft.

---

boutons (ga) contact the dendritic claws. C: Initial axonal segment of Purkinje cell. The base of the soma has basket axonal contacts (ba). Basket axons are separated from the Purkinje axon by glia but contact each other forming the pinceau of contacts between axons at their tips below this region. Scale: A = 5 μm; B = 3 μm; C = 1 μm. Micrographs courtesy of Dean Hillman and Suzanne Chen.

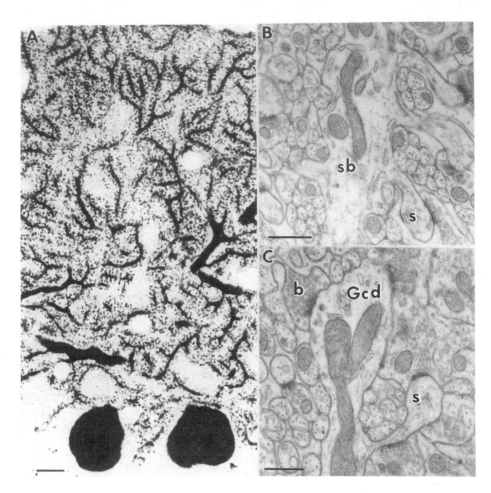

Fig. 7.6. Cerebellar molecular layer synaptic relationships of parallel fibers (granule cell axons) with Purkinje cells and interneurons. **A:** Immunoreaction of a Purkinje cell showing the detail of spine density on spiny branchlets (Calbindin antibody on a 1-μm plastic section.) The profiles of two Purkinje cell somata are seen with segments of the main dendritic arbor and numerous spiny branchlets. Emerging spines and profiles of spine heads dot the field, revealing the high density of Purkinje-cell spine synapses with parallel fibers. Longitudinal sections of spiny branchlets show that the interspace interval of spines along the dendrite is near the diameter of the spine head. Note that the larger main branches have few spines. **B:** Electron micrograph of a Purkinje cell spiny branchlet (sb) that is longitudinally sectioned and has spines (s) emerging from the dendritic shaft in contact with a parallel fiber bouton. Bergmann glial projections shroud the spine shaft and junctional site. **C:** Golgi cell dendrite (Gcd) with parallel fiber (b) synapses. Spine (s) emerges from the dendritic shaft with parallel fiber synapse on the head and the shaft. Parallel fiber boutons (b) synapse directly on the dendrite. Scale: A = 10 μm; B = 1 μm; C = 1 μm. Micrographs courtesy of Dean Hillman and Suzanne Chen.

Modulation of Excitatory Synapses. In addition to the excitatory action of climbing and parallel fibers on Purkinje cells (see page 275) and their intrinsic roles in Purkinje cell integration, other functions related to their temporal interaction have been proposed. Ito et al. (1982) reported that simultaneous low-frequency activation (1–4 Hz) of these two inputs such that climbing fibers precede parallel fiber activation (induction) reduces subsequent parallel fiber action on Purkinje cells when both inputs are again stimulated (expression). Thus, following such pairing, the parallel fiber EPSP or EPSC amplitude is reduced by 20–50%; this effect is maximal after 5–10 min. It lasts as long as it has been studied, usually 1–2 hr, and is called *long-term depression* (LTD). Comparable phenomena induced by low-frequency stimulation have been found in other regions of the brain (cf. Chaps. 10–12).

The order and temporal sequence for the generation of this depression were initially proposed on theoretical grounds by Albus (1971) as the basis for his hypothesis that the cerebellar cortex may be the seat of motor learning. Ito et al. (1982) interpreted their results as a confirmation of Albus's theory, but this is a matter of controversy. The phenomenon has since been studied largely in cerebellar slices, dispersed Purkinje cells, and more reduced preparations (Narasimhan and Linden, 1996). With these in vitro preparations, the cellular mechanism underlying this form of "memory" has become an area of active research (Linden and Connor, 1993) and discussion (Llinás and Welsh, 1993).

An important issue with LTD has been its apparent specificity. Since climbing fiber activation stimulates the entire dendritic tree, the specificity is determined by the parallel fiber synapses. That is, only Purkinje cells that respond to those parallel fibers that were coactivated with climbing fiber input during the induction phase would presumably show a decrease in parallel fiber activation. This would mean that the input from a small group of granule cells would be selectively depressed, modifying the "computational" power of each Purkinje cell.

However, it has been recently shown that the opposite order of stimulation—parallel fiber activation preceding climbing fiber activation of Purkinje cells—can also lead to LTD (Chen and Thompson, 1995) and that parallel fibers in their own right can also activate such a process (Hartell, 1996). Indeed, parallel fibers alone can activate calcium entry on spines of Purkinje cells (Denk et al., 1995). Thus, a new hypothesis as to how LTD may relate to motor function must be developed since Albus's learning hypothesis was quite specific on the nature and order of climbing fiber–parallel fiber interaction.

From a molecular biological point of view, it has been proposed that LTD induction is associated with activation of voltage-gated calcium channels following climbing fiber activity and of metabotropic glutamate receptors (mGluR1) and AMPA glutamate receptors following parallel fiber activity. Climbing fiber activation of Purkinje cells leads to the opening of voltage-gated calcium channels and the generation of calcium spikes in the dendrites. The resulting increased intracellular concentration of calcium is necessary for LTD induction. Direct Purkinje cell depolarization can be substituted for climbing fiber activation. Activation of the metabotropic glutamate channels leads to phospholipase C–mediated production of diacylglycerol and inositol-1,4,5-triphosphate. The AMPA receptors are linked to Na^+ selective channels and sodium entry through the AMAP channels is necessary for the induction of LTD (Linden et al., 1993). Ionophoresis of glutamate can be substituted for parallel fiber stimulation. The ultimate expression of LTD is thought to be due to desensitization of AMPA-receptor function (Linden, 1994).

We can summarize what is known about the induction of LTD in the cerebellar cortex as follows. (*1*) Climbing fiber stimulation leads to increased intracellular concentration of calcium through voltage-gated channels and to increased cGMP, possibly through NO and guanylate cyclase. Parallel fibers also increase, in their own right, calcium concentration in these dendrites. (*2*) Parallel fiber activation leads to activation of metabotropic glutamate receptor–linked channels, which in turn leads to increased diacyglycerol and inositol-1,4,5-triphosphate. (*3*) Parallel fiber activation leads to activation of glutamic receptors and inflow of sodium and calcium via the ligand-dependent channels and of calcium to voltage-gated channels. (*4*) The expression of LTD is through desensitization of specific, parallel fiber-activated Purkinje cell AMPA receptors. The physiological role of LTD as well as its mode of generation is still a matter of debate. Indeed, placing LTD in the context of cerebellar function awaits further studies carried out under physiological conditions.

Plasticity of Purkinje Cell Connectivity. In the Purkinje cell dendritic tree, the climbing fiber input is normally proximal to the parallel fiber input (Fox et al., 1967). When damage to the climbing fibers occurs in the adult animal, however, spines proliferate in large numbers on Purkinje cell smooth dendrites. These are promptly invaded by newly formed parallel fiber contacts (Sotelo et al., 1975), indicating a tug of war or a territoriality between the two systems. Also, destruction of the parallel fibers promotes multiple climbing-fiber innervation (Mariani et al., 1977), indicating that a true competition for a Purkinje-cell dendritic tree exists between parallel and climbing fiber afferents and even between climbing fiber afferents themselves. It also indicates that a single climbing fiber cannot provide all the necessary input, since Purkinje cells do become innervated by climbing fibers after parallel fiber damage.

Quantitative studies have been made of the changes in the parallel fiber–Purkinje cell synapse localized after lesioning of the parallel fiber input. In one set of experiments, the parallel fibers were sectioned and the molecular layer was undercut (to destroy the granule cells) (Hillman and Chen, 1984). The number, size, and average contact area of the parallel fiber–Purkinje cell synapses were evaluated 2 to 3 weeks after the lesion and compared with control values from unlesioned animals. It was found that the number of parallel fibers contacting a Purkinje cell was reduced in relation to the extent of the lesion, but that the area of synaptic contact of the surviving synapses was proportionally increased. Thus, there was a change in the position and size of the synapses in response to perturbations, but the total area of synaptic contact remained stable. Change in the size of the presynaptic boutons was not accompanied by a change in the presynaptic grid densities or the number of synaptic vesicles (Hillman and Chen, 1985a). This suggests that as the size of the boutons increased, there was a parallel increase in the morphological correlates of the neurotransmitter release machinery. Stabilization of the total synaptic area has also been seen in other areas of the CNS (see Hillman and Chen, 1985b).

Other Connectivity in the Molecular Layer. In addition to Purkinje cells, the dendrites of stellate, basket, and Golgi cells receive inputs in the molecular layer (see Fig. 7.3C). The stellate cells in turn make inhibitory synapses into Purkinje-cell dendritic shafts. Parallel fiber swellings make excitatory synapses onto stellate-cell dendritic spines. The basket cells receive excitatory synaptic connections from climbing fibers and parallel fibers and are inhibited by Purkinje-cell axon collaterals. Parallel and climbing fibers make the same *en passant* synapses with basket cell dendrites as with Purkinje cell dendrites. Finally, Golgi cell dendrites receive excitatory synapses from the parallel fibers. These axodendritic synapses are by far the largest number of synapses onto Golgi cells.

CEREBELLAR NUCLEI

Five different types of synaptic terminals have been distinguished on the basis of the characteristics of their membrane attachment and shape of synaptic vesicles. Both axosomatic and axodendritic synapses are found. The presynaptic terminals are made by mossy and climbing fibers, and by Purkinje cell axon collaterals (Palkovits et al., 1977). Purkinje cell axons have 2 to 3 branches which arborize extensively in the nucleus, describing a narrow cone. Synapses are formed at the terminals and at *en passant* thickenings along the length of the axon. Synapses are usually formed with dendritic thorns or spines of nuclear cells, although some synapses are axosomatic. The thickenings and terminals have dispersed ovoid vesicles, usually found where they contact the dendrites of nuclear neurons. It has been calculated that a Purkinje cell may contact as many as 35 nuclear cells, but most contacts are made with 3 to 6 Purkinje cells. In addition to this divergence, there is convergence since there are about 26 nuclear cells for each Purkinje cell. There are about 860 Purkinje cell axons for each nuclear cell.

Complex synaptic combinations such as serial and triadic synapses are found in the cerebellar nuclei (Hámori and Mezey, 1977), as seen in the retina (Chap. 6) and thalamic nuclei (Chap. 8). These imply a quite complex interaction between the afferents and nuclear cells. In these synapses the first presynaptic element may be a Purkinje-cell axon terminal, a brainstem afferent terminal (climbing or mossy fibers), or an axon terminal collateral. The last ones probably involve projecting nuclear-cell axon collaterals. The second terminal in the sequence, which is both pre- and postsynaptic, derives from the cerebellar nuclear cells themselves; they are either axon collaterals of projecting neurons or Golgi type II interneurons. Although such synapses are a regular feature of the nuclei, they do not form as large a percentage of synapses as in some sensory systems.

BASIC CIRCUIT ORGANIZATION

There are three main circuits in the cerebellum, two circuits in the cortex, which include afferent fibers as shown in Fig. 7.3 and one circuit in the deep nuclei. They are diagrammed in Fig. 7.7.

MOSSY FIBER CIRCUIT

The sequence of events that follows the stimulation of mossy fibers was first suggested by János Szentágothai of the Semmelweis University School of Medicine in Budapest:

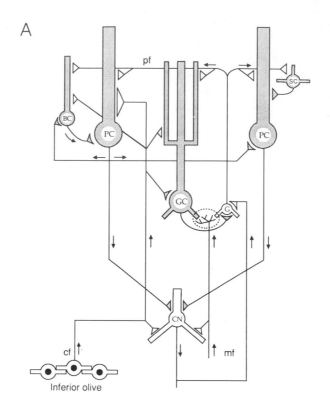

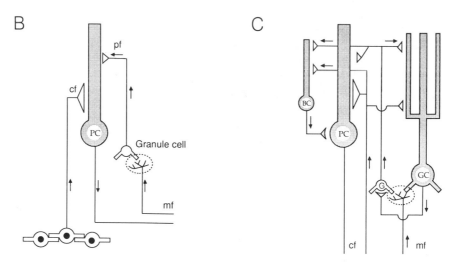

Fig. 7.7. Diagram of the basic circuit in the mammalian cerebellum. **A:** This circuit includes all the elements making specific synaptic connections in the cerebellar cortex and nuclei. **B,C:** Simplified diagrams of cerebellar cortex showing the afferent circuits (B) and the intrinsic neurons (C). BC, basket cell; cf, climbing fiber; CN, cerebellar nuclear cell; G, granule cell; GC, Golgi cell; mf, mossy fiber; PC, Purkinje cell; pf, parallel fiber; SC, stellate cell.

the stimulation of a small number of mossy fibers activates, through the granule cells and their parallel fibers, an extensive array of Purkinje cells and all three types of inhibitory interneurons. Subsequent interactions of the neurons tend to limit the extent and duration of the response. The activation of Purkinje cells through the parallel fibers is soon inhibited by the basket cells and the stellate cells, which are activated by the same parallel fibers. Because the axons of the basket and stellate cells run at right angles to the parallel fibers, the inhibition is not confined to the activated Purkinje cells; those on each side of the beam or column of stimulated Purkinje cells are also subject to strong inhibition. The effect of the inhibitory neurons is therefore to sharpen the boundary and increase the contrast between those cells that have been activated and those that have not.

At the same time, the parallel fibers and the mossy fibers activate the Golgi cells in the granular layer. The Golgi cells exert their inhibitory effect on the granule cells and thereby quench any further activity in the parallel fibers. This mechanism is one of negative feedback: through the Golgi cells the parallel fiber extinguishes its own stimulus (Fig. 7.7A). The net result of these interactions is the brief firing of a relatively large but sharply defined population of Purkinje cells.

CLIMBING FIBER CIRCUIT

Stimulation of a group of climbing fibers produces a powerful excitation of Purkinje cells. The stimulus elicits prolonged bursts of high-frequency potentials. The climbing fibers also activate Golgi cells, which inhibit the input through the mossy fibers (Fig. 7.7A). Thus, when climbing fibers fire, their Purkinje cells are dominated by this input. The climbing fiber input to basket and stellate cells sharpens the area of activated Purkinje cells.

CEREBELLAR CORTEX–DEEP NUCLEI CIRCUIT

Electrical activation of mossy fiber inputs to the cerebellar system generates an early excitation in the cerebellar nuclei since the collaterals terminate directly on the cerebellar nuclear cells (Fig. 7.7A). The same information then proceeds to the cerebellar cortex, which in turn produces an early excitation of Purkinje cells to be translated into inhibition at the cerebellar nucleus. This inhibition is followed by a prolonged increase in excitability of the cerebellar nuclear (CN) cells. The increased excitability is the result of two actions: (*1*) disinhibition due to reduced Purkinje cell activity, which in turn results from the inhibitory action of basket and stellate cells after the initial activation of Purkinje cells; and (*2*) CN cell intrinsic properties (see below). The Purkinje cell inhibition is also due indirectly to the inhibitory action of the Golgi interneuron, which, by preventing the mossy fiber input from reaching the molecular layer, reduces the excitatory drive to Purkinje cells. The CN projecting neurons themselves send axon collaterals to cortical inhibitory interneurons including basket cells, which thus provide recurrent inhibition of the CN neurons, as seen in spinal motoneurons (Chap. 4).

INTRINSIC MEMBRANE PROPERTIES

In Chap. 2 it was emphasized that the functional characteristics of a neuron are the outcome of a complex interplay between its intrinsic membrane properties and its synaptic interactions. In no part of the brain is this exemplified more vividly than in the cerebellum. Indeed, as already mentioned in Chap. 2, the Purkinje cell is one of the best known models for demonstrating these properties. Because of this importance, we will consider the intrinsic membrane properties separately in this section before addressing the synaptic actions of the system.

PURKINJE CELLS

The intrinsic membrane properties of cells may be considered independent of synaptic input, although interaction of synaptic potentials with intrinsic membrane properties shapes the activity of the cell. Intrinsic properties are usually studied by determining the response to direct activation, that is, to depolarizing or hyperpolarizing current injected into the cell, usually into the soma. Purkinje-cell electrical activity may be recorded under in vivo or in vitro conditions; however, since the most reliable recordings are obtained in vitro, our understanding of the electrical properties of the mammalian Purkinje cell membrane has come mainly from studies of cerebellar slices (Llinás and Sugimori, 1978, 1980a,b). Antidromic activation of a Purkinje cell is characterized by a large spike having an initial segment–soma dendritic (IS–SD) break that is in many ways similar to that obtained in vivo from motoneurons and other central neurons.

Direct stimulation of Purkinje soma via the recording microelectrode demonstrates that these cells fire in a way that is quite different from that seen in other neurons. Indeed, square current pulses lasting about 1 sec (Fig. 7.8A) produce, at just threshold depolarization, a repetitive activation of the cell. That is to say, with long pulses the neuron fires, but a single isolated spike cannot be generated by this type of stimulation. This burst of activity is produced by a low-threshold, sodium-dependent conductance that does not inactivate within several seconds and serves to trigger the fast action potentials. This sodium conductance is different from that responsible for the fast action potentials seen in virtually all nerve cells: it is activated at a lower voltage and does not inactivate. With increased stimulation the onset of the repetitive firing moves earlier. Also, at the end of the initial pulse of firing, a reduction in the amplitude of the spikes is followed by a rhythmic bursting, as marked by arrows in Fig. 7.8B.

Pharmacological studies in cerebellar slices have shown that the fast action potentials and the bursting have different ionic mechanisms. Removal of extracellular sodium or the application of tetrodotoxin (TTX, a sodium-conductance blocker) to the bath causes a complete abolition of the fast action potentials seen in Fig. 7.8A and B but leaves a late, slow-rising burst potential intact, as shown in Fig. 7.8C. This slow bursting of Purkinje cells has been found to be generated by a voltage-activated calcium conductance followed by a calcium-dependent potassium conductance increase. We know the spikes are calcium dependent because they are seen in the absence of sodium and because they are blocked by the removal of calcium from the extracellular medium or by ions that block the slow calcium conductance (cobalt, cadmium, manganese), as shown in Fig. 7.8D. When the calcium in the bathing solution is replaced by barium, the afterhyperpolarization is reduced and the bursting response is converted into a prolonged single action potential. This demonstrates the presence of a calcium-activated potassium conductance, since it is known that barium does not activate the calcium-activated potassium conductance. All electroresponsiveness is gone following calcium

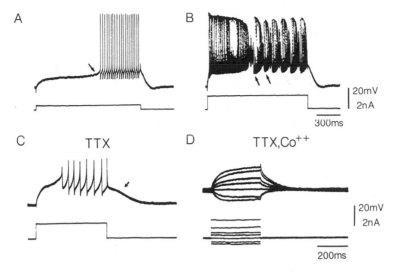

Fig. 7.8. Intrinsic properties of mammalian Purkinje cells recorded in vitro. **A:** A prolonged, threshold current pulse injected into the soma of a Purkinje cell elicits a train of action potentials after an initial local response (arrow). **B:** Increased current strength elicits high-frequency firing and oscillatory behavior (arrows). **C:** After addition of TTX to the bath, the fast action potentials are blocked, and the slowly rising action potentials underlying the oscillations seen in B are revealed. A slow after-depolarization may also be seen. **D:** Addition of cobalt chloride (Co^{2+}) to the TTX perfusate removes all electroresponsiveness, indicating that the slow action potentials in C were calcium dependent. [Modified from Llinás and Sugimori, 1980a, with permission.]

and sodium blockade, as shown by the application of both tetrodotoxin (TTX) and cobalt to the extracellular medium (see Fig. 7.8D). Thus, at the somatic level, Purkinje cells have not one, but three main mechanisms for spike generation: (*1*) a sodium-dependent spike similar to that seen in other cells, which is blocked by the absence of extracellular sodium or by the application of TTX; (*2*) a low-threshold, non-inactivating sodium spike; and (*3*) a calcium-dependent action potential, which has a slow rising time and a rather rapid return to baseline.

The distribution and properties of voltage-gated channels in the dendrites will be discussed below (Dendritic Properties).

CEREBELLAR NUCLEAR CELLS

The electrical properties of cerebellar nuclear (CN) neurons were first studied in detail in in vitro preparations (Jahnsen, 1986a,b; Llinás and Mühlethaler, 1988b). Like Purkinje cells, CN cells have a collection of ionic conductances that give them complex firing abilities. CN cells have a non-inactivating sodium conductance similar to that described in Purkinje cells, in addition to the usual sodium- and potassium-dependent conductances that generate fast action potentials. The firing of CN cells depends on their resting potential. If a cell is depolarized with a current pulse from the resting potential as in Fig. 7.9A, the cell fires a train of action potentials. However, if the same current pulse is injected when the cell is held hyperpolarized from the rest-

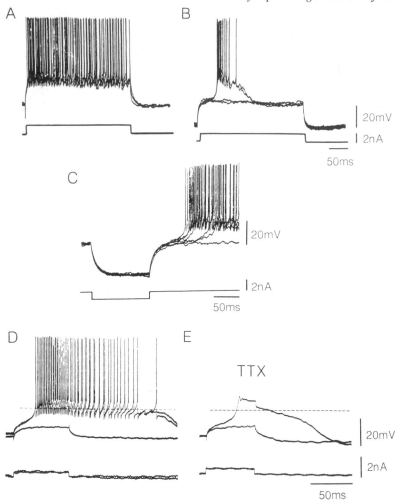

Fig. 7.9. Intrinsic properties of cerebellar nuclear neurons. **A:** A depolarizing current injection from resting potential elicits tonic firing. **B:** When the same strength current pulse is delivered from a hyperpolarized membrane level, an all-or-none burst response is elicited. **C:** Hyperpolarizing current injection from the resting potential elicits a strong rebound burst of action potentials from a slow depolarization. **D:** Response to current injection from a hyperpolarized level (resting potential marked by broken line). **E:** Addition of TTX to the perfusate blocked the fast action potentials, revealing a slowly rising, prolonged depolarization and after-depolarization; these responses were then blocked by addition of Co^{2+} to the bath. [Modified from Llinás and Mühlethaler, 1988b, with permission.]

ing potential, all-or-nothing bursts are seen, as shown in Fig. 7.9B and D. Also, if a hyperpolarizing current pulse is injected into a CN neuron, a burst of action potentials is seen at the end of the current injection (Fig. 7.9C).

This "rebound response" following hyperpolarization is important in CN cell function. This is easily understood since Purkinje cells are inhibitory and generate inhibitory postsynaptic potentials (IPSPs) in CN cells. The ionic basis for these burst responses

was determined by pharmacological studies. Thus, after eliminating the fast sodium conductance by application of TTX, although the fast action potentials seen in Fig. 7.9D are blocked, a slowly rising spike is elicited from the hyperpolarized membrane potential (Fig. 7.9E). The threshold for these spikes is lower than that for the fast sodium-dependent action potentials; they are therefore called *low-threshold spikes* (LTS). They are calcium dependent since they are blocked after addition of cobalt or removal of calcium from the bath, and are insensitive to TTX. The presence of a LTS is probably of major functional significance in these neurons because climbing fiber activation of Purkinje cells following such bursts can easily be elicited following the powerful IPSPs produced by this input (see Fig. 7.15; Llinás and Mühlethaler, 1988b).

SYNAPTIC ACTIONS

CLIMBING FIBER ACTION ON PURKINJE CELLS

Although for the most part, a one-to-one relationship exists between a climbing fiber and a given Purkinje cell (each Purkinje cell receives one climbing fiber), the cell of origin of this afferent (the inferior olivary neuron) is probably capable of producing more than one climbing fiber afferent and probably as many as ten. One of the most powerful synaptic junctions in the CNS is that between the climbing fiber afferent and the dendrite of a Purkinje cell. This has been called a *distributed synapse* since a single presynaptic fiber makes contact with the postsynaptic cell at many points throughout the Purkinje cell dendritic tree, and the synapse is distributed over a large surface area. This is in contrast to more typical synapses, as between a 1a terminal and motoneuron, where there are only a few, relatively localized points of contact (see Chap. 4). Eccles et al. (1966a) demonstrated electrophysiologically that stimulation of the inferior olive produces a powerful activation of the Purkinje cell. This synaptic excitation is characterized by an all-or-nothing burst of spikes that shows little variability from one activation to the next. These are called *complex spikes*. Several complex spikes recorded from an isolated preparation are superimposed in Fig. 7.10A and B. It is now known that the spikes on the broad EPSP are produced at the dendrite by a voltage-activated calcium conductance (see below) and at the somatic and axonic levels by the usual Hodgkin-Huxley sodium–potassium spikes (Llinás and Sugimori, 1978, 1980b).

Climbing fiber responses in Purkinje cells may be elicited by placing a stimulating electrode in the white matter near the midline. This "juxtafastigial" stimulation activates inferior olivary axons in the white matter. Following a juxtafastigial stimulus, climbing fiber synapses are activated simultaneously and produce a very large unitary EPSP in the postsynaptic dendrite. This unitary synaptic potential usually has an amplitude of 40 mV and lasts 20 msec. The all-or-nothing character of the climbing fiber burst actually represents the all-or-nothing character of the presynaptic spike in the climbing fiber. If the Purkinje cells are hyperpolarized far enough to prevent the cell from spiking, the all-or-nothing character of the EPSPs may be seen (Fig. 7.10C).

Under conditions in which the sodium- and calcium-dependent spikes are prevented, the chemical nature of the synapse may be studied in detail and its distributed character clearly demonstrated. Depolarization of the soma or dendrite can produce a reduction in amplitude and an actual reversal of the sign of the climbing fiber EPSP, as

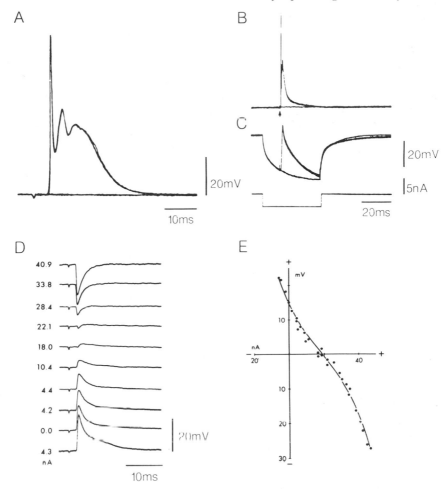

Fig. 7.10. Climbing fiber activation of mammalian Purkinje cells in vitro. **A:** All-or-none complex spikes in a Purkinje cell evoked by white matter stimulation are superimposed. **B:** In another Purkinje cell, five threshold white-matter stimuli (arrow) evoke very uniform complex spikes on four occasions. **C:** If threshold stimuli are delivered when the cell is hyperpolarized (to prevent action potential firing), the all-or-none climbing fiber EPSP may be seen. **D:** Reversal of climbing fiber EPSP. Notice that, as expected in a distributed synapse, the reversal is biphasic, with the early portion of the potential reversing at lower levels of injected current than the late part; this may be seen at 18, 22, and 28 nA. **E:** Plot of the voltage–current relation for the EPSP reversal shown in D. [Modified from Llinás and Nicholson, 1976, and Llinás and Mühlethaler, 1988a, with permission.]

shown in Fig. 7.10D. A large increase in the EPSP amplitude is seen when the membrane potential is moved in the hyperpolarizing direction (lower traces in D). The reversal in sign (shown in Fig. 7.10D, 22.1 nA) is then necessary and sufficient evidence to indicate that a synaptic junction is chemical in nature (see Chap. 2).

The fact that different parts of the EPSP (the peak and falling phase) reverse at different levels of depolarization (see biphasic reversal at 22.1 nA in Fig. 7.10D) indi-

cates that the synapse occurs at multiple sites having different distances from the site of recording in the soma (Llinás and Nicholson, 1976). Because a current point source, a microelectrode, is utilized to change the membrane potential, the potential change along the dendrite is maximum near the site of impalement and decreases with distance. Because the synapses closest to the site of recording generate most of the rising phase of the recorded EPSP, this component is the first to reverse. Those synapses located at a distance generate the slowest components (owing to the cable properties of the dendrites) and are less affected by the current injection. Recordings similar to those obtained in vitro can also be obtained in vivo.

Activation of the climbing fiber afferents generates a burst of action potentials at the Purkinje cell axon. The frequency of this response is high, generally 500/sec. Indeed, it is higher normally than that seen after parallel fiber stimulation, suggesting that one of the possible functions of the climbing fiber system is to produce a discharge of distinct bursts of action potentials. As discussed later, climbing fiber activation also produces very sharp IPSPs in the target neurons of Purkinje cells.

PARALLEL FIBER ACTION ON PURKINJE CELLS

As discussed above, mossy fiber inputs activate Purkinje cells via the parallel fiber–Purkinje cell synapse (Eccles et al., 1966b). Early investigators named these responses *simple spikes*. Purkinje cell responses to spontaneous activity in the parallel fibers are illustrated in Fig. 7.11A; notice that during this recording period, two complex climbing fiber spikes were also recorded. This circuit can be activated by direct parallel fiber stimulation of the cerebellar surface or via the mossy fiber–granule cell–parallel fiber pathway from white matter stimulation. Both types of stimulation generate short-latency EPSPs in Purkinje cells.

This postsynaptic potential differs from that generated by the climbing fiber in two ways. First, it is graded as shown by the response to juxtafastigial stimuli of increasing intensity (Fig. 7.11B,C). Second, it is generally followed by an IPSP (see trace, Fig. 7.11B). The IPSP is generated by activation of the inhibitory interneurons of the molecular layer. The parallel fiber synaptic depolarization can generate action potentials at the somatic level as well as dendritic calcium spikes if the stimulus is large enough (see below). Because parallel fiber activation of Purkinje cells is followed by a disynaptic inhibition, this synaptic sequence is reviewed in detail in conjunction with the inhibitory systems in the next section.

INHIBITORY SYNAPSES IN THE CORTEX

Inhibitory neurons are organized in the cerebellar cortex into two main categories: those that reside in the molecular layer are the basket and stellate cells, whereas those that reside in the granular layer are the Golgi cells.

Granular Layer. In the granular layer, the main inhibitory system is the Golgi cell axonic plexus. This plexus releases GABA, inhibiting granule cell dendrites within the granule cell glomerulus. Indeed, while mossy fibers activate the terminal dendritic claws of the granule cells, the Golgi cell axons also distribute their contacts on the dendrites of the granule cells and may block the synaptic action of the mossy fibers by the re-

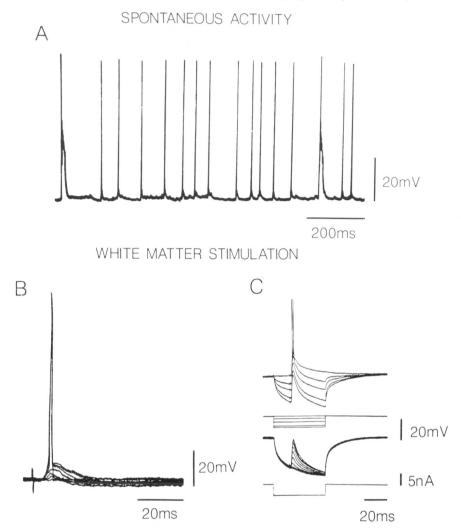

Fig. 7.11. Mossy fiber activation of mammalian Purkinje cells in vitro. **A:** Spontaneous activity in the mossy fiber–parallel fiber system gives rise to fast, simple spikes in Purkinje cells, which are in contrast to the two broad, climbing fiber–evoked complex spikes in the trace. **B:** White matter stimulation of increasing strength evoked graded EPSP–IPSP sequences due to mossy fiber–parallel fiber activation. **C:** When such stimulation is delivered during hyperpolarizing pulses of increasing amplitude (middle trace), the parallel fiber–mediated EPSP may be seen (top trace); the bottom trace illustrates the graded nature of the synaptic potential. [Modified from Llinás and Mühlethaler, 1988a, with permission.]

lease of GABA. The inhibition that ensues is so powerful as to totally block the parallel fiber input to the cerebellar cortex (Eccles et al., 1966d).

Molecular Layer. In the molecular layer, inputs from a climbing fiber and from the parallel fibers represent the two types of excitatory afferents terminating on a Purkinje cell. The Purkinje cell, however, receives input from three inhibitory systems as well: one subserved by the basket cell, the second by the stellate cell, and the third by the catecholamine system arising from the locus coeruleus (Bloom et al., 1971; Pikel et al.; 1974). Activation of the *basket cells* generates a graded inhibition at each side of the activated bundle of parallel fibers (Andersen et al., 1964; Eccles et al., 1966b,c). This can be seen clearly when recordings are made lateral to the beam of stimulated parallel fibers. In this case, at low stimulus intensity, only the IPSP is seen; however, if the stimulus intensity is increased, more Purkinje cells are excited by the parallel fibers and an EPSP–IPSP sequence is seen (Fig. 7.12A). The basket cell IPSP is generated by a membrane conductance increase to chloride, most probably by the release of gamma-aminobutyric acid (GABA, see below). The second inhibitory system is that represented by the *stellate cells*, which synapse mainly on Purkinje cell dendrites. Electrophysiologically they have the same pattern of inhibition as that of basket cells.

Monoaminergic inhibition. The third inhibitory system in the molecular layer is that of the locus coeruleus; its catecholamine-mediated inhibition generates a large, prolonged hyperpolarization in Purkinje cells (Hoffer et al., 1973). Although intriguing questions arise about the function of this system, it is possible (because of its rather widespread character) that it is related to the general state of wakefulness of the animal rather than to specific cerebellar functions. Indeed, morphologically, the system consists of rather thin filamentous afferents that reach the cerebellar cortex and bifurcate widely to cover not only the neuronal elements but probably also the vascular system (Bloom et al., 1971).

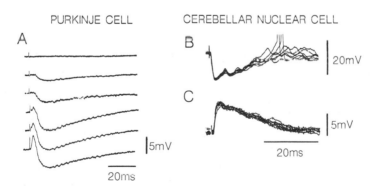

Fig. 7.12. Inhibitory synaptic potentials in Purkinje cells and cerebellar nuclear cells. **A:** Here, the stimulating electrode was placed on the cerebellar surface lateral to the recorded Purkinje cell because under such conditions, powerful IPSPs could be recorded in the Purkinje cell. As the stimulus intensity was increased (lower traces), the band of activated parallel fibers became wider, and finally the parallel fibers synapsing on the recorded Purkinje cell were themselves activated; thus an EPSP preceded the IPSP. **B:** IPSPs recorded in a cerebellar nuclear cell. Stimulation of the white matter between the cerebellar cortex and nuclei may elicit graded EPSPs and IPSPs. For particular locations and amplitudes of stimulation, IPSPs may be elicited in the absence of an early EPSP, as shown here. These IPSPs are very regular, often triggering rebound firing of the cell, as seen here. **C:** That these large potentials are synaptic potentials is shown by their reversal upon injection of a hyperpolarizing current.

PURKINJE CELL ACTION ON CEREBELLAR NUCLEAR CELLS

Perhaps one of the most surprising findings in the physiology of the cerebellum is the fact that the only output of the cerebellar cortex, the Purkinje cells, exercises an inhibitory input onto the cerebellar nuclear neurons (Ito et al., 1964). This finding indicates that the cerebellar cortex is the most sophisticated inhibitory system in the brain, not only because of its refinement of connectivity and the integrative ability of these neurons but also because of the extent of information reaching the cerebellar cortex. Indeed, there are as many neurons in the cortex (5×10^{10}) as there are neurons in the rest of the brain. The powerful GABA inhibition of the Purkinje cells on the cerebellar nuclei also demonstrates the rich biochemistry of the system (Obata et al., 1967). The Purkinje cells project in a radial pattern onto the nuclei as discussed previously (see Neuronal Elements).

Electrical stimulation of the cerebellar white matter can elicit quite complex sequences of EPSPs and IPSPs in CN cells. Here we will consider the simplest case— where white matter stimulation is limited to the Purkinje cell axons. In this case, only IPSPs are recorded. The records shown in Fig. 7.12B were made from a CN cell in a cerebellum–brainstem preparation isolated from adult guinea pig (Llinás and Mühlethaler, 1988b). In the example shown in Fig. 7.12C, several IPSPs were elicited; it can be seen that their onset and amplitude are very reliable (four traces are superimposed) and that they can be easily reversed in sign by current injection, as in this example. The response of CN cells to white matter stimulation is not always so straightforward, as will be discussed below (Functional Circuits).

NEUROTRANSMITTERS

GLUTAMATE

Several indirect lines of evidence indicate that glutamate is the neurotransmitter in granule cells. It depolarizes Purkinje cells when applied ionophoretically to the dendrites (Krnjević and Phillis, 1963; Curtis and Johnston, 1974; Sugimori and Llinás, 1981) and the dendrites are more sensitive than the soma to the glutamate. Further, naturally occurring L-glutamate is more potent than the D-glutamate isomer (Chujo et al., 1975; Crepel et al., 1982). In frog Purkinje cells, the reversal potential of the glutamine-elicited EPSP is close to that for parallel-fiber-evoked EPSPs (Hackett et al., 1979).

Neurochemical studies have shown that the glutamate content is lower than normal in cerebella in which the number of granular cells has been reduced by X-irradiation (Valcana et al., 1972; McBride et al., 1976), by virus infection (Young et al., 1974), or by mutation (Hudson et al., 1976; Roffler-Tarlov and Turey, 1982). Also, compared to control values, glutamate uptake is reduced in synaptosomal preparations from cerebella in which the granule cell number has been reduced (Young et al., 1974; Rohde et al., 1979). Quantitative localization of glutamate immunoreactivity has shown that parallel and mossy fiber terminals have significantly higher levels of glutamate than do Golgi or Purkinje cells (Somogyi et al., 1986).

Finally, glutamate release from synaptosomal preparations of rat cerebellum is reduced in synaptosomes prepared from X-irradiated agranular cerebella. The release is dependent on calcium, antagonized by increased magnesium, and stimulated by membrane depolarization caused by elevated levels of potassium. These characteristics mimic those essential for neurotransmitter release (Sandoval and Cotman, 1978).

GABA

The most likely candidate for the neurotransmitter liberated from basket cells and Purkinje cells is GABA.

Basket cell inhibition or Purkinje-cell electrical activity is blocked by application of agents known to block GABA receptors, such as bicuculline or picrotoxin. This effect has been demonstrated in several ways, involving a reduction in the ability of basket cell activation to (*1*) depress Purkinje cell spontaneous firing (Curtis and Felix, 1971), (*2*) depress Purkinje cell antidromic field potentials (Bisti et al., 1971), or (*3*) elicit IPSPs in Purkinje cells (Dupont et al., 1979). Also, ionophoretic application of GABA inhibits Purkinje cell spontaneous activity (Kawamura and Provini, 1970; Okamoto et al., 1976; Okamoto and Sakai, 1981). Finally, immunocytochemical studies have demonstrated the presence of the GABA-synthesizing enzyme glutamic acid dehydrogenase (GAD) in basket cell terminals around Purkinje cell somata (McLaughlin et al., 1974; Chan-Palay et al., 1979; Oertel et al., 1981). Basket cells also take up radioactive GABA (Ljungdahl and Hökfelt, 1973; Sotelo et al., 1972).

Although the inhibitory transmitter of stellate cells has not been decisively established, it may be taurine (Frederickson et al., 1978).

The inhibitory nature of Purkinje cells was first demonstrated in Deiters' nucleus. Ionophoretic application of GABA hyperpolarizes Deiters' neurons (Obata et al., 1967), a target of Purkinje cell axons. IPSPs following Purkinje cell activation, as well as GABA-induced potentials, reverse near the same membrane potential and are mediated by an increased conductance to chlorine (Obata and Shinozaki, 1970; ten Bruggencate and Engberg, 1971). Picrotoxin blocks both Purkinje cell IPSPs and GABA potentials in Deiters' neurons. A reduction in GAD activity in the interpositus cerebellar nucleus is associated with destruction of the cerebellar hemisphere of the same side. Immunocytochemical studies have associated GAD activity with Purkinje-cell axon terminals (Fonnum et al., 1970). In fact, GAD activity in Purkinje-cell axon terminals is very high; 350–1000 mM GABA can be synthesized per hour (Fonnum and Walberg, 1973).

MONOAMINERGIC AFFERENTS

In addition to the inhibition produced by local circuit neurons, elements of the cerebellar cortex (in particular, the Purkinje cells) may be inhibited by release of norepinephrine following activation of the locus coeruleus (see Foote et al., 1983). This form of inhibition, first demonstrated by Bloom and collaborators (Siggins et al., 1971b), suggests that Purkinje cell excitability may be depressed for protracted periods by the release of norepinephrine from terminals arising from the brainstem neurons. The terminals, rather than synapsing at specific points, seem widespread within the cortex. Their activation apparently produces a widespread release of catecholamines that hyperpolarize the Purkinje cells. Such hyperpolarization seems to be mimicked by application of cyclic adenosine-3′,5′-monophosphate (cAMP) (Siggins et al., 1971a,c), and norepinephrine may function by the activation of an electrogenic sodium pump similar to those in other central neurons (Phillis and Wu, 1981). Indeed, the possibility that an electrogenic sodium pump may be activated by norepinephrine is indicated, since the hyperpolarization is accompanied by a decreased ionic conductance change (Siggins et al., 1971c).

There is also evidence for dopaminergic cerebellar afferents projecting to the cerebellar nuclei, and to the Purkinje and granular cell layers of the cortex (Simon et al., 1979). The raphe nuclei, which synthesize and release serotonin, project fibers to all parts of the cerebellar nuclei and cortex (Takeuchi et al., 1982). These terminate at mossy fiber rosettes diffusely throughout the granular layer; in the molecular layer they bifurcate like parallel fibers and synapse with the intrinsic neurons (Chan-Palay, 1977). In the molecular and granular layers, beaded fibers with fine varicosities have been labeled with serotonin-specific antibodies (Takeuchi et al., 1982).

MOSSY FIBERS

No neurotransmitter candidates have been clearly identified to be liberated from mossy fibers. There is some indirect evidence for several candidates, however. For example, among the peptides, somatostatin-immunoreactive fibers have been shown to enter the cerebellum (Inagaki et al., 1982); these probably end as mossy fibers. Acetylcholine (ACh) is present in some mossy fiber terminals isolated as synaptosomes (Israël and Whittaker, 1965), and some mossy fibers contain acetylcholinesterase (Phillis, 1968). Choline acetyltransferase, the enzyme for ACh synthesis, has been demonstrated on mossy fibers and glomeruli by using immunocytochemistry (Kan et al., 1978, 1980). However, a role for ACh as a transmitter has not been supported by pharmacological or physiological studies.

DENDRITIC PROPERTIES

MICROELECTRODE RECORDINGS

That dendrites are capable of electroresponsive activity and are not simple, passive cables was first shown in Purkinje cells. The earliest recordings indicating that the dendrites are active were made from alligator cerebellum. Here, intradendritic recordings revealed large dendritic spikes in response to parallel fiber stimulation (Llinás and Nicholson, 1971). Injection of hyperpolarizing current allowed these spikes to be dissected into several all-or-none components. From these early studies it was proposed that there are several "hot spots" in the dendrites that are capable of spike generation, and that dendritic spikes travel toward the soma in a discontinuous manner. Subsequent intradendritic recordings from pigeon Purkinje cells showed that dendritic spikes are calcium dependent (Llinás and Hess, 1976). It was not until cerebellar slice preparation was used, however, that the dendritic properties of Purkinje cells were revealed in all their complexity.

The types of spontaneous action potentials that may be seen at different levels in a mammalian Purkinje cell soma and dendrites are illustrated for an in vitro experiment in Fig. 7.13. A typical bursting is seen at the somatic level (B). Recordings obtained at different levels in the dendritic tree are shown in C, D, and E. The decrease in amplitude of the fast spike which occurs as recordings are made further from the soma

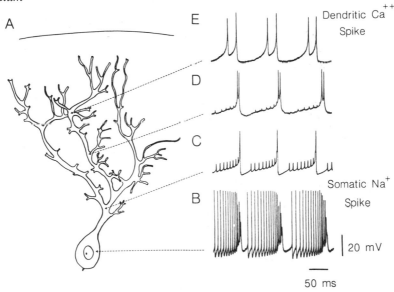

Fig. 7.13. Composite illustration of recordings made from different regions of a Purkinje cell in vitro. **A:** Drawing of typical mammalian Purkinje cell. **B:** Fast action potentials dominate this recording, with slower membrane oscillations. **C–E:** As the electrode moves away from the soma, (*1*) the amplitude of the fast, Na-dependent action potentials progressively decreases until they are not seen in the most distal branches; and (*2*) the slow, prolonged, calcium-dependent action potentials increase in amplitude and become distinct in the distal branches. Although the dendritic spikes are discontinually propagated toward the soma, the somatic spikes do not actively invade the dendrites. [Modified from Llinás and Sugimori, 1980a, with permission.]

indicates clearly that the fast sodium action potentials seen at the soma do not actively invade the dendrites. Rather, they are electrotonically conducted and can be detected only to about mid-dendritic level, their amplitude decrementing rather quickly with distance.

The bursting calcium-dependent spike, on the other hand, is large and rather prominent in the upper dendrites, indicating a differential distribution for sodium and calcium conductances. Furthermore, direct stimulation of dendrites after application of TTX, as shown in Fig. 7.14A, produces two types of calcium-dependent electroresponsiveness. A small stimulus can generate a plateau-like response and a burst of action potentials. Because both responses can be blocked by cobalt, cadmium, or D600 (see Fig. 7.14B), it must be concluded that the dendrites of the Purkinje cell are capable of generating calcium-dependent spikes, which may be either of a prolonged plateau form or clear, all-or-nothing action potentials.

The Purkinje cells thus demonstrate the following set of voltage-dependent ionic conductances. As discussed earlier, in the soma there are (*1*) a rapid, inactivating Hodgkin-Huxley sodium current that generates a fast spike; (*2*) a fast voltage-activated potassium current that generates the afterhyperpolarization following a fast spike; and (*3*) a calcium-activated potassium conductance. In addition, the somatic membrane displays a non-inactivating, voltage-activated sodium conductance capable of generating

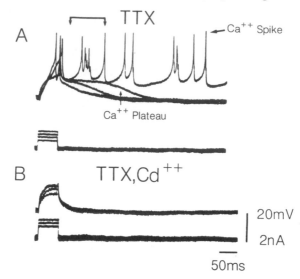

Fig. 7.14. Purkinje cell dendritic recordings in vitro. **A:** Intradendritic recording in the presence of TTX. Short depolarizing pulses elicit Ca-dependent plateau potentials and Ca spikes. As the current amplitude is increased, the plateau responses increase in duration, and full spike bursts are generated. **B:** The calcium dependence of both the plateau and the spike bursts is demonstrated by their complete abolition after Cd^{2+} has been added to the TTX bathing solution.

repetitive firing of the Purkinje cell following prolonged depolarization. At the dendritic level, on the other hand, excitability seems to be due mainly to a voltage-activated calcium conductance increase. This conductance may generate a low plateau potential or calcium spikes (Fig. 7.14A), and the spikes may be followed by potassium activation from an increase of both voltage-activated and calcium-activated conductances to potassium.

It is therefore clear that the complex electrical responses observed in these cells after direct stimulation or activation of climbing or parallel fibers are largely due to the electroresponsive properties of the Purkinje cells themselves.

OPTICAL RECORDING

Optical probes have been used to mark the spatial distribution of voltage-sensitive ionic channels in Purkinje cells. The sodium conductance is restricted to the soma and axon as visualized by using fluorescently labeled TTX (Sugimori et al., 1986).

Mapping of the distribution of an increase in intracellular calcium concentration ($[Ca^{2+}]_i$) during spontaneous and evoked Purkinje cell activity allows visualization of the probable location of calcium channels in the somatodendritic membrane. This has been done in experiments using Arsenazo III absorption (Ross and Werman, 1986), and Fura-2 as a calcium indicator. Experiments using the fluorescent Ca^{2+} indicator Fura-2 have shown that during spontaneous bursting, the $[Ca^{2+}]_i$ increases first in the fine dendritic branches, where the increase is also the largest (Tank et al., 1988). The $[Ca^{2+}]_i$ is later seen to increase in the dendritic trunk, and by this time it has begun to subside in the fine dendrites. The $[Ca^{2+}]_i$ in the soma increases very little. This temporal sequence of increased calcium activity, first in the distal and then in the proximal dendrites, supports the electrophysiological description of the two calcium conductances—the low-threshold plateau and all-or-none calcium-dependent dendritic spikes (see Fig. 7.13). The presence of voltage-activated calcium channels in the spiny branchlets provides a mechanism whereby parallel fiber EPSPs can be enhanced by slow local increases in calcium conductance. In contrast, when the synaptic activity is in the larger dendritic branches, full calcium-dependent dendritic spikes can be generated in the main dendritic tree. Climbing fiber synapses tend to depolarize the main dendritic tree, producing full dendritic spikes. Thus, the distribution of calcium channels over the dendritic tree is a critical element in the fine tuning of the electrophysiological sophistication of this most remarkable cell.

If a cell loaded with Fura-2 is depolarized by somatic current injection, the increased $[Ca^{2+}]_i$ in the dendrites is not uniform. Rather, there are well-localized areas of marked increases, supporting the earlier hypothesis of "hot spots" of calcium influx (Llinás and Nicholson, 1971).

FUNCTIONAL CIRCUITS

We have seen that there are two main types of afferents to Purkinje cells: (*1*) the climbing fiber–Purkinje cell system (Fig. 7.2A), which is organized into groups of specifically and synchronously activated Purkinje cells having quite different spatial locations (Armstrong, 1974); and (*2*) the mossy fiber–granule cell–parallel fiber–Purkinje cell system (Fig. 7.2B), in which Purkinje cells are activated at given loci in very specific geometrical patterns owing to the particular spatial relationship between the parallel fibers and the Purkinje cells dendrites. In the latter case, instead of the one-to-one relationship seen between the Purkinje cell and its climbing fiber afferent, a many-to-many relationship is present. Moreover, the directionality of the parallel fibers has been shown to be all-important in determining the peculiar orthogonal organization of these fibers with respect to the lateral spread of the Purkinje cell dendritic tree. Thus, in the climbing fiber mode of activation, specific Purkinje cells may be activated, whereas with mossy and parallel fiber input, large numbers of Purkinje cells are activated in rows.

In considering the functional circuit of the cerebellum, the cerebellar nuclear cells must be included, for what the cortex ultimately does is to help determine the firing of these cells. CN cells are regulated in three ways:

1. By excitatory input from collaterals of the cerebellar afferent systems.
2. By inhibitory inputs from Purkinje cells activated over the mossy or climbing fiber pathways. Mossy fiber activation should generate a *tonic inhibition* in Purkinje cells, due to simple spikes firing synchronously at 30–40 Hz (Bell and Grimm, 1969), as well as a *transient inhibition* following a specific mossy fiber volley.
3. By the climbing fiber system, which originates in the inferior olivary nucleus, where the neurons are known to have powerful pacemaker properties and to be electrotonically coupled (Llinás and Yarom, 1986). This system generates rhythmic and synchronous activation of Purkinje cells, and thus not surprisingly, *rhythmic inhibition* of CN neurons.

Let us consider more closely this last circuit, which includes the inferior olive, cerebellar nuclei, and Purkinje cells (Figs. 7.15 and 7.16). If the activity of the circuit is taken to start at the inferior olive, the axons of these cells may be followed to the cortex as climbing fibers or to the CN as collaterals. As recorded from the soma of a CN cell, activation of this pathway by white matter stimulation generates the complex response shown in Fig. 7.15 right. This response may be considered as having five parts as shown in the figure: (*1*) antidromic excitation of the CN cell (1 in Fig. 7.15); (2) direct excitation of Purkinje cells, which is seen in the CN as a small IPSP (2 in Fig. 7.15); (*3 and 4*) a second EPSP–IPSP sequence (3 and 4 in Fig. 7.15) with a latency of 3–4.5 msec. The EPSP results from climbing fiber collateral activation of the CN cells, and the IPSP is generated following synaptic activation of the Purkinje cells. Finally, (*5*) a rebound response is recorded, which is due to the intrinsic membrane properties of the CN cells themselves (Fig. 7.15). Thus, the response in Fig. 7.15 is a combination of the properties of the synaptic circuit and the intrinsic properties of the Purkinje cells and CN cells.

In fact, in this circuit the membrane properties of CN neurons are particularly important because the punctate and rather powerful synaptic EPSP–IPSP sequences are often followed by a rebound spike burst, as is seen in Fig. 7.15 right. This means, then, that if a sufficient number of inferior olivary neurons, having a common rhythmicity, are activated synchronously at any particular time, a large and equally synchronous activation of Purkinje cells will occur. In fact, this is what occurs when harmaline, a

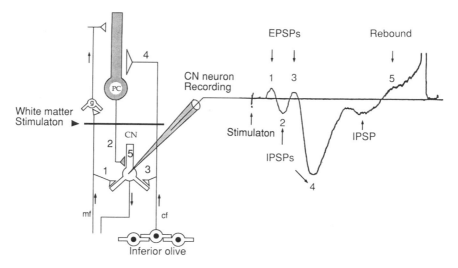

Fig. 7.15. Response of cerebellar nuclear cells to white matter stimulation. **A:** Drawing of elements activated after white matter stimulation. **B:** White matter stimulation activates mossy fibers, climbing fibers, and Purkinje cell (PC) axons. The first response (1), a graded EPSP, is due to activation of the mossy fiber collaterals; the second (2), a small IPSP, is due to direct stimulation of Purkinje cell axons. The third response (3), a graded EPSP, is due to activation of climbing fiber collaterals. Finally (4), the powerful IPSP and smaller IPSPs follow climbing fiber activation of Purkinje cells. Although the cell is at the resting potential, the hyperpolarization is often sufficient to elicit a rebound response in the cerebellar nuclear cell (5).

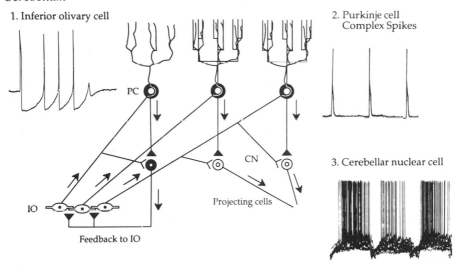

Fig. 7.16. Diagram of the circuit involved in the production of rhythmic activity in the olivo-cerebellar system. (1) Rhythmic activity in the inferior olivary neurons is transmitted to the Purkinje cells (PC), where it is transformed to complex spikes (2) to the cerebellar nuclear projecting cells (white somata) and inhibitory cells (filled soma) eliciting EPSPs. Complex spikes trigger high-frequency firing of Purkinje cell axons that impinge on the cerebellar nuclear cells with powerful IPSPs and rebound firing (3). Thus bursts of spikes are transmitted to the rest of the nervous system including the cerebellum (as mossy fibers). The cerebellar nuclear cells projecting to the inferior olive (IO) are inhibitory and synapse in the glomeruli. (Filled synaptic terminals are inhibitory and open synaptic terminals are excitatory.)

tremorgenic agent known to act directly on the inferior olive (de Montigny and Lamarre, 1974; Llinás and Volkind, 1973; Llinás and Yarom, 1986), is administered. Such activation would be reflected in the CN as inhibition followed by a rebound activation. The activity in the circuit in the presence of harmaline is shown in the diagram in Fig. 7.16. This activity has been shown in vitro and is probably also the case in vivo, as indicated by multiple-electrode recording studies of Purkinje cell activity in the rat cortex (Llinás, 1985). The climbing fiber system generates rostrocaudal bands of synchronous Purkinje cell activation, and Purkinje cells within such bands (which are about 200 μm across) fire with the same frequency, and at intervals as close as 0.5–1.0 msec, indicating that the olivocerebellar system is quite tightly organized.

Spontaneous background inhibitory potentials recorded from CN neurons indicate that Purkinje cells also fire with some degree of synchronicity in the absence of harmaline. The powerful rebound excitation following these IPSPs is in turn transmitted to the rest of the CNS as an excitatory input and to the inferior olive as an inhibitory input (via the GABAergic nucleoolivary pathway) (Mugnaini and Oertel, 1981; Sotelo et al., 1986). This pathway is important since it seems to have a decoupling effect on the electrotonic junction in the inferior olive (Sotelo et al., 1986; Llinás and Sasaki, 1989; Lang et al., 1996). In short, the olivocerebellar system would serve as an oscillatory circuit capable of generating timing sequences such as those observed in tremor and in the organization of coordinated movements (Llinás, 1985). The mossy fiber–

parallel fiber system provides a continuous and very delicate regulation of the excitability of the cerebellar nuclei, brought about by the tonic activation of simple spikes in Purkinje cells, that ultimately generates the fine control of movement known as motor coordination. The fact that the mossy fibers inform the cerebellar cortex of both ascending and descending messages to and from the motor centers in the spinal cord and brainstem gives us an idea of the ultimate role of the mossy fiber system; it informs the cortex of the place and rate of movement of limbs and puts the motor intentions generated by the brain into the context of the status of the body at the time the movement is to be executed.

Because the Purkinje cell is an inhibitory neuron, the entire output of the elaborate cerebellar cortical neuronal network produces an organized, large-scale inhibition of neurons in the cerebellar nuclei. It should be recalled that of all the cells residing in the cortex only the granule cells are excitatory; all the rest are inhibitory. As illustrated in Figs. 7.15 and 7.16, an understanding of their membrane properties and synaptic interactions provides fundamental insight into the functioning of the cerebellar cortex.

8

THALAMUS

S. MURRAY SHERMAN AND CHRISTOF KOCH

The thalamus is the gateway to neocortex, and as such these two main components of the vertebrate telencephalon have evolved in close relation to each other. Virtually all routes to cortex are relayed via the thalamus, although inputs from other subcortical sites exist, such as brainstem, basal forebrain, and the claustrum. Our conscious perception of the world around us depends on information reaching cortex and being analyzed there, and thus the thalamus represents a key link in this process.

However, as well shall see in this chapter, the thalamus does much more than merely act as a passive and machine-like relay of information to cortex. Instead, the ability to pass through this gateway is determined by specialized neuronal circuitry: the gate can be completely open, which results in the relay of all information to cortex; completely closed, which cuts off cortex from the outside world; or partially open, which permits certain information to reach cortical levels. Also, the special properties of relay cells can strongly influence the nature of the thalamic relay. Thus the thalamus filters and transforms the flow of information to cortex and as such is an important neuronal substrate for many forms of attention (Singer, 1977; Sherman and Koch, 1986; Sherman, 1988, 1993; Steriade and Llinás, 1988; Steriade et al., 1993; Sherman and Guillery, 1996).

OVERALL ORGANIZATION

The thalamus is most highly developed in mammals and especially so in primates. All sensory systems pass through the thalamus on their way to neocortex. This includes somatosensory information from the muscles, deep tissues, and skin; visual information from the eyes; auditory information from the ears; and gustatory information from the taste buds. Each part of the thalamus, in turn, receives fibers from the area of cortex to which it projects (Jones, 1985).

The main exception to this pattern is the relay of olfactory information because the initial stages of olfactory processing represent phylogenetically very old circuitry that probably predates the evolution of thalamocortical pathways. Cells in the nasal epithelium project directly to the olfactory bulb (see Chap. 5), which then projects to the primary olfactory cortex (see Chap. 10). This cortex is paleocortex. It has three layers and evolved before neocortex (see Chap. 10), which has six layers. The olfactory pathway can then be followed from olfactory paleocortex into the mediodorsal nucleus of the thalamus, from which it is relayed to the insular and orbital cortex, which is neocortex. Later in this chapter, we reconsider the olfactory pathway in the context of first- and higher-order thalamic relays.

The thalamus can be divided on the basis of connectivity and embryological origin into three main divisions: *dorsal thalamus*, *ventral thalamus*, and *epithalamus*. The dorsal thalamus, which is the largest division, has massive reciprocal connections with cerebral cortex and striatum; in fact, virtually the whole cortex receives a projection from the dorsal thalamus. People often mean "dorsal thalamus" when they refer simply to "thalamus." The ventral thalamus does not innervate cortex. However, it does receive innervation from cortex, and most of its subnuclei, collectively known as the *thalamic reticular nucleus* (TRN; also known as the *nucleus reticularis thalami* or the *reticular nucleus of the thalamus*), have reciprocal connections with specific nuclei in the dorsal thalamus (Jones, 1985; Ohara and Lieberman, 1985). The epithalamus lacks direct afferent or efferent connections with cortex and is actually more closely associated with hypothalamus; it will not be considered further here.

The dorsal thalamus can be divided into a number of discrete nuclei. Figure 8.1 and Table 8.1 illustrate the major thalamic nuclei that relay subcortical information to the cerebral cortex, and in some cases, to the basal ganglia as well. We now recognize that

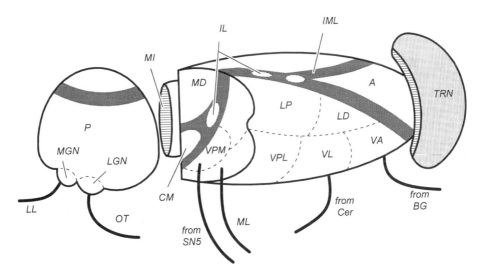

Fig. 8.1. Schematic three-dimensional view of right thalamus with many of its major nuclei. A cut is placed in the posterior part to reveal a representative cross section. Some of the important ascending afferents are also shown. To prevent obscuring the dorsal thalamus, only the rostral tip of the thalamic reticular nucleus (TRN) is shown. Other abbreviations: A, anterior; BG, basal ganglia; Cer, cerebellum; CM, centromedian; IL, intralaminar nuclei; IML, internal medullary lamina; LD, lateral dorsal; LL, lateral lemniscus; LP, lateral posterior; LGN, lateral geniculate nucleus; MGN, medial geniculate nucleus; MD, mediodorsal; MI, midline nuclei; ML, medial lemniscus; OT, optic tract; P, pulvinar; SN5, main sensory and spinal nuclei of the 5th nerve; ST, spinothalamic; VA, ventral anterior; VL, ventrolateral; VPL, ventral posterolateral; VPM, ventral posteromedial. See Jones (1985) for details of connectivity of these nuclei. [Redrawn from Brodal, 1981, with permission.]

Table 8.1. Thalamic Nuclei Relaying Subcortical Inputs

Nucleus	Major subcortical input	Projection
Pulvinar (Pu)*	Superior colliculus, pretectum	Visual cortex (dense)
Medial Geniculate Nucleus (MGN)	Lateral lemniscus	Auditory cortex (dense)
Lateral Geniculate Nucleus (LGN)	Optic tract	Visual cortex (dense)
Midline Nuclei (MI)	Spinal cord, cerebellum, basal ganglia	Cortex (diffuse) and basal ganglia
Central Medial Nucleus (CM)	Spinal cord, cerebellum, basal ganglia	Cortex (diffuse) and basal ganglia
Intralaminar Nuclei (IL)	Spinal cord, cerebellum, basal ganglia	Cortex (diffuse) and basal ganglia
Medial Dorsal Nucleus (MD)	Olfactory cortex, amygdala	Frontal cortex (diffuse)
Ventral Medial Nucleus (VM)	Substantia nigra	Cortex (diffuse)
Ventral Posteromedial Nucleus (VPM)	Trigeminal nerve	Somatosensory cortex (dense)
Ventral Posterolateral Nucleus (VPL)	Medial lemniscus	Somatosensory cortex (dense)
Posterior Nucleus (Po)	Superior colliculus, spinal cord	Insular cortex (dense)
Lateral Dorsal Nucleus (LD)	Fornix	Cingulate cortex (dense)
Ventral Lateral Nucleus (VL)	Cerebellum	Motor cortex (dense)
Ventral Anterior Nucleus (VA)	Cerebellum, basal ganglia	Cortex (diffuse)
Anterior Nuclei (A)	Subiculum, mammilary body	Olfactory cortex (dense)

Parenthetic abbreviations refer to locations of the nuclei in Fig. 8.1.

many, and perhaps all, of these nuclei have unique functional correlates, with specific input and output routes. Three generalizations can be made about these connections. First, all dorsal thalamic nuclei project to neocortex, but some tend to project *diffusely* to large, ill-defined cortical regions, terminating largely in layer 1 of cortex, while others project *densely* to more restricted, well-defined regions, terminating mostly in layer 4 (see Table 8.1). Second, these outputs of dorsal thalamic nuclei are limited to the same hemisphere, since no contralateral efferent connections involving any thalamic nucleus have been found. Third, no connections between dorsal thalamic nuclei have yet been described.

An exhaustive survey of all dorsal thalamic nuclei is beyond the scope of this chapter (for a more thorough account, see Jones, 1985), but examples of the best-studied nuclei follow. The *lateral geniculate nucleus* (LGN) relays input from the retina to visual cortex. There are two LGN divisions: the dorsal division, which is part of the dorsal thalamus, projects to cortex, and, unless otherwise specified, is what we mean by "LGN"; and the ventral division, which is part of the ventral thalamus and also receives retinal input but projects only subcortically, mostly to the midbrain. The *medial geniculate nucleus* (MGN) receives auditory input from the *inferior colliculus* and projects to auditory cortex. The *ventral posterolateral nucleus* (VPL) transmits somatosensory input from the body, providing the cortex with information about touch, pressure, joint position, temperature, and pain; its contiguous companion is the *ventral mediolateral nucleus* (VPM), which transmits somatosensory information from the head. The VPL receives ascending input from the spinal cord and dorsal column nuclei in the medulla, while the VPM receives input from the 5th cranial nerve via the main sensory and spinal nuclei of this nerve. The *basal ventral medial nucleus* receives gustatory input relayed from the pons and projects to primary somatosensory cortex. The *ventral lateral nucleus* receives most of its input from the deep cerebellar nuclei and projects to primary motor cortex. The *ventral anterior nucleus* is innervated by the basal ganglia and projects both to motor cortex and the basal ganglia. The *pulvinar* is a particularly interesting example. It has several divisions, and these are not yet completely understood or agreed upon. Much of its primary input that is related to cortex emanates from the superior colliculus and the pretectum, but another important source of such input derives from cortex itself. This relay of cortical information back to cortex exemplifies a newly appreciated type of thalamic nucleus; this is considered more fully near the end of this chapter.

THE LGN AS THE PROTOTYPICAL THALAMIC NUCLEUS

At the level of synaptic circuitry, more is known about the LGN than about any other thalamic structure, and this nucleus has been more thoroughly studied in the cat than in any other species. It seems likely that many of the organizational principles of the cat's LGN apply generally to other dorsal thalamic nuclei across mammals, although our present knowledge of most other such nuclei is too sparse for us to be completely comfortable with this generalization. Nonetheless, many of the specific examples for the functional organization of the thalamus derive from the cat's LGN, and most of the discussion of thalamus below refers to the LGN. It is thus worth briefly introducing this nucleus to the reader.

Figure 8.2 illustrates the laminar patterns of the cat's LGN (see Sherman and Spear, 1982; Sherman, 1985; Sherman and Koch, 1986). It is comprised of several laminae, most of which are innervated by one or the other retina. In addition to the segregation based on ocular origin, axons from neighboring retinal loci innervate neighboring geniculate zones, thereby setting up an orderly point-to-point map of visual space within the LGN. This is known as a *retinotopic map*, and analogous maps representing other sensory modalities exist within other thalamic nuclei, such as the VPL, VPM, and MGN (Jones, 1985). Most is known about the *A-laminae* (laminae A and A1) of the LGN, which form a reasonably matched pair, with lamina A innervated by the contralateral retina and lamina A1 innervated by the ipsilateral retina. The other main geniculate zones are the C-laminae and medial interlaminar nucleus, which, despite its name, is really just a part of the LGN. For details of these other LGN regions in the cat and how this relates to LGNs in other species, the reader can consult various reviews (Sherman and Spear, 1982; Stone, 1983; Sherman, 1985; Shapley and Perry, 1986; Hendry and Yoshioka, 1994; Casagrande and Norton, 1996); the remainder of our treatment will be limited to the A-laminae of the cat.

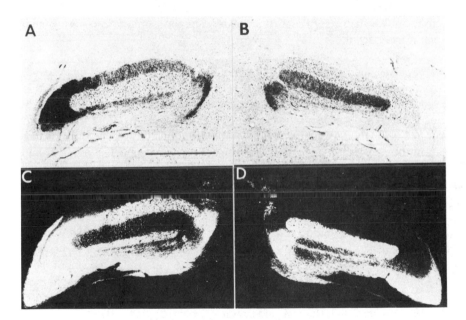

Fig. 8.2. Photomicrographs of left (**A,C**) and right (**B,D**) LGN of the cat as seen in coronal view near the middle of the nucleus. The sections were treated for autoradiography after retinogeniculate terminals from the right eye were labeled by injecting that eye with tritiated proline. The labeled terminals are dark, and this permits visualization of the various laminae innervated by one or the other eye. Lamina A is innervated by the contralateral eye, and lamina A1, by the ipsilateral eye. Lamina A is the most dorsal lamina, and lamina A1 is just beneath it. Thus the left lamina A and right lamina A1 are dark due to the autoradiographic labeling of terminals from the right eye. Other laminar zones below and medial to the A-laminae can also be seen, but these are not considered further here (see Sherman, 1985; for a fuller account of these laminae.) Although not labeled, the TRN lies just above lamina A. A,B, bright-field, C,D dark-field photomicrographs. [Revised from Sherman, 1985, with permission.]

NEURONAL ELEMENTS OF THE THALAMUS

The neuronal elements of the thalamus can be divided into three components: the *extrinsic afferent inputs* to the nucleus, the *relay cells* (or principal neurons) that project to cortex, and the *interneurons* (or intrinsic neurons).

INPUTS

Figure 8.3 schematically illustrates the major afferents for a typical dorsal thalamic nucleus. We can divide the inputs into two broad classes: *driving* and *modulatory* inputs. The driving input represents the primary information to be relayed to cortex, such as retinal input to the LGN. The modulatory input is all other input, and this serves to modulate or control the relay of information from the driving input to cortex. Modulatory input can be further subdivided into cortical modulatory inputs and brainstem modulatory inputs. Seen in this perspective, the retinal or driving afferents to LGN relay cells are one class among several and, at least in terms of number of synapses formed on these relay cells, are a minority input. The modulatory afferents include long pathways from the cortex and brainstem plus local inputs from TRN cells and interneurons. Figure 8.3 indicates both the inputs to thalamus and the neurotransmitters they use, but we shall return later to consider neurotransmitters and postsynaptic receptors in more detail.

Retinal or Driving Afferents. The driving input is the best characterized input to a dorsal thalamic nucleus. This input is glutamatergic, meaning it uses the amino acid glutamate or a similar compound as a neurotransmitter (Kemp and Sillito, 1982; Moody and Sillito, 1988; Salt, 1988; Scharfman et al., 1990; Kown et al., 1991; Salt and Eaton, 1996). For the LGN, this input arises from the ganglion cells of the retina, whose axons form the *optic nerve* and *tract*. The number of retinogeniculate axons from each retina varies with species; it is slightly under 100,000 in cats and is roughly 1 million in monkeys and humans (Rakic and Riley, 1983; Williams et al., 1983). Comparable input to the VPL and MGN derives, respectively, from the *medial lemniscus* and *lateral lemniscus*.

In cats, the retinal ganglion cells that innervate the A-laminae can be divided into two physiologically and morphologically distinct classes: *X cells* (also known as *β cells*) and *Y cells* (also known as *α cells*). See Chap. 6 for a fuller account of these and other retinal ganglion cell classes. Most details of the differences in morphology and receptive fields of X and Y cells do not concern us here (for details, see Sherman and Spear, 1982; Stone, 1983; Rodieck and Brening, 1983; Shapley and Lennie, 1985; Sherman, 1985, 1988), but subtle differences in the sort of visual information they carry do exist. This exemplifies an important principle for thalamic relays: the same nucleus can relay different sorts of signals to cortex in parallel. Other mammals, including primates, have comparable retinal ganglion cell classes (Stone, 1983; Rodieck and Brening, 1983; Shapley and Lennie, 1985; Sherman, 1985, 1988; Levey et al., 1987). Such parallel processing seems to be a feature of all sensory systems (Sherman and Spear, 1982; Stone, 1983; Dykes, 1983; Rodieck and Brening, 1983; Jones, 1985; Shapley and Lennie, 1985; Sherman, 1985, 1988). Every X and Y cell innervates the LGN and branches to innervate other targets in the midbrain (Bowling and Michael, 1984; Sur

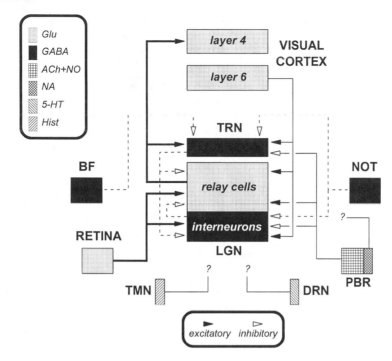

Fig. 8.3. Schematic summary of main inputs to thalamic relay cells, using the LGN as a proto-typical example. The main sensory input arrives from retina via the optic tract. Local GABA-ergic inhibitory input is provided by interneurons and cells of the thalamic reticular nucleus (TRN). Other main inputs emanate from layer 6 of visual cortex, from the parabrachial region (PBR), from the dorsal raphé nucleus (DRN), from the tuberomamillary nucleus (TMN) of the hypothalamus, from the basal forebrain (BF), and from the nucleus of the optic tract (NOT). The key indicates the neurotransmitters used by the various inputs: Glu, glutamate; GABA, γ-aminobutyric acid; ACh, acetylcholine; NO, nitric oxide; NA, noradrenaline; 5-HT, serotonin; Hist, histamine. [Redrawn from Sherman and Koch, 1986, with permission.]

et al., 1987; Tamamaki et al., 1994). Furthermore, within the LGN, these retinal cell types each innervates a unique geniculate cell type, thereby establishing relay X and Y classes of geniculate cells and parallel, functionally distinct X and Y pathways.

Cortical Afferents. A major input to thalamus originates among layer 6 pyramidal cells of the cortex (see Fig. 8.3). In fact, there seems to be at least an order of magnitude of more corticothalamic axons than thalamocortical ones. Thus in cats roughly 4,000,000 axons from visual cortex innervate the geniculate relay cells of the A-laminae (Sherman and Koch, 1986). Each cortical axon innervates many thalamic neurons, thereby establishing considerable divergence and convergence in the corticothalamic pathway. Like retinal (or driving) axons, these cortical axons are excitatory and appear to be glutamatergic (Giuffrida and Rustioni, 1988; McCormick and Von Krosigk, 1992; Montero, 1994). Strong reciprocity exists in thalamocortical connections, because the cortical input for each thalamic nucleus generally, but not always, originates from the same cortical area that is innervated by the thalamic nucleus in question. Thus for the LGN, this cortical pathway emanates from visual cortex (mostly areas 17, 18, and 19), and roughly half of these layer 6 cells contribute to the corticogeniculate pathway. Likewise, somatosensory and auditory cortex project back, respectively, to the VPL and MGN.

The corticothalamic pathway faithfully adheres to the map established in the thalamic nucleus (see above). For instance, the corticogeniculate pathway conforms to the retinotopic map in the LGN. However, there is some question as to the precision of this map due to recent evidence that, in the cat, the spread of an individual corticogeniculate axon arbor can be quite extensive, having a maximal extent of 1.5 mm, although the central core is about 0.4–0.5 mm in diameter, which was taken to mean that each geniculate cell can be influenced by events far outside its classical receptive field (Murphy and Sillito, 1996). However, due to two other features of relay cells, it is also possible that individual corticogeniculate arbors even up to 1–2 mm across might still represent precise retinotopic connections. First, the dendritic arbor of a typical relay cell can have a diameter of roughly 0.4–0.5 mm. Since the corticogeniculate terminals contact peripheral dendrites, a single cortical axon contacting a single relay cell would have a terminal arbor of 0.4–0.5 mm across. However, it is likely that each corticogeniculate axon contacts many relay cells, and this raises the second point. Sanderson (1971) showed that relay cells representing the same receptive field location in visual space are not located along a single "projection" line through the LGN but rather scatter around that line with a spread of perhaps 1–2 mm, depending on the location of the receptive fields within the visual field. Thus a single corticogeniculate axon contacting many relay cells with closely matched receptive field locations might well spread up to 1–2 mm across, thereby adhering to an accurate and precise retinotopic map.

Another issue related to the corticogeniculate (and thus corticothalamic) feedback concerns the precision of these retinotopic patterns. Only a subset of pyramidal cells in layer 6 actually comprises the corticogeniculate pathway, the remainder innervating the claustrum, and these corticogeniculate cells tend to be located in the top half of layer 6 (Lund et al., 1975; Katz, 1987; Usrey and Fitzpatrick, 1996). These layer-6 corticogeniculate cells also project into that part of layer 4 that is supplied by geniculocortical input (Lund et al., 1975; Usrey and Fitzpatrick, 1996), implying that these layer 6 cells not only control the relay of information through LGN but may also modulate the flow of LGN input into cortex. It is interesting that, unlike some other intrinsic cortical circuits, the layer 6 projection to layer 4 is very limited in horizontal extent (Katz, 1987), thereby limiting the retinotopic spread of information. This allows for information to cycle between the visual cortex and the LGN in a precise retinotopic manner, allowing for the establishment of reverberatory loops.

Finally, corticogeniculate neurons seem to be heterogeneous and probably represent several functional classes (Tsumoto and Suda, 1980; Katz, 1987), although they have not yet been properly classified and it is not clear to what extent other corticothalamic pathways contain functional subsets of axons.

Brainstem Afferents. Other inputs to the thalamus emanate from various brainstem sources. The mix and relative strength of these brainstem inputs can vary both with species as well as with specific thalamic nuclei (Fitzpatrick et al. 1989). Afferents from the pons and midbrain (see Fig. 8.3) include cholinergic neurons (i.e., using acetyl-

choline as a neurotransmitter) of the *parabrachial region* (the cells of origin are located near the brachium conjuctivum; this is also known as the *pedunculopontine
tegmental nucleus*), noradrenergic neurons (i.e., using noradrenalin; also known as *norepinephrine*) of the *locus coeruleus*, and serotonergic neurons (i.e., using serotonin) of
the *dorsal raphé nucleus*. These inputs can either excite or inhibit thalamic neurons
(see Chap. 2 and below). By far the most numerous of these inputs to the lateral geniculate nucleus of the cat is the cholinergic input, representing perhaps 90% of the brainstem input (Smith et al., 1988; Bickford et al., 1993). In many species, the cholinergic cells of the parabrachial region or pedunculopontine tegmental nucleus and
noradrenergic cells of the locus coeruleus are distinct and separate. In others, such as
the cat, they overlap extensively. Thus while the cells can be distinguished by their
neurotransmitters, they may not always occupy distinct and separate nuclei.

Figure 8.3 also indicates other smaller and less well-studied brainstem inputs (Harting et al., 1986; Fitzpatrick et al., 1988; Cucchiaro et al., 1991, 1993; Uhlrich et al.,
1993; Bickford et al., 1994). The *tuberomammilary nucleus* of the hypothalamus provides a histaminergic input. A GABAergic input (i.e., it uses γ-aminobutyric acid, or
GABA, as a neurotransmitter) exists from the *basal forebrain* to the TRN, and while
this input does not directly innervate dorsal thalamus, it can influence relay properties
indirectly through the TRN. Finally, the LGN receives additional, although sparse brainstem inputs that may be unique to the visual pathways. These include afferents from
the *superior colliculus* and *parabigeminal nucleus* of the midbrain and from the pretectal *nucleus of the optic tract* (NOT). The parabigeminal input is cholinergic, that for
the pretectum is GABAergic, and that for the superior colliculus is thought to be glutamatergic. There is evidence that the GABAergic input from the NOT does not innervate relay cells directly but instead innervates TRN cells and interneurons, which
would presumably disinhibit relay cells.

Inputs From the TRN. A final extrinsic source of innervation to each dorsal thalamic nucleus derives from the TRN (Jones, 1985; Ohara and Lieberman, 1985; Cox et al.,
1996; Sherman and Guillery, 1996). The TRN forms a shell anteriorly and dorsally
around the dorsal thalamus (see Fig. 8.1). Generally, each dorsal thalamic nucleus (e.g.,
the LGN, VPL, MGN, etc.) has a subnucleus of the TRN associated with it, and reciprocal connections are formed between them (Jones, 1985; Sherman and Guillery,
1996). That is, relay cell axons en route to cortex pass through the appropriate TRN
zone, where they emit collateral terminals, and the TRN cells in turn project axons
back into the dorsal thalamic nucleus. Figure 8.4D shows a representative TRN cell.
It is worth noting that corticothalamic axons from layer 6 also pass through the appropriate TRN zone en route to their thalamic destination, and they also provide collateral innervation to these TRN cells. (However, see below for the pattern for layer 5
corticothalamic axons.) Finally, the TRN is also innervated by the same regions of
brainstem that innervate the dorsal thalamus. The TRN cells are GABAergic and inhibit their dorsal thalamic targets.

RELAY NEURONS

Relay (or projection) neurons, which represent roughly 75% of the cells in most thalamic nuclei (but see below), are the only output of a dorsal thalamic nucleus. They

project to cortex with a collateral innervation of the TRN en route. Relay cells in intralaminar thalamic nuclei also project to the basal ganglia (see Fig. 8.1 and Table 8.1). An important feature of thalamic nuclei is that different classes of relay cell can exist within a nucleus to provide parallel streams of thalamocortical relay through each nucleus (Stone, 1983; Dykes, 1983; Rodieck and Brening, 1983; Jones, 1985; Sherman, 1985). This feature is best appreciated in the A-laminae of the cat's LGN and is considered in more detail below. However, other processing streams exist in other portions of the cat's LGN and in other thalamic nuclei and in other species.

X and Y Cells. Roughly 300,000 relay cells reside in each of the A-laminae of the cat's LGN (Sanderson, 1971); relay X and Y cells are illustrated in Fig. 8.4A,B. These are fairly representative of thalamic relay cells in other nuclei. The relay X cells receive retinal input nearly exclusively from β cells, and the relay Y cells, from α cells (see Chap. 6 for a description of these retinal ganglion cell types; see also Sherman and Spear, 1982; Stone, 1983; Rodieck and Brening, 1983; Shapley and Lennie, 1985; Sherman, 1985). It is likely that a similar relationship holds for other species as well, although knowledge of relay cell types and their retinal inputs is not as complete as for the cat. For example, in the monkey's (and human's) LGN, the main laminae are divided into a dorsal set of smaller cells known as the *parvocellular* laminae, and a ven-

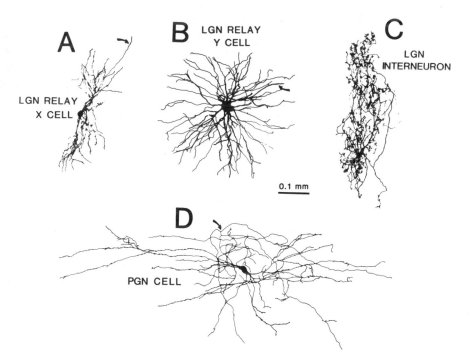

Fig. 8.4. Tracing of four representative neurons from the cat's LGN and TRN. Each of the cells was first studied physiologically and then labeled intracellularly with horseradish peroxidase. Where obvious, the axon is indicated by an arrow. **A:** Relay X cell. **B:** Relay Y cell. **C:** Interneuron. **D:** TRN neuron from the perigeniculate nucleus (PGN), a part of the TRN. [Redrawn from Sherman and Koch, 1986, with permission.]

tral set of larger cells known as the *magnocellular* laminae. These laminae are innervated by distinct retinal cell types (see Chap. 6): $P\beta$ (for primate β; also known as P for parvocellular) innervate the parvocellular laminae, and $P\alpha$ (for primate α; also known as M for magnocellular) innervate the magnocellular laminae. Although there is still considerable debate on the subject, it seems likely that the parvocellular and magnocellular pathways are homologous, respectively, to the X and Y pathways in the cat. It also seems likely that comparable and perhaps homologous pathways exist for other species as well (Stone, 1983; Rodieck and Brening, 1983; Shapley and Lennie, 1985; Sherman, 1985; Irvin et al., 1993; Hendry and Yoshioka, 1994).

The projection of relay cells concentrates in layer 4 of the cortical target area, with a smaller terminal zone in layer 6. In the cat, geniculate cells of the A-laminae project both to cortical areas 17 (striate cortex or V1) and 18 (V2). The relay X cells project exclusively to area 17, while the relay Y cells project to both areas. However, the homologous relay cells in primates project only to area 17. Similar relationships hold for other thalamic nuclei, since multiple projections from VPL to somatosensory cortex and MGN to auditory cortex have been described.

Lagged and Nonlagged Cells. Mastronarde (1987) described a new type of relay cell in the cat's LGN, which he termed *lagged*, and this is distinguished from the conventional type, called *nonlagged*. This new classification has received considerable attention (Humphrey and Weller, 1988; Saul and Humphrey, 1990, 1992; Heggelund and Hartveit, 1990; Lu et al., 1995). Essentially, nonlagged cells retain the same basic receptive field properties of the input retinal X or Y axons; they respond briskly and with short latency to visual stimuli. Lagged cells respond more sluggishly and with longer latency. One suggestion is that these represent two different temporal relay channels that can be used by cortex to create such features as directional selectivity for moving stimuli (Saul and Humphrey, 1990, 1992), but the specific significance of these cell types remains unclear (Lu et al., 1995). It is also not yet clear the extent to which lagged and nonlagged cell types are seen in other species or in other thalamic nuclei. Nonetheless, this observation of lagged and nonlagged relay cells holds promise to become a key feature of thalamic relays.

INTERNEURONS

Roughly 25% of the cells in most thalamic nuclei are local interneurons. However, as an example of the bewildering variation in relative numbers of relay cells and interneurons, the cat's LGN and VPL plus the rat's LGN have roughly a 3-to-1 relay cell-to-interneuron ratio, but the rat's VPL and other thalamic nuclei have practically no interneurons (Ohara et al., 1983; Ralston, 1983; Spreafico et al., 1983; Fitzpatrick et al., 1984; Jones, 1985). Thus analogous nuclei in the same animal (e.g., the rat's LGN and VPL) can vary in this regard, as can homologous nuclei across species (e.g., the VPL of cats and rats). Arcelli et al. (1997), in a recent study of the variation of GABAergic interneurons across nuclei and species, argued that this variation could be an index of "complexity" in the evolution of intrathalamic processing.

Interneurons have been best described for the LGN, but they seem basically similar in other thalamic nuclei. Geniculate interneurons have small cell bodies with long, thin, and sinuous dendrites (Fig. 8.4C). The dendrites are notable for giving rise to bulbous appendages connected to the stem dendrite by long (10 μm or more), thin (usually less than 0.1 μm in diameter) processes; these appendages usually occur in clusters. Overall, the dendrites with their bulbous appendages look like the terminal arbor of an axon, and thus Guillery (1966) referred to these dendrites as *axoniform* in appearance. In fact, these bulbous appendages represent a major synaptic output of the cell, since they are synaptic terminals that are both presynaptic and postsynaptic to other elements in the geniculate neuropil (Guillery, 1969a,b; Ralston, 1971; Famiglietti and Peters, 1972; Hamos et al., 1985; Ralston et al., 1988). Most of the synapses from interneurons are thus dendritic in origin.

These interneurons usually have a conventional axon that arborizes locally, typically within the dendritic arbor (Hamos et al., 1985; Montero, 1987), although axonless interneurons may exist (Ralston et al., 1988). In the cat's LGN, interneurons seem to be mostly associated with the X pathway, since they receive retinal input only from X axons, and their dendritic outputs contact mostly only relay X cells (Sherman and Friedlander, 1988). Evidence for interneuronal influences on relay Y cells also exists (Lindström, 1982), and this may reflect the axonal output. All interneurons are GABAergic, and both their dendritic and axonal outputs inhibit their postsynaptic targets.

As noted above, the TRN is a source of nonretinal or modulatory afferents to the dorsal thalamus. TRN cells do not project beyond the thalamus and instead provide local, GABAergic, inhibitory input to thalamic relay cells. They are thus functionally in many ways similar to interneurons, and many investigators group them with interneurons as local inhibitory cells. It is not yet clear what, if any, fundamentally different role in the relay of driving inputs is played by the TRN cells and interneurons.

SYNAPTIC CONNECTIONS

TYPES OF SYNAPTIC TERMINAL

The synaptology of both relay cells and interneurons has been described on the basis of electron microscopic studies. Most of these studies have concentrated on the LGN and VPL with rather similar results (Guillery, 1969a,b; Wilson et al., 1984; Hamos et al., 1985; Jones, 1985; Montero, 1987; Ralston et al., 1988). The following description derives from the A-laminae of the LGN.

Four major types of synaptic terminal exist there (Guillery, 1969a,b), and their origins are for the most part known. *RLP* terminals (*r*ound vesicles, *l*arge profiles, and *p*ale mitochondria) form asymmetrical synapses. They derive from retina and are glutamatergic. While it had been thought that perhaps 10–20% of all terminals in the LGN are retinal in origin, newer evidence suggests that this percentage may be much smaller (Van Horn et al., 1997). *RSD* terminals (*r*ound vesicles, *s*mall profiles, and *d*ark mitochondria) also form asymmetrical synapses and are the most numerous, comprising roughly half of all terminals. Roughly half of the RSD terminals derive from cortex and are glutamatergic, and roughly half derive from brainstem sources (Erişir et al., 1997b). Most of these brainstem terminals are cholinergic, although some are noradrenergic or serotonergic. A few (probably less than 5%) of the terminals that otherwise resemble RSD terminals are relatively large and might be considered to be *RLD* terminals (*r*ound vesicles, *l*arge profiles, and *d*ark mitochondria). These mostly emanate from the parabrachial region of the midbrain and are cholinergic. *F* terminals (flattened vesicles) form symmetrical synapses and represent a little more than one quarter of the terminals in the LGN. These are GABAergic. Two subtypes, *F1* and *F2*, have been recognized. Although a constellation of features can distinguish them, the most salient are that F1 terminals derive from axons and are strictly presynaptic, whereas F2 terminals are dendritic in origin and are both presynaptic and postsynaptic. F1 terminals arise from axons of TRN cells, interneurons, and, in the case of LGN, from axons of NOT cells; F2 terminals derive from dendrites of interneurons.

INPUTS TO RELAY CELLS

Reconstructions at the electron microscopic level reveal that geniculate relay cells in the cat receive roughly 4000 synapses, nearly all onto their dendrites with rare contacts on their somata (Wilson et al., 1984). Figure 8.5 schematically summarizes the

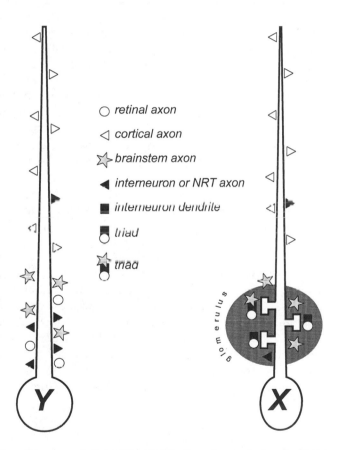

Fig. 8.5. Schematic representation of the distribution of synaptic terminals onto a typical dendrite of a relay X and Y cell. For simplicity, only a single, unbranched dendrite is shown for each neuron. Each type of synaptic terminal, as well as the synaptic triad, is indicated by a unique symbol. The density (synapses/μm of dendritic length) of each terminal type is also represented by the relative number of synaptic terminals. Dendritic appendages are denoted by the T-shaped attachments to dendrites, and the glomerulus related to the X cell is shown. See text for details. [Redrawn from Wilson et al., 1984, with permission.]

distribution of various types of synaptic input on the dendritic arbors of these relay X and Y cells. Relay cells in other thalamic nuclei probably have a comparable pattern of synaptic inputs. For both relay X and Y cells, inputs from retinal and F terminals concentrate in the proximal region of the dendritic arbor, whereas cortical RSD input dominates distal dendrites, and there is little or no overlap in these zones (Erişir et al., 1997a). Parabrachial RSD and RLD terminals are found proximally, among retinal terminals. However, major differences between relay X and Y cells exist in the types of F terminal present and in the detailed nature of the retinal input. To explain these differences, first a description of the *glomerulus* and the *synaptic triad* is required.

A glomerulus is a complex synaptic structure (Fig. 8.6). Glomeruli seem to be related to interneurons, and it is interesting that the rat's VPL, which lacks interneurons (see above), also lacks glomeruli (Ralston, 1983). For the A-laminae of the cat's LGN, glomeruli include a major set of inputs to proximal dendrites of relay X cells, but they associate rarely with the Y pathway (Wilson et al., 1984; Sherman, 1988; Sherman and Friedlander, 1988). Glomeruli are common in other thalamic nuclei, but the pattern of specificity for functional types outside of the LGN is presently unknown (Jones, 1985; Ralston et al., 1988). Glomeruli have terminals of all four types noted above, and these terminals interrelate with each other in a complex arrangement. Virtually all glomeruli in the LGN include a retinal terminal, which is typically located at or near the glomerular center and is surrounded by a number of other terminals. Thus the glomerulus represents an important morphological feature of retinogeniculate transmission. Other common terminals found in glomeruli are F terminals (both F1 and F2) and terminals from brainstem. Cortical terminals rarely if ever innervate glomeruli (Erişir et al., 1997a).

This retinal terminal in the glomerulus contacts two different postsynaptic elements: an F2 terminal that derives from dendritic appendages of interneurons, and a dendrite (or its appendage) of a relay X cell. The retinal terminal usually contacts several F2 terminals within a glomerulus, and all of the synapses formed by the retinal terminal are asymmetrical. The interneuron's F2 terminals, in turn, make symmetrical synaptic contacts onto the same postsynaptic element of the relay X cell, be it dendritic appendage or shaft, contacted by the retinal terminal. Since three terminal types are involved, this special neuronal circuit within the glomerulus is known as a *triad* (for a detailed hypothesis concerning the role of these triadic circuits, see Koch, 1985). Figure 8.7 illustrates a triad involving RLP and F2 terminals and a dendritic appendage of a relay X cell. A retinal terminal is usually the common presynaptic element in the triad, but occasionally other terminals, such as those from the brainstem, can serve this function. Both a retinal terminal and brainstem axon can

---

Fig. 8.6. Reconstruction of a glomerular zone in the geniculate A-laminae of the cat's LGN, showing the F2 terminals from an intracellularly labeled interneuron, the postsynaptic cluster of appendages from a relay X cell, and the location of synaptic contacts; each scale bar represents 1.0 μm. **a:** Labeled processes from the interneuron. A thin stem dendrite (d) emits an extremely fine process (open arrow) that arborizes into 12 F2 terminals connected by extremely fine processes. These terminals are postsynaptic to retinal or RLP terminals (circles), unlabeled F terminals (triangles; most or all of these may be F1 terminals, but they were not sufficiently reconstructed to be certain), and an RSD terminal (star). The labeled F2 terminals also form synap-

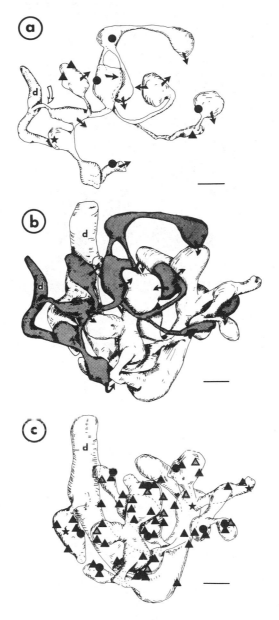

tic outputs (solid arrows). **b:** Combined reconstruction of the labeled interneuron's processes from a (stippled area) and unlabeled postsynaptic processes from c (open area). The synapses from the F2 terminals onto the relay X cell's appendages are illustrated (solid arrows; these represent the same solid arrows as in a). **c:** Unlabeled postsynaptic dendrite (d) from a relay X cell with 8 appendages that receive all of the neuron's synaptic input in the reconstructed zone. These include 9 synapses from RLP or retinal terminals (circles), 9 from F2 terminals of the labeled interneuron (stippled triangles; these correspond to the solid arrows in a and b), 40 from unlabeled F terminals (solid triangles), and 3 from RSD terminals (stars). The 16 triadic synaptic arrangements are illustrated by overlapping pairs of symbols for synapses from RLP and F terminals. [From Hamos et al., 1985, with permission.]

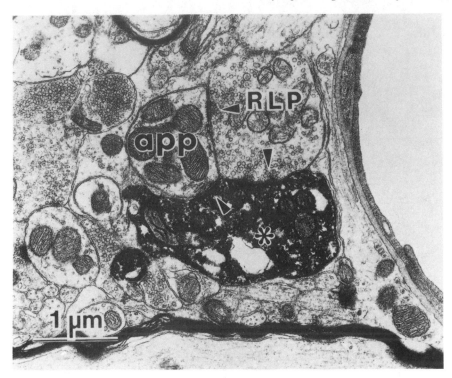

Fig. 8.7. Electron micrograph of a triadic synaptic relationship from the A-laminae of the cat's LGN. An interneuron was labeled with horseradish peroxidase, which creates an electron-dense reaction product, and its labeled F2 terminal is dark in this micrograph. A retinal terminal (RLP) contacts both the labeled F2 terminal and the dendritic appendage (app) of a relay X cell. The labeled F2 contacts the same appendage. Synaptic contacts are indicated by arrowheads. Scale: 1.0 μm.

share the same F2 terminal and postsynaptic relay X cell process in triadic circuitry within a glomerulus.

The vast majority of retinal input to relay X cells is filtered through this complicated circuitry of the glomerulus. Retinal input to relay Y cells is simpler and involves conventional asymmetrical synapses onto proximal dendritic shafts (Wilson et al., 1984; Sherman, 1988). F2 terminals are nearly always limited to glomeruli, and the lack of glomeruli associated with the Y pathway results in very few such terminals contacting relay Y cells. More than 90% of the F input to these cells is of the F1 variety, while roughly two-thirds of F input onto relay X cells is of the F2 variety.

INPUTS TO INTERNEURONS

As with our previous examples, most of our detailed knowledge of interneurons stems from studies of the LGN, but comparable studies in other thalamic nuclei, especially the VPL, reveal basically similar properties for thalamic interneurons (Ralston et al., 1988). In the LGN, many retinal, RSD, and F1 terminals contact interneurons (Hamos et al., 1985). Much of this input is focused onto their dendritic appendages, which are the presynaptic F2 terminals. Input is also formed onto dendritic shafts and somata, and these are the only geniculate neurons that seem to receive significant retinal input onto their somata.

BASIC NEURONAL CIRCUIT

Enough is known about the cat's LGN to provide a schematic circuit diagram, including a fair estimate of the numbers of neuronal elements present. Of course, many of the specific features of this diagram remain somewhat uncertain, but the broad outlines seem clear. It seems likely that these broad outlines apply as well to other thalamic nuclei.

COMPONENT POPULATIONS

Each of the A-laminae of the cat's LGN contain roughly 400,000 neurons (Sanderson, 1971). Of these, perhaps 300,000 are relay cells and 100,000 are interneurons. The interneurons have two outputs, the major one being dendritic via F2 terminals and the minor one being axonal via F1 terminals. The dendritic output of interneurons seems to target relay X cells nearly exclusively, but the target nature of the axonal output is unclear. Slightly more relay X cells (150,000–200,000) than relay Y cells (100,000–150,000) seem to exist (Sherman, 1985). These geniculate neurons are innervated by a slightly fewer than 100,000 retinogeniculate axons and by more than 4,000,000 corticogeniculate axons (Sherman and Koch, 1986), although the details of how these latter axons innervate relay X and Y cells plus interneurons are not yet clear. We also still lack estimates for the number of afferent axons from the TRN and various brainstem sites, and such estimates are only partly available for other species.

INTRINSIC CIRCUITRY

The basic organization of major inputs to the cat's LGN is summarized schematically in Fig. 8.8. Many of the details of this circuit, including the differences between the X and Y pathways, have been described above. These relay cells also receive input from cortex and from the brainstem. Major inhibitory input derives from local GABA-ergic cells, which are the interneurons and TRN cells. Both of these GABAergic cells are innervated by cortex and by the brainstem parabrachial region. In addition, TRN cells are innervated by axon collaterals from the relay cells, and interneurons receive input from retinal X axons. TRN cells also receive a GABAergic input from the basal forebrain. Not included for simplicity are lesser known and probably smaller inputs described above from the hypothalamus (histaminergic), pretectum (GABAergic), the parabrachial region or locus coeruleus (noradrenergic), and the dorsal raphé nucleus (serotonergic).

Although much of the circuitry outlined in Fig. 8.8 is sketchy, the following conclusions can be tentatively drawn. Much of this repeats earlier points, but it is offered here as a concise summary. Relay cells receive retinal input onto proximal dendrites in close association with GABAergic and parabrachial input. The GABAergic input derives from TRN cells and interneurons. Distal dendrites are dominated by cortical input, and, at least for LGN relay cells, these inputs are limited to dendritic locations more distal than those of retinal inputs (Guillery, 1969a,b; Wilson et al., 1984; Erişir

A: *X pathway*   ## B: *Y pathway*

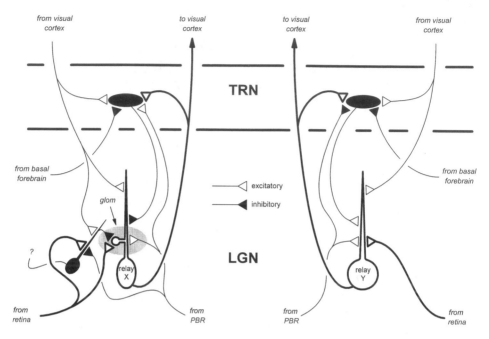

Fig. 8.8. Schematic view of X and Y circuits for the A-laminae of the cat's LGN. **A:** X pathway. Much of the input to relay X cells (open profile), including inputs from retina, from dendrites of interneurons (filled profile), from the thalamic reticular nucleus (TRN; filled profiles), and from the parabrachial region (PBR) is filtered through glomeruli (glom; stippled region). Retinal terminals engage in triadic relationships with terminals from the interneuron's dendrites and dendritic appendages on the relay cell. Cortical input dominates the peripheral dendrites of the relay cell. The interneuron is also innervated from retina, cortex, and the PBR; the target of the interneuron's axon remains unknown, except that it is extraglomerular. The TRN cell is innervated from geniculocortical axons, corticogeniculate axons, PBR axons, and axons from the basal forebrain. **B:** Y pathway. This pathway is much simpler, because interneurons do not appear to provide many inputs from their dendrites. The retinal axon contacts the relay cell (open profile) on proximal dendritic shafts among terminals from PBR axons. Other inputs to the relay and TRN cells are similar to that shown in A.

et al., 1997a). Some GABAergic inputs can also be seen on distal dendrites, although most are found proximally. However, the electrotonic compactness of relay cells implies that even the distal inputs can be quite important functionally.

   Figure 8.8 also summarizes some differences between the X and Y pathways, and perhaps this can be taken as a reflection of the kinds of variation present throughout thalamic circuitry. Three main differences exist: the nature of retinal input, the presence of glomeruli, and the role of interneurons. Retinal input to relay Y cells is fairly straightforward, innervating proximal dendritic shafts in simple contact zones. Retinal input to relay X cells is much more elaborate, since it involves complicated triadic relationships that include dendritic terminals of interneurons. Glomeruli are also a ma-

jor feature of X but not Y circuitry, and the glomerulus may be viewed as a major filter of retinogeniculate transmission (see above). Finally, interneuronal dendritic outputs also seem to be intimately related to X but not Y circuitry. The axonal targets of interneurons largely remain a mystery; however, the axons use F1 terminals and contact extraglomerular dendritic shafts, whereas the dendritic outputs use F2 terminals and contact dendritic appendages in glomeruli.

It should be emphasized that the circuit schematically represented by Fig. 8.8 is preliminary and greatly simplified. Many questions still remain. For example, what is the interrelated pattern of innervation involving single cortical axons, TRN cells (or interneurons), and relay cells? The implication of this last question is illustrated in Fig. 8.9 by showing two extremes of possible functional circuits involving inputs to relay cells and the local, GABAergic inhibitory cells. This adheres to our superficial knowledge of interconnections among these cell populations and makes the point that in many cases we still cannot even determine if activation of these circuits excites or inhibits relay cells. For instance, Fig. 8.9A shows a true feedback inhibitory circuit in which an axon collateral from a relay cell (cell b) excites a TRN cell (cell 2) that in turn inhibits this same relay cell. Figure 8.9B depicts a very different picture: now relay cell b excites TRN cells 1 and 3, but not 2, and TRN cells 1 and 3 do not inhibit relay cell b, but rather inhibit its neighbors (cells a and c). Since cells a and c excite the TRN cell (cell 2) that inhibits relay cell b, the net result of the circuit depicted in Fig. 8.9B is that activity in relay cell b results in its further *disinhibition*, which is precisely the opposite of the feedback inhibition resulting from Fig. 8.9A. Likewise, the circuits shown in Fig. 8.9C,D have opposite effects when the corticogeniculate axon is activated: that in Fig. 8.9C results in feedforward inhibition of relay cell b, while that in Fig. 8.9D results in feedforward disinhibition of this same cell. The message here is that the details count, particularly for connections of individual neurons, and we are not yet sufficiently certain of many of the details that enable us even to determine the final effect on relay cells of activating certain inputs or local circuits. It should be noted that the circuits depicted here are probably extreme examples, and combinations of each type probably exist.

DENDRITIC CABLE PROPERTIES

RELAY CELLS

Both X and Y classes of relay cell are electrically rather compact, with dendritic arbors extending for roughly one length constant (Bloomfield et al., 1987; Bloomfield and Sherman, 1989). In practice, this means that even the most distally located synaptic input can have significant effects on the soma and axon, with attenuation of postsynaptic potentials never exceeding one-third to one-half (see Fig. 8.10). One of the reasons for the electrotonically restricted dendritic arbors of relay X and Y cells is the nature of their dendritic branches. These branches closely adhere to Rall's *3/2 branching rule* (Bloomfield et al., 1987). This states that the diameters of the daughter dendrites each raised to the 3/2 power and summed equals the diameter of the parent dendrite raised to the 3/2 power (Rall, 1977; discussed in Johnston and Wu, 1995; Segev, 1995; Shepherd, 1998). Such branching matches impedance on both sides of the branch point and permits efficient current flow across these branches in *both* directions. This

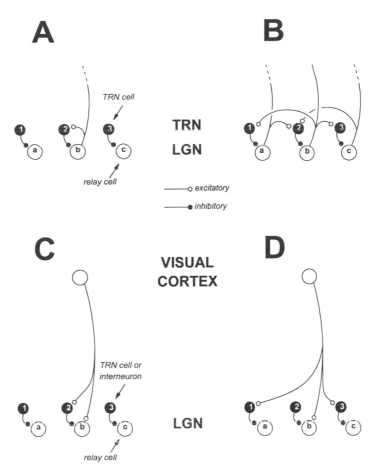

Fig. 8.9. Schema showing examples of different types of inhibitory circuits involving geniculate relay cells. Excitatory cells and their synaptic outputs are shown as open circles, and inhibitory (GABAergic) cells and their outputs are shown as solid circles. **A:** Circuit beginning with relay cell axon that represents feedback inhibition. A collateral of the axon from relay cell b excites TRN cell 2 that then inhibits cell b. **B:** Circuit beginning with relay cell axon that does not represent feedback inhibition. Here, axon collaterals from relay cell b excite TRN cells 1 and 3. These TRN cells then inhibit relay cells a and c, but do not directly influence relay cell b. There is thus no feedback inhibition. However, note that the inhibition of relay cells a and c reduce their excitatory effect on TRN cell 2, resulting in less inhibition from this TRN cell onto cell b. Thus, instead of feedback inhibition seen in A, this circuit represents feedback disinhibition, which is the opposite. **C:** Circuit beginning with cortical axon that represents feedforward inhibition. A cortical axon innervates relay cell b and directly excites it, but a collateral of this same axon excites a TRN cell or interneuron 2 that then inhibits relay cell b. **D:** Circuit beginning with cortical axon that does not represent feedforward inhibition. The main difference in D is that, while the cortical axon still directly innervates and excites relay cell b, its collaterals excite TRN cells or interneurons 1 and 3, which then inhibit relay cells a and c. There would be no inhibitory effect on relay cell b.

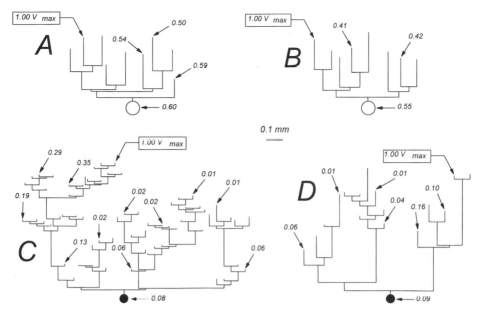

Fig. 8.10. **A–D:** Cable modeling of attenuation of single voltage injection (i.e., the activation of a single synapse) within the dendritic arbors of the two relay X cells and two interneurons from the A-laminae of the cat's LGN. The site of voltage injection is indicated by the boxed value labeled 1.00 V_{max} (maximum voltage). Voltage attenuation at various terminal endings within the arbor and soma is indicated by arrows and given as fractions of V_{max}. Note that voltage never falls below 0.5 of its maximum value anywhere within the dendritic arbor or soma for either relay cell. However, considerable voltage attenuation is evident for the interneurons so that very little of the synaptic current will reach the soma. [From Bloomfield and Sherman, 1989, with permission.]

maximizes the transmission of distal postsynaptic potentials to the soma. This also implies that a potential generated anywhere in the dendritic arbor or at the soma will be efficiently transmitted throughout the dendritic arbor. Among other things, this means that the discharge of an action potential will depolarize the entire dendrite arbor by tens of millivolts, and this could have significant effects on voltage-dependent processes in the dendrites (see below).

INTERNEURONS

Unlike relay cells, interneurons are not electrically compact (Bloomfield and Sherman, 1989). This is partly because their dendrites are thinner and longer than those of relay cells. More importantly, the dendritic branch points of interneurons violate the 3/2 branching rule, because daughter branches tend to be too thin. This limits the current flowing across these branch points. As a result, *providing that there are no major active conductances in the dendritic arbor of interneurons,* much of the synaptic circuitry in distal dendrites, including that involving the F2 terminals, would be functionally isolated from the soma and axon (Fig. 8.10). We emphasize the proviso here concerning the assumption of no significant Ca^{2+} and Na^+ conductances in the dendrites, and this

attribute remains unknown. Ralston (1971) proposed some time ago that synaptic input onto the F2 terminals of interneurons in the cat's VPL would also be isolated from
the soma. Other examples of this property are found in the olfactory bulb (see Chap.
5) and retina (see Chap. 6).

Computational modeling based on these observations with the assumption of passive cable properties suggests an interesting mode of operation for these interneurons (Sherman, 1988; Bloomfield and Sherman, 1989), which is schematically depicted by Fig. 8.11. Clusters of dendritic appendages, which are major sites of input

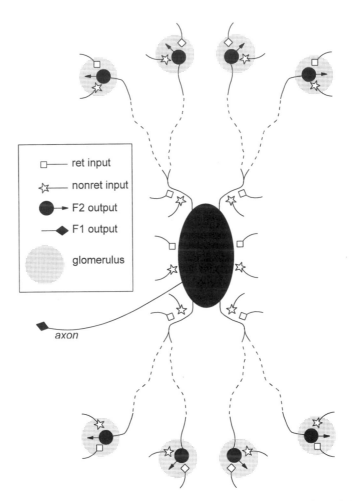

Fig. 8.11. Schematic view of hypothesis for functioning of interneurons in the cat's LGN. Retinal and nonretinal inputs are shown both to the glomeruli as well as to the proximal dendrites
and soma. The glomerular inputs are acted upon and lead to F2 outputs from the dendrites,
whereas the inputs to the proximal dendrites and soma lead to F1 outputs from the axon. The
dashed lines indicate the electrotonic isolation between glomeruli and the proximal dendrites
plus soma. This isolation suggests that the two sets of synaptic computations, peripheral for the
glomerular F2 outputs and proximal for the axonal F1 outputs, transpire in parallel and independently of one another. Most glomeruli are also functionally isolated from one other.

and output, represent local circuits whose computations are largely independent of activity in other clusters and in the soma. In contrast, the axonal output is controlled in a more orthodox manner by input to the soma and proximal dendrites. This output appears to be mediated by conventional action potentials (Sherman and Friedlander, 1988). Also, while the dendritic F2 outputs innervate relay X cells through glomeruli, the axon forms F1 terminals that innervate dendritic shafts of unknown origin outside of glomeruli (Hamos et al., 1985; Montero, 1987; Sherman and Friedlander, 1988). This suggests that the interneuron simultaneously does double duty: integration of the axonal F1 outputs via action potentials depends on one set of proximal inputs and involves one type of postsynaptic target, while integration of the dendritic F2 outputs depends on local inputs and involves a different postsynaptic target. Examples of electrotonic properties governing similar operational modes are discussed in other chapters.

MEMBRANE PROPERTIES

INTRINSIC CONDUCTANCES

The intrinsic electrophysiological properties of neurons play a great role in determining their integrative characteristics (see Chap. 2). We can no longer view a thalamic cell as being a simple response element that linearly sums its synaptic inputs to determine its axonal output. Thus cable modeling as described above is only a beginning toward explaining how a neuron responds to various synaptic inputs. In reality, these cells have a variety of active membrane conductances. Many of these are controlled in a conventional manner by ligand-binding of neurotransmitters, including effects of second-messenger pathways activated by metabotropic receptors, but some are controlled by membrane voltage, and others are controlled by concentration levels of certain ions, such as Ca^{2+}.

Both in vitro and in vivo experiments directed at different thalamic nuclei across several mammalian species have revealed a surprising plethora of intrinsic membrane conductances present in all thalamic neurons, both in the dorsal thalamus nuclei as well as within TRN neurons (Steriade et al., 1987; Steriade and Llinás, 1988; Huguenard and McCormick, 1992; McCormick and Huguenard, 1992). These conductances all lead to currents that alter the membrane potential. The number of active conductances described for thalamic neurons continues to grow. Which conductances are active can greatly affect the nature of the thalamic neuron's relay of its input to cortex. Conductances found in thalamic neurons are generally found in many other brain cells as well; for the most part, these have been described in detail in Chap. 2. The major and best-understood ones operating in thalamic neurons are listed below (see also Chap. 2).

Na⁺ Conductances. Two voltage-dependent Na^+ conductances have been described. The fast, inactivating Na^+ conductance, similar to the one described by Hodgkin and Huxley for the squid giant axon, is voltage dependent and subserves the conventional action potential. The other Na^+ conductance is persistent and non-inactivating. This creates a plateau depolarization that serves to inactivate certain currents, such as I_A and I_T (see below).

Ca²⁺ Conductances. There are at least two voltage-dependent Ca^{2+} conductances. One has a high threshold and is most likely located in the dendrites; rather little is known about this conductance. The other has a lower threshold and plays a dramatic role in retinogeniculate transmission (and the transmission of other driving inputs in other nuclei). It is often known as the *low-threshold Ca^{2+} conductance* and is described more fully below. This leads to Ca^{2+} entry into the cell, thereby depolarizing it and producing the *low-threshold spike.* The low-threshold spike occurs both in TRN cells and thalamic relay neurons, but preliminary evidence suggests that, at least for the LGN, this conductance normally plays little role in interneurons (see below).

Apart from those underlying the generation of conventional action potentials, the low-threshold Ca^{2+} conductance is probably the most important conductance for relay cells. The activation state of this conductance controls which of two distinct response modes, *tonic* or *burst*, is operative when a thalamic relay cell responds to afferent input (Jahnsen and Llinás, 1984a,b; Crunelli et al., 1989; McCormick and Feeser, 1990; Lo et al., 1991; Guido et al., 1992; Guido and Weyand, 1995; Mukherjee and Kaplan, 1995). "Tonic" used in this sense refers to a response mode of a geniculate relay cell, and here it is paired with "burst." X and Y cells, the relay cell types found in the A-laminae of the cat's lateral geniculate nucleus, display both response modes. This should not be confused with another, obsolete use of "tonic" when paired with "phasic" to refer to a cell type: "tonic" for X and "phasic" for Y (Sherman, 1985). Throughout this account, we shall use "tonic" only to refer to response mode and not to cell type.

During the tonic mode of firing, this Ca^{2+} conductance is inactive, and the neuronal response to a depolarizing input is characterized by a steady stream of action potentials of a frequency and duration that increase monotonically with increases in the strength and duration of the depolarizing stimulus (see below). During the burst mode, when this Ca^{2+} conductance is activated, the neuronal response to such an input consists of brief bursts of action potentials separated by silent periods. It is worth emphasizing that this bears no resemblance to the known firing patterns of afferent inputs: for instance, retinogeniculate axons show no evidence of burst firing (Lo et al., 1991).

The activation state of this Ca^{2+} conductance is dependent on membrane voltage, and when activated, this conductance produces the low-threshold spike (Jahnsen and Llinás, 1984a,b; McCormick and Feeser, 1990; Lo et al., 1991; Huguenard and McCormick, 1992; McCormick and Huguenard, 1992). Figure 8.12A–C illustrates its voltage dependency. This actually depicts a simple experiment during which a standard depolarizing current pulse (bottom trace) was injected into the cell through the intracellular recording electrode, and the variable is the initial V_m, which differs among the three examples of Fig. 8.12A–C. When the cell starts off relatively depolarized (Fig. 8.12A), the current pulse depolarizes the cell beyond its action potential threshold, and a stream of unitary, conventional action potentials is discharged for as long as the cell is sufficiently depolarized. When the cell is hyperpolarized slightly from this level (Fig. 8.12B), the same depolarizing pulse is no longer sufficient to drive the cell to threshold, and a purely ohmic response occurs. However, when the cell is further hyperpolarized (Fig. 8.12C), the depolarizing pulse now activates a large triangular depolarization (the low-threshold spike) that is sufficient to drive the cell briefly above its threshold, thereby producing a high-frequency burst typically of 2–10 conventional ac-

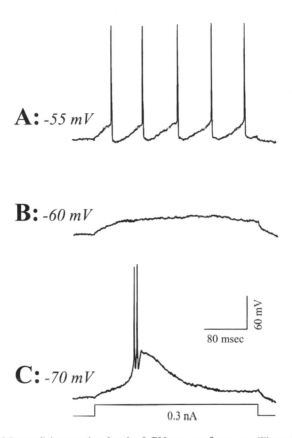

Fig. 8.12. Tonic and burst firing modes for the LGN neuron from cat. The cell was recorded intracellularly in an in vitro slice preparation and was held at different initial membrane voltages as shown by adjusting current injected into the cell through the recording electrode. Each of the three upper, recording traces shows the response to the same depolarizing 0.3 nA current pulse (bottom trace) injected into the cell, also via the recording electrode. **A:** Tonic response. When the cell is relatively depolarized (−55 mV), the current injection produces a membrane depolarization sufficient to evoke a stream of conventional action potentials. **B:** No response. At a middle level of polarization (−60 mV), the injected current pulse depolarizes the cell insufficiently to evoke action potentials, resulting in a purely ohmic response. **C:** Burst response. When the cell is relatively hyperpolarized (−70 mV), the same depolarizing pulse now triggers a low-threshold Ca^{2+} spike. Riding the crest of this low-threshold Ca^{2+} spike is a burst of two conventional action potentials (the number of action potentials in the burst can vary up to about 10). The low-threshold Ca^{2+} has a voltage dependency that prevents it from being activated from the more depolarized levels of A and B (see text for details).

tion potentials. This burst has briefer interspike intervals (≤4 msec) than is seen during tonic firing (≥4 msec).

The behavior illustrated in Fig. 8.12 is explained by the voltage dependency of the Ca^{2+} conductance underlying the low-threshold spike: it is *inactivated* by membrane depolarizations more positive than about −60 mV (Fig. 8.12 A,B), but it is *de-inactivated* at more hyperpolarized levels from which it can be *activated* by a suitably large depolarization (Fig. 8.12C), such as an EPSP. The membrane current resulting from the low-threshold Ca^{2+} conductance is known as I_T, because it represents an influx of Ca^{2+} ions via membrane pores known as *T channels*. This influx leads to a spike-like depolarization due to Ca^{2+} entry, and this produces the low-threshold spike. Thus the low-threshold Ca^{2+} conductance, low-threshold spike, and I_T all refer to closely related phenomena.

Activation of the low-threshold spike is quickly followed by repolarization of the membrane to its former, hyperpolarized level by the rapid inactivation of the T current (for a detailed account of I_T and related currents in thalamic neurons, see Jahnsen and Llinás, 1984a,b; Huguenard and McCormick, 1992; McCormick and Huguenard, 1992). In addition, there is an activation of various K^+ conductances (see below), including one that is voltage-dependent and one that is activated by the Ca^{2+} entry that occurs during the low-threshold spike. This repolarization serves partially to de-inactivate the low-threshold spike, but there is also a time dependency for de-inactivation: complete de-inactivation requires that the hyperpolarization be maintained, generally for ≥ 100 msec. This can be thought of as a sort of refractory period for the low-threshold spike. Thus a very brief hyperpolarization followed by depolarization will not produce a low-threshold spike, and the frequency of low-threshold spiking rarely exceeds 10 Hz. Between the low-threshold spikes and associated bursts of conventional action potentials, the cell is relatively silent.

The low-threshold spike provides an amplification that permits a hyperpolarized cell to generate action potentials in response to a moderate EPSP. The spike-like depolarization resulting from the Ca^{2+} conductance has an activation threshold. In many ways, this spike behaves like a conventional Na^+/K^+ action potential: both have an activation threshold and lead to voltage spikes. However, compared with the Na^+/K^+ spike, the threshold for the Ca^{2+} spike is less sharp and its amplitude is more graded. Nonetheless, its threshold and spike-like behavior mean that the amplification represented by the low-threshold spike is nonlinear. That is, the limited time course of the low-threshold spike limits the firing of action potentials to a brief burst typically lasting <20 msec even when an activating depolarization is sustained for much longer periods. Since these action potentials are the only response relayed to cortex, the time course of this response does not faithfully represent that of the input: both a very brief depolarization and one that lasted much longer would elicit similar responses relayed to cortex. Another feature of this nonlinearity is the representation of amplitude. The spike-like depolarization resulting from the activated Ca^{2+} conductance means that the low-threshold spike has a very compressed dynamic range. This means that, as an activating stimulus increases in amplitude, it will rapidly evoke the maximum low-threshold spike (and thus maximum burst of action potentials) so that further increases in stimulus amplitude cannot be represented. Indeed, it is not clear that the actual number of conventional action potentials in the burst riding the low-threshold spike codes for any stimulus variable. In contrast, the tonic response mode is much more linear in its stimulus/response relationship. Temporally, the duration of elevated firing during tonic mode lasts as long as the activating depolarization (see Fig. 8.12A), so time is well represented. Although not shown in Fig. 8.12A, during tonic firing there is also a relatively linear transformation between stimulus amplitude and response frequency. Thus tonic firing represents a much more linear transformation than does burst firing.

K$^+$ Conductances. A number of voltage and/or Ca^{2+} dependent K$^+$ conductances exist that give rise to various membrane currents (see Chap. 2). The best known is the *delayed rectifier* (I_K), which is part of the action potential and repolarizes the neuron following the Na$^+$ conductance. Several others (I_A, I_C, and possibly I_{AHP}) hyperpolarize the neuron for varying lengths of time following a conventional action potential. The amount of this hyperpolarization determines the cell's relative refractory period, which limits its maximum firing rate. Finally, thalamic cells exhibit a variable K$^+$ "leak" current.

I_A and its relationship with I_T is particularly interesting. The voltage dependencies of these two currents are generally similar in that both are inactive at depolarized V_m and can be activated by depolarization from relatively hyperpolarized V_m. However, while I_T leads to depolarization due to Ca^{2+} entry, I_A leads to hyperpolarization due to K$^+$ leaving the cell. Since I_A is activated by depolarization, this means that it will oppose that depolarization, making it smaller and slowing it down. However, for most relay cells, the activation and inactivation curves of I_T are offset by at least 10 mV in the hyperpolarized direction with respect to those of I_A (Pape et al. 1994). This means that when a relay cell is hyeprpolarized sufficiently to de-inactivate both currents and is then depolarized, I_T will activate before I_A, and the resultant spike-like depolarization will rapidly inactivate I_A before it has a chance to develop. It may thus be uncommon to activate I_A in relay cells under most conditions. However, there is a narrow window of V_m in which I_T is largely inactivated and I_A is largely de-inactivated, and depolarization that occurs within this limited membrane voltage range will activate I_A but not I_T.

This pattern is different in interneurons (Pape et al., 1994), because the voltage dependencies of I_T and I_A largely overlap. Thus I_A and I_T will tend to be activated together, but the effect of I_A in offsetting and slowing the depolarization will prevent full expression of I_T. The result is that interneurons rarely express I_T (Pape et al. 1994).

Hyperpolarization Activated Conductance. A conductance that is activated by membrane hyperpolarization and inactivated by depolarization is often associated with the low-threshold Ca^{2+} conductance. This *hyperpolarization-activated cation conductance*, leads, via influx of cations, to a depolarizing current, which is called I_h (McCormick and Pape, 1990). Activation is slow, with a time constant of >200 msec. The combination of I_T, the above-mentioned K$^+$ conductances, and I_h helps to support rhythmic bursting, typically at 3–10 Hz for the low-threshold spikes, which is often seen in recordings from in vitro slice preparations of thalamus (see also below). Hyperpolarizing a cell will activate I_h, but so slowly that I_T fully de-inactivates. Once I_h is activated, it will depolarize the cell, thereby activating I_T. This in turn inactivates both I_h and I_T while activating K$^+$ conductances, resulting in repolarization. The cycle then repeats. This leads to prolonged rhythmic bursting. This bursting can be interrupted only by a sufficiently strong and prolonged depolarization to produce tonic firing, and appropriate membrane voltage shifts can effectively switch the cell between rhythmic bursting and tonic firing. The significance of these different response modes in thalamic function is considered more fully below.

SYNAPTIC TRANSMISSION

GLUTAMATERGIC INPUTS

The retinal and cortical inputs to thalamus are both glutamatergic (see above).

Retinogeniculate (and Other Driving) Inputs. Retinogeniculate axons innervating relay cells (and driving inputs innervating relay cells in other nuclei) activate *ionotropic* receptors, meaning that there is a fairly direct and simple link between the postsynaptic receptor and the gated ion channel (see Chap. 2). The ionotropic glutamate receptors involved in retinogeniculate transmission include *NMDA* (*N*-methyl-D-aspartate) and *non-NMDA* types, the latter represented by *kainate* and *AMPA* ([±]-α-amino-3-hydroxy-5-methylisoxazole-4-propionic acid) types (Kemp and Sillito, 1982; Moody and Sillito, 1988; Salt, 1988; Scharfman et al., 1990; Kwon et al., 1991; Salt and Eaton, 1996). The EPSP from NMDA activation is slower than that from AMPA/kainate activation and faster than that from metabotropic activation. Also, the NMDA receptor has the interesting property of being both voltage- and transmitter-dependent (Mayer and Westbrook, 1987). At relatively depolarized V_m levels, activation of the receptor increases the conductance of Na^+ and other cations (mostly Ca^{2+} and some K^+). However, at increasing membrane hyperpolarization, Mg^{2+} ions can clog the ion channel and reduce the conductance. The range over which membrane depolarization can increase conductance of the channel associated with the NMDA receptor seems to vary across cells, but it can extend from $-140mV$ to $-40mV$. Thus, in order for an EPSP to be generated via an NMDA receptor, two events must occur simultaneously: the presynaptic presence of a glutamate-like neurotransmitter coupled with a postsynaptic depolarization sufficient to unblock the channel. As pointed out in Chap. 1, this enables the NMDA receptor complex to act as a sort of molecular *AND* gate (Koch, 1987).

Less is known about the pharmacology of retinal or driving input onto interneurons. Studies of the LGN in vitro suggest that the retinogeniculate EPSP controlling action potentials in interneurons involves only ionotropic glutamate receptors (Pape and McCormick, 1995). However, the retinal input onto dendritic terminals of interneurons, an input that may not greatly affect action potential generation (see above), may activate a metabotropic receptor (Zhou et al., 1994; Godwin et al., 1996b).

Corticogeniculate Inputs. Corticogeniculate axons onto relay cells appear to activate the same types of ionotropic receptors as do retinogeniculate axons. However, in addition to these, the axons from cortex also activate a *metabotropic* glutamate receptor on relay cells, and such a receptor is not activated by retinogeniculate axons (McCormick and Von Krosigk, 1992). Metabotropic receptors as a class are interesting, because they act indirectly on ion channels via second-messenger pathways, and activation of these pathways can lead to other cellular responses in addition to any effects on ion channels. The metabotropic receptor activated by corticogeniculate axons produces a very slow and long-lasting EPSP due to reduction of a K^+ "leak" current (McCormick and Von Krosigk, 1992). This longer time course of the metabotropic compared with ionotropic response is ideal for switching relay cells from burst to tonic response mode, and observations from both in vitro and in vivo indicate that such switching does readily occur as a result of activation of the metabotropic glutamate receptors (Godwin et al., 1996a).

Cortical axons appear not to activate metabotropic glutamate receptors on interneurons (Pape and McCormick, 1995), but virtually nothing is known of the nature of glutamate receptors activated by these axons on TRN cells.

GABAERGIC INPUTS

Thalamic relay cells receive an inhibitory, GABAergic input from TRN cells and interneurons. The postsynaptic response to these inputs involve both $GABA_A$ and $GABA_B$ receptors (see Chap. 2). The former is ionotropic, and the latter, metabotropic. Activation of the $GABA_A$ receptor increases a Cl^- conductance, whereas activation of the $GABA_B$ receptor increases a K^+ conductance. Since the reversal potential for K^+ is much more negative (at roughly -100 mV) than that for Cl^+ (at roughly -70 mV), $GABA_B$ activation results in more hyperpolarization than does $GABA_A$ activation. However, the neuronal conductance increase and thus the decrease in neuronal input resistance is much greater with $GABA_A$ than with $GABA_B$. As a result, $GABA_A$ inhibits more by clamping the membrane at a subthreshold level and thus *shunting* EPSPs, while $GABA_B$ inhibits more by hyperpolarizing the membrane. The $GABA_A$ response is thus much more nonlinear, acting more like a voltage multiplication, while the $GABA_B$ response is more linear, acting like simple voltage subtraction (see Chap. 1). Also, the $GABA_A$ response is faster than is the $GABA_B$ response.

BRAINSTEM INPUTS

Parabrachial Inputs. In cats, most of the input to the lateral geniculate nucleus from the brainstem derives from the parabrachial region (de Lima et al., 1985; de Lima and Singer, 1987; Fitzpatrick et al., 1988; Smith et al., 1988; Raczkowski and Fitzpatrick, 1989; Fitzpatrick et al., 1989, Bickford et al., 1993). Activation of this input in relay cells produces an excitatory postsynaptic potential due primarily to activation of two different receptors (McCormick and Prince, 1987a; McCormick, 1989a, 1992). The first is an ionotropic nicotinic receptor that produces a fast excitatory postsynaptic potential by permitting influx of cations. The second is a metabotropic muscarinic receptor, an M1 type, that triggers a second-messenger pathway ultimately leading to a reduction in a K^+ conductance. This muscarinic response is a very slow, long-lasting excitatory postsynaptic potential. It seems remarkably similar to the metabotropic glutamate response seen from activation of corticogeniculate input (see above), and the possibility exists that both metabotropic receptors may be linked to the same second-messenger pathway and K^+ channels. As is the case for cortical input, both in vitro and in vivo studies suggest that activating this cholinergic input switches the response mode of thalamic relay cells from burst to tonic (McCormick and Prince, 1987a; McCormick, 1989a, 1992; Lu et al., 1993).

Activation of the cholinergic inputs from the parabrachial region generally inhibits interneurons and reticular cells (Dingledine and Kelly, 1977; Ahlsén et al., 1984; McCormick and Prince, 1987a; McCormick and Pape, 1988). This is interesting, because individual parabrachial axons branch to innervate these cells as well as relay cells and, as noted above, these axons excite relay cells. This is accomplished by yet another type of muscarinic receptor, a type other than M1, that dominates on these GABAergic targets (McCormick and Prince, 1987a; Hu et al., 1989a,b; McCormick, 1989a, 1992). Activation of this receptor increases a K^+ conductance, leading to hyperpolarization. However, cells of the thalamic reticular nucleus also respond to this cholinergic input with another, nicotinic receptor that leads to fast depolarization (Lee and McCormick, 1995). Nonetheless, the main effect of cholinergic stimulation of these cells seems dominated by the muscarinic, inhibitory response (Dingledine and Kelly, 1977; McCormick and Prince, 1987a; McCormick and Pape, 1988; Hu et al., 1989a,b; McCormick, 1989a, 1992). Since these interneurons and reticular cells inhibit relay cells, activation of this cholinergic pathway thus disinhibits relay cells (see Fig. 8.9).

In addition to ACh, these axons appear to colocalize *nitric oxide* (NO; Erişir et al., 1997a; Bickford et al., 1993), a neurotransmitter or neuromodulator with a widespread distribution in the brain (Schuman and Madison, 1991, 1994; Bredt and Snyder, 1992; Snyder, 1992). Relatively little is known concerning the action of NO in the thalamus, but recent studies suggest that its release from parabrachial terminals serves two possible roles in the lateral geniculate nucleus: to switch response mode from burst to tonic (Pape and Mager, 1992), perhaps complementing the role of acetylcholine (ACh) in this regard; and to promote the generation of NMDA responses from retinal inputs (Cudeiro et al., 1994a,b, 1996). A recent study suggests that NO may also serve to enhance NMDA receptor activation in TRN cells, although the source of inputs to activate these receptors has not been identified (Rivadulla et al., 1996). Nothing is as yet known about the action of NO on interneurons.

Other Brainstem Inputs. Other less well understood brainstem inputs to thalamus include noradrenergic axons from cells in the parabrachial region, serotonergic axons from cells in the dorsal raphé nucleus, and histaminergic axons from cells in the tuberomammillary nucleus of the hypothalamus; other inputs unique to specific thalamic nuclei may also occur, such as the GABAergic input to the LGN from cells from the pretectum (see above for details).

Noradrenalin seems to increase excitability of relay cells in the lateral geniculate nucleus. Like ACh, noradrenalin promotes tonic firing (McCormick, 1989a, 1992; Pape and McCormick, 1989; Funke et al., 1993). This neurotransmitter depolarizes TRN cells by reducing a K^+ conductance (McCormick and Wang, 1991), but has no clear effect on interneurons (Pape and McCormick, 1995). Effects of serotonin are complex. Ionophoresis onto relay cells in vivo generally inhibits them, but in vitro studies suggest that this is the consequence of direct excitation that is stronger for local GABAergic cells than for relay cells (McCormick, 1989a, 1992). Serotonin depolarizes TRN cells by blocking a K^+ conductance (McCormick and Wang, 1991), and it produces a slight depolarization of some interneurons, not clearly affecting others (Pape and McCormick, 1995). Finally, histamine application to relay cells generally excites them (McCormick, 1992). Histamine also depolarizes interneurons, but apparently through unknown presynaptic mechanisms and not through any direct effect on these cells (Pape and McCormick, 1995). It should be noted that these observations of effects on interneurons represent recording from the cell body and axon and thus may be limited to axonal output without reflecting effects on dendritic output (see above).

GATING AND OTHER TRANSFORMATIONS IN THE THALAMIC RELAY

The rich array of membrane properties of thalamic relay cells plus their complex ensemble of inputs from various sources suggest that the relay of peripheral information to cortex is not a simple, trivial affair. Instead, it is a complex process that we are just beginning to understand. This is a marked change from earlier views of, for instance, the LGN, which was thought to provide a simple, machine-like relay of retinal information to cortex with minor processing added. This will be considered in more depth here, both in terms of the different burst and tonic response modes introduced above and the role they play in the thalamic relay, and in terms of what we are just beginning to learn about the role of cortical and brainstem inputs in this relay.

BURST AND TONIC RELAY RESPONSE MODES

Signal Transmission During Burst and Tonic Firing. Burst and tonic modes clearly represent two very different types of response to afferent input and thus two very different forms of thalamic relay. In fact, earlier studies suggested that tonic firing represented the only true relay mode and that burst firing, when it occurred, was always characterized by *rhythmic* bursting that was synchronized across large regions of thalamus. This functionally disconnected the relay cell from its primary afferent input, thereby interrupting the relay (McCarley et al., 1983; Steriade and Llinás, 1988; McCormick and Feeser, 1990; Steriade and McCarley, 1990; Steriade et al., 1990a,b, 1993; McCormick and Bal, 1994; Steriade and Contreras, 1995). The idea was that switching between these modes was accomplished by inputs that changed V_m. Rhythmic bursting was often seen in vitro, and the first in vivo studies of the response modes in cats demonstrated that, when the animal entered quiet or non-REM sleep, thalamic relay cells began to burst rhythmically, and that such rhythmic bursting was not seen during awake, alert states (Livingstone and Hubel, 1981; McCarley et al., 1983; Steriade and Llinás, 1988; Steriade et al., 1990a,b, 1993; Steriade and McCarley, 1990; Steriade and Contreras, 1995).

However, more recent data in anesthetized and awake, behaving cats makes clear that cells can burst arrhythmically and asynchronously, and they can still respond well to visual stimulation (Lo et al., 1991; Guido et al., 1992, 1995; Guido and Weyand, 1995; Mukherjee and Kaplan, 1995; Sherman, 1995; Godwin et al., 1996a). That is, during spontaneous activity, the cells may often discharge a low-threshold spike with a burst response, but these burst discharges occur irregularly. When the cell is then stimulated visually, the cell may produce a burst in response to each presentation of the stimulus, and the bursting under these conditions clearly reflects the external stimulus rather than any intrinsic pacemaker (Guido et al., 1992, 1995; Guido and Weyand, 1995; Mukherjee and Kaplan, 1995; Sherman, 1995; Godwin et al., 1996a). There thus seem to be three different response modes: rhythmic bursting, arrhythmic bursting, and tonic firing. The first occurs during quiet or non-REM sleep, perhaps during drowsiness, and might also occur during epileptic episodes (McCarley et al., 1983; Steriade and Llinás, 1988; McCormick and Feeser, 1990; Steriade et al., 1990a,b, 1993; Steriade and McCarley, 1990; McCormick and Bal, 1994; Steriade and Contreras, 1995); this seems to be associated with an interruption of the relay through thalamus. The last two occur during active vision, meaning that both burst and tonic modes can be effective relay modes.

What, then, are the differences in the relay between burst and tonic firing modes? Figure 8.13 shows a representative example of an LGN relay cell in a lightly anesthetized cat responding to a visual stimulus, which is a sinusoidal luminance grating drifting through its receptive field. The same cell responds in tonic mode when depolarized (Fig. 8.13A) and in burst mode when hyperpolarized (Fig. 8.13B); both spontaneous activity (upper histograms) and visually evoked responses (lower histograms) are shown. Two main differences are evident. First, note that the response to the sinusoidal visual stimulus appears to be much more sinusoidal during tonic firing than during burst firing. This is because tonic mode displays greater linear summation than does burst mode (Guido et al., 1992, 1995; Mukherjee and Kaplan, 1995; Sherman, 1995). This is probably due to the nonlinear amplification of the low-threshold spike, which provides a similar response regardless of the amplitude or duration of any suprathreshold stimulus (see above). The signal relayed to cortex is thus less distorted when the relay is in tonic mode, and this mode would thus be superior for accurate analysis by cortex of sensory stimuli. Second, note that while the visual response during both modes is robust, the spontaneous activity is much higher during tonic firing. The latter is actually an important feature of the linear summation during tonic firing,

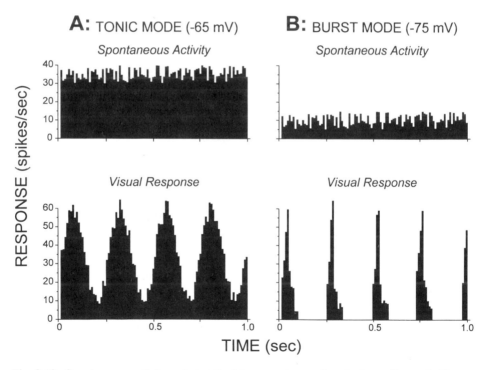

Fig. 8.13. Spontaneous activity and visually driven responses of geniculate cell recorded in a cat in vivo during tonic and burst modes. The cell was recorded intracellularly, and current injection was used to adjust mean membrane voltage to either −65 mV, which was sufficiently depolarized to inactivate I_T and promote tonic responses, or −75 mV, which was sufficiently hyperpolarized to de-inactivate I_T, allowing it to be activated and promote burst responses. The upper row of histograms shows spontaneous activity, and the lower row shows responses to four cycles of a sinusoidal grating drifted through the receptive field. A: Tonic mode. B: Burst mode.

because the higher background discharge minimizes nonlinearities due to half-wave rectification. Furthermore, burst firing provides a much higher signal (visual response)-to-noise (spontaneous activity) ratio than does tonic firing, implying that burst mode may be superior for detecting the presence of a stimulus (Guido et al., 1995). In fact, relay cells in burst mode are able to detect stimuli far better than when these same cells are in tonic mode (Guido et al., 1995; Sherman, 1995).

Perhaps burst mode is used during visual search or maybe during periods when attention is directed elsewhere (e.g., to another sensory modality or to another part of visual space) as a sort of "wake-up" call for novel and potentially interesting or dangerous stimuli. This idea is in some ways similar to the "searchlight" hypothesis for burst firing (Crick, 1984). However, while burst firing may be ideal for signal detection, the nonlinear distortion during this relay mode means that the stimulus will not be accurately analyzed. Tonic mode, with its more linear relay, would permit more faithful signal analysis.

Control of Response Mode. From the preceding discussion, one can imagine that relay cells can be switched via nonretinal inputs between modes. This may occur in a state-dependent fashion based on the requirements of the visual system regarding signal detection or analysis. For this to work, there must be a ready means for nonretinal inputs to control these response modes. This may be accomplished chiefly through effects on the membrane potential of relay cells, since the low-threshold Ca^{2+} conductance underlying the burst mode is voltage-dependent. Both parabrachial and cortical inputs appear to be able to do this.

Electrical activation of the parabrachial region in vivo causes dramatic switching of geniculate relay cells from burst to tonic mode (Lu et al. 1993). Likewise, in vitro application of ACh, the chief transmitter used by parabrachial inputs to the lateral geniculate nucleus, eliminates low-threshold spiking, causing bursting cells to fire in tonic mode (McCormick, 1989a, 1992). NO, which is colocalized with ACh in the parabrachial terminals may also promote tonic firing (Pape and Mager, 1992). The role of corticogeniculate input in control of response mode has been more difficult to assess in vivo, because electrical activation of this pathway also usually activates geniculocortical axons antidromically, obscuring the interpretation of any effects. Also, as can be appreciated from Fig. 8.3, any global activation or inactivation of cortex will both excite relay cells directly and inhibit them indirectly (via interneuron and TRN activation), and thus these cruder attempts to modulate corticothalamic inputs may produce weak or inconsistent results. However, because corticogeniculate but not retinogeniculate inputs use a metabotropic glutamate receptor (see above), it is possible to mimic activation of the corticogeniculate input onto relay cells fairly specifically by applying agonists for this receptor to geniculate relay cells. When this is done in vivo, geniculate cells switch firing mode from burst to tonic (Godwin et al. 1996a). Also, in vitro application of agonists to this metabotropic receptor switches firing from burst mode to tonic mode (McCormick and Von Krosigk, 1992).

OTHER EFFECTS OF NONRETINAL OR MODULATORY INPUTS ON THE THALAMIC RELAY

Although we have focused so far on the role of brainstem and cortical afferents to thalamus in terms of their ability to affect response mode, other roles may be played by these and other inputs regarding thalamic relay properties.

TRN Inputs. Although thalamic neurons may switch between relay and burst modes at any time during awake, alert behavioral states, the burst mode dominates during less alert periods, including drowsiness and quiet or non-REM sleep (McCarley et al., 1983; Steriade and Llinás, 1988; Steriade et al., 1990a,b, 1993; Steriade and McCarley, 1990; Steriade and Contreras, 1995). During such inattentive periods, the EEG in all mammals, including humans, becomes highly synchronized, and fast, rhythmic spike-like electrical phenomena known as *spindles* can be seen (see Fig. 8.14). These spindles have a frequency of 7–14 Hz.

This dominant feature of the synchronized EEG is generated in the thalamus (Steriade and Llinás, 1988). Studies of thalamic neurons have shown that all TRN cells can spontaneously generate rhythmic discharges at a rate of approximately 10 Hz. The

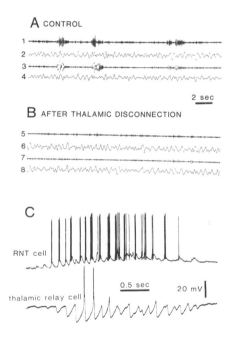

Fig. 8.14. Relationship of thalamus to spindle activity in the cortical electroencephalogram (EEG) of cats. **A,B:** Effect on the EEG of rostral thalamic transections that disconnect the thalamus from the cortex. The numbering of traces is as follows: 1 and 5, higher-frequency EEG (7–14 Hz) for right hemisphere; 2 and 6, lower-frequency EEG (0.5–4 Hz) for right hemisphere; 3 and 7, higher-frequency EEG (7–14 Hz) for left hemisphere; 4 and 8, lower-frequency EEG (0.5–4 Hz) for left hemisphere. Normally (**A,** before transection), each hemisphere shows activity in both the higher (7–14 Hz) and lower (0.5–4 Hz) filtered traces. After transection (**B),** the higher frequencies are selectively eliminated from the EEG. **C:** Activity of thalamic neurons during an EEG spindle. During the spindle, the TRN neuron (top) undergoes a long-lasting, slow depolarization that elevates its firing rate. In contrast, a thalamic relay cell (bottom) is hyperpolarized rhythmically, and the rebound from these hyperpolarizations often leads to low-threshold Ca^{2+} spikes. The elevated firing in the TRN cell seems to cause the rhythmic hyperpolarizations in the relay cell. [A,B revised from Steriade et al. 1987; C revised from Steriade and Llinás, 1988, with permission.]

low-threshold spike appears to be a key feature of this endogenous bursting behavior, and the oscillations can be generated within individual TRN cells. Also, groups of deafferented TRN neurons can generate such synchronized oscillatory activity in the absence of external input (Steriade et al., 1987; Steriade and Llinás, 1988). TRN neurons are extensively connected to other TRN cells via collaterals of the axon that innervates dorsal thalamus, and these connections could serve to synchronize entire TRN regions; dendrodendritic synapses may also exist among TRN neurons to further synchronize these cells.

Since TRN neurons provide an inhibitory, GABAergic input to thalamic relay cells, the TRN entrains its oscillatory activity onto these relay cells. That is, the synchronized bursts of TRN activity would lead to waves of hyperpolarization among relay cells; this would de-inactivate low threshold spikes in the relay cells, and they would synchronously enter the burst mode. By themselves, neurons in the LGN or VPL do not spontaneously generate spindle rhythmicity, since disconnecting the projection cells from the TRN via surgical or chemical means abolishes the oscillations (Steriade et al., 1987; Steriade and Llinás, 1988). Thus this feature of synchronized, rhythmic bursting among relay cells, which is associated with inattentive and unconscious states and interruption of the thalamic relay, depends critically on the TRN.

Brainstem Inputs. Non-REM sleep and spindle activity is associated with quiescence among many of the cholinergic inputs to the thalamus from the parabrachial region (Steriade and Contreras, 1995). It thus seems plausible that increasing activity among these inputs will serve to terminate the synchronized, rhythmic activity and restore relay cell responses to tonic or arrhythmic burst firing. This has yet to be demonstrated empirically, but it is consistent with other evidence presented above. While the effects of the various brainstem inputs is complex, many strongly inhibit TRN cells, and such inhibition may well serve to break up the functional network that synchronizes these cells. In any case, there is ample evidence that activity in brainstem afferents is associated with more alert behavioral states.

There is also evidence that eye movements can affect the geniculate relay (Büttner and Fuchs, 1973; Noda, 1975; Bartlett et al., 1976; Lal and Friedlander, 1989; Guido and Weyand, 1995). Both saccades and passive movement of the eye can have such effects. While the details for this have yet to be worked out, it seems likely that these effects are accomplished via brainstem afferents to thalamus.

Cortical Inputs. As noted above, the corticogeniculate input is both massive and heterogeneous. It is thus plausible that it subserves several distinct functions. Perhaps this is why earlier attempts to identify any *single* function for this "feedback" pathway have led to confusing and conflicting conclusions. For instance, some studies suggest that the corticogeniculate pathway facilitates relay cell firing, whereas other suggest the opposite (Kalil and Chase, 1970; Baker and Malpeli, 1977; Schmielau and Singer, 1977; Geisert et al., 1981; McClurkin and Marrocco, 1984; McClurkin et al., 1994). The large number of layer 6 inputs suggests that this feedback could be highly specific to receptive field location, orientation, direction of motion, and ocularity. Mumford (1994) has developed a detailed framework, based on ideas from machine vision, in which the detection of weak or incomplete stimuli under noisy conditions (think of a gray mouse at dusk) would be enhanced via such feedback. In this context, it should be pointed out that the vast majority of experiments carried out in the LGN have involved anesthetized animals stimulated with single bars or gratings on a blank background, not a situation that might be expected to activate the type of feedback function suggested by Mumford (1994). Schmielau and Singer (1977) have proposed that corticogeniculate input is important to binocular functions, such as stereopsis. Several studies have identified a role for the corticogeniculate input in controlling inhibitory surrounds of geniculate relay cells (Sillito et al., 1993; Cudeiro and Sillito, 1996). More recent studies have suggested that the pathway affects temporal properties of relay cell discharges (McClurkin et al., 1994) or establishes correlated firing among nearby relay cells with similar receptive field properties (Sillito et al., 1994). Above we suggest that this input serves to control response mode, tonic or burst, of the relay cells. Given the likelihood that the corticogeniculate pathway is heterogeneous, these different suggestions for its function are not incompatible, and more functions may yet emerge.

FIRST- AND HIGHER-ORDER THALAMIC RELAYS

Every thalamic nucleus appears to receive afferents from layer 6 of the relevant cortical region or regions, such as visual cortex for LGN (Jones and Powell, 1968; Rinvik, 1972; Kunzle, 1976; Updyke, 1977; Berson and Graybiel, 1983). These layer 6 corticothalamic terminals have RSD morphology, are located on distal dendrites, and are rarely if every found in glomeruli (Jones and Powell, 1969a,b; Morest, 1975; Majorossy and Kiss, 1976a,b; Somogyi et al., 1978; Liu et al., 1995).

However, some thalamic nuclei also receive an input emanating from pyramidal cells of layer 5 (Mathers, 1972; Robson and Hall, 1977; Ogren and Hendrickson, 1979; Hoogland et al., 1991; Schwartz et al., 1991; Bourassa et al., 1995; Guillery, 1995; Sherman and Guillery, 1996). Examples of nuclei receiving layer 5 input are pulvinar, the mediodorsal nucleus, and the dorsal division of the medial geniculate nucleus, but a complete survey of nuclei receiving such input remains to be done. Interestingly, the pattern of innervation of these layer 5 inputs is more like that of primary afferents. That is, the innervation pattern of these layer 5 axons is more like that of retinal axons in the LGN than of layer 6 axons there. These layer 5 axons are relatively coarse and terminate in richly branched arbors, like retinal axons. This is unlike the finer layer 6 axons that terminate more simply. Like retinal axons, these layer 5 axons branch to innervate other brainstem targets, whereas the layer 6 axons terminate exclusively in thalamus. These layer 5 axons also end with large terminals, much like RLP terminals in the LGN, that contact proximal dendrites, often in triadic arrangements in glomeruli, whereas the layer 6 axons end with RSD terminals distally outside of glomeruli and without triadic arrangements. Finally, although both layer 5 and 6 axons pass through TRN en route to their dorsal thalamic target, the layer 5 axons do not seem to innervate TRN with a collateral, whereas layer 6 ones do. This, too, is like the primary input, since, for example, driving or retinal inputs do not innervate TRN.

These morphological observations suggest that corticothalamic axons from layer 5 may act as primary afferents for some of the thalamic nuclei that have few if any other primary afferent axons. It is noteworthy in this context that these thalamic nuclei known to receive a layer 5 input lack a clearly defined or major subcortical input that could be regarded as primary. A consideration of the effects that cortical lesions or inactivation have upon the receptive fields of cells in the thalamic nuclei we are considering provides indirect evidence in support of this view that the primary input for these thalamic nuclei derives from layer 5 of cortex. For a nucleus innervated by primary subcortical afferents, such as LGN or VPL, cortical inactivation has relatively little effect on the receptive fields of the thalamic cells (Kalil and Chase, 1970; Baker and Malpeli, 1977; Schmielau and Singer, 1977; Geisert et al., 1981; McClurkin and Marrocco, 1984; Yuan et al., 1986; Diamond et al., 1992; McClurkin et al., 1994). In stark contrast to this, receptive field properties of cells in nuclei that receive layer 5 afferents from cortex are greatly affected after cortical inactivation (Bender, 1983; Diamond et al., 1992).

The layer 5 innervation pattern suggests that certain thalamic nuclei receive their primary afferents from the cortex rather than subcortically and they relay this afferent cortical activity to other cortical areas. This provides the thalamus with a much more extensive role in corticocortical communication than previously considered (Kaas, 1978; Van Essen and Maunsell, 1983; Van Essen, 1985; Zeki and Shipp, 1988; Van Essen et al., 1990; Felleman and Van Essen, 1991; Knierim and Van Essen, 1992; Young, 1992; Nakamura et al., 1993; Preuss et al., 1993; DeYoe et al., 1994; Salin and Bullier, 1995). There are thus at least two functionally distinct corticothalamic systems. One derives from layer 6 and serves to modulate the relay properties of its thalamic target. The other derives from layer 5 and represents the primary information to be relayed by its target thalamic cells. Note that these latter thalamic relay cells are also under the modulatory influence of layer 6 input, which is ubiquitous for all thalamic nuclei.

By the same sort of logic, we can now recognize two types of thalamic nucleus one receiving its primary afferents from subcortical sources and the other, from cortical sources. The former have been called *first-order* relay nuclei, and the second, *higher-order* relay nuclei because they receive their primary inputs from cortex that has already received and acted on information from its first-order thalamic relays (Guillery, 1995; Sherman and Guillery, 1996). This organization is summarized schematically in Fig. 8.15.

The first-order relay may be viewed as the initial transfer of peripheral information to cortex for further processing, and the higher-order relay may be viewed as the relay of information already processed somewhat by cortex. It is interesting in this context to reconsider the olfactory pathway, which has always stood out among sensory pathways as not having a primary thalamocortical component. In a sense, we can view the projection from the olfactory bulb to olfactory paleocortex as analogous to a first-order relay without a thalamic component, perhaps because it evolved before thalamus and neocortex. Then the projection from olfactory paleocortex through the mediodorsal thalamic nucleus to insular and orbital neocortex looks very much like a higher-order relay. Such a consideration of the olfactory pathway may provide some insights into evolution of thalamus and neocortex.

While we know very little about detailed properties of these higher-order thalamic nuclei, it seems parsimonious to suggest for now that they are similar to those we have described above, including the same sorts of cellular properties (including burst and

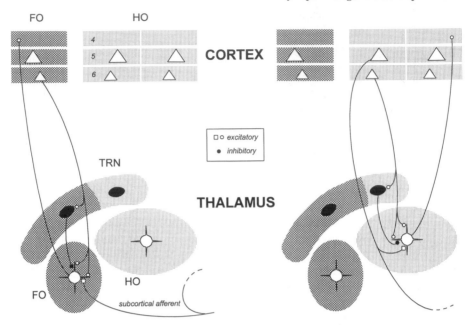

Fig. 8.15. Schematic representation of first-order (FO) and higher-order (HO) thalamic relays. Both types of relay receive a modulatory cortical input from layer 6 (only cortical layers 4, 5, and 6 are shown) that contacts distal dendrites of the relay cells with small terminals. These cortical axons also branch to innervate TRN. The first-order relay (left) receives its primary input from a subcortical afferent that contacts proximal dendrites with large terminals, often in glomeruli (not shown). This information is relayed to layer 4 of cortex. Note that the subcortical input branches to innervate other subcortical structures, but does not innervate TRN. The higher-order relay (right) receives its primary input from layer 5 of cortex, and this contacts proximal dendrites with large terminals, often in glomeruli (not shown). This information is relayed mainly to another area of cortex, terminating chiefly in layer 4. Note that the layer 5 input branches to innervate other subcortical structures, but does not innervate TRN. Thus in many ways the layer 5 input is like the subcortical input of a first order relay, but unlike the modulatory input from layer 6 of cortex. See text for details.

tonic firing), intrinsic circuits, and cortical and brainstem inputs. That is, both first- and higher-order thalamic relay nuclei have a "dominant" or "driving" input, which, for instance, derives from retina for the lateral geniculate nucleus and from cortical layer 5 for higher-order relays. This driving input is always modulated by a massive layer 6 cortical input as well as by various brainstem inputs.

An important implication of this view of thalamocortical interactions is that it permits a much richer avenue of communication among cortical areas. These areas can communicate through the thalamus, with some thalamocortical inputs relaying to their target cortical areas the output, via layer 5, of another cortical area. Furthermore, other cortical areas, via their layer 6 outputs, can modify this thalamic route of corticocortical communication.

FUNCTIONAL SIGNIFICANCE OF THALAMIC CIRCUITS

Noted above is the observation that each geniculate cell receives the vast majority of its retinal input from one or very few retinal ganglion cells of the same type (left or right retina, on or off center, X and Y). Thus the spatial receptive field of each geniculate cell is nearly identical to that of its retinal input: geniculate cells display circular receptive fields organized into concentrically arranged, antagonist centers and surrounds. Subtle differences have been described between receptive fields of geniculate cells and those of their retinal inputs, and these mostly involve greater inhibition seen postsynaptically (reviewed in Sherman and Spear, 1982; Shapley and Lennie, 1985; Sherman, 1985). Preliminary data suggest a similar resemblance in spatial receptive field properties between MGN or VPL cells and their driving inputs. For the purposes of the present discussion, we conclude that significant receptive field transformation occurs rarely if at all at the level of thalamus.

This absence of a major receptive field transformation across the retinogeniculate synapse stands in stark contrast to the obvious transformations seen when progressing through the synaptic zones of retina or cortex or across the geniculocortical synapse. Comparable transformations exist as well in other parts of the visual system, such as the superior colliculus and extrastriate visual cortex. Similar transformations also exist outside the thalamus in other sensory systems, such as the spinal cord and cortex for the somatosensory system, and the inferior colliculus and cortex for the auditory system. These other, extrathalamic transformations represent obvious, functional roles for these other regions of sensory systems: synaptic zones there clearly form more complex receptive field properties as the hierarchy is ascended, and this provides a basis for these sensory systems to extract information about stimuli in the world outside.

It is this absence of any clear spatial change in receptive fields across the retinogeniculate synapse (or across the synapse from driving inputs elsewhere) that has prompted many investigators to think of specific sensory thalamic nuclei as merely passive relay stations for signals from the periphery to cortex. However, such a trivial function belies morphological data presented above for the LGN that only a minority of the synapses present in the neuropil and onto relay cells is retinal in origin. This minority of synaptic terminals is only 10–20% by most accounts (Guillery, 1969a,b; Sherman and Koch, 1986; Sherman and Guillery, 1996), although newer data suggest that the value may be much less (Van Horn et al., 1997). The function of the vast majority of synaptic input seems invisible to conventional receptive field approaches. In fact, evidence accumulated over the past decade strongly suggests that this nonretinal input serves to gate retinogeniculate transmission or transform it in ways, such as the control of burst or tonic response modes, that will serve different behavioral needs of sensory processing.

This provides a unique role for the thalamus: it is not merely a passive relay nor is it primarily involved in receptive field elaboration; instead, it actively filters the flow of information to cortex, and the nature of the filtering is dependent on the animal's state of consciousness and alertness. This active filtering has not been revealed by the usual receptive field studies, but recording in unanesthetized animals has revealed considerable state-dependent variation in responsiveness of geniculate neurons. We are now beginning to gain insights into how certain nonretinal or modulatory inputs to thalamus, such as from cortex or brainstem, control this filtering process. While it seems clear what general role the LGN and other thalamic nuclei play, it is neither clear how many different types of filtering exist for retinal and other driving inputs nor precisely how these filtering functions are achieved. Finally, there is new evidence that the relay function served by thalamus is not limited to transferring peripheral information (e.g., from retinal or spinal cord) to cortex, but that certain thalamic nuclei serve chiefly to relay information from cortex to cortex, and this role of thalamus may prove crucial to cortico-cortical interactions.

9

BASAL GANGLIA

CHARLES J. WILSON

The basal ganglia are a richly interconnected set of brain nuclei found in the forebrain and midbrain of mammals, birds, and reptiles. In many species, including most mammals, the forebrain nuclei of the basal ganglia are the most prominent subcortical telencephalic structures. The large size of these nuclei, and their similarity in structure in such a wide range of species, make it likely that they contribute some very essential function to the basic organizational plan of the brain of the terrestrial vertebrates. However, the assignment of a specific functional role for the basal ganglia has been difficult, as it has been for other brain structures that have no direct connections with either the sensory or motor organs.

The most widely accepted views of basal ganglia function are based on observations of humans afflicted with degenerative diseases that attack these structures. In all cases these diseases produce severe deficits of movement. None of the movement deficits is simple, however, or easily described. In some, such as Parkinson's disease, movements are more difficult to make, as if the body were somehow made rigid and resistive to changes in position. In others, such as Huntington's disease, useless and unintended movements interfere with the execution of useful and intended ones. In general, these symptoms affect only voluntary, purposive movements, with reflexive movements being relatively unaffected. These clinical observations have led most investigators to view the basal ganglia as components of a widespread system that is somehow involved in the generation of goal-directed voluntary movement, but in complex and subtle aspects of that process.

The anatomical connections of the basal ganglia link it to elements of the sensory, motor, cognitive, and motivational apparatus of the brain. These connections are best appreciated within the context of the arrangement of the several nuclei that make up the basal ganglia. A diagram showing the arrangement of the most prominent of these nuclei as they appear in a frontal section of the human brain is shown in Fig. 9.1. The major structures are the caudate nucleus, putamen, globus pallidus, substantia nigra, and subthalamic nucleus. Also seen in the diagram are the two largest sources of input to the basal ganglia, the cerebral cortex and the thalamus.

Several of the major connections between these structures are shown in Fig. 9.1. In dealing with this complexity, it is helpful to focus on the overall direction of information flow. Most of the input to the basal ganglia from other brain structures arrives

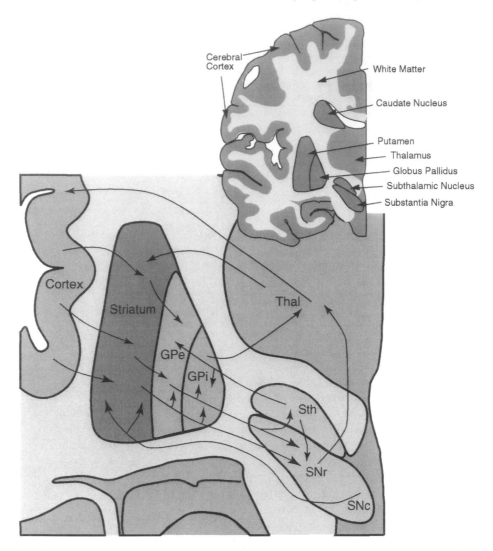

Fig. 9.1. Schematic representation of a transverse section through a human brain hemisphere showing the sizes and locations of several important components of the basal ganglia and connections among them. GPe, globus pallidus, external segment; GPi, globus pallidus, internal segment; Thal, thalamus; Sth, subthalamic nucleus; SNr, substantia nigra, pars reticulata; SNc, substantia nigra, pars compacta.

in the *neostriatum*, which consists of the caudate nucleus, putamen, and nucleus accumbens. Within the caudate nucleus and the putamen, inputs from sensory, motor, and association *cortical* areas converge with inputs from the *thalamic* intralaminar nuclei, dopaminergic inputs from the *substantia nigra pars compacta* (SNc), and serotoninergic inputs from the *dorsal raphé* nucleus (not shown). Not shown are analogous connections arising from the limbic cortex and hippocampus and formed in a third structure, the nucleus accumbens. These three input structures of the basal ganglia (caudate nucleus, putamen, and nucleus accumbens) are very similar in their internal structure. In the connectional diagram in Fig. 9.1, the putamen has been used to represent the entire neostriatum.

The output from the neostriatum projects almost exclusively to other basal ganglia structures. The main targets of these axons are three nuclei, the *external segment* of the *globus pallidus* (GPe), the *internal segment* of the *globus pallidus* (GPi), and the *pars reticulata* of the *substantia nigra* (SNr). These three structures are very similar in their cellular organization. Two of them, the internal segment of the globus pallidus and the substantia nigra pars reticulata, project to structures outside the basal ganglia and provide the main output pathways for the results of neuronal operations performed within the nuclei. Their targets are primarily in the *thalamus* (mostly in the ventral tier thalamic nuclei which project to frontal cortex), *lateral habenular nucleus*, and in the deep layers of the *superior colliculus*. For simplicity, only the thalamic projections are shown in Fig. 9.1. The external segment of the globus pallidus projects mainly to the *subthalamic nucleus*, a small but important component of the basal ganglia that, like the neostriatum, receives input from the cortex and projects to the globus pallidus and substantia nigra.

Several overall features of these connections should be recognized. First, whereas inputs from outside the basal ganglia can enter the system at several points, including the subthalamic nucleus, substantia nigra, and globus pallidus, by far the most inputs enter at the level of the neostriatum. The neostriatum has reciprocal projections with the substantia nigra, but not with its other major sources of afferents. That is, there are no direct projections of the neostriatum back to the cortex or the thalamus. Second, the projections of the neostriatum form two major pathways through the basal ganglia. One of these, called the *direct pathway*, is formed by neurons that have direct projections to the internal segment of the globus pallidus or to substantia nigra, and so gain immediate access to the output of the basal ganglia. The other neostriatal efferent pathway, called the *indirect pathway*, is formed by neurons projecting no farther than the external segment of the globus pallidus. These neurons can affect the basal ganglia output by way of the subthalamic nucleus and its projections to the internal segment of the globus pallidus and the substantia nigra, or by the projections of the GPe to the output neurons. Of course, there is a variety of even more indirect pathways and loops, but this distinction between the direct and indirect pathway is important because it emphasizes the dual nature of the neostriatal output. Finally, the neostriatum is the natural focus of our attention in the basal ganglia because it is the largest of the basal ganglia structures, the recipient of most of its afferent input, and the origin of the two major pathways through the basal ganglia. Thus, it has been the object of most basal ganglia research, and its organization will be the main topic of this chapter.

NEURONAL ELEMENTS

The neostriatum consists mainly of the principal neurons and the afferent fibers. Despite the numerical preponderance of principal neurons, however, the interneurons of the neostriatum are rich in variety and complexity. The major neuronal elements are shown in simplified form in Fig. 9.2, in the standard scale to facilitate comparison with

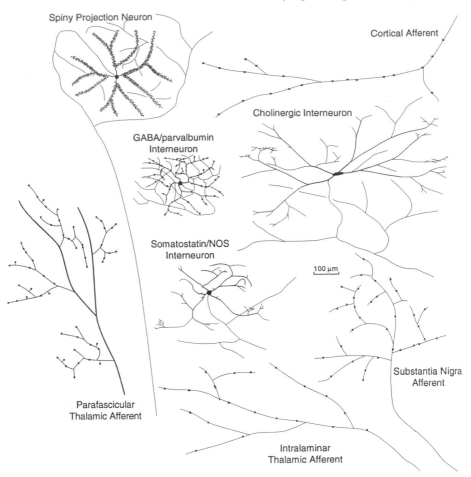

Fig. 9.2. The afferent fibers and neuron types of the neostriatum, shown at the standard scale.

other brain regions. Camera lucida drawings of some of the elements are shown in Fig. 9.3 at expanded magnification, to show their structure in greater detail.

INPUTS

As already indicated, input fibers to the neostriatum arise primarily from the cerebral cortex, the intralaminar nuclei of the thalamus, the dopaminergic neurons of the substantia nigra (pars compacta), the serotoninergic neurons of the dorsal raphé nucleus, and the basolateral nucleus of the amygdala. Less numerous inputs also arise from the external segment of the globus pallidus and from the substantia nigra, pars reticulata (see review by Graybiel and Ragsdale, 1983).

Cortical Afferents. Until recently, the arborization patterns of afferent fibers in the neostriatum were studied almost exclusively using the Golgi method. Whereas the Golgi method provides an excellent image of the stained fibers, the origin of a stained axon

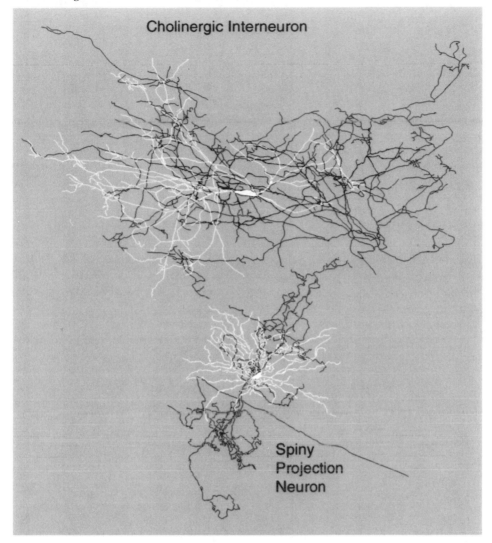

Fig. 9.3. Camera lucida drawings of a spiny projection neuron, and a cholinergic interneuron. The dendrites are shown in white and the axons in black.

is often indeterminant because it usually cannot be followed all the way back to its cell body of origin in a distant part of the brain. Investigators using the Golgi techniques to study the neostriatum were able to identify afferent fibers by tracing them to the internal capsule, but they could not be certain which fibers were from cerebral cortex, which were from substantia nigra, and so on. More recently, the morphology of identified axons has been studied using axonal staining with the lectin *Phaseolus Vulgaris* Leucoagglutinin (PHA-L) or with biotinylated dextran amine (BDA). Either marker is injected extracellularly in an afferent structure, and stains a group of neurons around the injection site. After a period of 1–2 weeks, the tracer will have moved, either by diffusion or by axonal transport, so that the axons of some of those neurons will be completely and diffusely stained over very long distances. The selectivity and intensity of staining compares favorably with the Golgi method, and these techniques have the advantage of experimental choice of the group of neurons whose axons are to be stained. Even more precise are the methods that allow single neurons to be labeled, either by intracellular injection of a marker or by injection of a marker molecule so close to a single neuron that only one cell is stained. Such methods have been used for many years to study the dendritic morphology of neurons and their local axonal arborizations, but introduction of biocytin and related molecules (Horikawa and Armstrong, 1988) has increased the sensitivity of this method to allow axons to be traced over many millimeters and has revealed axonal arborizations in dramatic detail.

Golgi studies showed that afferent fibers to the neostriatum arborize mostly in the pattern described by Cajal as *cruciform axodendritic* (Fox et al., 1971). This pattern is illustrated for cortical and some thalamic afferents in Fig. 9.2. *Cruciform axodendritic* means that the fibers take a relatively straight course through the tissue, crossing over dendrites and making synapses with them *en passant*. The implication of this kind of arborization pattern is that individual fibers cross the dendritic fields of many neurons, but do not make many synapses with any given cell. Conversely, neostriatal neurons can be expected to receive inputs from a large number of afferent fibers, but not to receive many synapses from any one of them. The reader will recognize that these are the same rules that govern the input connections in several other regions: from granule cell parallel axons to cartwheel and pyramidal cells in the dorsal cochlear nucleus (Chap. 4); from parallel fibers to Purkinje cells (Chap. 8), and from lateral olfactory tract fibers to olfactory pyramidal neurons (Chap. 10). So far, at least, there seems to be no input pathway in the neostriatum that can be compared with the climbing fibers of the cerebellar cortex. However, recent studies employing single axonal staining have shown that cortical and thalamic fibers do not all arborize in a highly extended fashion. Axons from the parafascicular nucleus of the thalamus (Deschênes et al., 1996), and a subset of corticostriatal axons (Cowan and Wilson, 1994) arborize by forming several small and separate focal arborizations. This sort of afferent arborization is represented by the parafascicular axon shown in Fig. 9.2.

Even in the focal arborizations, the density of synaptic contacts from any one axon is small compared with the overall density of synaptic inputs from the cortex or thalamus. Thus, at the level of single neurons, convergence of many different axons seems to be the dominant pattern of axonal arborization in the neostriatum. It is therefore fundamental to determine the distribution of neurons in the cortex and elsewhere that converge onto a single neostriatal neuron, and most theories of basal ganglia organization can be reduced to statements about the functional patterns formed by the convergence of afferents. So far, there is no experimental method for specifically staining all the cells that make synaptic contact on one neuron. Instead, investigators have attempted to infer features of axonal convergence, especially that of cortical fibers, from studies of the spatial patterns formed by axonal arborizations. Studies using modern axonal tracing methods have established that the projections arising from even a very small region of the cerebral cortex may extend through a large region of the neostriatum, being especially extensive in the rostrocaudal direction (e.g., Selemon and Goldman-Rakic, 1985; Flaherty and Graybiel, 1994). Although it has not yet been experimentally confirmed, most investigators presume that single cortical afferent fibers correspondingly extend over large portions of the neostriatum. If so, one might conclude that it is geometrically necessary that inputs from wide areas of the cortex would have access to a common pool of neostriatal neurons, and that no cortical area could exercise exclusive control of any neostriatal neuron. This scheme suggests a sort of combinatorial logic circuit in the neostriatum, in which a striatal neuron may only be excited if there is convergent input from the correct combination of cortical (and perhaps other) pathways.

If this is even approximately correct, it becomes very important to learn which areas of cortex send axons to each area of the neostriatum. One particularly wants to know if some cortical areas overlap greatly in their projections to the neostriatum, while fibers from other cortical areas never converge. Initial studies of the arborization patterns of selected cortical areas yielded the provocative suggestion that cortical regions interconnected by strong corticocortical connections (and therefore likely to be functionally related) project to similar, perhaps overlapping, portions in the neostriatum, whereas functionally unrelated cortical areas had nonoverlapping domains in the neostriatum (Yeterian and Van Hoesen, 1978). Subsequent, more detailed examination of the axonal projection patterns, however, revealed that the axonal arborizations possess a rich internal patterning (e.g., Flaherty and Graybiel, 1994). Within the rather large general area of neostriatum occupied by fibers from a specific cortical region there are areas of relative concentration and rarefaction of inputs. Another cortical area projecting to this same region may exhibit either a similar or a complementary pattern of fiber arborization. In some cases, it has been shown that functionally related regions (for example the motor and sensory cortical representations of a single body part) specifically converge on a particular region of the striatum (Flaherty and Graybiel, 1991). Such experiments provide a strong suggestion that disparate cortical representations of sensory stimuli and movements may converge to form a single representation in the neostriatum, although convergence at a cellular level has not yet been demonstrated.

In the study of axonal innervation patterns, it is often forgotten that the postsynaptic neurons have dendrites that can reach across the domains created by the axonal arborizations and sample from more than one of them. This introduces still more complicated possibilities for the convergence of synaptic inputs. It is typical of brain organization that some cells restrict their dendritic fields to correspond to the geometry of axonal arborizations, while others create a higher order level of organization by reaching out to receive combinations of nonoverlapping but adjacent inputs. The possible input combinations are determined by both the pattern of axonal arborizations and the patterns of dendritic branching. It is therefore important not only which axons actually overlap with others in the target zone, but also which are neighbors and which never are. Axonal domains that are not adjacent are unlikely to converge on any cells, regardless of their dendritic fields, whereas neighboring axonal arborizations are likely to converge on some cells even if they do not overlap.

In summary, the rules governing the spatial organization of cortical afferent fiber arborizations in the neostriatum are beginning to be worked out and will continue to be an important area for future anatomical study of the neostriatum. It will be necessary to interpret this organization within the context of the dendritic fields of each of the neostriatal cell types and in relation to the mosaic clusters of neostriatal cells (see below).

Other Afferents. Many of the characteristics of corticostriatal afferent fibers are also shared by thalamic, nigral, and amygdalar afferents, although they have been studied in much less detail. Like the corticostriatal axons, inputs from these structures also project to large areas within the neostriatum, and do so in the cruciform axodendritic pattern. Like the corticostriatal axons, their terminal arborizations are not of uniform density but show a clustered fine grain organization suggestive of complex patterns of convergence within larger input domains.

PRINCIPAL NEURON

Most of the neurons in the neostriatum are principal neurons. This stands in contrast to brain structures such as the retina or cerebellar cortex, where the principal neurons are few in comparison to interneurons. The neostriatal principal neurons are called *spiny neurons* because of the large numbers of dendritic spines that cover their dendrites (e.g., DiFiglia et al., 1976; Wilson and Groves, 1980). As shown in Figs. 9.3 and 9.4, the cell bodies of these cells range from 12–20 μm in diameter, and they give rise to a small number of dendritic trunks with diameters of 2–3 μm. The cell bodies and the initial dendritic trunks are usually free of spines. The smooth trunks divide within 10–30 μm of their origins to give rise to spiny secondary dendrites that may branch one or two more times. A spiny neuron generally has 25–30 dendritic terminal branches, which radiate in all directions from the cell body to fill a roughly spherical volume with a radius of 0.3–0.5 mm (300–500 μm). The density of dendritic spines increases rapidly from the first appearance of spines at about 20 μm from the soma to a peak at a distance of about 80 μm from the soma. The peak spine density can be as high as 4–6 per 1 μm of dendritic length, making the neostriatal principal neuron one of the most spine-laden cells in the brain (in density, not total spine number). The spiny dendrites taper gradually in diameter from about 1.5 μm to only 0.25 μm at the tips, and the spine density likewise tapers gradually, reaching about half the peak value at the dendritic tips (Wilson et al., 1983b). The total number of spines and the implications of spines for the function of the spiny neuron are discussed below.

The axon of the spiny cell arises from a well-defined initial segment on the soma or a proximal dendritic trunk. The main axon emits several collaterals before leaving the vicinity of the cell body, and these give rise to a local collateral arborization. The local axonal arborizations of spiny neurons are so rich that they caused many earlier investigators using the Golgi method to conclude that these cells must be interneurons. The spiny cells were among the first cells to be studied by intracellular injection of horseradish peroxidase (HRP) (see Kitai et al., 1976a), which revealed that their collateral axonal arborizations were even more elaborate than when visualized using the Golgi method. A drawing of a spiny projection neuron with its complete local collateral field is shown in Fig. 9.3, and a photomicrograph of an intracellularly stained spiny neuron from the rat is shown in Fig. 9.4. Originally believed to be an interneuron, the spiny cells were identified as projection cells in the 1970s. Recent studies using intracellular labeling have shown that all the spiny cells project outside the neostriatum as well as contributing to the axonal plexus in the region around the cell body (Chang et al., 1981; Kawaguchi et al., 1990). Furthermore, spiny neurons fall into two general classes depending upon their axonal targets. One class of spiny neurons (approximately half) forms the origin of the indirect pathway, projecting to the external segment of

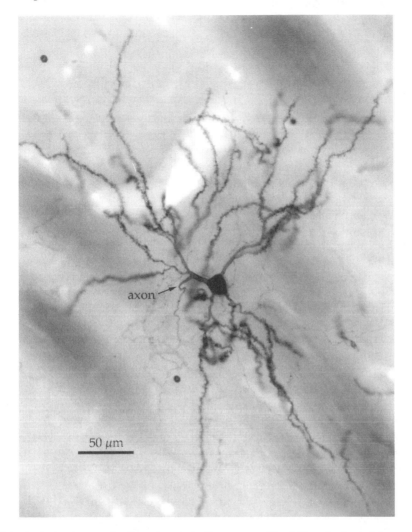

Fig. 9.4. A photomicrograph of a spiny projection neuron. Dendritic spines can be seen on all but the most proximal portions of the dendrites. The axon initial segment is indicated by the arrow, and some fine branches of the local axonal arborization are visible. [From Wilson and Kawaguchi, 1996, with permission.]

the globus pallidus and to no other target, while the remaining spiny neurons have highly collateralized axons, projecting to some combination of striatal targets, the internal and external segments of the globus pallidus, and substantia nigra. These neurons form the direct pathway from the neostriatum.

A second kind of principal neuron has been described, although this cell is much less common (DiFiglia et al., 1976; Bolam et al., 1981). It is characterized by a much lower dendritic spine density, a larger soma with occasional dendritic spines, and fewer but longer and less branched dendrites. This cell has been shown to project to the substantia nigra, but due to its relative rarity, there is little more known about it.

INTERNEURONS

Golgi studies of the neostriatum have revealed a great diversity of aspiny neuron morphology. The number of cell types that can be described on morphological grounds may be as high as eight or nine, and in most schemes there are still neurons that cannot be categorized (e.g., Chang et al., 1982). Taken together, these cells only account for a small proportion of the cells in the neostriatum, and it is not at all clear what the existence of so many different kinds of rare interneurons could mean. Moreover, it is not necessarily the case that each morphological category of neuron represents a functionally distinct cell type. Whereas little progress was made in the study of neostriatal interneurons for many years, recently, great progress has been made by using the combination of intracellular recording and staining, and immunocytochemical identification of neuron types based on the content of neurotransmitters and neuromodulators. For purposes of this discussion, as for most other practical purposes at this time, it is enough to describe only three interneuron types that have been examined in sufficient detail to be characterized as functionally and structurally separate categories. These are (*1*) the giant cholinergic interneuron (*2*) the GABA/parvalbumin-containing basket cells; and (*3*) the somatostatin/NOS–containing interneurons. The morphological characteristics of these cells are shown in Fig. 9.2 and the cholinergic interneuron is shown in detail in Fig. 9.3.

Cholinergic Interneuron. Although representing less than 2% of all the cells in the neostriatum, the largest cells in the tissue have long fascinated students of the basal ganglia. These cells were originally recognized as interneurons by Kölliker in the late 1800s. Because they are few and large, however, many later investigators have assumed (by analogy with so many other brain structures) that they are the principal cells, and that the numerous small neurons are interneurons. In recent years, the discovery that most or all of the largest cells are cholinergic and that acetylcholine-containing axons do not participate in the efferent projections to globus pallidus and substantia nigra has led to a general acceptance of the interneuronal status of the giant cell of Kölliker.

These cells have been described in Golgi-stained sections (e.g., DiFiglia and Carey, 1986), through immunocytochemistry for cholinacetyltransferase (e.g., Bolam et al., 1984), and using intracellular staining (Wilson et al., 1990; Kawaguchi, 1992). A camera lucida drawing of one of these cells is shown in Fig. 9.3. They usually have an elongated cell body, up to 50 or 60 μm in length, but commonly only 15–25 μm in its shortest diameter. A few stout dendrites arise from the soma and branch in a radiating fashion, with some dendrites extending 0.5–0.75 mm (500–750 μm) from the soma. The distal dendrites exhibit some irregularly shaped appendages and varicosities. The axons of these neurons arise from dendritic trunks. They may be myelinated initially, but they lose their myelin in the reductions of axonal diameter that occur in repeated bifurcations. The axon branches many times in the fashion classically associated with interneurons, i.e., with daughter branches being approximately equal in size and forming approximately 120° angles with each other and with the parent branch. The resulting arborization consists of a dense plexus of extremely fine axonal branches that fill the region of the dendritic field (commonly up to 1 mm from the soma) and sometimes go beyond, but do not leave, the neostriatum.

GABA/Parvalbumin-Containing Interneurons. An interneuron with a strong capacity for uptake of exogenous GABA, and staining intensely for both the GABA-synthesizing enzyme glutamate decarboxylase and for GABA itself was characterized in studies by Bolam and collaborators in the 1980s (Bolam et al., 1983). The morphological characteristics of the cell were identified by the combination of Golgi staining with GABA uptake or immunocytochemistry, and it was established to be an aspiny neuron of medium diameter. Because the spiny projection neurons are also GABAergic, further studies of these cells awaited the discovery that they can be identified by the presence of the cadmium-binding protein parvalbumin (Gerfen et al., 1987; Kita et al., 1990; Cowan et al., 1990). Most parvalbumin-containing cells are medium sized, that is, with somata about the same size as the spiny neurons; some cells are larger than this, but smaller than the giant cell of Kölliker. Perhaps they should be called medium and large cells, but they are usually referred to simply as *medium cells.* They have round somata and smooth, often varicose dendrites, and an intensely branching axonal arborization that often forms baskets on the somata of the spiny neurons. Thus they are close relatives of the GABA- and parvalbumin-containing basket cells of the hippocampus and cerebral cortex, which they also resemble in their firing pattern and physiological properties (see below). These cells represent only 3–5% of the total cell number in the neostriatum, and so they are usually widely spaced apart. But their dendrites are connected by gap junctions, and so they may interact electrically to form a network larger than a single neuron's dendritic and axonal tree (Kita et al., 1990). Intracellular staining studies (Kawaguchi, 1993; see Fig. 9.11) have shown that the cells can be divided into two subgroups according to whether their dendrites and axons ramify strictly locally (within 100–150 μm of the soma) or more extended (up to 300 μm).

Somatostatin/NOS-containing Inteurons. A second group of medium-sized aspiny interneurons identified on the basis of their neurotransmitter content was first recognized as positive in the histochemical reaction for NADPH-diaphorase. At the time, the significance of this enzymatic activity was unknown, but a small subset of neurons was seen to be diffusely and beautifully stained (Vincent et al., 1983b). Recently, this enzymatic activity has been shown to be due to a neuronal form of nitric oxide synthase (NOS), the enzyme that produces the neuromodulator nitric oxide. In addition, the neurons staining for NADPH-diaphorase and NOS have been shown to be identical to those staining for two other known striatal neuromodulators, somatostatin and neuropeptide-Y. These neurons represent 1–2% of the total population of neurons and are medium sized with longer and less branched dendrites and a more extented axonal field than the GABA/parvalbumin interneurons (Kawaguchi et al., 1995). The axons of these cells do not make pericellular baskets around the spiny neurons. Whereas the somata of these neurons are not intensely stained for GABA or GAD, their axon terminals contain GABA, and it is likely that they too are GABAergic interneurons (Kawaguchi et al., 1995).

Calrentinin-containing Interneurons. A third group of aspiny GABAergic interneurons contains the calcium-binding protein calretinin (Bennett and Bolam, 1993). These cells have not yet been studied in intracellular staining experiments, and so their morphology is not known in detail, and they are not shown in Fig. 9.2.

EFFERENT AXONS

The axons of spiny neostriatal neurons are gathered into small fiber fascicles that perforate the gray matter of the neostriatum, giving it the striated appearance for which it is named. Although these axons form a major fiber system of the forebrain, they are not large or heavily myelinated. In rats, the axons are near the threshold diameter for myelination (about 0.25 μm) and may or may not be myelinated. Some axons are myelinated briefly near the cell body but lose their myelin thereafter (Chang et al., 1981). In primates, the axons are larger and more consistently myelinated, although the gradual tapering in axonal diameter that occurs over the course of these axons is accompanied by a thinning and partial loss of the myelination in these species as well (Fox and Rafols, 1976). The two subpopulations of spiny neurons that give rise to the direct and indirect pathways are both GABAergic, forming GABA-containing synapses in the neostriatum, globus pallidus, and substantia nigra. In addition to GABA, these axons contain peptide neurotransmitters, with indirect pathway axons containing enkephalin, whereas the axons of the direct pathway contain substance P and dynorphin (e g., Gerfen and Young, 1988, Flaherty and Graybiel, 1994).

In the globus pallidus and substantia nigra, the axons of neostriatal spiny neurons arborize in a very characteristic *longitudinal axodendritic* pattern. This pattern, which contrasts sharply with that of afferent fibers in the neostriatum, is characterized by individual neostriatal efferent axons running parallel to dendrites of the pallidal and nigral target neurons, making multiple synaptic contacts that almost completely ensheath the dendrites of the postsynaptic cells (e.g., DiFiglia and Rafols, 1988).

CELL POPULATIONS

According to studies of Nissl-stained sections which show all cell bodies, there are approximately 111 million neurons in the neostriatum of the human (Fox and Rafols, 1976). Principal neurons make up the largest population, representing about 77% of cells in monkeys. The principal neurons are responsible for a larger proportion of the total cell population in cats, rats, and mice, accounting for perhaps as much as 95% of all cells (Graveland and DiFiglia, 1985a). The remaining cells, about 3–4% in carnivores and rodents and perhaps as many as 23% in primates, are divided among the various types of interneurons. There are approximately 540,000 neurons in the lateral segment of globus pallidus and 170,000 cells in the internal segment. On the basis of these numbers alone, there must be an impressive convergence of inputs from the neostriatum onto the output cells of the globus pallidus. Approximately half of neostriatal projection neurons project exclusively to the globus pallidus. The other half also make some synaptic contacts, but only considering those that project exclusively to GPe, there would be about 55,000,000 neostriatal neurons contributing to the innervation of 540,000 cells in the external segment of the globus pallidus, and a minimal convergence ratio of 100 to 1. Even higher ratios would be obtained for the internal segment of the globus pallidus and the substantia nigra, pars reticulata, which contain fewer neurons and have more collateralized projections.

In view of the longitudinal axodendritic synaptic arrangement in these structures, the influence of neostriatal output on the cells of these structures must be very strong. Of course, this does not imply a random mixing of neostriatal information in the globus pallidus and substantia nigra, and it does not imply that all GP neurons receive the same inputs. In fact, this convergence ensures that, in principle, each neuron of the globus pallidus could receive a unique combination of neostriatal inputs. Extracellular recording studies have shown that correlations among the neurons of globus pallidus are few in awake behaving animals, which suggests that even nearby cells do not tend to fire together; they probably would if they shared a large proportion of their sources of input (Nini et al., 1995). Anatomical data employing transneuronal axonal tracing with viruses also show that the spatial arrangement of inputs in these structures is very specific, and that spatial patterns of activity in the neostriatum may be expected to be preserved in the output structures (Hoover and Strick, 1993).

Because the arrangement of neostriatal cell bodies and the arborization patterns of afferent axons do not follow any simple geometrical arrangement, quantitative estimates of the degree of convergence and divergence are not easily obtained for neostriatal afferents. The evidence currently available indicates that all the asymmetric synapses formed on the heads of dendritic spines arise from afferent fibers (although not all afferent synapses are of this type; see below). This suggests that we can derive a lower limit to the number of afferent synapses formed onto individual spiny neurons by counting the number of dendritic spines per cell. Counts of spine density have been made in several species, and they are generally in agreement. Although spine density is somewhat lower in humans and monkeys than in rats and cats, the dendrites are slightly longer as well, making the number of spines per dendrite approximately the same (Graveland and DiFiglia, 1985b). The integrated spine density in the rat has been measured, and it varies among cells from about 300 to 500 per dendrite (Wilson et al., 1983b). Since there are 25–30 dendrites per spiny neuron, this yields a count of about 7500–15,000 spines per spiny neuron. Each dendritic spine gets at least one presumed excitatory synapse, which means that each spiny neuron has at least this many excitatory inputs. Electron-microscopic stereological measurements in rats have shown that the neostriatum of that animal contains approximately one asymmetrical synapse (nearly all on dendritic spines) per cubic micron of tissue (Ingham et al., 1996) and light microscopic cell counts in rats yield a density of about 140,000 cells per square millimeter (Oorschot, 1996). An estimate of average synaptic input of about 7100 asymmetric synapses per cell (of any type) is available from the combination of these two measurements. This is in reasonable agreement with the calculation above made by counting spines. It is remarkable, in view of this large excitatory innervation, that most spiny neurons are electrophysiologically silent most of the time. How this comes about requires analysis of the functional organization of the spiny neuron and its dendritic tree (see below).

SYNAPTIC CONNECTIONS

The typical synaptic connections of the neostriatum are shown in Fig. 9.5. We will describe briefly each of the main types of connections.

CORTICAL AND THALAMIC CONNECTIONS

The most noticeable feature of the neostriatum as seen in the electron microscope is the large number of small axons forming asymmetrical synapses (Gray's type I; see Chap. 1) on the heads of dendritic spines. This kind of synapse accounts for about 85%

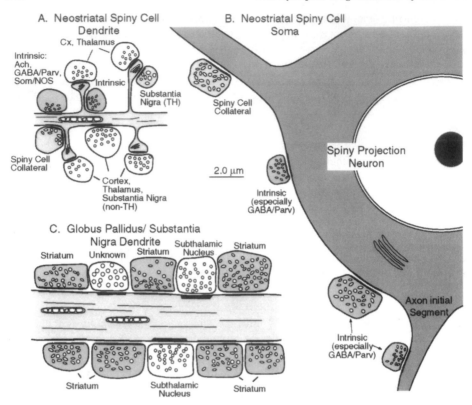

Fig. 9.5. The major synaptic types of the neostriatal spiny neuron and the neurons in the sub-stantia nigra and globus pallidus that receive input from it. **A:** The distal spiny dendrites of the spiny neurons. Inputs with round synaptic vesicles form asymmetrical inputs primarily on den-dritic spines, but occasionally on the shafts of the dendrites. These arise mostly from afferent fibers, especially from the cerebral cortex (Cx) and thalamus, but also from other structures, such as the non-TH-staining axons from the substantia nigra. Spiny cell collaterals, TH-stain-ing axons from the substantia nigra, and intrinsic intrastriatal connections (from aspiny neurons) form symmetrical synapses with pleomorphic and flattened vesicles on the stalks of dendritic spines, on the proximal part of the spine heads, and on dendritic shafts. Axodendritic synapses are overrepresented so that all the synapse types could be shown. Most of the surface of the dendritic shaft is free of synaptic input. **B:** The inputs to the proximal surface of the spiny neu-rons are from interneurons and collateral arborizations of the spiny neurons. They form sym-metrical synapses with pleomorphic or flattened synaptic vesicles at very low density on the as-piny initial portion of the dendrites, the somata, and axon initial segments. **C:** Synaptic types observed on dendrites in the globus pallidus and substantia nigra.

of all synapses in the neostriatum (Kemp and Powell, 1971a). It is the characteristic synaptic type formed by afferents from cerebral cortex, and from parts of the in-tralaminar nuclei of the thalamus (e.g., Kemp and Powell, 1971b). The axons from the cerebral cortex and thalamus are similar in morphology, both exhibiting small, round synaptic vesicles. A smaller number of cortical afferent synapses are made onto den-dritic shafts and somata of neostriatal neurons. Some of these are formed on dendritic shafts of spiny projection neurons, and others are on the somata and dendrites of the aspiny neurons. One area of the thalamus has been shown to form preferentially axo-dendritic rather than axospinous synapses (Dubé et al., 1988; Xu et al., 1991).

SUBSTANTIA NIGRA CONNECTIONS

The nigrostriatal projection has been more intensely studied because it has presented an interesting and puzzling inconsistency. There are several ways to label a pathway so that its axons can be identified in the electron microscope. For example, there is an EM variant of the axonal tracing technique employing extracellular injections of radioactive amino acids, which are taken up by cells and converted to proteins and transported down the axons. Through this method, axons arising from one part of the brain can be identified in electron micrographs of sections taken from another area, in which they terminate. Another approach is to destroy the neurons in one area and use the characteristic changes that accompany axonal degeneration to identify the axons in a distant, otherwise unharmed brain area. Still another is to label the axons that form a particular projection by making use of a biochemical marker that is characteristic of the projection. In the case of the dopaminergic neurons of the nigrostriatal pathway, this is especially easy because they have a very large complement of the enzyme tyrosine hydroxylase (TH), which is essential for the synthesis of dopamine. Immunocytochemistry using antibodies to TH is therefore an excellent way to demonstrate which axons are from the substantia nigra. Two other methods take advantage of special properties of the dopaminergic axons. One is destruction of these axons with the selective neurotoxin 6-hydroxydopamine, which is believed to kill specifically dopaminergic axons in the neostriatum. The degenerating axons can be identified by the characteristic appearance of degenerating neuronal tissue. The second is the labeling of dopaminergic neurons with another dopamine analog, 5-hydroxydopamine. This does not kill dopaminergic axons but is specifically absorbed by them, and is directly visible in the electron microscope in tissue fixed in the conventional way.

The reason for describing all of these methods is that although they are all well-proven tools in other systems, in the nigrostriatal pathway they produce different, apparently inconsistent results. For example, after autoradiographic labeling of the nigrostriatal pathway, or selective destruction of that pathway using either conventional lesions of the substantia nigra or treatment with 6-hydroxydopamine (e.g., Hattori et al., 1973), the axons that are labeled in the neostriatum appear similar to those of the corticostriatal or thalamostriatal projections. That is, they are of Gray's type I in that they contain small round synaptic vesicles and form asymmetrical synapses on the heads of dendritic spines. If the TH method is used instead, a different kind of axon is labeled, which contains larger, more variably shaped synaptic vesicles, and it forms symmetrical synapses on dendritic shafts, somata, and the stalks of dendritic spines (e.g., Freund et al., 1984). Both experiments have been repeated several times, and there is no readily available explanation, other than to reject arbitrarily one of the two sets of observations. In the diagram shown in Fig. 9.5, two nigrostriatal endings are shown, one labeled TH, and the other non-TH. It remains to be seen whether both of them are really there. One point that can be made from this is that trusted experimental technique sometimes produce inconsistent findings. It is permissible to postpone judgement on such difficult issues while awaiting the new insight that will provide an explanation.

AXON COLLATERAL CONNECTIONS

The boutons that arise from the local collaterals of spiny neurons contain large synaptic vesicles of variable shape and form symmetrical synapses onto the stalks of dendritic spines, dendritic shafts, somata, and initial segments of axons (Wilson and Groves, 1980; Bishop et al., 1981; Somogyi et al., 1981). These synapses are similar in appearance to those stained positively with TH. Like the TH synapses, local spiny cell collaterals that end on dendritic spines share that spine with some other input, often a cortical fiber. Some of the terminals of spiny cell axons form synapses with dendrites, somata, and initial axonal segments of other spiny neurons, but some are definitely made with these portions of the aspiny cells, including the cholinergic interneuron (Bolam et al., 1986).

INTERNEURON CONNECTIONS

Synapses formed by the axons of the cholinergic interneuron, and those of the other interneuron types (DiFiglia and Aronin, 1982; Takagi et al., 1983; Bolam et al., 1984; Phelps et al., 1985) contribute to a third major morphological synaptic type in the neostriatum. These synapses have small, flattened vesicles and form symmetrical synapses on the stalks of dendritic spines, dendritic shafts, somata, and initial segments; they therefore fall into Gray's type II (see Chap. 1). They are common on spiny neurons, and axons from both cholinergic interneurons and both types of GABAergic interneurons have been shown to terminate in this way on identified spiny cells. Terminals of this type, and the terminals with large pleomorphic synaptic vesicles, form the primary synaptic types found on the somata and proximal dendritic surface of the spiny cell.

Inputs to the cholinergic interneuron are of the same three major morphological types, but they do not show the specific localization on the cell surface that is observed on the spiny neurons (Chang and Kitai, 1982; DiFiglia and Carey, 1986). Boutons with small, round vesicles form asymmetrical synapses on dendrites of all sizes, and even on the somata of aspiny neurons. Likewise, symmetrical synapses formed by boutons with large pleomorphic vesicles, and by boutons with small, flattened synaptic vesicles, are seen on all parts of these cells. The synaptic density on the cholinergic neuron is much lower as well, with large parts of the surface area of the cell being free of synapses. It is likely that despite its large size, the giant interneuron receives many fewer synaptic contacts than the spiny cell. Attempts to show synaptic input to the cholinergic neuron from the cerebral cortex have not met with great success, whereas the thalamic input makes easily demonstrable synaptic contacts on cholinergic cells (Lapper and Bolam, 1992). This preference for thalamic input by the cholinergic cell may account in part for their difference in the activity of these cells during behavior (see below).

OUTPUT CONNECTIONS

The output axons of the spiny neurons form synapses in the substantia nigra and globus pallidus that are similar in morphology to the synapses formed by their local axonal terminals (Chang et al., 1981). In both the globus pallidus and substantia nigra, the dendrites of most neurons are completely encased in a quiltwork of synaptic terminals. Most of those terminals are derived from the neostriatal efferent fibers. A second kind of terminal found on these dendrites, containing small, round vesicles and forming asymmetrical contacts, is derived from the subthalamic nucleus (Kita and Kitai, 1987), while a third type, containing larger round vesicles and also forming asymmetrical contacts, is from an unidentified source.

BASIC CIRCUIT

The known connections between elements in the neostriatum are summarized in Fig. 9.6. Although this diagram is no doubt incomplete, especially in its portrayal of the connections of interneurons, it does show the most well-established connections among the cells. Two identical spiny cells are shown in the diagram, but only to indicate that they are more common than the other cells. The spiny neurons receive input from every element in the neostriatum, including each other (although this connection between spiny cells is not shown). A GABA/parvalbumin interneuron, and a GABA/somatostatin/NOS neuron are shown as intrinsic inhibitory elements, making synapses primarily with the principal cells. Although the direct effects of interneurons on neostriatal spiny neurons have not yet been observed directly in experiments, these cells are shown as inhibitory on the basis of the distribution and morphology of the synapses they make, as well as the presence of GABA in their presynaptic terminals. The somatostatin/NOS neurons presumably release somatostatin and nitric oxide as transmitters, in addition to GABA, and their functions cannot be characterized as simply excitatory or inhibitory (see below). Both the GABA/parvalbumin neurons and cholinergic interneurons have been shown to make synaptic contacts with striatal spiny neurons (Izzo and Bolam, 1988; Kita et al., 1990; Bennett and Bolam, 1994). The former interneuron is almost certainly a powerful inhibitory influence in the striatum (Kita, 1993), whereas the postsynaptic effect of acetylcholine in the neostriatum is uncertain. To indicate this uncertainty, the synapses made by the giant aspiny interneurons are shown gray.

Afferent inputs go to all of the neostriatal cell types, where most make excitatory synapses predominantly on the dendritic spines of the spiny neurons. Included in this category are inputs from cerebral cortex, the thalamic nuclei, and amygdala, and perhaps TH-negative inputs from the substantia nigra. The TH-containing axons are shown separately in Fig. 9.6. These axons end upon spine stalks and dendritic shafts, rather than spine heads, and do not make the classical Gray's type I synapse formed by other neostriatal afferent fibers. Because the physiological action of these fibers does not allow for a simple classification as excitatory or inhibitory, these terminals are also marked gray.

Regardless of the uncertainty about the action of some interneurons, the neostriatum is unusual in that the principal neurons, as well as many of the interneurons, are inhibitory. In this regard, it is similar to the cerebellar cortex (Chap. 7). The next neuron in the output pathway, the principal neuron of the globus pallidus and substantia nigra, is also shown in Fig. 9.6; it is also inhibitory. Excitatory influences in the basal ganglia arise mostly from incoming fibers.

Appreciation of the operation of this mostly inhibitory circuit requires a knowledge of the firing patterns of the neurons involved. This will be described in a later section, but for the present purposes it is important to understand that neostriatal spiny cells fire very rarely and in episodes that last for only about 0.1 to 3 sec. Most interneurons

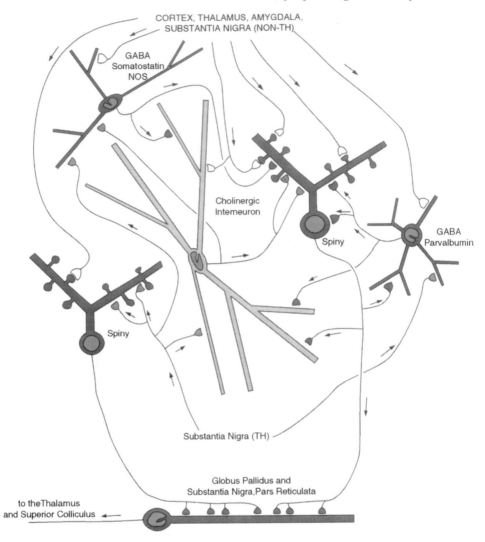

CORTEX, THALAMUS, AMYGDALA,
SUBSTANTIA NIGRA (NON-TH)

GABA
Somatostatin
NOS

Cholinergic
Interneuron

Spiny

GABA
Parvalbumin

Spiny

Substantia Nigra (TH)

Globus Pallidus and
Substantia Nigra,Pars Reticulata

to theThalamus
and Superior Colliculus

Fig. 9.6. Simplified basic circuit of the neostriatum and its outputs. Excitatory afferent input from several sources is received by all cell types. Because of their large numbers and heavy afferent innervation, most of these are formed on spiny neurons. Spiny cells contribute inhibitory input to all cell types. The interneurons regulate activity through the direct pathway consisting of the afferent fibers and the spiny projection neurons. The output of the spiny neurons converges on the dendrites of target cells in the substantia nigra and globus pallidus, which themselves project to the thalamus and superior colliculus.

likewise do not fire impulses continually. Thus, tonic intrinsic inhibitory interactions between the neurons are probably not important contributors to the membrane potential of the spiny neuron under resting conditions, but instead limit firing during episodes of excitation that arise because of activity in excitatory inputs. The cells in the globus pallidus and substantia nigra, on the other hand, fire tonically at very high rates. Their tonic firing produces a constant inhibition of neurons in the thalamus and superior colliculus. The firing of spiny neostriatal neurons can cause a transient pause in that tonic inhibition, releasing thalamic and superior colliculus neurons to respond to excitatory inputs that would otherwise be subthreshold. Thus the neostriatum acts to disinhibit neurons in the thalamus and superior colliculus in response to excitation in its afferent fibers, and the interneurons of the neostriatum help to regulate the duration, strength, and spatial pattern of that disinhibition.

MOSAIC ORGANIZATION OF THE NEOSTRIATUM

In the human neostriatum, and in the neostriatum of some primates, the neurons can be seen to be clustered into groups of high density separated by areas of lower cell density. No such internal organization can be seen in most other animals. Despite the apparent cell clusters of primates, the neostriatum has long been believed to be structurally homogeneous. This stood in contrast with the cerebral and cerebellar cortices, olfactory bulb, and other brain structures that possess a very prominent layered organization.

It is now evident that the clusters of cells in the primate neostriatum, originally called *cell islands*, represent a fundamental feature of the organization of this structure and are present in a less visible, perhaps less differentiated, form in all mammals. Unlike layered structures, however, this mosaic organizational plan does not separate the tissue into many compartments, but rather, only two. In primates, these are clear enough; they are called *cell islands* and *matrix* (Goldman-Rakic, 1982). The matrix is the somewhat less cell-dense neostriatal tissue between the cell islands. A very important finding for the interpretation of this organization was the observation that afferent fibers, particularly fibers of cortical origin, observe these tissue compartment boundaries (e.g., Goldman and Nauta, 1977; Graybiel et al., 1981). Certain cortical areas project preferentially to the matrix and mostly avoid the islands. This observation encourages a search for traces of cell islands and matrix in other animals, like the cat or the rat, who have no visible clustering of the neurons to indicate the boundaries of the mosaic. When this is done, cortical axons that should project to the matrix are seen to fill a space in the neostriatum that is perforated with many small, irregularly shaped spaces that seem to correspond to the islands seen in primates. Although it is now well established that these are the same thing, they are given a slightly different name. They are called *striosomes*, or sometimes just *patches* (Graybiel et al., 1981; Herkenham and Pert, 1981).

In the rat and monkey, some areas of the cerebral cortex have been shown to project preferentially to the striosomes as well (e.g., Gerfen, 1984; Eblen and Graybiel, 1995). This preferential projection is not absolute however, but reflects areal differences in the distribution of various types of corticostriatal neurons (Gerfen, 1989). Many cortical areas in the rat have been shown to project to both patches and matrix, with projections from more deeply situated neurons providing the input to the patches and more superficial ones projecting to the matrix. The laminar distribution of corticostriatal neurons varies among cortical regions corresponding to their preference for patches and matrix (Wilson, 1987). On this basis, it might be expected that the axons of cortical cells projecting to patch and matrix would arborize differently in the neostriatum. Axons from corticostriatal neurons have been shown to arborize in two distinctly different patterns—one that extends over a large distance and one that consists of one or more small focal clusters of boutons confined to an area about the same size as the striosomes (Cowan and Wilson, 1994; Kincaid and Wilson, 1996). Each corticostriatal neuron gives rise to one or the other of these patterns, but apparently no cell makes both kinds of arborization. Whereas the cortical projections to striosomes arise mostly from the cells that make focal projections, some of the focal projections fall into the matrix. Thus there may be an internal structure to the connections made in the matrix, with small, striosome-sized regions in the matrix distinguished from the surrounding tissue by their cortical connections and perhaps by other features. This proposal of discontinuous compartments within the matrix termed *matrisomes* (Flaherty and Graybiel, 1994) will likely be examined intensively in future studies.

Other afferent pathways also observe the boundaries between striosomes and matrix. Thalamic projections from the midline nuclei have been reported to project specifically to striosomes, whereas the anterior and posterior intralaminar groups, the rostral ventral tier nuclei, and parts of the posterior lateral nuclear complex, project preferentially to the matrix (Ragsdale and Graybiel, 1991). Individual thalamostriatal axons have been stained by a variant of the intracellular staining method by Deschênes and co-workers (1996). This method, called the *juxtacellular staining method* because the cell is never impaled but only approached very closely, allows complete staining of single neurons in vivo, even in regions of the brain where intracellular recording has proven too difficult. The studies using this method have shown that thalamic axons, like those from the cerebral cortex, arborize either in an extended pattern or in a focal pattern, and that the focal arborizations can occur in the matrix. They further showed that the projections from the parafascicular nucleus arborize in a more focal pattern than those from the intralaminar nuclei. Remember that these two parts of the thalamostriatal projection also differ in their postsynaptic targets, with parafascicular projections going mainly to dendritic shafts, while the intralaminar nuclei project to dendritic spines.

The dopaminergic inputs from the substantia nigra also observe the boundaries between striosomes and matrix. In the rat, there are two different sets of nigrostriatal dopaminergic neurons, one that innervates the patch (striosome) compartment, and one that innervates the matrix (Gerfen, 1985; Langer and Graybiel, 1989). So far, there have been no descriptions of the individual axonal branching patterns of nigrostriatal axons.

The observation that afferent axons respect the boundaries of internal neostriatal tissue compartments has no immediate functional implications. Because most afferent fibers make synapses on the dendrites of neostriatal neurons, afferents that are confined to the matrix could easily be making synapses with neurons of the striosomes if those cells send their dendrites into the matrix (see Neuronal Elements, above). A similar uncertainty holds for the internal interconnections among neostriatal neurons. It is important, therefore, whether the dendritic and axonal fields observe the boundaries and to determine this for each of the cell types. In the past few years, this information has become available for all of the major cell types; it is shown schematically in Fig. 9.7. The overall result is that afferent fibers, the local axons of spiny neurons, and their dendritic fields observe compartmental boundaries (Kawaguchi et al., 1989), whereas the dendrites of interneurons cross compartmental boundaries (Chesselet and Graybiel, 1986; Cowan et al., 1990; Kawaguchi, 1992). The relation of axonal fields

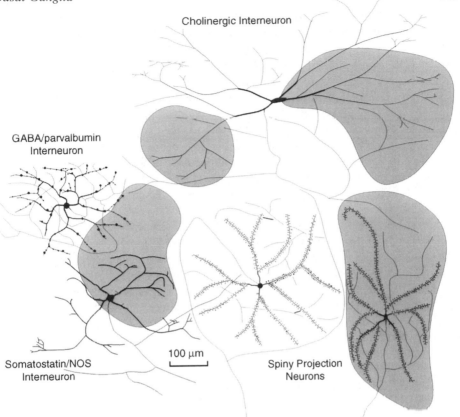

Fig. 9.7. The mosaic internal organization of the neostriatum in relation to the dendritic fields of the major cell types, drawn at the same scale. The striosomal compartment of the neostriatum is shown stippled, while the matrix is white. Two different populations of spiny neurons, one associated with the striosomes and one with the matrix are represented by the two spiny cells. Their dendrites and local axonal fields are mostly confined to the compartment containing the cell body. The aspiny interneurons, however, have dendritic fields that cross compartment boundaries.

of interneurons to the compartmental boundaries is an interesting topic that has not been fully explored. Axons of both acetylcholine and somatostatin/NOS neurons are more dense in the matrix than in the striosomes (Gerfen, 1985; Graybiel et al., 1986; Chesselet and Graybiel, 1986), but the somata of these two cell types are approximately evenly distributed in the two compartments, and their dendrites do not have any apparent preference for either compartment. The axons of these cells must somehow arborize more profusely in the matrix. A preference for the matrix is apparent in the axonal arborizations of some cholinergic neurons stained intracellularly (Kawaguchi, 1992).

Given that the striosomes and matrix receive different synaptic inputs, it is natural to wonder whether they might have different output targets. Such a difference does exist for the projections to the substantia nigra. There, striosomes project preferentially to the substantia nigra pars compacta, where the dopaminergic nigrostriatal neurons are located, whereas the matrix projects to pars reticulata, where nondopaminergic neurons projecting to the thalamus and superior colliculus are found (Gerfen, 1985, Jimenez-Castellanos and Graybiel, 1989).

These observations indicate that the most direct pathway through the neostriatum, going from afferent fibers to the principal neurons and out to the target structures, consists of two parallel and independent pathways, one from the striosomes and one from the matrix. These dichotomy is not to be confused with the direct and indirect pathway, which are present in both compartments (see below). Communication between compartments may be a major role of the interneurons in the neostriatum.

A particularly exciting development has been the discovery that neostriatal compartments can be distinguished on the basis of their cytochemical characteristics (e.g., Graybiel et al., 1981). Cells in the striosomes and matrix, although similar in many respects, are sufficiently different biochemically to allow demonstration of the compartments using many standard cytochemical methods. For example, in many species the concentration of acetylcholinesterase is detectably higher in the matrix, allowing visualization of the striosomes as acetylcholinesterase-poor zones in sections stained for the presence of this enzyme (e.g., Graybiel et al., 1981). Another useful biochemical marker is the mu opiate receptor, which is present in much higher concentration in the neuropil of the striosomes (e.g., Herkenham and Pert, 1981). The peptides met-enkephalin and substance P, both very abundant in the neostriatum, are also differentially localized, but in a more complex way. In some parts of the neostriatum, the striosomes are richer in these substances, whereas other parts preferentially express them in the matrix. The functional meaning of these differences is not known. Their existence proves, however, that we cannot consider the mosaic organization of the neostriatum to be a simple topographical relationship, representing nothing more than the arrangement of afferents and efferents. The differences between the two compartments run deeper than that.

DIRECT AND INDIRECT PATHWAYS

The use of the peptides enkephalin and substance P as cytochemical markers to distinguish the striosomal and matrix compartments of the neostriatum was instrumental in the discovery of another major organizational principle of the basal ganglia, the direct and indirect neostriatal efferent pathways. In early intracellular staining studies in rats it was shown that about half of spiny neurons had dense and elaborate projections to the external segment of the globus pallidus, and that these cells did not project to the substantia nigra, as assessed using antidromic stimulation (Chang et al., 1981). Double retrograde tracing studies later showed that neurons heavily labeled by injections of tracers in the substantia nigra or GPi were rarely heavily labeled by injection in the GPe (e.g., Parent et al., 1984). At the same time, studies of the cellular localization of the peptides enkephalin and substance P showed that these were specific markers for mostly nonoverlapping subpopulations of striatal spiny projection neurons (e.g., Penny et al., 1986). GABA, on the other hand, coexists with these peptides, since it is present in all subclasses of spiny neurons (Kita and Kitai, 1988). Moreover, the external pallidal segment was found to contain many striatal axon terminals staining for enkephalin, whereas substance P was common in neostriatal axons terminating in the internal pallidal segment and the substantia nigra. Subsequent intracellular staining studies have confirmed that about half of spiny neurons project to the external segment of the globus pallidus and nowhere else, while the remaining half of the cells have smaller collateral projections to the external pallidal segment but primarily project to the internal pallidal segment, the substantia nigra, or both (Kawaguchi et al., 1990). These two populations of neurons and their connections are seen superimposed upon the mosaic organization of the neostriatum in Fig. 9.8.

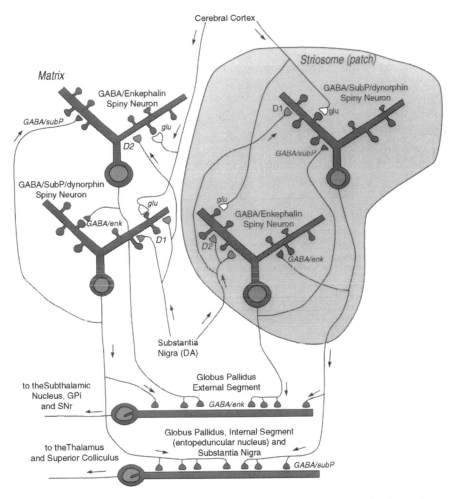

Fig. 9.8. The direct and indirect pathways, arising from both the striosomal and matrix compartments. These consist of separate sets of GABAergic spiny neurons, with the indirect pathway neurons containing the co-transmitter Enkephalin (enk), while the direct pathway neurons contain substance P (subP) and dynorphin. Separate dopaminergic axons innervate the striosomes and matrix, but the direct and indirect pathway neurons in each compartment express different dopamine receptors. Whereas indirect pathway spiny neurons innervate only the external pallidal segment, the direct pathway neurons project both to the external segment, and either the internal pallidal segment, substantia nigra pars reticulata, or both.

Because enkephalin and substance P differentially stain the striosome and matrix compartments, there were initial suspicions that these pathways may be yet another reflection of the mosaic organization of the neostriatum. Quantitative studies of the distribution of spiny neurons projecting primarily to the substantia nigra versus external pallidum have shown that, although these are the substance P and enkephalin-containing spiny cell subpopulations, they are not differentially located in the striosome and matrix compartments (Gerfen and Young, 1988). Instead, these two subpopulations of spiny neurons are intermingled throughout both compartments and in all regions of the neostriatum. Spiny neurons of the direct and indirect pathways also make direct synaptic connection among each other, as well as within each subgroup (Yung et al., 1996).

The reason that enkephalin and substance P differentially stain the striosomes and matrix, and the complex nature of the pattern of staining seen using these markers, continue to be a mystery. This probably reflects a quantitative difference in the level of expression of peptides within the cells of the two compartments.

Morphologically, the spiny neurons forming the direct and indirect pathways are very similar, except for the difference in their axonal projections (see above). This explains why the distinction between them was not apparent until recently, as axons of spiny cells are not well stained by Golgi impregnation. Studies employing cytochemical methods have revealed a number of other differences. One of these that may be of particular importance is a difference in the dopamine receptors expressed on the surfaces of the two groups of cells. Although there are a number of different dopamine receptor subtypes present in the neostriatum and elsewhere, they can be generally grouped into two classes, the D1 class and the D2 class. The most common of the D1 class in the neostriatum, D1a, is preferentially expressed by the substance P–containing cells of the direct pathway; the D2 receptor is specifically expressed on enkephalin containing spiny neurons (e.g., Gerfen et al., 1990; Surmeier et al., 1996).

SYNAPTIC ACTIONS

SPINY NEURON

The neurotransmitter of the spiny neuron has long been believed to be GABA. At their target neurons in the substantia nigra and globus pallidus, the spiny neurons have a powerful inhibitory effect, mediated by GABA acting mainly at $GABA_A$ receptors (e.g., Precht and Yoshida, 1971). By analogy, it has long been assumed that the spiny neurons powerfully inhibit each other. A large proportion of the synapses made by the collaterals of spiny neurons is made on dendritic spines or can otherwise be identified as having a spiny neuron as the postsynaptic element (Wilson and Groves, 1980; Yung et al., 1996). Thus the network of the spiny neurons and their recurrent collaterals has the appearance of a mutually inhibitory network of principal neurons, and many influential theories of the neostriatum have been based on the assumption that the spiny cells exert a powerful mutual inhibition.

Recently, a direct test of the strength of mutual inhibition among spiny neurons failed to produce any evidence of it (Jaeger et al., 1994). This test employed two different techniques. In the first, spiny neurons were antidromically activated by electrical stimulation of either the substantia nigra or the external segment of the globus pallidus. The stimulation was set near the threshold for antidromic action potential generation for a single neuron recorded intracellularly. This means that there was an antidromic action potential in response to the stimulus about half the time, and about half the time the stimulus failed to evoke an antidromic action potential. Under these circumstances, it is expected that about half of the spiny neurons are antidromically activated in response to any one stimulus presentation. Even on the trials in which there was no antidromic activation of the recorded neuron, about half of the neighboring spiny neurons can be expected to respond to the stimulus. This assumption was confirmed by the presence of a field potential generated by the antidromic action potentials in the spiny neurons which did not vary from stimulus to stimulus. If the spiny neurons strongly inhibited their neighbors, a powerful (half maximal) IPSP should be generated in the recorded neuron in response to this stimulus, even on those stimulus presentations in which there was no antidromic action potential to mask the synaptic response. This is the method that was used to demonstrate the powerful Renshaw inhibition of motoneurons in the spinal cord (see Chap. 3). When employed in the neostriatum, no IPSP could be detected at all. In the second method, pairs of nearby spiny neurons were recorded intracellularly in slices. In no case could action potentials generated in one of the neurons by injection of depolarizing current produce any detectable synaptic potential in the other spiny cell. An example of results of such an experiment is shown in Fig. 9.9.

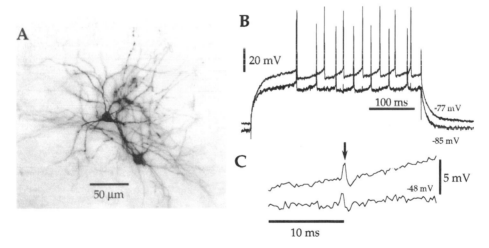

Fig. 9.9. Intracellular recordings of a pair of nearby striatal spiny neurons in vitro, showing the method for searching for inhibition between these cells. **A:** Both neurons, stained by intracellular injection of biocytin in the slice. The cells are located within each other's dendritic and axonal fields. **B:** Repetitive action potentials generated in both cells by intracellular current pulses. **C:** Spike-triggered averages for both neurons. For each cell, the membrane potential was averaged for a period immediately before and immediately after an action potential in the other neuron (indicated by the arrow). The capacitative coupling between the electrodes appears as a brief (approximately 1 ms) transient exactly aligned with the arrow. An IPSP would appear as a hyperpolarization to the right of the transient and lasting for 10–50 ms. [From Jaeger et al., 1994, with permission.]

These experiments do not rule out synaptic inhibition among spiny neurons, but they make it very unlikely that this is a central organizing principle of the neostriatum. They also point out a weakness in qualitative approaches to the study of synaptic circuitry. Because synapses could be observed to occur among spiny neurons, and because the axon collaterals of spiny neurons are a prominent feature of their morphology, it was assumed that mutual inhibition was much stronger than it proved to be. Nothing in the morphological literature allowed an estimate of the number of synapses formed by a spiny neuron upon its neighbors, and even now there is no quantitative estimate of the connectivity of spiny neurons. However, despite these negative results, GABAergic inhibition is demonstrable in the neostriatum, and the absence of strong inhibition via the output neurons has drawn attention to the role of interneurons.

INTERNEURONS

With the exception of the cholinergic interneuron, all of the well-studied interneurons in the neostriatum contain GABA and presumably release it as a synaptic neurotransmitter. Like the subtypes of spiny neurons, the various interneuron subtypes can be distinguished by the presence or absence of peptides also believed to be involved in neurotransmission. One class of aspiny interneurons that has not been shown to contain any other neurotransmitter is the GABA/parvalbumin neuron. These neurons are easily distinguished from the spiny cells by their especially high concentration of GABA, which causes them to stand out from other GABAergic neurons in immuno-cytochemical studies (Bolam et al., 1983), and by their content of the calcium-buffering protein parvalbumin (Cowan et al., 1990, Kita et al., 1990). Parvalbumin is present in some, but not all, classes of GABAergic neurons in various parts of the brain, including the cerebral cortex, hippocampus, and thalamus. In the basal ganglia, it is found in the GABAergic principal cells of the substantia nigra and globus pallidus, as well as in the strongly GABA-positive aspiny interneurons in the neostriatum. In all cases, it appears to be concentrated in cells that are capable of maintaining high rates of firing.

The physiological properties of the GABA/parvalbumin interneuron in the neostriatum have been described by Kawaguchi (1993b). In slices of the neostriatum in vitro, cell bodies of neurons were visualized using interference optics, and likely interneurons were identified by their somatic shape and size. These neurons were recorded using the whole-cell method under visual control and their physiological properties characterized by their responses to injected current pulses. The cells were then stained by intracellular injection of biocytin, and the slices were fixed and prepared for immunocytochemical staining. The morphological features of the interneurons were determined by intracellular staining, and the identity of the cells was confirmed by immunocytochemical staining of the same cells using antibodies for parvalbumin, choline acetyltransferase, GABA, or somatostatin. This allowed the first physiological studies of unequivocally identified neostriatal interneurons. The parvalbumin-containing interneurons in the neostriatum, like those in the cortex and hippocampus, were fast-firing neurons with short-duration action potentials and very short but powerful spike afterhyperpolarization. These properties, which allow the neurons to sustain high firing rates without substantial spike-frequency adaptation, are probably not due to the presence of parvalbumin, but are simply correlated with it. Instead, these properties result from the complement of ion channels expressed by these neurons. The function of parvalbumin in these neurons and its possible relation to their firing pattern are not known.

The GABA/parvalbumin interneurons receive powerful excitation from the cerebral cortex and are unlikely to act as a feedforward inhibitory pathway in parallel with the direct connection from the cortex to the principal neurons (Kita, 1993). The dendritic and axonal fields of these neurons are compact, but the presence of gap junctions connecting these neurons together suggests the possibility that the inhibitory effects of these cells may spread over a wider area than that of the excitation. Much of the inhibition observed in the aftermath of cortical excitation in the neostriatum is probably attributable to these neurons.

The somatostatin/NOS interneuron likewise contains (and presumably releases) GABA, but unlike the GABA/parvalbumin neuron, its soma does not stain heavily for GABA or its synthetic enzyme, GAD. This neuron has been thought not to be GABAergic, which set it apart from similar neurons in the cerebral cortex and hippocampus that were known to contain GABA as well as somatostatin. After treatment of the neostriatum with colchicine, which blocks axonal transport, somatostatin-containing striatal interneurons were shown to become GABA and GAD positive, suggesting that these substances may not be present in the soma and dendrites because they are efficiently transported into the axons of the cells (Kubota et al., 1993). However, the possibility that this treatment was actually inducing expression of GAD could not be eliminated. Recently, electron-microscopic immunocytochemical studies of the axon terminals of these neurons have shown that they contain GABA as well as somatostatin in the absence of any colchicine treatment (Kawaguchi et al., 1995). These cells probably represent another GABAergic interneuron in the neostriatum. The combined physiological, morphological, and immunocytochemical studies of Kawaguchi (1993b) have shown that these cells have a unique response to depolarization, consisting of slow, regular firing accompanied by pronounced spike-frequency adaptation and plateau potentials. These neurons, like the GABA/parvalbumin interneurons, receive a direct cortical input. The axons of these neurons extend much father than their dendritic fields, perhaps 1 mm or more in many cases. Like the other interneurons, these make synapses primarily with the principal neurons and secondarily with other interneurons. These cells also release somatostatin, neuropeptide Y, and nitric oxide. The effects of these substances on striatal neurons can be expected to attract intense study in the next few years. Nitric oxide, which can diffuse across cell membranes, has already been shown to have profound effects on the release of glutamate, GABA, acetylcholine (ACh), and dopamine by axons in the neostriatum (Kawaguchi et al., 1995).

Although cholinergic neurons are few in number, their axonal arborizations are very large and dense, and they provide a very rich cholinergic innervation to the neostriatum. This is another good example of the error that is committed if we judge the importance of a cell type purely by the number of cells. The cholinergic neurons of the neostriatum and the system of cholinergic synapses that they give rise to in the neostriatal neuropil are known to exert a powerful influence on the firing of the spiny neurons and the final output of the neostriatum. Pharmacological treatments for many human disorders, including Huntington's disease, Parkinson's disease, and even schizophrenia, often rely upon manipulation of transmission at cholinergic synapses in the neostriatum. The action of the giant cholinergic interneurons on the spiny cells of the neostriatum are mostly known through studies of the direct application of ACh to neurons in vitro. Multiple ACh receptors are known to exist in the neostriatum, and the relative contributions of each to synaptic transmission between the neurons is unknown. In early experiments, nicotinic cholinergic receptors have been reported to contribute to the fast EPSP evoked in neostriatal neurons by local stimulation in slices, and nicotinic receptors are present in the neostriatum. In situ hybridization studies of nicotinic receptor mRNA have shown that these receptors are expressed in the cerebral cortex, the thalamus and the substantia nigra, but not by most striatal neurons (Wada et al., 1989). Thus nicotinic receptors in the neostriatum are most likely to be present on afferent fibers rather than on the spiny neurons. Muscarinic receptors, which are plentifully expressed by neostriatal neurons, are probably responsible for most of the postsynaptic effects of acetylcholine. Muscarinic agonists have been reported to underly slow depolarizations or hyperpolarizations, the first probably due to a decrease in potassium conductance, and in either case, simultaneously causing a decrease in the amplitude of fast EPSPs elicited by intrastriatal stimulation (Dodt and Misgeld, 1986; Calabresi et al., 1993). The muscarinic effects of ACh do not indicate a classical neurotransmitter function, but rather a way of altering the membrane properties of the spiny neuron, and thereby its responsiveness to other inputs. For example, muscarinic receptor activation has been shown to reduce high voltage–activated calcium currents (L, N, and P type currents) in the principal cells of the neostriatum by way of the m1 and m4 muscarinic receptors (Howe and Surmeier, 1995). These currents are activated whenever a spiny neuron fires an action potential, and they have been shown to regulate repetitive firing in spiny cells by way of a calcium-dependent potassium conductance (Pineda et al., 1992). Thus, by reducing spike afterhyperpolarization of spiny neurons, cholinergic interneurons could increase their responsiveness to inputs, and especially their ability to fire rapidly to sustained depolarization.

INPUT FIBERS

A variety of evidence indicates that the neurotransmitter in the corticostriatal pathway is glutamate (e.g., McGeer et al., 1977). The thalamostriatal pathway is less clear, but is likely to be glutamate as well, because virtually all excitatory responses evoked in spiny neurons by local stimulation are abolished by application of excitatory amino acid receptor blockers (Jiang and North, 1991; Kita, 1996). The nigrostriatal projection is almost entirely dopaminergic, and the input from the raphé contains serotonin.

Because the neostriatum is a central structure, several synaptic relays removed from the direct sensory input pathways, it is not possible to analyze its synaptic actions by natural stimulation, as in so many other regions considered in this book. Analysis of synaptic actions therefore must rely on activation of neostriatal input and output pathways by electrical stimulation. We shall summarize the evidence for the main types of excitatory and inhibitory actions that control the activity of the striatal neurons as revealed by this experimental approach.

ACTIONS OF CORTICAL AND THALAMIC INPUTS

Stimulation of the cerebral cortex in intact animals sets up a synchronous volley of impulses in a subset of the corticostriatal axons, which evokes a large-amplitude EPSP in the spiny neurons of the neostriatum (e.g., Wilson, 1986a). The latency of this EPSP matches that of the fastest corticostriatal axons, and shows a constant latency despite changes in stimulus intensity or frequency, as expected for a monosynaptic EPSP. The behavior of this EPSP suggests that it represents the action of many synapses, each of whose effect at the soma is very weak. Its amplitude is finely graded with stimulus intensity. That is, very small changes in stimulus intensity produce correspondingly small changes in EPSP amplitude. Likewise, the EPSP shows no minimal threshold amplitude. Thus the synaptic potential components contributed by individual axons are too small to detect in a conventional intracellular recording, and the EPSP that is recorded must be composed of many such small EPSPs.

This initial EPSP is followed by a long-lasting hyperpolarization, and upon its termination, by a period of depolarization and increased synaptic noise. These components of the response are illustrated in Fig. 9.10Aa. Among these late components of

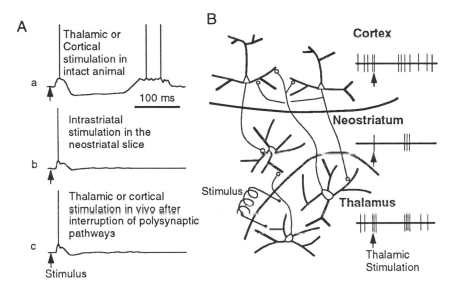

Fig. 9.10. Synaptic potentials evoked in spiny neurons by stimulation of the cerebral cortex and the thalamus, and their interpretation. **A:** Synaptic potentials in three different preparations. The trace shown in **a** shows the response evoked by stimulation of the cortex or thalamus (the response is the same for either site) in an intact animal. There is an initial large EPSP, which can trigger an action potential, followed by a long period of membrane hyperpolarization and inhibition of synaptic responses. This period is followed by a period of rebound excitation. The trace labeled **b** shows the response evoked by local stimulation in neostriatal slices, part of which is probably due to stimulation of cortical and thalamic afferents. The trace labeled **c** shows the response to cortical or thalamic stimulation in an animal in which the polysynaptic pathways shown in B have been interrupted experimentally. **B:** A diagram showing some of the synaptic connections between the cerebral cortex, thalamus, and neostriatum that contribute to the long-lasting inhibition and rebound excitation observed in spiny neostriatal neurons after cortical or thalamic stimulation. Typical responses of a cortical, striatal, and thalamic neuron upon stimulation of the thalamus are illustrated at the right. Stimulation of the cortex produces similar responses, due to activation of the same circuits.

the response we should find the effects of recurrent collaterals of the spiny neurons that fired action potentials in response to the initial EPSP and the effects of interneurons excited by the stimulus. The complexity of the response observed in the in vivo preparation suggests that it would be useful to carry out further analysis in a simplified preparation, such as slices of neostriatum. Such experiments have not usually been performed using cortical stimulation because it is difficult to get any significant piece of the corticostriatal pathway intact in a slice. They have instead used intrastriatal stimulation or stimulation of the subcortical white matter. Because of the nature of current spread from stimulation sites, these two kinds of stimulation are probably the same thing. They stimulate not only the corticostriatal fibers but all afferent fibers, the axons of spiny neurons, and striatal interneurons. Nonetheless, the response to this kind of stimulation is very informative. As shown in Fig. 9.10Ab, excitatory inputs in vitro never produce the pronounced, long-lasting inhibition or rebound excitation seen in the intact animal. Instead, the EPSP, which looks similar to that observed in vivo, is followed by only a small and short-lasting IPSP. Similar results have been obtained using cortical stimulation in a slice prepared to maintain the integrity of a portion of the corticostriatal projection (Kawaguchi et al., 1989). The IPSP component seen after cortical or local stimulation in slices probably is not due to recurrent axon collaterals of the spiny neurons but rather to inhibitory interneurons excited by the stimulus (Kita, 1993).

The short-duration monosynaptic component of the corticostriatal EPSP is mediated by glutamate, primarily acting at non-NMDA receptors (e.g., Calabresi et al., 1996). However, neostriatal spiny neurons possess NMDA receptors in abundance, but in most experimental preparations, their contribution to evoked EPSPs is prevented by the voltage-dependent magnesium block of the NMDA ion channel. When spiny neurons are depolarized by passage of transmembrane current, or the block is relieved by removal of extracellular magnesium, an NMDA component of the EPSP is readily demonstrated. Like most glutamate-mediated synapses, those on neostriatal spiny neurons can undergo long-lasting changes in effectiveness after tetanic stimulation. Tetanic local stimulation in striatal slices under experimental conditions that minimize NMDA receptor activation leads to long-term depression (LTD) of glutamatergic synaptic transmission. The same stimulation, applied in the absence of extracellular magnesium, so that NMDA receptors are active, will give rise to long-term potentiation (LTP) (Calabresi et al., 1996; Kita, 1996). A unique feature of these use-dependent changes in synaptic strength in the neostriatum is their dependence upon dopamine. Induction of LTD in the neostriatum absolutely depends upon the presence of dopamine. Moreover, coapplication of dopamine at the time of tetanic stimulation has been reported to be sufficient to induce LTP, even under conditions that would otherwise produce LTD (Wickens et al., 1996).

Stimulation of the thalamus in intact animals produces effects that are very similar to those of cortical stimulation (e.g., Wilson et al., 1983a). It is important to note in such experiments that when stimulating one area, we are often engaging the activity of many structures indirectly. This is illustrated for the thalamo-cortico-striatal system in Fig. 9.10B. We cannot stimulate thalamostriatal cells without also stimulating thalamic neurons that project to cortex, and stimulation of these thalamocortical fibers has profound effects on cortical activity. Also, some cortical neurons projecting to the thalamus are stimulated antidromically, and their recurrent collaterals in the cortex are activated. It is important to attempt to separate these polysynaptic effects from the direct response to stimulation by experimentally interrupting the polysynaptic pathways. When such experiments are performed, the cortical and thalamic responses are greatly simplified, and they display almost identical EPSPs (Fig. 9.10Ac). Although it is usually assumed that the corticostriatal input is more powerful than the thalamic one, there is no indication of this in a comparison of the sizes of the responses that can be produced by stimulation of the two structures. Their maximal EPSP amplitudes are approximately equal.

The results of the experiments described above indicate that the late components of the responses seen in intact animals are not due to the action of intrastriatal circuits. If the long-lasting hyperpolarization and late depolarization components of the response do not result from intrastriatal circuitry, then to what could they be due?

Measurement of the effect of hyperpolarizing and depolarizing currents and of conductance changes that accompany the membrane potential change can help to provide an answer. The long-lasting hyperpolarization is slightly increased in amplitude when the cell is hyperpolarized, and decreased with membrane depolarization. The effect is approximately equal in magnitude to the effect of the same manipulation on the EPSP. This suggests that the ionic currents responsible for the long-lasting hyperpolarization resemble those responsible for the EPSP. Secondly, measurement of whole-cell input resistance (R_N) during the long-lasting hyperpolarization shows that the cell has a net increase in resistance during this time. This measurement is difficult because of the large anomalous rectification of spiny neurons in this voltage range (see below) which has to be compensated out of the analysis. When this is done, the long-lasting hyperpolarization is seen to be accompanied by a decrease in conductance (increase in the resistance) of the cell. This is what would be expected if the long-lasting hyperpolarization were a disfacilitation, that is, the removal of an excitatory input

This interpretation is strengthened by examination of the behavior of neurons in the cerebral cortex and thalamus after stimulation of either structure. It has long been known that stimulation of the thalamus produces an initial excitatory effect in the cerebral cortex, which is followed by a long-lasting inhibitory period. The inhibitory period is itself followed by a "rebound" excitation (see Thalamus, Chap. 9; Neocortex, Chap. 12). A similar pattern of excitation and inhibition is observed in both the cortex and thalamus after application of a stimulus to the cortex. This pattern is precisely what is required if the long-lasting hyperpolarization and subsequent excitatory period in the neostriatum were due to a removal and subsequent reassertion of tonic excitatory influences from the cortex and thalamus. This scheme for the generation of the long-lasting effects of cortical or thalamic stimulation is illustrated in Fig. 9.10B.

Giant aspiny interneurons, almost certainly cholinergic cells, are directly excited by cortical and thalamic stimulation (Wilson et al., 1990). These cells exhibit simple EPSPs, with fast rise times and little or no late response components. The maximal amplitudes of the EPSPs are much smaller than they are for the spiny neurons (see below). It is possible, however, to detect discrete components in the EPSPs in these neurons, especially with low-intensity stimuli. Thus the EPSPs evoked in the aspiny neurons appear to consist of the action of fewer axons than those in the spiny neurons, with each synaptic contact creating a larger EPSP as observed from the soma. These properties are consistent with there being relatively fewer excitatory afferent synapses on these neurons, and with the placement of these synapses on relatively proximal dendritic shafts and even somata. In vivo intracellular recordings of the responses of a cell that is probably the GABA/parvalbumin neuron have been reported by Kita (1993). These cells responded to cortical stimulation with a very powerful EPSP that gave rise to a burst of action potentials.

The synaptic effects of local striatal stimulation on each of the interneuron types has been studied in slices by Kawaguchi (1993b). Examples showing the responses of the major cell types are shown in Fig. 9.11. Cholinergic interneurons respond with a small, discrete EPSP, which can evoke a single action potential. GABA/parvalbumin neurons respond with an EPSP capable of evoking one or a burst of action potentials. Synaptic activation of the somatostatin/NOS neurons by local stimulation in slices can trigger a regenerative calcium-dependent, low-threshold response (LTS) that can develop into a self-sustained plateau potential, greatly outlasting the synaptic conductance. During the plateau potential, the cells are capable of generating repetitive fast action po-

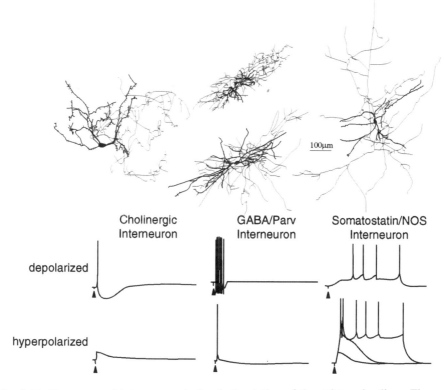

Fig. 9.11. Responses of interneurons to local stimulation of the striatum in slices. The upper traces are responses evoked when the cells were experimentally depolarized near spike threshold using constant current. The lower traces are responses evoked at more hyperpolarized levels. The three different responses shown for the somatostatin/NOS cell at hyperpolarized levels are for three different stimulus intensities, to show the development of the LTS and plateau potential. Examples of each neuron type is shown above the traces. Two different examples of the GABA/parvalbumin neuron are shown, one with a larger and one with a smaller dendritic field. The axons are shown in gray. [From Kawaguchi, 1993b, with permission.]

tentials. Thus, unlike any of the other neostriatal cells, these neurons have the capacity to set up a long-lasting response to relatively brief synaptic inputs.

ACTIONS OF SUBSTANTIA NIGRA INPUTS

Responses of spiny neurons to stimulation of the nigrostriatal afferents have been difficult to characterize. The nigrostriatal fibers are notoriously resistant to electrical stimulation, and they lie very close to other fiber systems that can produce large excitatory responses in the neostriatum (e.g., cortical efferent fibers in the cerebral peduncle and internal capsule). Simple stimulation of the nigrostriatal pathway therefore produces results that are difficult to interpret.

Early studies employing stimulation of substantia yielded mixed results. Using extracellular recordings, both excitatory and inhibitory responses were observed. It was difficult to prove in these studies that the responses observed in extracellular recording experiments were really due to the direct effect of the nigrostriatal axons, rather than indirect polysynaptic pathways within the neostriatum and between the neostriatum and related structures. Intracellular recordings were more consistent in showing excitation (see review by Kitai, 1981). Intracellular recordings provide a more direct measurement of the effect of stimulation because they allow visualization of subthreshold responses and a more direct view of the response to synaptic activation. The latency of the responses is also more accurately measured, because the synaptic responses are directly visible, rather than inferred from the latency of action potentials that may follow it by a variable additional delay. In these ways, the results of the intracellular recording experiments were more reliable, but when the antidromic conduction time of nigrostriatal neurons was measured, it was discovered to be much longer than the latency of the EPSP observed in striatal neurons after stimulation of the substantia nigra. Further analysis of the EPSPs observed in the intracellular recordings of nigrostriatal responses revealed that a large proportion of these were actually due to activation of fibers of passage (Wilson et al., 1982). This is shown schematically in Fig. 9.12A and B. Stimulation of the substantia nigra excites cortical axons passing through and near that region. Some of these give off collaterals in the striatum, producing a monosynaptic excitation when excited, and they can also excite other corticostriatal neurons, giving rise to a polysynaptic excitation of the neostriatal neurons. The polysynaptic excitation is removed if the cortex is removed acutely, but the direct axon collateral remains. Thus one can get a very simple monosynaptic response in the neostriatum upon substantia nigra stimulation in the acutely decorticate animal, but it is caused by corticostriatal, not nigrostriatal axons. Chronic decortication, which causes all cortical axons to degenerate after several days, allows stimulation of the nigrostriatal axons without the complication of cortical axons. Under these conditions (Fig. 9.12Ac), usually no clear synaptic response is seen at all. Thus, a synaptic response owing purely to the nigrostriatal pathway is difficult to demonstrate in an unambiguous way, even after removal of the confounding fibers of passage.

In parallel with these efforts to understand the nigrostriatal input, other investigators performed experiments employing ionophoretic application of dopamine and dopamine agonists to neostriatal neurons in vivo. These studies likewise produced mixed results. In most experiments, changes in firing rate due to dopamine application were recorded extracellularly, and the effect of dopamine on the cell was inferred from

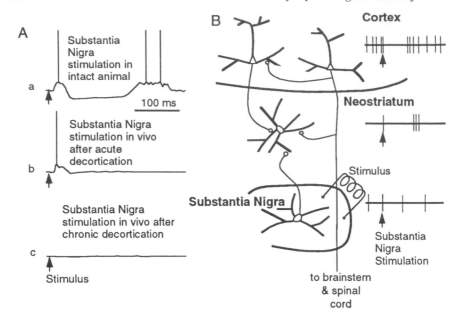

Fig. 9.12. Synaptic potentials evoked in spiny neurons by stimulation of the substantia nigra. **A:** Synaptic potentials in three different preparations. The trace in **a** shows the response evoked in intact animals, which resembles the response to cortical or thalamic stimulation. Immediately after removal or deactivation of cortical polysynaptic circuits, substantia nigra stimulation no longer evokes the late components of the response. After loss of cortical axons by degeneration after chronic cortical lesions, no reliable PSP response to substantia nigra stimulation is seen. **B:** The arrangement of cortical axons explains the responses in A. Substantia nigra stimulation evokes a monosynaptic excitation via axon collaterals of cortical neurons projecting to the brainstem and inadvertently excited by substantia nigra stimulation. These cells also evoke polysynaptic responses via their intracortical connections. The nigrostriatal projection axons, while present, produce no PSP in the striatal spiny neurons.

the firing rate changes. In these studies, some neurons increased their firing rate, while others decreased. In a smaller number of experiments, the effects of dopamine were observed more directly by intracellular recording. These experiments (Kitai et al., 1976b; Herrling and Hull, 1980) usually revealed depolarizations, often accompanied by a decrease in neuronal excitability and a decrease in firing rate. Understanding such unusual responses requires an analysis of the ionic mechanisms underlying them, and this analysis cannot be performed in the in vivo preparation.

For this reason, studies of the effects of the nigrostriatal input on neostriatal neurons have recently concentrated on the direct application of dopamine or dopaminergic agonists onto striatal neurons in vitro. These studies have not revealed an ionic conductance in spiny neurons that can be directly gated by dopamine. Even the D2 receptor, which in dopaminergic neurons of the substantia nigra can be shown to mediate a fast IPSP, owing to a potassium conductance increase (Lacey et al., 1987), has no such direct effects on spiny neurons (of the indirect pathway) that possess the D2 receptor. Instead, dopamine receptors, like muscarinic receptors on spiny neurons, act indirectly by altering the voltage-gated ion channels that are responsible for action potentials and for the dendritic properties of the cells. These effects do not lead to fast changes in membrane potential (hence the absence of PSPs in response to substantia nigra stimulation) and they are often not easily categorized as either excitatory or inhibitory. For example, D1a receptor activation raises the threshold for action potentials on spiny neurons (of the direct pathway) that possess this receptor by altering the availability of sodium channels responsible for action potentials (Surmeier et al., 1992). Because this will cause the cell to be less likely to fire action potentials, it could be considered to be a kind of inhibition. However, D1a receptor agonists also reduce the amplitude of a voltage-dependent potassium current that is activated by depolarization (Surmeier and Kitai, 1993). This slowly inactivating potassium conductance (I_{As}, see below) would normally oppose depolarization, so its reduction should make the spiny neuron more sensitive to synaptic depolarization. D2 receptor agonists produce opposite effects on spiny neurons, enhancing the voltage-sensitive potassium current and increasing the availability of sodium channels. Both D1a and D2 receptors reduce high voltage–activated calcium channels in spiny neurons (Surmeiter et al., 1995).

This diversity of effects is quite different from the direct effects of neurotransmitter-gated conductances that are generally thought to be associated with fast synaptic transmission. Two general points about these neuromodulatory effects of dopamine should be emphasized. First, the diversity of the neuromodulatory effects of dopamine produces a computationally rich kind of intercellular communication. This is no requirement that all of the effects of any one dopamine receptor should combine to create a simple net increase or decrease in excitability. Instead, this mechanism is capable of producing conditional changes in excitability that depend upon the presence of another input or the past history of synaptic excitation and inhibition. Second, it should be noted that this diversity is possible because these effects of dopamine are indirect, being mediated by intracellular signaling pathways (such as cyclic AMP and phospholipase C) that can interact with a variety of ion channels and other molecules, including the receptors for other neurotransmitters. Indeed, there is evidence that dopaminergic receptor activation can alter the sensitivity of glutamate receptors in the neostriatum. In slices of the rat neostriatum, dopamine acting at D1a receptors has been reported to reduce the sensitivity of neurons to non-NMDA glutamate agonists, while increasing the sensitivity to NMDA (e.g., Levine et al., 1995). The reader will recognize the possible relationship between this effect and the already described effects of dopamine on LTD and LTP in the neostriatum.

DENDRITIC PROPERTIES

The properties of dendrites constitute a theme running through most of the chapters of this book, and perhaps nowhere are they more important than in the spiny neurons of the neostriatum. In the analysis of the linear properties of dendrites, three electrophysiological parameters are particularly important: the input resistance (R_N), the membrane time constant (τ), and the electrotonic length of the dendritic tree (L). We will discuss how the spiny neuron has served as a case study for the experimental determination of these properties. This will give the student a greater appreciation for the crucial importance of the dendrites in determining the input–output characteristics of the spiny neuron.

For many neurons, one observes much higher input resistances when the cells are recorded in tissue slices than when recorded in intact animals. Two arguments are usually presented to explain this fact. First, tonic synaptic activity, which is generally lost in the preparation of the slices, will act to lower apparent input resistance by the opening of synaptic ionic conductance channels. Second, the damage done by the microelectrode is probably somewhat less under the mechanically more stable conditions of the in vitro recording chamber.

In the case of neostriatal spiny neurons, the input resistance recorded in slices is 20–60 Mohm, which in fact matches very well with that obtained in vivo (Sugimori et al., 1978; Kita et al., 1984; Bargas et al., 1988). This is probably because the most important influence on input resistance in spiny neurons is neither damage done by the electrode nor synaptic activity. The biggest determinant is instead the action of a fast anomalous rectification. This rectification can be seen by passage of current pulses of different amplitudes through the spiny neuron (Fig. 9.13). If the cell were to show no rectification, the input resistance (the ratio between the size of the voltage shift and the amplitude of the injected current that causes it) would remain constant regardless of the size of the current pulse (dotted line in the graph on the right in Fig. 9.13); i.e., increasing the size of the current pulse in constant steps would produce voltage deflections that also increase by constant steps. In contrast, the usual behavior of spiny neurons is illustrated by the curve shown on the right in Fig. 9.13. These cells show a marked anomalous rectification over their entire subthreshold range of membrane potentials. In anomalous rectification (also called inward rectification; see Chap. 2), input resistance decreases with increasing membrane polarization. In the voltage range near the resting potential and going more negative, the rectification is due to the action of a potassium conductance called g_{IRK}, which increases as the cell is hyperpolarized. Anomalous rectification also is apparent with current injections that move the membrane potential in the depolarizing direction; in this case it appears as a slowly developing depolarization (arrow in Fig. 9.13) superimposed upon the linear charging curve to depolarizing currents.

This ramp-like depolarizing response results from a combination of the slow inactivation of a voltage-dependent potassium conductance that is turned on as the cell is depolarized, and the activation of sodium conductance I_{Na} near spike threshold (Nisenbaum and Wilson, 1995). This can be seen in intracellular recording experiments employing the ion channel poison tetrodotoxin (TTX), which poisons sodium channels, and 4-amino pyridine (4-AP), which poisons the inactivating potassium channels found in spiny neurons. The effects of these drugs on the ramp-like depolarization are shown in Fig. 9.13 (bottom trace). TTX greatly reduces the ramp, indicating that a portion of the current causing it is carried by sodium channels (Chap. 2). A residual ramp-like response to depolarization is retained even when all sodium channels are blocked. Blockade of potassium channels with 4-AP totally blocks the ramp-like depolarization, whether it is given alone or in the presence of TTX. In addition, however, the early part of the response to depolarizing current is enhanced by 4-AP, and a distinct sag in the response is observed (Fig. 9.13). There are at least three voltage-dependent potassium conductances contributing to the subthreshold response of spiny neurons to depolarizing currents (Nisenbaum et al., 1996). They differ in their voltage-dependence and also in their time courses. One of the most important differences is their rate of inactivation. Two of the conductances, called g_{As} and g_{Af}, are transient in nature, due

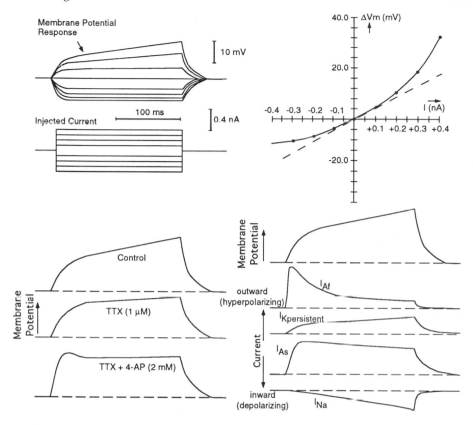

Fig. 9.13. The response of the neostriatal neuron to application of transmembrane current pulses through an intracellular microelectrode. At top left are shown the membrane potential response and injected current waveforms for current pulses of eight different but equally spaced intensities. The arrow in the largest response indicates the onset of the slow depolarizing membrane response, which is superimposed upon the linear portion of the response to depolarizing currents. At top right, a steady-state current-voltage relationship is shown. The dotted line indicates the behavior that would be expected of a linear neuron. The deviations from this line, both in the depolarizing and hyperpolarizing directions, are typical of that seen in neostriatal spiny neurons. At lower left are responses to large depolarizing currents, comparing control responses to those after poisoning of sodium channels with tetrodotoxin (TTX) and a combination of TTX and a selective blockade of inactivating, depolarization-activated potassium currents using 4-amino pyridine (4-AP). At lower right are the time courses of currents activated by a depolarizing current pulse in the absence of blockers.

to inactivation. These two differ in the rate of inactivation, with g_{Af} inactivating rapidly (tens of milliseconds) and g_{As} inactivating slowly (hundreds of milliseconds). The other conductances (called $g_{Kpersistent}$) are persistent, either not inactivating or inactivating with a time course of several seconds. As a group, they activate as the cell membrane approaches the action potential threshold, and they work together to cause the membrane resistance to decrease as the cell approaches spike threshold. The currents flowing through each of the conductances in response to a constant current pulse (as seen in computer simulations) are shown at bottom right in Fig. 9.13. Because some of these conductances inactivate, the membrane resistance decreases gradually over time after the cell is depolarized. This inactivation causes the gradual ramp-like depolarization seen with depolarizing current pulses. Thus the inactivation of the potassium conductance is the *cause* of the ramp depolarization, but much of the charge is carried by the sodium current, which is beginning to turn on in this same voltage range. Thus the rectification in the depolarizing direction is not apparent immediately after the onset of the current injection, but increases with time. In fact, the responses in the depolarizing direction do not really achieve steady state, but grow gradually until the neuron fires an action potential. In the hyperpolarizing direction, the onset of anomalous rectification in neostriatal spiny neurons is fast relative to the time constant of the neuron, so it affects the entire time course of the charging curve. (Anomalous rectification is not really an anomaly. It is actually quite common. It is called anomalous because it was not expected on the basis of the original biophysical theory of membranes.)

It is difficult to apply the linear cable theory to such a nonlinear cell. Certainly, the time constant of the cell cannot be a constant if the membrane resistivity is altered by any shift in membrane potential. It is therefore perhaps not surprising that there has been some disagreement about the time constants of the cells. Recent experiments in tissue slices using small current pulses (to minimize the effects of anomalous rectification) have yielded values near 5 ms for the time constant under these circumstances. It is quite possible to increase the time constant to 10 or 15 ms by depolarizing the cells slightly (Nisenbaum and Wilson, 1995), and longer time constants have been obtained with small changes in the extracellular potassium concentration (Bargas et al., 1988).

Again, using small current pulses in cells recorded in vitro, the electrotonic length of the equivalent cylinder of the dendrites has been measured to be about 1.5–1.8 length constants. This electrotonic length seems very long, and it is especially surprising in view of the relatively short dendrites of these cells (about 200 μm). This result is predicted by cable theory, however, because of the spiny nature of the dendrites. The dendritic spines create a very large surface area. Measurement of this area is made difficult by the small dimensions of the spines. These structures cannot be accurately measured in the light microscope (remember that the resolution of the light microscope allows measurements to the nearest 0.25 μm or thereabouts, while the stalks of dendritic spines can be as small as 0.1 μm).

Estimation of the surface areas of neostriatal spiny neurons has been accomplished using a combination of reconstruction of serial sections from electron micrographs and high-voltage electron microscopy (HVEM) of thick (5 μm) sections (Wilson, 1992). These measurements have shown that the dendritic field of spiny neurons cannot be approximated as a cylinder, or even a tapered cylinder. Its surface area is dominated by the dendritic spines, which are greatest at about 80 μm from the soma, where the dendritic spine density is highest, and taper off slowly to the tips of the dendrites. This distribution of surface area is shown in Fig. 9.14. Because the dendritic diameter does not change in proportion to the surface area, the leakage of current from the dendrites of the spiny neuron and the low-pass filtering effect of the dendrites are both increased dramatically by the presence of spines. This effect is shown in Fig. 9.15 for a spiny

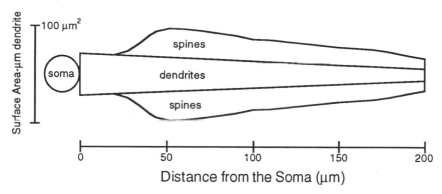

Fig. 9.14. The distribution of membrane on the neostriatal spiny neuron as a function of distance from the soma. The total somatic membrane is represented by the diameter of the circle marked soma. The remaining membrane area is shown as a density (square μm per μm of linear distance from the soma), and the contributions of the spines and dendrites are indicated. [From Wilson, 1986b, with permission.]

dendrite with different spine densities. It is clear that the addition of dendritic spines has a very large effect on the electrotonic length of the dendrites, even in neurons with very high membrane resistivities. When this is taken into account for the neostriatal spiny neurons, the measurements of time constant (t), electrotonic length (L), and input resistance (R_N) of the cells can be seen to agree on a membrane resistivity (R_M) ranging from about 5000 to 15,000 ohm-cm^2, depending on the state of the anomalous rectification (which itself depends upon membrane potential).

We are now in a position to pull together these considerations of dendritic properties and understand how they contribute to the input–output operations of the spiny neuron. The small amplitudes of individual synaptic responses on spiny neurons are probably due to their placement on dendritic spines and on the electrotonically long dendrites. The electrotonic length of the dendrites is actually not constant, but variable, due to the action of the voltage-sensitive conductances. When the cell is very hyperpolarized, the membrane conductance is dominated by the fast inwardly rectifying potassium conductance g_{IRK}. The membrane resistance is low because of this conductance and as a result, the electrotonic length of the dendrites is long. In computer simulations of the spiny neuron, isolated synaptic inputs have little effect at the soma under these circumstances (Wilson, 1992). The large maximal amplitude of the EPSPs evoked by afferent stimulation can be explained by the large number of inputs converging on each cell and by the nonlinear behavior of the neostriatal spiny neuron when depolarized by large inputs. When large numbers of synapses depolarize the neuron, the hyperpolarization-activated potassium current turns off, raising the membrane resistance. The effect of this will be to shorten the dendrites electrotonically and make the cell more sensitive to subsequent inputs, which will cooperate to depolarize the cell more, until the cell membrane escapes the influence of the hyperpolarization-activated potassium current by depolarizing beyond its activation range. As the membrane potential leaves the range dominated by g_{IRK}, it enters the membrane potential range in

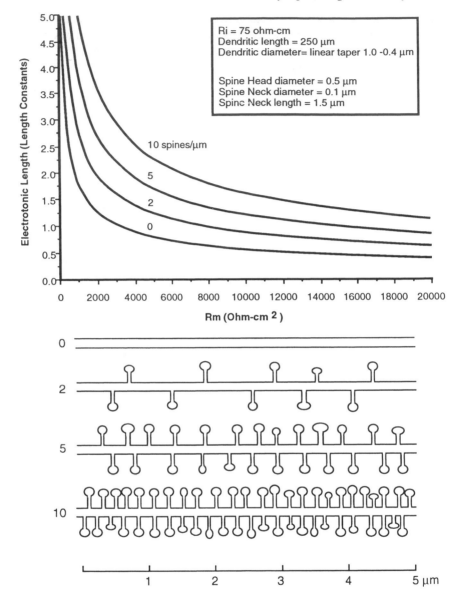

Fig. 9.15. Effect of dendritic spines on the relationship between membrane resistivity and electrotonic length for dendrites. Spine densities for each of the curves are indicated below. [Modified from Wilson, 1988, with permission.]

which the depolarization-activated potassium conductances turn on. The electrotonic length of the dendrites will increase again as the membrane potential approaches threshold, and the effects of individual synapses decreases.

These changes in electrotonic length and membrane potential during an episode of synaptic excitation are shown schematically in Fig. 9.16. An increase in excitatory synaptic input would then result in a small depolarization, which would evoke more potassium current, which in turn would oppose the synaptic excitation. A decrease in excitation would produce a corresponding decrease in potassium current. Thus the depolarization-activated potassium current acts to maintain the synaptic potential in a just subthreshold range, unless the synaptic excitation (like the depolarizing current injection in Fig. 9.13) is maintained for long enough to allow inactivation of the potassium conductance. Thus different sets of potassium channels dominate the dendritic properties of the spiny neurons at different membrane potentials. Near the resting potential, the cell is dominated by a potassium channel that increases when the cell is hyperpolarized; the dendrites are electrotonically long, but the neurons are extremely sensitive to depolarizing inputs if they are large enough to overcome the low membrane resistance and short length constant and escape the effects of the potassium conductance. Because of the electrotonic contraction that results from depolarization in this membrane potential range, all synaptic inputs placed more distal to a powerful input would be enhanced in importance. Once the membrane potential begins to approach the spike threshold however, other membrane conductances will be engaged. Unless

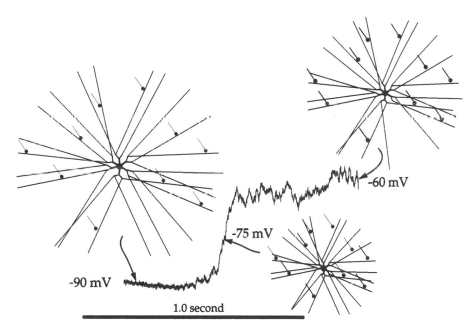

Fig. 9.16. Electrotonic expansion and contraction of the spiny cell dendritic tree during the course of synaptic excitation. During periods of relative synaptic quiescence, the electrotonic structure of the cell is extended due to the action of anomalous rectification. In the course of excitatory input, depolarization deactivates the rectification, causing an electrotonic collapse of the cell and a resulting increase in synaptic effectiveness. As the cell depolarizes rapidly, depolarization-activated potassium conductances cause the electrotonic structure of the cell to expand, and the cell achieves a relatively constant membrane potential at a level determined by the equilibrium between synaptic currents and the resulting potassium currents. This equilibrium point is on average below the spike threshold.

the depolarization is maintained for a long period (as in the case of injected current pulses), the input resistance of the cells will be dominated by the depolarization-activated potassium conductances. As these conductances are activated, they lead to another electrotonic expansion of the dendrites. Strong synaptic inputs will result in depolarization to a membrane potential at which the synaptic current is balanced by the potassium current. The membrane potential at which this will occur is determined by the voltage sensitivity and strength of the potassium conductance, and the strength of the synaptic excitation.

FUNCTIONAL OPERATIONS

It is clear that progress is being made toward a complete analysis of the synaptic connections, membrane properties, and cell morphology of the neostriatal spiny neuron. We turn finally to consider the insight this information provides into the firing patterns that underlie the normal functions of the neostriatum. In the case of the spiny neuron, a knowledge of its dendritic properties and their voltage-dependence is essential for the explanation of their natural pattern of firing.

NATURAL FIRING PATTERNS

Neostriatal spiny neurons exhibit a very characteristic firing pattern. Even in unanesthetized and behaving animals, the cells are usually silent. Occasionally, the cells fire a train of several action potentials that lasts from 0.1 to 2.0 sec, and then become silent once again (see Fig. 9.17, top). The train of action potentials is not really stereotyped enough to be called a burst. The discharge rate during the episode of firing usually does not become greater than 40/sec, and the cells usually do not fire rhythmically during the episode (suggesting that firing rate is not limited by spike afterpotentials). In behaving animals, these episodes of firing are sometimes locked to the onset of movements (e.g., DeLong, 1973; Kimura et al., 1984).

Why are the cells silent so much of the time? The answer to this question evaded investigators employing extracellular recording but was readily obtained when intracellular recordings in vivo became routinely available. Intracellular recording experiments show that when spiny neurons do fire, the train of action potentials arises from a prolonged episode of depolarization accompanied by an increased synaptic noise (Wilson and Groves, 1981). The depolarizing episodes also show several other revealing characteristics. They cannot be triggered by depolarizing current pulses; they cannot be terminated by hyperpolarizing current pulses; and they do not disappear when the cell is hyperpolarized below spike threshold by passage of current into the soma. In these ways, the depolarizing episodes are reminiscent of the period of depolarization that follows the long-lasting hyperpolarization after stimulation of neostriatal afferent pathways (see Figs. 9.10 and 9.12). This similarity suggests the possibility that the naturally occurring episodes of depolarization are caused by an increase in synaptic input to the neuron. When excited electrically, large numbers of afferent fibers are excited synchronously. Under more natural conditions, such large-scale synchrony in the corticostriatal or thalamostriatal pathway is unlikely. In anesthetized animals, and perhaps also in waking animals, there may, however, be local corticostriatal and thalamostriatal synchrony—that is, correlations in firing of small converging subsets of

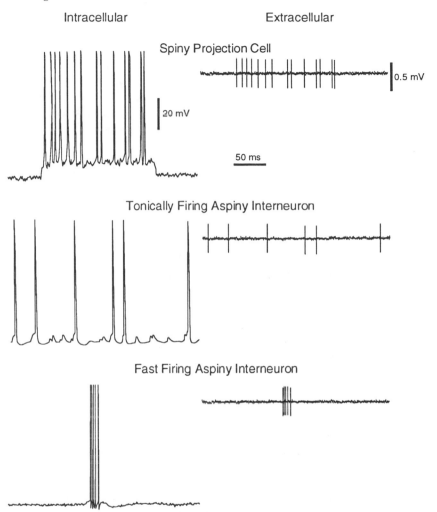

Fig. 9.17. Representative firing patterns of three kinds of neostriatal neurons. The patterns of activity as seen in extracellular recording are illustrated on the right, and the intracellular membrane potentials that lead to these firing patterns are illustrated on the left.

corticostriatal and thalamostriatal neurons that may be important for shaping the firing patterns of the cells.

Recently, in vivo intracellular recording experiments have revealed that the membrane potential achieved during the depolarizing episodes is not simply the envelope of converging synaptic input (Wilson and Kawaguchi, 1996). Blocking depolarization-activated potassium channels by intracellular injection of cesium caused the membrane potential during the depolarizing episodes to approach 0 mV (near the reversal potential for corticostriatal synapses). The membrane potential during the hyperpolarized episodes was almost unaffected. Of course, it was necessary to poison both sodium and calcium currents in the recorded neuron using intracellularly applied blockers, to prevent action potentials from interfering with the measurements. In the absence of subthreshold, voltage-dependent potassium currents, it was possible to measure the decrease in input resistance due to synaptic input during the depolarizing episodes. This showed that the depolarizations resulted from a very powerful synaptic input, and that the hyperpolarized episodes were periods of little or no synaptic input (either excitation or inhibition). The membrane potential during the depolarizations is held below spike threshold (on the average) by the potassium currents generated by synaptic excitation, rather than by synaptic inhibition. The mean subthreshold value of the membrane potential explains why the spiny neurons do not fire rhythmically during the depolarizations. Action potentials occur because of threshold crossings that occurred at unpredictable times during the depolarizations, and so interspike intervals in the depolarized state are highly variable. Still, while the membrane potential achieved and the firing rate maintained during the episodes of excitation does not accurately reflect the strength of the synaptic input, the timing and duration of the episodes of excitation are determined almost totally by the pattern of converging synaptic excitation on the spiny neurons.

Most neostriatal neurons are spiny cells, and nearly all recordings of single neurons that are obtained from the neostriatum are from spiny cells. It is therefore not always necessary to obtain anatomical verification of the cell type associated with responses that are common to most neurons. On the other hand, identification of firing patterns and synaptic responses of interneurons requires intracellular staining for the determination of interneuron type. Some recordings of identified *giant aspiny neurons*, almost certainly cholinergic interneurons, have been reported (Wilson et al., 1990). The firing pattern observed for these cells is illustrated in Fig. 9.17 (middle). They are tonically active cells, firing irregularly with average rates less than 20 hz. Action potentials from these cells arise from brief depolarizations that resemble unitary synaptic events. These vary in size, but are often as large as 5 mV. Action potentials arise from the largest of these, but often they are triggered by the summation of two or three. Thus in contrast to the spiny neurons, these cells may act to detect coincident activation in small numbers of afferent axons. At least some of these depolarizations are probably synaptic potentials evoked by afferent fibers, because stimulation of the cortex or thalamus can briefly increase the rate of their occurrence, whereas the rate falls during the period of long-lasting inhibition that is seen in spiny neurons. In extracellular recordings from behaving monkeys, neurons with firing patterns like that of the giant aspiny neuron have been reported to show a unique kind of response during execution of learned movements. Unlike the spiny neurons, which fire in relation to the movement itself, tonically firing neurons fire in relation to the sensory cue that triggers the movement (Kimura et al., 1984). This is not to say that the tonically active neurons are sensory cells. They do not respond to the same stimulus when it is not a signal for initiation of a movement, and the responses of these cells develop gradually during the acquisition of a learned movement (Graybiel et al., 1994). This firing pattern is also largely determined by the membrane properties of the neuron. Cholinergic neurons have resting membrane potentials (in the absence of input) within a few millivolts of the action potential threshold (Jiang and North, 1991; Kawaguchi, 1992). Contributing to this membrane potential is another kind of anomalous rectifier channel, the hyperpolarization-activated cation channel (h-channel). Because it conducts both potassium and sodium ions, this conductance gives rise to a current that reverses at a potential more depolarized than the normal resting potential (and more depolarized than spike threshold). This conductance turns on when the cell is hyperpolarized, however, and it does not inactivate. As a result, it contributes to the resting membrane potential, and has a net depolarizing effect. These cells also exhibit very large and long-lasting action potential hyperpolarizations. These tend to make the cell fire only once in response to EPSPs, and so contribute to the tendency of these cells to fire single spikes in response to discrete excitatory events. This combination of hyperpolarization-activated depolarizing current and large-spike afterhyperpolarizations is often associated with pacemaker cells, that is, cells capable of sustaining oscillations without rhythmic input. The cholinergic interneuron acts as a pacemaker in vitro, with only the application of a small amount of depolarizing current to get it started firing. In vivo, rhythmic firing is not common under most circumstances, presumably because the rhythm is interrupted by spikes evoked by synaptic potentials as described above.

Data on the firing patterns of the other interneurons in vivo are sparse. There are a few reports of bursting interneurons, and these cells have the morphological appearance of the GABA/parvalbumin neurons (Fig. 9.17, bottom). In slices, the GABA/parvalbumin interneuron has been shown to fire short-duration action potentials, to have powerful but short-lasting spike afterhyperpolarizations, and to fire at high frequencies with little spike-frequency adaptation in response to depolarization (Kawaguchi, 1993b). The other interneuron, the somatostatin/NOS neuron, has not been studied in vivo. The identification of these results in in vivo recordings and the description of their natural firing patterns, especially in behaving animals, are challenges for future work.

The end result of activity in the neostriatum must be expressed as a change in the activity of neurons in the globus pallidus and substantia nigra that receive an input from the neostriatum. Although the spiny neurons contain many peptides and other substances, physiological studies indicate that the primary fast effect of activity in spiny neurons is a GABAergic inhibition of the target cells. The cells in globus pallidus and in substantia nigra pars reticulata that are the target of this inhibition have very high rates of tonic activity. It is not clear whether excitatory input is required for these cells to fire as they do, but in any case, they usually fire rhythmically at a rate determined primarily by their own membrane characteristics (Nakanishi et al., 1991; Nambu and Llinàs, 1994). Inhibition exerted by (usually silent) neostriatal spiny neurons during their brief episodes of firing causes a momentary decrease in the rate of this tonic firing. The fast-firing cells of the globus pallidus and substantia nigra are themselves GABAergic neurons which exert a tonic inhibition on their target cells in the thalamus and superior colliculus (e.g., Deniau and Chevalier, 1985). Thus excitation of neostriatal spiny neurons leads to a disinhibition of the otherwise suppressed activity of neurons in the thalamus and superior colliculus.

COMPLEX INTEGRATIVE TASKS

Pauses in the firing of neurons in the globus pallidus and substantia nigra are observed in behaving animals, and the behavioral conditions that lead to their occurrence offer important clues to the function of the basal ganglia. An example from an experiment is shown in Fig. 9.18. In this experiment, the firing of substantia nigra neurons was

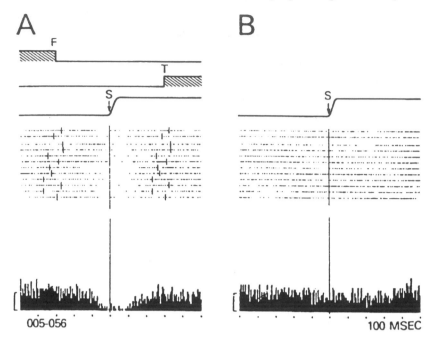

Fig. 9.18. The firing of a substantia nigra neuron during an eye movement to a remembered position as a part of a learned response (**A**), and during a comparable movement made spontaneously (**B**). [From Hikosaka and Wurtz, 1983, with permission.]

recorded simultaneously with eye movements in awake behaving monkeys. Responses to eye movements are shown under two conditions. In one, shown in Fig. 9.18A, the monkey has been trained to gaze at a point of flight (fixation point) until the light is turned off.

The timing of the fixation light is indicated by line F in Fig. 9.18A. After the fixation light is turned off, the monkey is to make a sudden eye movement (saccade) to a point at a new position, the target position. The target position must be remembered, because the target light is not turned on at the time that the eye movement is to be made. The target light is turned on later (at the time marked T in Fig. 9.18A), and the eye movement is made in the dark. In the other condition, there are no lights at all, and the monkey makes spontaneous movements. The experimenters selected trials in which the spontaneous movement was similar to the movements that occurred under the more controlled conditions. Responses under these conditions are shown in Fig. 9.18B. The firing of the neuron is indicated in two ways. In one it is shown as a series of horizontal raster lines, in which each line represents a single trial, and each point is a single action potential. All responses are aligned to the movement, with small vertical lines indicating the exact timing of the fixation and target lights for each trial. Below these is a histogram, in which the number of action potentials summed for all trials is plotted against time relative to the eye movement.

In both cases, eye movements occur in the dark, with no immediate sensory stimulus to trigger or guide them. The motor details of the eye movement are also the same in Fig. 9.18A and B. The responses of the neuron are dramatically different, however. In Fig. 9.18A, when the eye movement is to a remembered target and the performance of the eye movement is motivated by a reward, the substantia nigra neuron shows a profound pause in firing, almost certainly due to increased activity in the striatonigral pathway. In Fig. 9.18B, when the eye movement is unrelated to the task and unrewarded, the substantia nigra neuron shows no change in firing.

Although not all neurons responded in the way shown in Fig. 9.18, none of the substantia nigra responses studied by Hikosaka and Wurtz (1983) were readily categorized as strictly sensory or as motor. Instead, the responses of substantia nigra neurons during eye movements reflected more global circumstances of the experiment, including elements of what are usually considered cognitive and motivational, as well as sensory and motor, factors. These observations, and similar ones obtained in other nuclei of the basal ganglia, seem to give eloquent testimony to the convergence of afferent input from diverse cortical and thalamic regions and the processing of that information by the intrinsic circuits of the neostriatum.

10

OLFACTORY CORTEX

LEWIS B. HABERLY

The final three chapters will explore the neuronal circuitry of the cerebral cortex. This circuitry has a remarkable versatility that allows it to participate in brain functions as diverse as the recognition of faces, the perception of spatial relationships, the linking of smells with childhood memories, the comprehension of speech, the prediction of future events, and the generation of coordinated movement. Although such functions are not yet understood in terms of the operation of neuronal circuitry, the ongoing explosion in our knowledge of processes at the level of neurons and their connections is providing exciting clues concerning the nature of the underlying mechanisms. A feature of the cerebral cortex that has facilitated the analysis of neuronal processes is the presence of two phylogenetically old subdivisions whose architectures lend themselves to detailed morphological and physiological study. These are the *olfactory cortex* or *paleocortex*, and the *hippocampus* or *archicortex*. Although the *neocortex* forms the bulk of the human brain and subserves many of its more intriguing functions, its complexity makes analysis difficult. Fortunately, because all three types of cortex bear striking similarities in neuronal morphology, physiology, neurochemistry, and local circuitry, the hippocampus and olfactory cortex can be utilized as model systems for the study of certain questions of general interest for cortical function.

The olfactory cortex, with which our account of cerebral cortex will begin, is well suited for the analysis of questions related to mechanisms of sensory discrimination, including learning-related synaptic plasticity. It is also becoming widely used as a model to study epileptogenesis, to which it is highly susceptible. A particularly intriguing aspect of this cortex is its ability to process the exceedingly complex spatial and temporal patterns of neuronal activity that constitute the olfactory code (see Chap. 5), in spite of its comparatively simple structure. Other aspects of the olfactory cortex that have attracted interest are its similarity in architecture and other features to artificial "neural networks" with brain-like capabilities, and the presence of prominent oscillatory rhythms.

Olfactory cortex is usually defined as those areas that receive direct synaptic input from the olfactory bulb (Price, 1973). As in other types of cerebral cortex, many different olfactory cortical areas can be distinguished on the basis of anatomical differences (see reviews by Switzer et al., 1985; Price, 1987) (Fig. 10.1). The largest olfactory area, on which this chapter will focus, is the *piriform cortex* (also termed the

A. Olfactory bulb and cortex

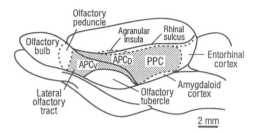

D. Prefrontal cortex, thalamus, hypothalamus

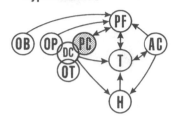

B. Olfactory bulb input

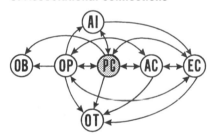

E. Hippocampal formation

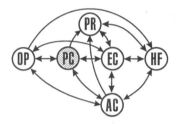

C. Associational connections

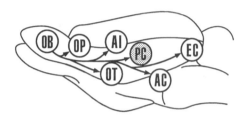

F. Cholinergic, Monoaminergic

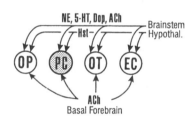

Fig. 10.1. Olfactory cortical areas and connections. **A:** Ventrolateral view of rat brain. The stippled area is the piriform cortex, the largest olfactory cortical area. APC_V, ventral part of anterior piriform cortex; APC_D, dorsal part of anterior piriform cortex; PPC, posterior piriform cortex. **B:** Projection areas of the olfactory bulb (OB). AC, amygdaloid cortex; AI, agranular insula; EC, entorhinal cortex; OP, olfactory peduncle (containing the anterior olfactory nucleus and other small olfactory cortical areas); OT, olfactory tubercle; PC, piriform cortex. **C:** Associational (cortico-cortical) connections between olfactory areas. **D:** Olfactory connections of the prefrontal (PF) cortex (orbital cortex and agranular insula), mediodorsal nucleus of the thalamus (T), and hypothalamus (H). DC, deep cells in PC, OT, and OP. **E:** Connections between olfactory cortex and the hippocampal formation (HF) and related areas. PR, perirhinal cortex. **F:** Cholinergic and monoaminergic inputs to olfactory cortex. NE, norepinephrine; 5-HT, serotonin; Dop, dopamine; Hst, histamine; ACh, acetylcholine. Double ended arrows in B–E indicate reciprocal connections that involve the same cortical subdivisions or nuclei.

primary olfactory cortex, pyriform cortex, and *prepyriform cortex*). Other cortical regions that receive direct olfactory bulb input include the *anterior olfactory "nucleus"* within the *olfactory peduncle,* the *olfactory tubercle,* the *entorhinal cortex,* the *agranular insula,* and cortical areas associated with the *amygdala* (Fig. 10.1B). Even though the agranular insula and entorhinal cortex are olfactory cortex as defined by olfactory bulb input, these areas are not paleocortex. They have a highly laminated structure like neocortex (5 or 6 layers, Krettek and Price, 1977a), and are considered to be transitional in form between neocortex and paleocortex.

NEURONAL ELEMENTS

CYTOARCHITECTURE

The piriform cortex, like hippocampal cortex, has been traditionally described in terms of three layers (Fig. 10.2). *Layer I* is a plexiform layer at the surface that contains dendrites, fiber systems, and a small number of neurons. It has been divided into a superficial part, *layer Ia,* that receives afferent fibers from the olfactory bulb by way of the *lateral olfactory tract* (LOT) (Fig. 10.1A), and a deep part, *layer Ib,* that receives *association* (cortico-cortical) *fibers* from other parts of the piriform cortex and other olfactory cortical areas (Price, 1973). *Layer II* is a compact layer of cell bodies. It can be divided into a superficial part, *layer IIa,* in which semilunar cells are concentrated, and a more densely packed deep part, *layer IIb,* that is dominated by pyramidal cell somata (Haberly and Price, 1978a). *Layer III* displays a gradient in structure from superficial to deep (Cajal, 1955; Valverde, 1965; Haberly, 1983). Its superficial part con-

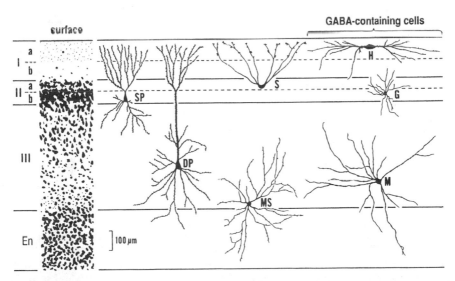

Fig. 10.2. Cytoarchitecture and major cell types of piriform cortex. SP, superficial pyramidal cell; DP, deep pyramidal cell; S, semilunar cell (pyramidal-type neuron without basal dendrites); MS, multipolar cell with spiny dendrites; M, multipolar cell with smooth dendrites; H, superficial horizontal cell, G, small globular-soma cell. MS and M cells are also found in the endopiriform nucleus (En); G cells are in all layers.

tains a moderately high density of pyramidal cells and large numbers of basal dendrites descending from pyramidal cells in layer II. With increasing depth, cell packing density falls, the density of myelinated axons increases, and multipolar cells become the predominant population. Layer III contains a high density of association axons that synapse on basal dendrites of pyramidal cells and other neuronal elements.

Deep to layer III is the *endopiriform nucleus*, which is interconnected with the overlying cortex. This nucleus, either alone or together with the deep part of layer III, has also been termed *layer IV* of the piriform cortex (O'Leary, 1937; Valverde, 1965). The predominant cell type in the endopiriform nucleus is a spiny multipolar neuron similar to those in the deep part of layer III (Tseng and Haberly, 1989a).

SUBDIVISIONS OF PIRIFORM CORTEX

Although the entire piriform cortex has the same basic three-layered organization, it is not homogeneous in structure. Many differences in both axonal connections and cytoarchitecture of different regions of piriform cortex have been described (Rose, 1928; Price, 1973; Haberly and Price, 1978a; Luskin and Price, 1983a; Behan et al., 1995). Although six or more regions could be readily differentiated on anatomical grounds, for the present account three subdivisions will be distinguished: the *posterior piriform cortex* (PPC), the *dorsal part of anterior piriform cortex* (APC_D), and the *ventral part of anterior piriform cortex* (APC_V). The LOT provides a convenient landmark for identification of these subdivisions. This tract covers the surface of the olfactory peduncle on emergence from the olfactory bulb, then narrows into a discrete band as it courses posteriorly over the surface of the ventral portion of piriform cortex (Fig. 10.1A). It ends at approximately the anterior to posterior midpoint of the piriform cortex. The PPC is the region posterior to the caudal end of the LOT, the APC_V is the strip of cortex that is deep to the LOT, and the APC_D is the strip that is lateral to the LOT (Fig. 10.1A). Architectural features that distinguish these subdivisions include a thick layer III in the PPC, a thick layer Ia and thin layer III in the APC_V, and a prominent layer IIa in the APC_D. Differences in connectivity are described in Basic Circuit, below.

In the neocortex there is much evidence that even subtle differences in cytoarchitecture and connections reflect functional specialization (Chap. 12). Although it can be speculated that the same is true for piriform cortex and other olfactory cortical areas, there has been no experimental analysis of this question.

INPUTS

The major source of *afferent input* to the piriform cortex is an uncrossed projection from mitral cells in the olfactory bulb. Cortical areas in the olfactory peduncle and the olfactory tubercle also receive a heavy projection from tufted cells in the olfactory bulb, but in piriform cortex this projection is substantial only to the anteroventral region (Haberly and Price, 1977; Skeen and Hall, 1977). Axons of mitral and tufted cells reach the piriform cortex and other olfactory areas by way of the LOT. Axons in this tract are predominantly myelinated but small in diameter (mean of 1.3 μm in the rat; Price and Sprich, 1975). Each LOT axon gives rise to many thin collaterals. These leave the LOT throughout its length and spread obliquely across the remaining surface of the piriform cortex and other olfactory areas (Devor, 1976). This mode of afferent input via tangentially spreading superficial fibers is shared by portions of the hippocampal formation, but contrasts with the neocortex where most input fiber systems enter from the deep white matter and terminate predominantly in spatially restricted "columns" (Chap. 12). However, so-called nonspecific thalamic afferents to neocortex do spread tangentially for long distances within layer I. Also, in the dorsal cortex of reptiles, which may be homologous to the neocortex of mammals, all afferent fibers spread tangentially in a superficial subzone of layer I, just as in the olfactory cortex (Hall and Ebner, 1970; Haberly, 1990a).

Central inputs to piriform cortex from subcortical structures originate in the basal forebrain, brainstem, thalamus, and hypothalamus (Haberly and Price, 1978a). Included are projections from areas that contain cholinergic, noradrenergic, sterotonergic, dopaminergic, and histiminergic cells (Fig. 10.1F); these are described in Neurotransmitters, below.

CONNECTIONS BETWEEN OLFACTORY CORTICAL AREAS

Extensive projections, termed *associational* fiber systems, link olfactory cortical areas on the same side of the brain (Fig. 10.1C). These include connections within and between the piriform cortex and other paleocortical areas that are detailed below (see Basic Circuit), and connections of the agranular insula and entorhinal cortex with paleocortical areas (Beckstead, 1979; Reep and Winans, 1982; Luskin and Price, 1983a,b). The olfactory tubercle is the only olfactory area that does not give rise to associational projections (Haberly and Price, 1978a). *Commissural* connections between olfactory areas on opposite sides are lighter and involve fewer areas than associational connections (Haberly and Price, 1978a,b; Luskin and Price, 1983a), but are sufficient to allow unilaterally delivered odors to drive unitary activity in the piriform cortex on the contralateral side (Wilson, 1997).

RETURN PROJECTIONS FROM OLFACTORY CORTEX TO OLFACTORY BULB

The piriform cortex and other olfactory cortical areas, with the exception of the olfactory tubercle, send projections back to the olfactory bulb (Figs. 10.1C, 10.5) (de Olmos et al., 1978; Haberly and Price, 1978a,b; Luskin and Price, 1983a; Carmichael et al., 1994). There has been no quantitative analysis of these projections, but like the return projections from sensory neocortex to thalamic nuclei, the reciprocal projections from olfactory cortex back to the olfactory bulb originate from a much larger number of cells than the afferent projection from the bulb to cortex. The reciprocal projections terminate primarily on granule cells that are inhibitory to mitral and tufted cells (Chap. 5). Although the functional roles of these pathway are unknown, an intriguing observation is that when they are blocked with a cooling probe in the olfactory peduncle, there are complex changes in the dynamics of oscillatory activity in the olfactory bulb (Gray and Skinner, 1988).

OUTPUTS

Many output pathways from the piriform cortex have been identified (Luskin and Price, 1983a; Price, 1985; Takagi, 1986; Price et al., 1991; Carmichael et al., 1994). The dominant pathways are heavy projections from pyramidal cells to other cortical areas (Fig. 10.1C–E). Cortical targets of these direct projections can be loosely grouped as areas implicated in certain forms of memory function (entorhinal cortex and perirhi-

nal cortex; see Staubli et al., 1986 and Chap. 11), prefrontal areas thought to be involved in complex discriminative processes (orbital and insular cortex; see Schoenbaum and Eichenbaum, 1995), amygdaloid areas that play a central role in the control
of emotions and visceral functions, and the olfactory tubercle, which has a close association with the striatum (Young et al., 1984).

Subcortical targets of the piriform cortex (Fig. 10.1D) include the hypothalamus
(Smithson et al., 1989) and the mediodorsal nucleus of the thalamus (Price, 1985, 1987).
A recent study has shown that the piriform cortex provides input by way of the
mediodorsal nucleus to the same prefrontal areas to which it projects directly (Ray and
Price, 1992). This projection originates from a relatively small number of predominantly deep cells that are concentrated in the medial part of the piriform cortex and the
olfactory tubercle (DC in Fig. 10.1D; Price, 1985; 1987). A light return projection from
the thalamus originates in the nucleus reuniens (Datiche et al., 1995).

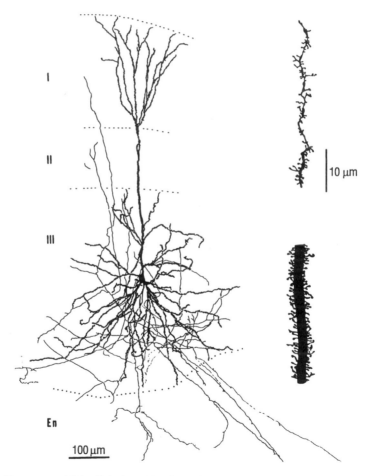

Fig. 10.3. Deep pyramidal cell in layer III of rat piriform cortex stained by intracellular dye injection. Fine processes are axon collaterals. Details of distal (top) and proximal apical dendrite
are at right. [Reproduced from Tseng and Haberly, 1989a, with permission.]

PRINCIPAL NEURON

Pyramidal cells are considered to be the principal neurons in all three types of cerebral cortex by virtue of their extensive dendritic trees and axons that project to other areas. As in the neocortex and hippocampus, pyramidal cells in the piriform cortex and other olfactory cortical areas have several distinctive features, as shown in Figs. 10.2, 10.3, and 10.4 (Haberly and Price, 1978a,b; Haberly, 1983; Haberly and Feig, 1983). At the light-microscopic level these include an *apical* dendritic tree that is directed toward the cortical surface, a *basal* tree that radiates from the cell body, a profusion of small *dendritic spines* on apical and basal dendrites, and an axon that is deep-directed at its point of origin. Pyramidal cells in all three types of cerebral cortex also display similar synaptic relationships, pharmacology, and physiological features.

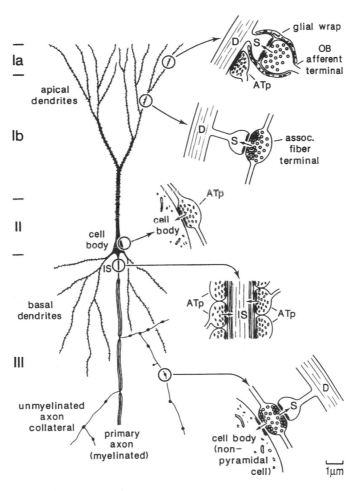

Fig. 10.4. Synaptic relationships of pyramidal cells in piriform cortex. AT$_P$, axon terminal with pleomorphic vesicles; D, dendritic shaft; IS, axon initial segment; OB, olfactory bulb; S, dendritic spine.

Two populations of pyramidal cells can be distinguished in the piriform cortex: *superficial pyramidal cells* (cell SP in Fig. 10.2), whose cell bodies are tightly packed in layer II, and *deep pyramidal cells* (cell DP in Fig. 10.2; see also Fig. 10.3), whose cell bodies are found in layer III at progressively lower density, with increasing depth from layer II. Morphologically, these two populations are virtually indistinguishable except for the lengths of their apical dendritic trunks. Physiologically, however, they display differences in membrane properties and synaptic responses as described below (Synaptic Actions).

The *apical dendrites* of most SP and DP cells arborize into secondary branches near the border between layers I and II. As a consequence, the lengths of apical trunks are determined by the depths of their somata. Most DP cells have single, long apical trunks (Fig. 10.3) whereas SP cells have short apical trunks (Fig. 10.2) or secondary dendrites that extend directly from cell bodies, as in layer II of the neocortex (Peters and Kaiserman-Abramof, 1970; Ghosh et al., 1988). The apical dendrites of SP and DP cells typically extend through both layers Ia and Ib to the cortical surface. *Basal dendrites* of SP cells are predominantly deep-directed and can extend for several hundred microns. The primary axons of pyramidal cells give rise to many thin collaterals that synapse in the vicinity of parent cells as well as at greater distances.

At the superficial border of layer II there are pyramidal-type neurons that resemble granule cells in the dentate gyrus (Chap. 11) and phylogenetically primitive pyramidal cells (Sanides and Sanides, 1972), by virtue of having apical but no basal dendrites (Calleja, 1893). Somata of these *semilunar* or forked cells are concentrated in layer IIa (Fig. 10.2; Haberly and Price, 1978a). Ultrastructurally, somata of semilunar cells resemble pyramidal cells (Haberly and Feig, 1983), and like pyramidal cells they have spiny dendrites and deep-directed axons. Semilunar cells, however, give rise to distinctive, large flattened spines in layer Ia (Haberly, 1983) that contrast with the tiny spines typical of pyramidal cells. An intriguing feature of semilunar cells is that they die within 24 hours following removal of the olfactory bulb (Heimer and Kalil, 1978).

INTRINSIC NEURONS

As in all parts of the cerebral cortex, studies with the Golgi staining method (O'Leary, 1937; Cajal, 1955; Valverde, 1965; Haberly, 1983) have revealed many different morphologically distinguishable types of nonpyramidal neurons in the piriform cortex. However, until these morphological data are combined with experimental data on connections, physiological properties, and neurochemistry, it will not be possible to determine how many functionally different neuronal populations are present. The present account will be restricted to a few distinctive types of nonpyramidal cells that clearly subserve different functions.

Multipolar Cells. In the deep part of layer III and the subjacent endopiriform nucleus, a large proportion of neurons have a multipolar appearance by virtue of dendrites that radiate in all directions and are thick at their origins (cells MS and M in Fig. 10.2). Cell bodies of these cells are on the same order of size as pyramidal cells (10–15 μm in mean diameter). Dendrites of many deep multipolar cells are several hundred microns in length, but only rarely extend superficial to layer III.

Several populations of deep multipolar cells can be distinguished. *Spiny multipolar cells* resemble DP cells in morphology and physiology—the only obvious difference being the lack of an apical dendrite (cell MS in Fig. 10.2). They give rise to a profusion of small spines (Tseng and Haberly, 1989a), probably use glutamate as a neurotransmitter (Hoffman and Haberly, 1993), and have voltage-dependent channels like those on DP cells (Tseng and Haberly, 1989b). Spiny multipolar cells in the endopiriform nucleus give rise to a dense axonal plexus (M. Behan, P. Sachdev, and L.B. Haberly, in preparation) that appears to extensively interconnect this cell population. Since these cells are excitatory, *regenerative positive feedback* can develop in the endopiriform nucleus when inhibition is compromised, leading to the generation of large, abnormal *epileptiform potentials* (Hoffman and Haberly, 1993). This circuitry may explain, in part, the high susceptibility of the nucleus and deep portion of the piriform cortex to the initiation of abnormal seizure activity (Piredda and Gale, 1985; Hoffman and Haberly, 1993).

A second population of deep multipolar cells has sparsely spiny, moderately varicose dendrites (cell M in Fig. 10.2). In Golgi material, axons from these cells have been observed to ascend to layers I and II of piriform cortex (O'Leary, 1937; Valverde, 1965). Indirect physiological (Satou et al., 1983a) and immunocytochemical evidence (Haberly et al., 1987; Kubota and Jones, 1992) suggests that they are GABAergic and participate in feedback inhibition of pyramidal cells.

Small Globular Cells. Small stellate cells with globular somata (cell G in Fig. 10.2) are found in all layers of the piriform cortex (Haberly, 1983). These cells mediate GABAergic inhibition as indicated by the presence of GABA and its synthetic enzyme, glutamic acid decarboxylase (GAD), as well as high-affinity GABA uptake (Haberly et al., 1987). Dendrites are fine in caliber, nearly spine-free, and originate abruptly from cell bodies, giving rise to the globular appearance. Intracellular injection of a small number of these cells in layer I has revealed unmyelinated, highly branched axons that arborize locally in layer I (Ekstrand and Haberly, 1995).

Superficial Horizontal Cells. Highly distinctive horizontal cells are found in layer Ia, almost exclusively in the vicinity of the LOT in the APC (cell H in Fig. 10.2). In the opposum, where these cells have been studied by Golgi impregnation, electron microscopy, and immunocytochemical staining (Haberly, 1983; Haberly and Feig, 1983; Haberly et al., 1987), they are the largest neurons in the cortex, give rise to the largest-diameter axons, have thick, horizontally directed dendrites that are largely confined to layer Ia, and large somatic spines. They all contain GABA and GAD, although unlike other populations of GABAergic cells in piriform cortex, they do not exhibit high-affinity uptake of GABA (Haberly et al., 1987). These cells bear a resemblance to Cajal-Retzius cells, which are numerous in embryonic neocortex, but largely disappear before adulthood. In the rat, the same population of cells is clearly recognizable by virtue of their location under the LOT and their large-caliber, superficially arborizing dendrites that are often bipolar in form, but they lack somatic spines (Ekstrand and Haberly, 1995; Ekstrand et al., 1996).

CELL POPULATIONS

The number of pyramidal cells in the piriform cortex has not been determined, but probably exceeds 10^6. This contrasts with the much smaller number of mitral cells (on the order of 5×10^4) that provide most of the afferent sensory input. In view of the highly branched nature of mitral cell axons (Scott, 1981; Luskin and Price, 1982; Ojima et al., 1984) and the spatially distributed projection pattern of the LOT (see Horizontal Organization, below), each mitral cell clearly provides synaptic input to a very large number of pyramidal cells, although again, there has been no quantitative analysis. This situation contrasts sharply with the olfactory receptor input to the olfactory bulb where unbranched axons from the exceedingly large number of receptor neurons converge onto a much smaller number of principal cells (Chap. 5).

SYNAPTIC CONNECTIONS

In general, synaptic relationships in the piriform cortex (Fig. 10.4) closely resemble those in both the hippocampal cortex and neocortex. As in these other areas, two major categories of synapses can be distinguished: those with *asymmetrical (Gray type I)* contacts with associated spherical vesicles, many of which use glutamate as an excitatory neurotransmitter (e.g., afferent and association fiber terminals in Fig. 10.4), and those with *symmetrical (Gray type II)* contacts with associated pleomorphic vesicles, many of which mediate GABAergic inhibitory postsynaptic currents (IPSCs) (ATp in Fig. 10.4).

On pyramidal cells, asymmetrical synapses are concentrated on *dendritic spines* and completely excluded from cell bodies and axon initial segments (Haberly and Feig, 1983; Haberly and Presto, 1986). The dendritic spines that receive these contacts have predominantly small terminal knobs, thin necks, and a *spine apparatus* (Haberly and Feig, 1983). Symmetrical synapses are found at high density on axon initial segments and at a lower density on cell bodies and the shafts of both apical and basal dendrites out to their distal ends (Haberly and Feig, 1983; Haberly and Presto, 1986). In spite of the relatively low density of symmetrical synapses on dendrites, the total number is much higher than on cell bodies and initial segments because of the much greater membrane area.

BASIC CIRCUIT

LAMINAR ORGANIZATION

A striking feature of piriform cortex, which is largely responsible for the relative ease with which its circuitry can be analyzed, is a precise organization of different fiber systems and other neuronal elements over depth. This is especially apparent in layer I where different fiber systems terminate in different sublayers (Fig. 10.5). Afferent axons arriving in the LOT synapse exclusively in layer Ia; association fiber systems from the piriform cortex synapse exclusively in layer Ib (Price, 1973). The sharply defined boundary between these two sublayers can be visualized with the Timm stain, which selectively stains layer Ib, in part at least, as a result of the presence of zinc in synaptic terminals of association fibers (Friedman and Price, 1984).

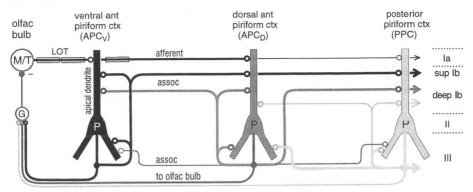

Fig. 10.5. Basic circuit for piriform cortex: excitatory connections of superficial pyramidal cells (P). Each schematic cell represents the entire population of superficial pyramidal cells within a subdivision. Line width denotes relative density of axonal projections. The small open circles represent excitatory synapses. Assoc, association axons; APC$_V$, ventral part of anterior piriform cortex that is deep to the lateral olfactory tract; APC$_D$, dorsal part of anterior piriform cortex; PPC, posterior piriform cortex; M/T, mitral and tufted cells in the olfactory bulb; G, granule cells in the olfactory bulb.

Afferent axons excite SP and DP cells through synapses on distal segments of their apical dendrites; association axons excite *the same pyramidal cells* through synapses on proximal and middle segments (Fig. 10.4; Haberly and Bower, 1984). Both afferent and association fibers also excite GABAergic cells in layer I (Ekstrand and Haberly, 1995). Semilunar cells are excited by afferent synapses on their distal apical segments; preliminary evidence indicates that they are also excited by association fibers (J.J. Ekstrand and L.B. Haberly, unpublished).

The relative thickness of layers Ia and Ib varies over a broad range in different parts of the piriform cortex and in different olfactory cortical areas (Price, 1973). Schwob and Price (1978) have provided evidence that the density of afferent terminals is proportional to the thickness of layer Ia, thereby greatly extending the range for relative strength of synaptic inputs from association and afferent fibers in different regions. This relative strength will be termed the *association-to-afferent-dominance ratio*. This ratio varies in rough proportion to distance from the LOT. Within the piriform cortex the ratio is lowest in APC$_V$ (deep to the LOT), intermediate in APC$_D$ (adjacent to the LOT), and increases from intermediate to high with increasing distance from the LOT in the PPC. In other olfactory cortical areas it is highest in the entorhinal cortex—the most distant area from the LOT, intermediate in the amygdaloid cortex that is near the caudal end of the LOT, and increases from intermediate in the lateral part of the olfactory tubercle that is adjacent to the LOT, to high in its medial part that is far-removed from the LOT.

Within layer Ib there is a further laminar organization: association fibers from different parts of the piriform cortex synapse at different depths (Figs. 10.5, 10.6; Luskin and Price, 1983a,b). Long association fibers from pyramidal cells in piriform cortex can also synapse extensively in layer III. As illustrated in Fig. 10.6, each projection to piriform cortex from an outside area has a distinctive laminar pattern of termination

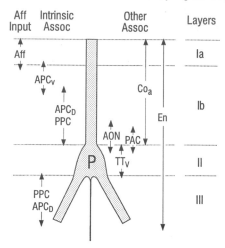

Fig. 10.6. Summary of the depth distributions of synaptic inputs to superficial pyramidal cells (P) in piriform cortex from afferent fibers (Aff Input, far left), intrinsic association fibers in piriform cortex (Intrinsic Assoc, left of cell), and associational inputs from other olfactory cortical areas and the endopiriform nucleus (Other Assoc, right of cell). The indicated distribution for each input is the depth of heaviest termination. APC_V and APC_D, ventral and dorsal subdivisions of the anterior piriform cortex; PPC, posterior piriform cortex; PAC, periamygdaloid cortex; AON, anterior olfactory "nucleus" (cortical area in the olfactory peduncle); Co_a, anterior cortical nucleus of the amygdala; En, endopiriform nucleus; TT_V, ventral tenia tecta.

(Luskin and Price, 1983a,b). Unlike the intrinsic associational connections of piriform cortex that are excluded from layer Ia and light in layer II, these projections can extend through the full depth of layer I or be concentrated in layer II.

The myelinated axons of pyramidal cells in piriform cortex typically give rise to many unmyelinated collaterals within a few hundred microns of their origin. These collaterals radiate through layer III, establishing a large number of synapses in the vicinity of the parent neuron. As described below, the extent to which association axons synapse in layer III over longer distances is a function of their sites of origin. Anatomical and physiological studies have provided evidence that association axons in layer III, both locally and at long distances, synapse on basal dendrites of SP cells (Haberly and Presto, 1986; Rodriguez and Haberly, 1989; Ketchum and Haberly, 1993a; Fig. 10.5). Electron microscopic observations on intracellularly stained neurons have revealed that these axons also synapse on nonpyramidal neurons in the vicinity of parent neurons, particularly in the deep part of layer III (Figs. 10.4, 10.7; Haberly and Presto, 1986). The extent to which association axons synapse on nonpyramidal cells over longer distances, and on DP cells at any distance, is unknown.

Semilunar cells (S in Fig. 10.2) also give rise to long associational projections, particularly to areas outside the piriform cortex, but they do not project to the opposite hemisphere or to the olfactory bulb (Haberly and Price, 1978a).

HORIZONTAL ORGANIZATION

Afferents. In contrast to the precise restriction of afferent fibers in depth, in the horizontal dimension (parallel to the cortical surface), the afferent input to piriform cortex

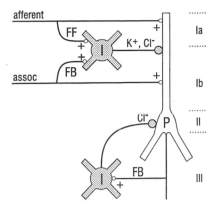

Fig. 10.7. Basic circuit for piriform cortex: inhibitory connections. I, GABAergic interneurons; P, superficial pyramidal cell; FB, excitatory input to interneuron mediating feedback inhibition; FF, excitatory input to interneuron mediating feedforward inhibition. Small open circles denote excitatory synapses; larger shaded circles denote inhibitory synapses. Cl⁻, postsynaptic inhibition mediated by GABA$_A$ receptors via increase in Cl⁻ conductance; K⁺, postsynaptic inhibition mediated by GABA$_B$ receptors via increase in K⁺ conductance; Assoc, association fibers.

from the olfactory bulb is highly distributed spatially. Rather than a systematic point-to-point topographical ordering as observed in the afferent input to sensory areas of neocortex (Chap. 11), single mitral cells project to broad regions of the olfactory cortex. Nevertheless, the distribution of afferents is not uniform, and ongoing studies continue to reveal an increasing degree of order.

One form of order has been revealed by the placement of small injections of retrograde axonal tracer in different olfactory cortical areas. From such injections, mitral cells are labeled in all parts of the olfactory bulb, but they are not evenly distributed (Haberly and Price, 1977; Scott et al., 1980). The labeled cells tend to be concentrated in broad, ill-defined regions.

A second form of order that has been observed in the horizontal dimension is a "patchiness" in the distribution of afferent arbors (Buonviso et al., 1991). In this study, in which injections of anterogradely transported tracer were limited to a small number of mitral cells (2–15), projections to the anterior portion of piriform cortex and other olfactory cortical areas included small, widely spaced patches of terminal branches. Similar patches had been previously observed in partially filled axonal arbors from intracellularly injected mitral cells (Ojima et al., 1984). These observations raise the possibility that the afferent input to certain parts of olfactory cortex may have a discontinuous distribution like that of inputs to primary sensory areas in neocortex (Chap. 11).

Association Fiber Systems. As in the case of the afferent system from the olfactory bulb, a remarkable feature of association fiber systems in olfactory cortex is their spatially distributed nature. Thus, small injections of retrogradely transported tracer label cell bodies over widespread areas in piriform cortex and other olfactory cortical areas (Haberly and Price, 1987a). Similarly, small injections of anterograde tracer label terminal arborizations that extend over broad areas, again with no hint of a systematic point-to-point "mapping" between regions (Luskin and Price, 1983a). However, as in the case of the afferent input, there is a broadly defined order in these systems. Each subdivision projects to a different combination of olfactory cortical areas and displays a unique laminar pattern for the cells of origin and the synaptic terminations of the association fibers to which it gives rise (Haberly and Price, 1978a,b; Luskin and Price, 1983a,b). Although many details are lacking and some of the supporting evidence is preliminary, the following principles of organization can be tentatively proposed.

First, the laminar pattern of termination of association fibers is determined by the area of origin and the cells of origin, not the area of termination. For example, the projection from SP cells in the APC_V is concentrated in the superficial part of layer Ib in the three subdivisions of piriform cortex and all other olfactory cortical areas (Behan et al., 1995).

Second, the synaptic terminations of association fibers from SP cells in the different subdivisions of piriform cortex are systematically ordered on the dendrites of other SP cells (Haberly and Price, 1978a; Luskin and Price, 1983b; Ketchum and Haberly, 1993a; Behan et al., 1995). This order follows the association-to-afferent-dominance ratio. As summarized in Fig. 10.6 (left side), association fibers from SP cells in the APC_V, where this ratio is lowest, synapse on mid-apical dendrites in *superficial Ib*, adjacent to the afferent input on distal segments in layer Ia. The associational input from the APC_D, where the ratio is intermediate, is concentrated on proximal apical dendritic segments in the mid to deep part of layer Ib (hereafter termed *deep Ib*) and in layer III at the depth of SP cell basal dendrites. Finally, the projection from the PPC where the ratio is the highest in piriform cortex, is concentrated in layer III, with a lighter component in deep Ib. A cortical area that has been termed *periamygdaloid cortex* (PAC) by Krettek and Price (1978), but considered as part of the piriform cortex by others (Paxinos and Watson, 1986), may constitute a fourth component of this system. The associational projection of this area to the piriform cortex is concentrated at the deep border of layer I (Fig. 10.6, right).

This laminar arrangement is potentially significant from a functional standpoint because of the systematic ordering of synaptic inputs both with respect to distance from cell bodies and to distance from the afferent input zone (Fig. 10.6). Since action potentials are initiated in the vicinity of the cell body in SP cells, the distance of excitatory inputs from the cell body would have an effect on their ability to influence cell output (see Dendritic Properties, below). Thus, excitatory current generated by synapses of association fibers from pyramidal cells in regions with a high association-to-afferent ratio would be expected to exert a stronger action on the generation of action potentials than current generated by synapses from pyramidal cells in regions where inputs are afferent dominated.

The position of a given association fiber input relative to the afferent input zone, and to inputs from other association fiber systems, could have a major impact in learning-related adjustments in synaptic efficacy. That is because the capacity for associative long-term potentiation is a strong function of the distance between simultaneously activated excitatory inputs (see Synaptic Actions, below). Thus, for example, under conditions where this process is enabled, a strong burst of activity in afferent fibers would potentiate synapses of weakly activated association fibers from the APC_V

to a greater degree than those from the APC$_D$ that are positioned further from the afferent input zone. Similarly, the simultaneous activation of synapses from the APC$_V$ and APC$_D$ would have a stronger mutually reinforcing action than the simultaneous activation of synapses from the APC$_V$ and PPC that are further removed spatially.

The third principle of organization is that associational connections between the subdivisions of piriform cortex display a marked anterior–posterior asymmetry. Whereas all three subdivisions have extensive *intrinsic* associational connections (i.e., projections to "themselves"), the associational connections between the APC and PPC are predominantly one-way. That is, both subdivisions of the APC project heavily to the PPC, but the return projection from the PPC is comparatively light (Haberly and Price, 1978a; Luskin and Price, 1983a). A similar organization is observed in the intrinsic connections of the endopiriform nucleus. This nucleus has extensive, long associational connections (Krettek and Price, 1977b), but like those in the overlying piriform cortex, the posteriorly directed component is heavier than the anteriorly directed one (M. Behan, P. Sachdev, L.B. Haberly, in preparation). The commissural connections of piriform cortex also display an anterior–posterior asymmetry: the PPC receives commissural input from the opposite APC, and the APC receives commissural input from the opposite anterior olfactory nucleus (Haberly and Price, 1978a).

The fourth principle of organization is that the anterior-posterior asymmetry in the intrinsic associational connections within piriform cortex may reflect a larger order for the entire olfactory cortex. The associational inputs to the cortical areas in the vicinity of the LOT from the anterior olfactory "nucleus" (AON), APC, PPC, and entorhinal cortex display an organization that, again, appears to be correlated with the association-to-afferent-dominance ratio (see Fig. 5 in Haberly and Price, 1978a). For example, the lateral part of the AON, where this ratio is low, projects to the APC$_V$ where the ratio is also low. In contrast, the PPC, where the ratio is high, avoids the APC$_V$, projects lightly to the APC$_D$ and lateral part of the olfactory tubercle where the ratio is intermediate, but projects heavily to strips of cortex that are further removed from the LOT that also have high ratios (the insular cortex and medial parts of the olfactory tubercle and peduncle).

Finally, single pyramidal cells in piriform cortex have multiple synaptic targets. Indirect evidence from studies with anatomical tracers (Haberly and Price, 1978a) and direct visualization by intracellular injection of single neurons (Haberly and Bower, 1984; D.M.G. Johnson, M. Behan, and L.B. Haberly, unpublished results) has revealed that individual cells can give rise to both associational and commissural fibers, and that associational projections from single cells can extend in both anterior and posterior directions and terminate in the piriform cortex, other olfactory cortical areas, and the olfactory bulb.

INHIBITORY SYSTEMS

Recent physiological studies have shown that synaptically mediated inhibitory processes in the piriform cortex, as in the other types of cerebral cortex, are diverse and complex (see Synaptic Actions, below). These studies have revealed inhibitory interneurons in feedforward and feedback loops, fast and slow inhibitory processes mediated by Cl^- and K^+, inhibitory inputs to dendrites as well as to cell bodies, and inhibition of inhibitory interneurons.

GABA-containing cells with dendrites in layer Ia are candidates for mediating *feed-forward inhibition*; i.e., inhibition that is tied to input as opposed to output fiber systems (Fig. 10.7). Both large superficial horizontal cells and small globular-soma cells (cells H and G in Fig. 10.2) could mediate feedforward inhibition. The large horizontal cells can be postulated to mediate inhibition at short latency because of their specializations that would decrease synaptic relay time: a position subjacent to myelinated afferent fibers in the LOT, afferent input to cell bodies, thick dendrites, and large-diameter myelinated axons. These cells give rise to many bouton-studded axon collaterals in layer I, which suggests that they synapse in this layer and mediate feedforward inhibition onto apical dendrites of pyramidal cells (Ekstrand et al., 1996).

Like large horizontal cells, superficially placed globular-soma cells have dendrites that are concentrated in layer Ia, indicating that they also mediate a relatively selective feedforward inhibition. Axons of these cells can arborize over a restricted depth range in layer I, perhaps allowing selective modulation of integrative or plastic processes in specific dendritic segments of pyramidal cells (Ekstrand and Haberly, 1995).

Since pyramidal cell axons are distributed to all layers with the exception of Ia, all but the most superficially placed GABA-containing cells are candidates for the mediation of *feedback (recurrent) inhibition*; i.e., inhibition that is tied to output and can therefore serve as an "auto-volume control" to regulate system excitability (Fig. 10.7). Biedenbach and Stevens (1969) first postulated that deep multipolar cells subserve this function. This hypothesis has been supported by additional indirect physiological evidence (Satou et al., 1983b), and by anatomical demonstrations that many of these cells are GABAergic (Haberly et al., 1987), that pyramidal cell axons synapse on their dendrites (Haberly and Presto, 1986), and that their axons ascend to layer II (O'Leary, 1937; Valverde, 1965) and give rise to GABA-containing boutons in "basket" arrays around pyramidal cell somata (Kubota and Jones, 1992). Globular-soma and small multipolar cells in layers Ib, II, and III may also contribute to feedback inhibition. Since many interneurons in layer I have dendrites that span both layers Ia and Ib (Haberly, 1983; Ekstrand and Haberly, 1995), it would appear that there are neurons that participate in both feedback and feedforward inhibition (Fig. 10.7).

Physiological evidence indicates that inhibitory interneurons synapse on other inhibitory interneurons in addition to pyramidal cells (Fig. 10.7; Satou et al., 1982; Ekstrand and Haberly, 1995). Symmetrical synapses and GABA-containing boutons have been observed on somata and proximal dendrites of GABAergic cells that may be the source of this inhibition (Haberly et al., 1987).

SYNAPTIC ACTIONS

It has been possible to study synaptic actions in the piriform cortex in considerable detail because the precise laminar organization allows selective shock stimulation of different fiber systems, and the visualization of synaptic currents in dendrites, by analysis of field potentials. The use of shock stimuli provides a powerful tool for the analysis of neuronal circuitry because of the synchronous, temporally ordered sequence of synaptic events that can be evoked at any point in brain slices as well as in intact systems. While such impulse stimuli are clearly artificial in nature, recent results described below suggest that findings obtained with this approach in the piriform cortex are directly applicable to understanding responses to natural stimuli.

SYNAPTIC POTENTIALS AND CURRENTS

Superficial Pyramidal Cells. In all three types of cerebral cortex, shock stimulation of excitatory pathways evokes an excitatory postsynaptic potential (EPSP) followed by Cl^--mediated, and slow, K^+-mediated inhibitory postsynaptic potentials (IPSPs) in pyramidal cells. Figure 10.8 illustrates this sequence for an SP cell in the piriform cortex. Since the Cl^--mediated IPSP is depolarizing at resting membrane potential in the piriform cortex (Scholfield, 1978b), it cannot be distinguished from the EPSP in intracellularly recorded voltage records under resting conditions (Fig. 10.8A, upper trace). However, its presence can be revealed by reversing the driving force on Cl^- by shifting the cell's membrane potential in the depolarizing direction (Fig. 10.8A, lower trace), or by measuring input resistance to reveal its associated conductance increase that is much larger at the cell body than that of the EPSP (Fig. 10.8B).

Deep Cells. In response to shock stimulation of afferent or association fibers, DP and multipolar cells in slices of piriform cortex display the same three synaptically mediated response components observed in SP cells (Tseng and Haberly, 1989a). However, in contrast to SP cells, the Cl^--mediated IPSP is hyperpolarizing in most deep cells in the resting state as a consequence of a more depolarized membrane potential.

In deep multipolar cells whose dendrites do not reach layer Ia, the EPSP evoked by stimulation of afferent fibers is disynaptic and therefore delayed with respect to the

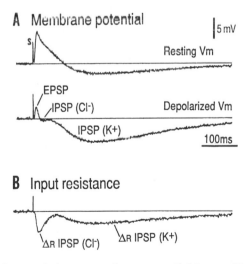

Fig. 10.8. Intracellularly recorded responses from a superficial pyramidal cell in a slice preparation of piriform cortex. Responses were evoked by shock stimulation of association fibers. **A:** Response at resting membrane potential (upper trace) and at a depolarized membrane potential induced by current injection (lower trace). S, shock artifact. **B:** Approximate time course of change in input resistance that accompanied the response in A. The response consists of an EPSP followed by a Cl^--mediated IPSP that is depolarizing at resting potential and a slow, K^+-mediated IPSP. [Modified from Tseng and Haberly, 1988, with permission.]

monosynaptic EPSP in pyramidal cells. As in SP cells, direct stimulation of association fibers in layer Ib or deeper layers monosynaptically evokes EPSPs in deep pyramidal and multipolar cells (Tseng and Haberly, 1989a).

Late Potentials and Epileptiform EPSPs in Deep Cells. In addition to short-latency postsynaptic potentials that resemble those in SP cells, deep cells also exhibit "late" synaptic potentials that are typically erratic in latency and amplitude (Tseng and Haberly, 1989a). After the application of convulsant drugs or other manipulations that have been used to model epileptic seizures, late potentials in deep cells become high in amplitude and exhibit an "all-or-none" quality as a result of a discrete threshold (Hoffman and Haberly, 1989). Below threshold the late epileptiform potential is absent; with increasing stimulus strength above threshold, latency decreases but amplitude remains relatively constant (Fig. 10.9). In the endopiriform nucleus of slices, it has been demonstrated that late potentials become epileptiform in character when a disruption in the normal balance between inhibition and excitation leads to synaptically mediated regenerative positive feedback in its population of extensively interconnected glutamatergic neurons (Hoffman and Haberly, 1991, 1993).

Synaptically Mediated Inhibitory Processes. The Cl^--mediated IPSP in piriform cortex is generated both in cell bodies and dendrites (Tseng and Haberly, 1988; Kapur et al., 1993) by the action of GABA on $GABA_A$ receptors. The slow, K^+-mediated IPSP is generated in dendrites by $GABA_B$ receptors (Tseng and Haberly, 1988; Kanter et al.,

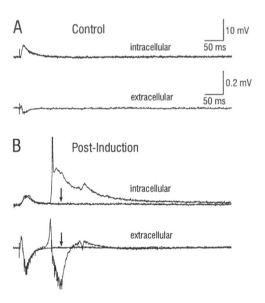

Fig. 10.9. Responses from the endopiriform nucleus to stimulation of association fibers under control conditions (**A**) and after the induction of epileptiform activity by a brief period of bursting resulting from transient exposure to bathing medium with no Mg^{2+}. The response in **B** consists of superimposed responses with and without (arrow) a late epileptiform component, both evoked by the same threshold-level stimulus.

1996). Recent studies with voltage-clamp recording have demonstrated that, as in the hippocampus (Pearce, 1993), GABA$_A$-mediated IPSCs in piriform cortex have fast and slow components, termed *GABA$_{A,fast}$* and *GABA$_{A,slow}$*, with time constants of decay on the order of 10 and 50 ms (Kapur et al., 1993 and in preparation). The GABA$_A$-mediated IPSC is slower in the distal apical dendrite than in the cell body as a consequence of a higher proportion of GABA$_{A,slow}$. Since the IPSCs in these distal dendritic and somatic regions can be evoked rather selectively by stimulation at different depths, it appears that they are mediated by different sets of interneurons.

The depolarizing GABA$_A$-mediated IPSC has an inhibitory action when a concomitantly occurring EPSP shifts the driving force on Cl$^-$ sufficiently in the depolarizing direction so that current through GABA$_A$ channels becomes outward (carried by inward movement of negatively charged chloride ions). This outward current opposes the generation of the EPSP by the inward EPSC. This nonlinear interaction between the EPSP and IPSP has been termed *shunting inhibition*—a term that has unfortunately led to a common misconception that excitatory current is directly shunted through GABA$_A$ channels, which is not possible due to their selective permeability to anions.

There is also evidence for presynaptic GABA$_B$-mediated inhibition of both excitatory (Tang and Hasselmo, 1994) and inhibitory (A. Kapur and L.B. Haberly, in preparation) inputs to SP cells. In both cases this presynaptic action is selective for particular inputs: it has a much stronger action on association fiber–mediated EPSPs than afferent-mediated EPSPs (Tang and Hasselmo, 1994) and on GABA$_{A,slow}$ than on GABA$_{A,fast}$ (A. Kapur and L.B. Haberly, in preparation). Since axo-axonic synaptic terminals are infrequent or absent in the piriform cortex (Haberly and Feig, 1983), presynaptic inhibition is mediated by the action of GABA on "autoreceptors" located on inhibitory synaptic terminals (GABA$_B$ receptors on the terminals from which GABA is released), and by diffusion of GABA through the extracellular space to excitatory synaptic terminals with GABA$_B$ receptors—a substantial distance in view of the separation of inhibitory to excitatory synapses on different dendritic elements. There is evidence that presynaptic GABA$_B$-mediated inhibition of GABA release plays a key role in the mediation of synaptic plasticity (Davies et al., 1991; Mott and Lewis, 1991).

VOLTAGE-DEPENDENT PROCESSES

Channels whose conductance is determined by voltage play a role in the integration of EPSCs and IPSCs in all parts of cerebral cortex. As described in Chap. 2, there are many types of such voltage dependent channels. To further complicate the analysis of their functional roles, different neurons display different mixtures of types, and many types are differentially distributed on the different elements of individual neurons.

As a result of voltage-dependent channels, the relationship between intracellularly injected current and the resulting voltage (I–V relationship; Fig. 10.10) displays nonlinearities in both depolarizing and hyperpolarizing directions for the three types of cells that have been examined in the piriform cortex: SP, DP, and deep multipolar cells (Scholfield, 1978a; Constanti and Galvan, 1983a; Tseng and Haberly, 1989b). Voltage-sensitive Ca^{2+}, Na$^+$, and K$^+$ channels shape these current-voltage curves. In the hyperpolarizing direction, at least two currents contribute to the observed nonlinearities: an M current (I$_M$) (Constanti and Galvan, 1983b) and a fast inward rectifier (I$_{f.i.r.}$) with unique properties (Constanti and Galvan, 1983a). Whereas I$_{f.i.r.}$ may be of lim-

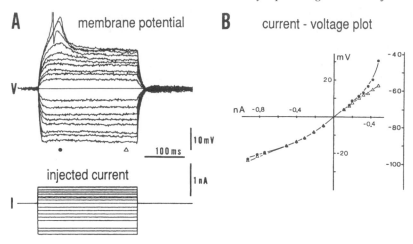

Fig. 10.10. Current-voltage relationship for deep pyramidal cell in piriform cortex. **A:** Voltage (V) responses to depolarizing (up) and hyperpolarizing (down) square pulses of intracellularly injected current (I). **B:** Plot of voltage as a function of current at the times indicated by solid circle and open triangle in A. The ordinate is potential relative to resting membrane potential; the scale at the right is absolute membrane potential. Note the nonlinear relationship that results from the opening and closing of voltage-sensitive channels. [Modified from Tseng and Haberly, 1989b, with permission.]

ited significance within the normal physiological range of potential and extracellular environment, I_M is tonically active at resting membrane potential and may contribute to accommodation of firing. In the depolarizing direction, transient low-threshold (I_T) and long-lasting, high-threshold (I_L) Ca^{2+} currents (Halliwell and Scholfield, 1984; Constanti et al., 1985; Tseng and Haberly, 1989b), and a "slow" Na^+ current (Tseng and Haberly, 1989b) appear to contribute to I–V nonlinearities.

The slow Na^+ current appears to underlie a long-lasting "regenerative" potential that can be triggered by depolarizing pulses in individual cells, or by synaptic stimulation when cells are held at a depolarized potential (Domroese and Haberly, 1996). Since this potential can evoke action potentials after a delay of 100 ms or longer, it has been speculated that it could be involved in the generation of long delays that can be the basis for the analysis of temporal patterns (Ketchum and Haberly, 1991). Based on the similarity in waveform of this regenerative potential to late epileptiform potentials in deep cells, it has also been speculated that it may play a role in epileptogenesis (Hoffman and Haberly, 1989). A long-lasting regenerative potential can also be generated by an unidentified high-threshold Ca^{2+} channel when current through this channel is increased by the addition of Ba^{2+} to the bathing medium (Tseng and Haberly, 1989b; Domroese and Haberly, 1996). This raises the possibility that under certain conditions, such as the activation of second-messenger systems that can alter the conductance of channels, both Na^+ and Ca^{2+} could participate in the mediation of regenerative potentials.

In a recent study, a transient K^+ current (I_A) has been identified that appears to contribute to the observed differences in response properties of SP and deep multipolar cells (Banks et al., 1996). In cells in the endopiriform nucleus, the steady-state inactivation curve for I_A (degree to which channels are inactivated as a function of membrane potential) is shifted by 10 mV in the depolarizing direction relative to SP cells. Modeling analysis suggested that this difference is sufficient to explain the more depolarized membrane potential of deep cells, and results in a 2-fold decrease in latency of the first spike evoked by depolarizing steps (Banks et al., 1996). Both of these factors could contribute to the greater susceptibility of the endopiriform nucleus to epileptogenesis.

There are also channels in pyramidal cells in piriform cortex that are activated by action potentials. These include fast and slow, and depolarizing and hyperpolarizing spike afterpotentials (Constanti and Sim, 1987a; Tseng and Haberly, 1988, 1989b). The most prominent of these is a K^+ current activated by Ca^{2+} influx (I_{AHP}). This current, which is substantial in most deep pyramidal and multipolar cells (Tseng and Haberly, 1989b), generates hyperpolarizing potentials that last for several seconds. In deep pyramidal and multipolar cells, I_{AHP} contributes to the rapid adaptation of firing that is observed during sustained depolarization. In SP cells, both I_{AHP} and I_M are weak at resting membrane potential in slices (Tseng and Haberly, 1988), but substantial at more depolarized potentials (Constanti and Sim, 1987a).

VISUALIZATION OF DENDRITIC PROCESSES BY CURRENT SOURCE–DENSITY ANALYSIS

A problem with the direct intracellular recording of membrane potentials and currents is that, for most neurons, this technique can only be applied at cell bodies and proximal dendrites. As a result, the power of intracellular recording is rather limited for the study of processes in dendrites. Fortunately, in highly ordered neuronal systems such as the piriform cortex, a technique termed *current source-density* (CSD) analysis allows the visualization of spatial and temporal sequences of membrane currents in dendrites (Mitzdorf, 1985). This information can be combined with data derived from intracellular recording to generate a detailed picture of the operation of integrative processes in dendrites.

Current source-density analysis involves a relatively simply mathematical manipulation carried out on the large *field potentials* that are generated when cortical systems are synchronously activated, as by shock stimulation of afferent fibers (Fig. 10.11). These potentials are generated by current passing through the extracellular space that links "active" current through membrane channels with passive "return" current. With CSD analysis, the distribution of net membrane current can be computed as a function of time and depth from sets of field potentials recorded at small depth increments. In the piriform cortex where different neuronal elements are segregated in depth, these net membrane currents can be interpreted in terms of sequences of synaptically mediated processes in specific dendritic segments and cell bodies of pyramidal cells (Haberly and Shepherd, 1973; Moyano et al., 1985; Rodriguez and Haberly, 1989; Ketchum and Haberly, 1993a,b; Biella and de Curtis, 1995).

AFFERENT STIMULATION EVOKES AN ORDERED SERIES OF POSTSYNAPTIC CURRENTS

Figure 10.12 illustrates net membrane currents derived by CSD analysis from the posterior piriform cortex in response to shock stimulation of the LOT. Inward current is represented as upward deflections in the surface plots (Fig. 10.12A,C) and as solid

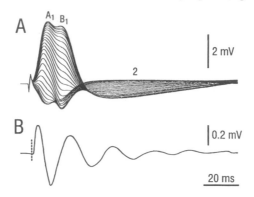

Fig. 10.11. Field potentials evoked in piriform cortex in vivo by strong (A) and weak (B) shock stimulation of afferent fibers. **A:** Superimposed responses recorded at small depth increments through the depth of the cortex in response to a strong stimulus. A_1, B_1, A and B components of period 1 of the field potential; 2, period 2 of field potential. **B:** 50 Hz oscillatory field potential evoked by a weak stimulus (dashed line). [A is reproduced from Ketchum and Haberly, 1993a; B is reproduced from Woolley and Timiras, 1965, with permission.]

lines in the contour plot (Fig. 10.12B). The response includes three peaks of inward current that have been identified as EPSCs: the large peak in layer Ia is the monosynaptic EPSC in distal apical dendrites; the immediately following large peak in superficial Ib is the disynaptic EPSC in mid-apical segments mediated by association fibers from the APC_V, and the small peak in deep Ib is a disynaptic EPSC in proximal dendritic segments mediated by association fibers that originate in the APC_D and other areas (see Fig. 10.5). In the APC, an EPSC in basal dendrites in layer III can also be visualized (Fig. 10.12C). This EPSC is obscured in the posterior piriform cortex by the outward return currents (downward deflections and dashed lines in Fig. 10.12A,B) associated with the large EPSCs in layer I.

Current associated with inhibitory processes overlaps in time with EPSCs, and in responses to strong afferent stimulation contributes comparatively little to net membrane current (see Dendritic Properties, below). The portion of the Cl^--mediated IPSC that remains following decay of the monosynaptic and disynaptic EPSCs can be seen as a small net inward current focused in layer II (II in Fig. 10.12B) that is coupled with outward current in layer I.

As illustrated in Fig. 10.12C, monosynaptic and disynaptic EPSCs can be separated by delivering a pair of shocks. The $GABA_A$-mediated IPSC evoked by the first shock blocks the generation of action potentials in response to the second shock, thereby resulting in an isolation of the monosynaptic EPSC.

TEMPORAL PATTERNS IN ACTIVATION BY AFFERENT FIBERS

A striking feature of the piriform cortex is a difference in the temporal pattern of activation of anterior and posterior parts by afferent fibers (Ketchum and Haberly, 1993a,b). Because the LOT passes over its surface, the entire APC is activated with near-synchrony relative to the time course of synaptic processes. By contrast, the PPC, which receives its afferent input via long collaterals from the LOT, is activated from

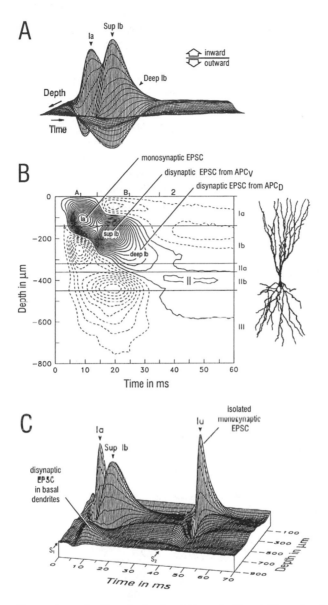

Fig. 10.12. Synaptic events evoked by shock stimulation of afferent fibers in rat piriform cortex in vivo as revealed by current source-density (CSD) analysis. **A:** Surface plot of net membrane current as a function of time and depth in *posterior* piriform cortex; inward current is upward. **B:** Same response presented as a contour plot with net inward current indicated by solid lines. Cortical lamination is indicated at the right. Time periods of the field potential (A_1, B_1, 2; see Fig. 10.11) are at the top. Response components are identified by the layers in which they are maximal (Ia, superficial Ib, deep Ib, and II; see text) and by the underlying synaptic events (e.g., monosynaptic EPSC). **C:** Response evoked in *anterior* piriform cortex by paired stimulation of afferent fibers. The response to the first shock (S_1 at lower left) is similar to that from the posterior piriform cortex in A with the exception of an inward current in basal dendrites in layer III. The response to the second shock (S_2) is an isolated monosynaptic EPSC (the disynaptic components are blocked when the IPSC evoked by S_1 prevents generation of action potentials by S_2). [Modified from Ketchum and Haberly, 1993a, with permission.]

rostral to caudal at a rate that is slow relative to synaptic processes. This is clearly seen when the isolated monosynaptic EPSC in PPC is recorded at a series of distances from the caudal end of the LOT (Fig. 10.13A,B).

DISPERSIVE PROPAGATION IN POSTERIOR PIRIFORM

In addition to the increase in latency, the monosynaptic EPSC in the PPC also increases in duration with increasing distance from the LOT (Fig. 10.13A,B). Analysis with phys-iological and modeling methods has shown that this increase in duration is a conse-quence of a spectrum in diameter of afferent axons that disperses the arrival times of action potentials (Fig. 10.13D) (Ketchum and Haberly, 1993b). An intriguing question is whether the spread in axonal diameter is a "deliberate," functionally significant fea-ture of this and other systems, or a result of inexact developmental processes with no

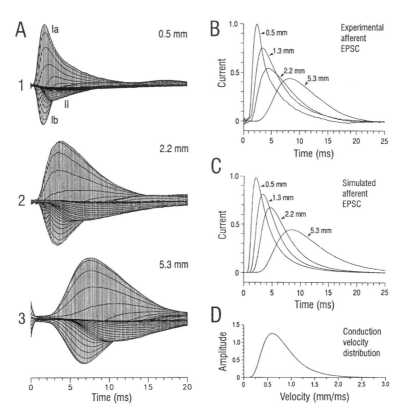

Fig. 10.13. "Dispersive propagation" of afferent-evoked response in posterior piriform cortex that results from a distribution in conduction velocity of afferent axons. Illustrated responses are net membrane current for the isolated monosynaptic component. A: Surface plots of net mem-brane current as a function of time. Amplitudes are normalized to emphasize the slowing of time course over distance. B: Inward current from A without normalization of amplitude. C: Simu-lation of response in B based on the assumption that conduction velocity in afferent axons is dis-tributed as illustrated in D (see text). [Modified from Ketchum and Haberly, 1993a,b, with per-mission.]

relevance to function. One effect of *dispersive propagation* is an increase in the capacity for associative interactions: it allows activity that originates over a larger area and over a broader range of latencies to arrive at the same time in areas of convergence. Since coincidence in arrival of convergent activity at a particular postsynaptic neuron would be related not only to which neurons in a projection area were active, but also to the temporal sequence of activity in those neurons, it could be the basis for the analysis of temporal patterns in the olfactory code (see model in Ketchum and Haberly, 1991). Dispersive propagation would facilitate the recall of temporal sequences stored through changes in synaptic efficacy that are triggered by coincidence (see Associative LTP and Functional Clues from Neuronal Circuitry, below).

TEMPORAL PATTERNS IN ACTIVATION BY ASSOCIATION FIBERS

Since association fibers in piriform cortex, like afferent fibers, spread parallel to the cortical surface, they also mediate sequential patterns of activation. However, unlike afferent fibers that may be activated quite synchronously during normal operation of the cortex as described below, natural patterns of activation by association fibers are complex as a consequence of their disynaptic relationship to afferent activity. For example, since the APC is activated with near synchrony by afferent volleys, activity in association fibers from this region originates rather synchronously over a broad area. A consequence of this distributed origin is that the spatial and temporal extents of propagating volleys within the PPC are relatively independent of distance (see Fig. 8 in Ketchum and Haberly, 1993b). This contrasts with volleys in afferent fibers that progressively increase in spatial and temporal extents within the PPC as a consequence of dispersive propagation (Fig. 10.13). Much additional study will be required to fully understand temporal aspects of the activation of olfactory cortex by the olfactory bulb.

A FAST (40–60 HZ) OSCILLATION MAY ORDER INTEGRATIVE PROCESSES IN
PYRAMIDAL CELLS

An important question is whether the highly ordered series of EPSCs observed in pyramidal cells in piriform cortex in response to shock stimulation also occurs during normal function of this system. Since natural odor stimulation has a time course that is slow relative to the shock-evoked sequence, it might be assumed that the precise spatial and temporal ordering of synaptic inputs observed by CSD analysis is an artifact of shock stimulation. However, odor stimulation induces a strong, 40–60 Hz *fast oscillation* (Adrian, 1942, 1953) that modulates the firing of afferents to piriform cortex into discrete bursts at the period of the oscillations (~20 ms) (Fig. 10.15B; Freeman, 1975; Eeckman and Freeman, 1990). Since 20 ms is a sufficient time for the full sequence of EPSCs to occur in piriform cortex, it can be postulated that the ordered sequence of postsynaptic events observed in response to strong shock stimulation occurs *within each cycle* of the fast oscillation evoked by odors. This hypothesis has been tested by application of CSD analysis to the fast oscillation evoked by single weak shocks to the LOT (Fig. 10.11B), which is believed to be generated by the same mechanism that generates the oscillatory response to odor (Ketchum and Haberly, 1993c). CSD analysis revealed that within each cycle of the fast oscillation initiated by a single weak shock, there is a monosynaptic EPSC in layer Ia, followed by a large disynaptic EPSC in layer Ib, as observed in response to strong shocks (compare A and B in Fig. 10.14). The disynaptic EPSC in each cycle follows the monosynaptic EPSC at nearly constant latency in anterior and posterior parts of piriform cortex. These EPSCs are followed by an inward membrane current in layer II that has been tentatively identified as the IPSC that generates the depolarizing, Cl^--mediated IPSP (II in Fig. 10.14).

Although confirmation will require a direct demonstration under more natural conditions, the results from this experiment suggest that there is a stereotyped spatial and temporal ordering of synaptic inputs to pyramidal cells during responses to odor stimuli that is enabled by the fast oscillatory rhythm (Fig. 10.15). The result would be a repetitive pairing of EPSCs at the period of the fast oscillation that might contribute to the induction of long-term potentiation (below). The Cl^--mediated IPSC might limit the integration of monosynaptic and disynaptic EPSCs to a recurring time window as illustrated in Fig. 10.15C.

SYNAPTIC PLASTICITY AND ITS REGULATION IN PIRIFORM CORTEX

NMDA-Dependent Homosynaptic LTP. A key question with regard to the operation of piriform cortex is whether it is involved in the learning of olfactory discriminations and associations, and if it is, what are the underlying mechanisms. There is growing evidence from behavioral studies that a form of activity-induced synaptic plasticity that requires the activation of NMDA receptors, termed *NMDA-dependent long term potentiation* (LTP), plays a role in a number of different learning processes including the acquisition of olfactory discriminations (Staubli et al., 1989). Recent demonstrations

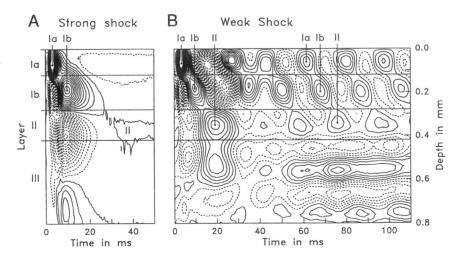

Fig. 10.14. Contour plots of net membrane current derived in vivo by CSD analysis of the nonoscillatory response to a strong shock (A) and the oscillatory response to a weak shock (B) (see Fig. 10.11). The response to the weak shock in B consists of a series of synaptic events that repeats within each cycle of the oscillatory response, each one of which resembles the response to the strong stimulus. Note that the monosynaptic EPSC (solid contours in layer Ia) is paired with the disynaptic association fiber–evoked EPSC (solid contours in layer Ib) within each cycle of the oscillatory response. Each cycle ends with an inward current in layer II that is believed to be the Cl^--mediated IPSC (inward when concomitant EPSPs are small). [Reproduced from Ketchum and Haberly, 1993c, with permission.]

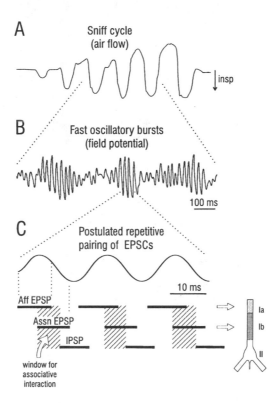

Fig. 10.15. Fast and slow oscillatory rhythms evoked by odor. **A:** Airflow through the nasal cavity of a rat during sniffing behavior triggered by odor presentation. Note the slow (4–8 Hz) oscillation that is correlated with the hippocampal theta rhythm. [Modified from Youngentob et al., 1987, with permission.] **B:** Field potential recorded from the piriform cortex of an unanesthetized rat during odor evoked sniffing. Each inspiratory cycle evokes an envelope of fast (50 Hz) oscillatory activity. [Modified from Woolley and Timiras, 1965, with permission.] Each inspiratory cycle evokes an envelope of fast oscillatory activity. **C:** Hypothesis derived from results of CSD analysis that monosynaptic and disynaptic EPSPs generated in adjacent dendritic segments are repetitively paired at 50 Hz during the fast oscillation. The cross-hatched area represents the time period wherein EPSPs overlap before onset of the IPSC.

of this form of synaptic plasticity in piriform cortex therefore support the involvement of this system in olfactory learning. NMDA-dependent LTP has been demonstrated in both afferent and association fiber systems in slices of piriform cortex (Fig. 10.16; Jung et al., 1990a; Kanter and Haberly, 1990; Carpenter et al., 1994; Collins, 1994) and in the afferent fiber system in anesthetized animals (Kapur and Haberly, 1991). As in the CA1 region of hippocampus, expression is primarily in the AMPA component of the EPSP (Jung and Larson, 1994), protein kinases are required for both induction and maintenance (Collins, 1994; Domroese and Haberly, 1995), and activation of metabotropic glutamate receptors in addition to NMDA receptors may be required for induction (Collins, 1994). This LTP can be induced by the "theta-burst" paradigm that consists of brief, high-frequency bursts of shock stimuli repeated at the frequency of the theta rhythm (4–8 Hz). Since odor-induced sniffing in rats (Fig. 10.15A) is corre-

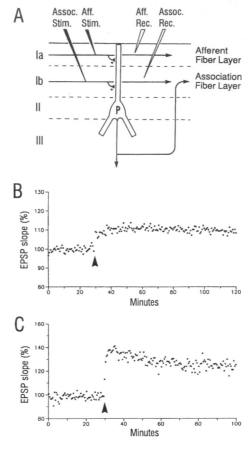

Fig. 10.16. Long-term potentiation (LTP) in a slice preparation of piriform cortex. **A:** Schematic of piriform cortex showing positions of stimulating (Stim.) and recording (Rec.) electrodes in afferent (Aff.) and association (Assoc.) fiber layers. **B:** Slope of the rising phase of the extra-cellularly recorded "population EPSP" evoked by stimulation of afferent fibers. At the arrow-head, a strong "theta-burst" stimulus applied to afferent fibers evoked a sustained potentiation. **C:** Same as B, but from stimulation of association fibers. [Modified from Kanter and Haberly, 1990, with permission.]

lated with the theta rhythm, and a burst of high-frequency oscillatory activity is evoked during each sniff cycle (Fig. 10.15B), this paradigm resembles naturally patterned activity in the olfactory system.

   In addition to LTP of monosynaptically evoked EPSPs, activity-dependent potentiation of a long-latency field potential component has been observed in the piriform cortex of unanesthetized rats. This process, termed *selective LTP*, is evoked by a series of brief, high-frequency shock trains applied to association fibers (Stripling et al., 1992; Galupo and Stripling, 1995). The potentiated component has a discrete threshold (Galupo and Stripling, 1995) that is reminiscent of late potentials in slices of piriform cortex as described above.

Associative LTP. An intriguing feature of NMDA-dependent LTP is that it provides a potential mechanism for various forms of associative learning (Brown et al., 1990). This capacity stems from the requirement of both neurotransmitter release and post-synaptic depolarization for activation of NMDA-mediated responses. As a result of this requirement, synaptic reinforcement can be restricted to simultaneously activated convergent inputs. The evidence that afferent and association fiber-evoked EPSCs are repetitively paired on adjacent dendritic segments at the frequency of the fast oscillation (Figs. 10.14, 10.15) suggests that this pairing plays a role in the induction of *associative LTP*. The same process could allow the reinforcement of simultaneously activated synapses of association fibers that originate from more than one location in piriform cortex or from other olfactory cortical areas.

The hypothesis that NMDA-dependent associative LTP occurs in the piriform cortex has been tested with the "weak–strong" paradigm developed in studies in hippocampus, where a weakly stimulated input is only potentiated during concomitant strong activation of an independent fiber system that terminates nearby (Levy and Steward, 1979; Barrionuevo and Brown, 1983). The results of similar experiments in the piriform cortex confirmed that NMDA-dependent associative LTP can be induced in either direction between afferent and association fiber inputs to pyramidal cells (Kanter and Haberly, 1993). The same result has also been obtained when two independent sets of association fibers are stimulated (Jung and Larson, 1994).

Since spatial proximity of the termination zones of different fiber systems is a key determinant of the capacity for associative LTP (White et al., 1990), predictions can be made concerning the extent to which the different excitatory systems in piriform cortex can interact in this fashion. As discussed earlier, it would be expected that the afferent fiber system would strongly interact with the association fiber system that originates in the APC$_V$ since these two systems terminate on adjacent apical dendritic segments, but would interact less with the systems from the APC$_D$ and PPC that synapse at greater distances from the afferent termination zone (Figs. 10.5, 10.6). Furthermore, association fiber systems that terminate on adjacent segments of pyramidal cells would have a greater propensity for plastic interaction. For example, association fiber synapses from the APC$_V$ in superficial Ib would be expected to strongly interact with those from the APC$_D$ in deep Ib, but not with those from the PPC that are concentrated on basal dendrites in layer III.

Role of Inhibition in Regulation of LTP. If LTP plays a role in learning and memory, then its occurrence or persistence must be regulated in order to avoid saturation of synaptic efficacies that would be inevitable if lasting potentiation occurs each time there is convergence and coincidence of neuronal activity. An elegant demonstration of such regulation in the piriform cortex is that lasting LTP can only be induced by weak theta-burst stimulation in behaving animals when the shock train is paired with reward (Roman et al., 1987, 1993). One process that has been shown to regulate LTP in piriform cortex (del Cerro et al., 1992; Kanter and Haberly, 1993; Collins, 1994) as originally demonstrated in the hippocampus (Wigstrom and Gustafsson, 1983) is the GABA$_A$-mediated IPSC. As described above (Synaptic Actions), this IPSC is mediated in dendritic and somatic regions by different interneurons. Because of its location and slower time course (Kapur et al., 1993, 1994, and in preparation), the dendritic IPSC has a much stronger action than the somatic IPSC on the NMDA component of afferent-evoked EPSCs (Fig. 10.17; Kanter et al., 1996). If centrifugal fiber systems that have been implicated in the regulation of learning and memory (see Neurotransmitters, below) were to selectively block this dendritic IPSC, NMDA-dependent LTP could be enabled without compromising the somatic-region IPSC. Preservation of negative feedback onto the somatic region would allow compensatory adjustments in system excitability, without which epileptiform bursting can develop. Since the somatic-region IPSC has little effect on the NMDA component (Kanter et al., 1996; A. Kapur et al., in preparation), these compensatory adjustments would have minimal effect on the induction of LTP.

NEUROTRANSMITTERS

GLUTAMATE

Findings with specific antagonists and a variety of other methods (reviewed by Haberly, 1990b) indicate that glutamate is the primary excitatory neurotransmitter in the piriform cortex as it is in the hippocampus (Chap. 11) and neocortex (Chap. 12). This is true for afferent and association fiber systems in piriform cortex (Jung et al., 1990b), as well as for intrinsic connections in the endopiriform nucleus (Hoffman and Haberly, 1993). As in the hippocampus and neocortex, glutamate mediates EPSCs via AMPA and NMDA receptors (Jung et al., 1990b). The AMPA receptor mediates a fast EPSC

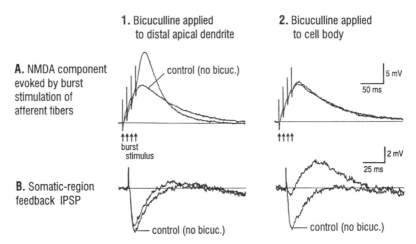

Fig. 10.17. The NMDA component of the EPSP evoked by burst stimulation of afferent fibers is potentiated by blockade of dendritic but not somatic GABA$_A$-mediated inhibition. Responses were intracellularly recorded from a superficial pyramidal cell in a slice preparation of piriform cortex with the AMPA component of the EPSP blocked by DNQX. **A:** Traces in the top row are intracellularly recorded responses to burst stimulation of afferent fibers. Responses after local application of bicuculline to the apical dendrite (left column) or cell body (right column) are superimposed on control responses. **B:** Somatic-region IPSP evoked by single shocks, immediately following responses in A. Note that dendritically applied bicuculline potentiated the NMDA component (A1) with little effect on the somatic-region IPSP (B1). [Modified from Kanter et al., 1966 with permission.]

via a nonspecific increase in cationic conductance with a reversal potential near zero mV. The NMDA receptor mediates an EPSC with a similar reversal, but with additional unique properties that underlie its role in various forms of activity-induced plasticity. These properties include a slower time course, a higher proportion of current carried by Ca^{2+}, and a requirement of postsynaptic depolarization to enable current flow. As described earlier, activation of the NMDA receptor is required for the induction of LTP in piriform cortex. In addition, activation of these receptors is required for the induction of epileptiform activity in slices of piriform cortex by bursting activity—a process that utilizes a different second-messenger pathway than LTP (Hoffman and Haberly, 1989; Domroese, 1995).

In addition to acting on AMPA and NMDA receptors that have integral channels, glutamate also acts on *metabotropic* receptors whose actions are mediated by way of second-messenger pathways (Chap. 2). Application of selective agonists for the metabotropic receptor evokes a long-lasting depolarization with accompanying spike discharge, and results in a long after-depolarization following large depolarizing pulses (Constanti and Libri, 1992). Metabotropic agonists have also been reported to induce a long-lasting increase in the afferent-evoked NMDA component (Collins, 1993).

GABA

Inhibitory processes in the piriform cortex also closely resemble those in the hippocampus and neocortex. Studies with a variety of methods have revealed that GABA is the predominant inhibitory neurotransmitter (reviewed by Haberly, 1990b). Its action is on postsynaptic $GABA_A$ receptors, and on $GABA_B$ receptors on both postsynaptic and presynaptic membrane as described above (see Synaptic Actions). $GABA_A$ receptors mediate an IPSC in cell bodies and dendrites through an increase in Cl^- conductance (Fig. 10.7). Postsynaptic $GABA_B$ receptors mediate a slowly developing, long-lasting IPSP in dendrites (Figs. 10.7 and 10.8A) via an increase in K^+ conductance.

PEPTIDES

Many neuropeptides or the mRNAs for their synthesis have been demonstrated in neurons in the piriform cortex and other olfactory areas, as in the hippocampus and neocortex. These include cholecystokinin (CCK; Westenbroek et al., 1987), corticotropin releasing factor (CRF; Bassett et al., 1992), gonadotropin releasing hormone (GnRH; Choi et al., 1994), neuropeptide Y (De Quidt and Emson, 1986), neurotensin (NT; Inagaki et al., 1983), somatostatin (Roberts et al., 1982), substance P (Ljungdahl et al., 1978), thyrotropin releasing hormone (TRH; Kubek et al., 1993), vasoactive intestinal peptide (VIP; Loren et al., 1979), and several opioids (Palkovits and Brownstein, 1985; Fallon and Leslie, 1986; Harlan et al., 1987). Evidence for the presence of receptors for CCK (Zarbin et al., 1983), oxytocin (Yoshimura et al., 1993), somatostatin (Senaris et al., 1994), vasopressin (Szot et al., 1994), and VIP (Magistretti et al., 1988) has also been provided. Unfortunately, there has been no analysis of the physiological roles of peptides in the piriform cortex.

ACETYLCHOLINE

As in other types of cerebral cortex, the piriform cortex and other olfactory cortical areas receive input from cholinergic cells in the basal forebrain (Fig. 10.1F) (Haberly and Price, 1978a; Gaykema et al., 1990). There is also a small number of bipolar neurons in the piriform cortex and certain other olfactory areas that contain choline acetyltransferase, and therefore probably use acetylcholine (ACh) as their neurotransmitter (Sofroniew et al., 1985).

Cholinergic agonists have been shown to exert a number of different actions on pyramidal cells in the piriform cortex, most of which were originally identified in the hippocampus. These include a presynaptic inhibition of intrinsic associational input to proximal apical dendrites with little effect on afferent input to distal dendrites (Hasselmo and Bower, 1992), a block of I_{AHP} and the accommodation of firing to which it contributes (Tseng and Haberly, 1989b; Barkai and Hasselmo, 1994), a block of I_M (Constanti and Sim, 1987b), a long-lasting depolarization with accompanying spike discharge (Constanti et al., 1993; Libri et al., 1994), the induction of a long-lasting after-depolarization evoked by large depolarizing pulses in deep cells (Constanti et al., 1993; Libri et al., 1994), and a modulation of long-term potentiation (Hasselmo and Barkai, 1996). Hasselmo and collaborators have used computer simulation to explore potential roles of cholinergic processes in olfactory learning and memory (Hasselmo et al., 1992; Hasselmo, 1994; Hasselmo and Barkai, 1996).

MONOAMINES

The piriform cortex receives projections from norepinephrine-, serotonin-, and dopamine-containing neurons in the brainstem, and histaminergic cells in the hypothalamus as do most other cortical areas (Fig. 10.1F). Evidence includes the presence of axons containing these monoamines (Björklund and Lindvall, 1984; Moore and Card, 1984; Inagaki et al., 1988; Datiche et al., 1996) and retrogradely labeled cells in the appropriate cell groups from injections of anatomical tracer in the piriform cortex and other olfactory cortical areas (Haberly and Price, 1978a).

A role for these neurotransmitters is suspected in many different functions. These include the regulation of learning, sleep, and emotions. In the piriform cortex as in the hippocampal formation, much of the analysis of mechanisms of action of monoamines has focused on their modulatory effects on inhibitory processes. In a series of studies, Aghajanian and collaborators have examined the actions of monoamines on a population of "fast-spiking" cells at the layer II–III border that appear to mediate GABAergic IPSPs in pyramidal cells. Serotonin, norepinephrine, and dopamine directly excite many of these interneurons with a concomitant increase in IPSPs in pyramidal cells (Sheldon and Aghajanian, 1991; Gellman and Aghajanian, 1993). This action of serotonin has been shown to be mediated by 5-HT2A receptors (Marek and Aghajanian, 1994, 1995). Recent studies have used this system to study the mechanism of action of antipsychotic agents (Gellman and Aghajanian, 1994).

DENDRITIC PROPERTIES

ELECTROTONIC STRUCTURE

The only detailed electrotonic analysis in the piriform cortex has been on superficial pyramidal cells. Parameters obtained by whole-cell patch recording and application of the method of Holmes and Rall (1992) to these data indicate that these cells are similar to pyramidal cells in the CA1 region of the hippocampus. Both cell types are electrotonically compact with a similar membrane time constant ($\cong$20 ms), input resistance ($\cong$ 100 MΩ), and membrane resistivity ($\cong 2 \times 10^4$ Ωcm^2) (Kapur et al., 1994, and in preparation).

INTEGRATIVE PROCESSES

The ease with which synaptically evoked membrane currents can be visualized as a function of time and depth by CSD analysis has afforded the opportunity for a detailed analysis of integrative processes in pyramidal cells in piriform cortex. This analysis has been carried out with a model for which the key parameters were well constrained by available morphological and physiological data (Ketchum and Haberly, 1993b). With this model the sequence of net membrane current computed by CSD analysis could be dissected into synaptic, capacitive, and resistive components, and membrane potential could be computed as a function of time and dendritic location. Results of this analysis are presented in Figs. 10.18 and 10.19 for the isolated monosynaptic EPSC and for the full sequence of postsynaptic currents evoked by afferent fiber stimulation.

Passive Return Current and the Electrotonic Spread of EPSPs. One of the more intriguing findings with this model was the complex nature of the passive outward return current associated with EPSCs, which is responsible for the electrotonic spread of EPSPs in dendrites. In a *steady-state* cable representation of a dendritic tree (cf. Rall, 1977) that is applicable to the study of electrotonic spread of slow synaptic potentials, all inward current through excitatory synaptic channels returns to the extracellular space through the membrane resistance (since no current passes through the membrane capacitance after potential reaches steady state). However, EPSCs in pyramidal cell dendrites are sufficiently fast that most of the return current passes through the membrane capacitance rather than resistive channels (compare C and D in Fig. 10.18). Since this outward capacitative current is carried by the removal of the hyperpolarizing charge on the resting membrane, it has a depolarizing (excitatory) effect on membrane potential. As seen in Fig. 10.19B, the outward capacitative current is concentrated in distal dendrites (downward peak in layers Ia and Ib) and falls off abruptly over distance so that the electrotonic spread of the EPSP that it drives is strongly decremental within the apical dendritic tree (Fig. 10.19D). Although the rate of falloff would be monotonic in a uniform cable model, CSD analysis (Ketchum and Haberly, 1993a,b) revealed that, in SP cells, a discontinuity develops when the spread of outward current reaches the cell-body layer (note the shoulder in outward current starting at a latency of 3 ms in Fig. 10.18A). Analysis of the isolated monosynaptic EPSC in which all membrane current deep to layer Ia is passive suggested that the discontinuity results from the abrupt increase in membrane area at the cell-body layer. For both the isolated monosynaptic (Fig. 10.18E) and full response (Fig. 10.19D), there is a corresponding discontinuity in the decrease in EPSP amplitude over depth at the junction between apical dendrites and cell bodies.

A surprising result was that, as the synaptic current decays over time, the capacitative current becomes inward with a depth profile that approximates that of the synaptic current (Figs. 10.18C and 10.19B). This inward current is associated with the *equalization* of potential in different parts of the neuron that follows the termination of active currents (Ketchum and Haberly, 1993b). A technical consideration for those employ-

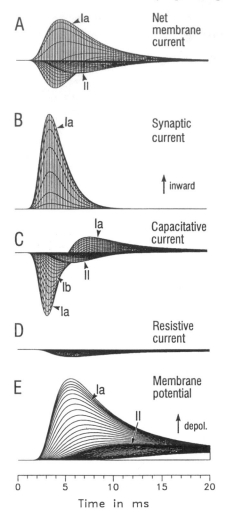

Fig. 10.18. Synaptic current, passive "return" current and membrane potential for the monosynaptic, afferent-evoked response, computed with a cable representation of the pyramidal cell population. The monosynaptic component was isolated as illustrated in Fig. 10.12C. **A:** Net membrane current determined by CSD analysis. **B:** Synaptic current (monosynaptic EPSC). Note that the EPSC is faster and larger than the net membrane current. **C:** Capacitative component of the passive return current associated with the EPSC. **D:** Resistive component of return current. Depths of selected components are indicated by the arrowheads. [Modified from Ketchum and Haberly, 1993b, with permission.]

ing CSD analysis is that the net inward membrane current computed with this technique can be substantially slower and smaller than the synaptic current because of this inward tail of capacitative current, together with the outward capacitative current at shorter latency (compare A and B in Fig. 10.18). As a result of an increase in the size of the current dipole arising from the spread of outward return current as described above, the discrepancy in time course of field potentials relative to the underlying

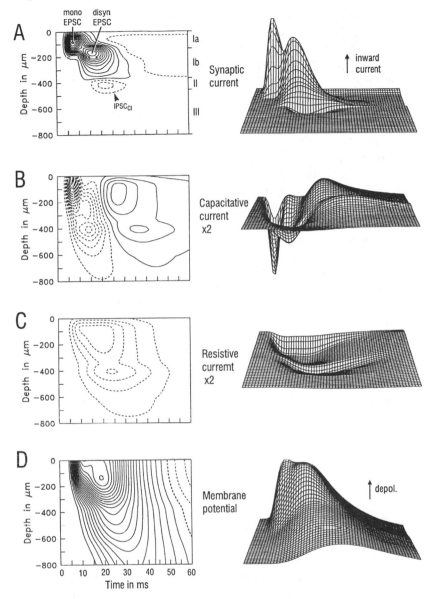

Fig. 10.19. Same as in Fig. 10.18, but for the complete response to stimulation of afferent fibers. [Modified from Ketchum and Haberly, 1993b, with permission.]

synaptic currents can be much greater than the discrepancy in net membrane current (see Fig. 7 in Ketchum and Haberly, 1993a).

Effects of Electrotonic Spread in Dendrites on the Amplitude of EPSPs. A central issue for understanding the integrative processing of synaptic inputs is the extent of falloff in EPSP amplitude from sites of synaptic input on dendrites to the site or sites where the cell's output is determined by the generation of action potentials that enter its axon. Although recent studies suggest that action potentials in certain pyramidal cells can originate in the dendritic tree, there is much evidence that the primary site of origin is near the cell body—probably in the unmyelinated *initial segment* of the axon.

In simulations with the model, peak amplitude of the monosynaptic EPSP in cell bodies was approximately 25% of that in distal dendrites (Fig. 10.19D). This compared with 50% and 80% of peak amplitude, respectively, for the disynaptic EPSPs generated in superficial and deep parts of layer Ib. It follows from this analysis that despite the small amplitude of the EPSC in deep Ib, the EPSP it generates has an effect on output comparable to that from the much larger inputs at more distal sites. A surprise was that the small separation between the monosynaptic EPSC and the disynaptic EPSC in superficial Ib (approximately 75 μm between peaks, Fig. 10.12B) resulted in a 2-fold difference in the extent of falloff of the resulting EPSPs at the soma.

Effects of Electrotonic Spread on the Timecourse of EPSPs. A key parameter governing the operation of neuronal circuitry is the delay from the time that action potentials arrive in presynaptic axons to the time of initiation of action potentials in the postsynaptic neuron. For most neurons in the central nervous system the delay at the synapse, which is less than 1 ms, makes an insignificant contribution to the total delay. Analysis with the model revealed that the primary source of delay in SP cells is the slow time course of electrotonic spread of EPSPs to the cell body. For the monosynaptic EPSP, peak depolarization at the cell body required approximately 6 ms following peak depolarization at the afferent input zone in layer Ia. This compares with a 2-ms latency from the peak of the EPSC to the peak of the EPSP in layer Ia.

As a consequence of the slow time course of electrotonic spread, the EPSP at the cell body resulting from sequential monosynaptic and disynaptic EPSPs has a monophasic time course (note that the 2 peaks in layer Ia in Fig. 10.19D coalesce into a single peak in layer II). It had been previously speculated that the single peak observed by intracellular recording in cell bodies is a consequence of a shunting of the disynaptic EPSP by GABA$_A$-mediated inhibition. However, when this inhibitory process was omitted, the somatic EPSP remained monophasic.

Integration of Multiple EPSPs. As seen in Figs. 10.12B and 10.14B, the disynaptic EPSC occurs at a substantial latency following the monosynaptic EPSC (Ketchum and Haberly, 1993a,c). An important question is whether this slow sequencing, much of which is a consequence of the membrane parameters that underlie the slow electrotonic spread, is dictated by functional considerations. The extent to which this delay influences the integration of the monosynaptic and two disynaptic EPSCs was investigated with the CSD-derived model. The results showed that when all three EPSCs were applied simultaneously, peak potential at the cell body was only 2% greater than the peak potential generated by the largest EPSC when presented alone. However, when the three EPSCs were presented in the natural sequence, peak amplitude increased to 50% greater than the largest individual EPSC, suggesting that the long latency of disynaptic EPSCs may substantially increase the extent of summation between monosynaptic and disynaptic inputs. This increase in summation is primarily a consequence of the delay in disynaptic EPSCs until the peak depolarization from the monosynaptic EPSC is achieved at the cell-body layer (compare Fig. 10.18E with Fig. 10.19A).

Interaction of EPSPs and IPSCs. The final issue investigated with the model was the extent of current shunting by somatic $GABA_A$-mediated inhibition on the generation of EPSPs (see Synaptic Actions, above). As seen in Fig. 10.19A, the outward current carried by Cl^- through $GABA_A$ channels in layer II was small in comparison with excitatory synaptic current, even when the conductance of these channels was set at the maximum value at which the observed current and voltage responses could be reproduced. The outward Cl^- current was small because the depolarization achieved in cell bodies during EPSCs was near the equilibrium potential for Cl^-. Only when membrane potential was shifted by 10 mV or more in the depolarizing direction did the driving force on Cl^- at the cell body become sufficiently strong that its shunting action on the EPSP could be visualized with the model, as in intracellular recordings (Fig. 9 in Ketchum and Haberly, 1993b). Although dendritically localized $GABA_A$ inhibition, which is now known to be present in piriform cortex (Kapur et al., 1993; Kanter et al., 1996), could provide a stronger shunting action because of the higher level of depolarization achieved in dendrites during EPSCs, CSD analysis revealed that summation of monosynaptic and disynaptic EPSCs is nearly linear when this IPSC is present, suggesting that shunting is minimal (Ketchum and Haberly, 1993a). This modest effect of $GABA_A$-mediated inhibition on fast, AMPA receptor–mediated EPSPs contrasts with the strong effect of dendritically localized $GABA_A$-mediated inhibition on the NMDA component of EPSPs as described earlier (see Fig. 10.17 and Synaptic Plasticity and its Regulation in Piriform Cortex).

FUNCTIONAL OPERATIONS

RESPONSES TO ODOR STIMULATION

Extracellularly recorded action potentials (*single units*) evoked by odor in the piriform cortex have been examined in unanesthetized monkeys and rats. In a study of unit responses in the macaque to "passive" odor stimulation (no odor-related training), more than 50% of units responded to at least 1 out of the 8 odorants presented and 44% responded to 2 or more (Fig. 10.20; Tanabe et al., 1975). A similar result was obtained by Schoenbaum and Eichenbaum (1995) from a large sample of units in the rat during *performance* of a previously learned odor discrimination task. Most units were found to be "coarsely tuned," displaying responses that differed in degree to several of the 8 odors that were presented. However, in a study by McCollum and co-workers (1991) in which units were studied during *acquisition* of an olfactory discrimination involving 7 odorants, most units were found to be broadly tuned in naive rats, but only 4 out of 62 continued to respond after completion of discrimination training. Possible sources of the discrepancies in results between these studies include methodological differences that could have differentially biased the populations of neurons that were studied, or differences in the locations of neurons that were studied. In view of the marked differences in connectivity between subdivisions, differences in response properties for neurons at different locations would be expected.

Responses of olfactory cortex to odors have also been examined by visualizing spa-

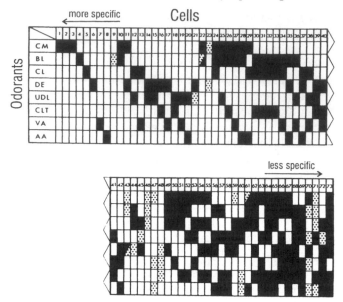

Fig. 10.20. Responses of 73 single units in piriform and amygdaloid cortex of the macaque to 8 odorants. Solid shading, excitatory response; stippling, inhibitory response; open areas, no response. Results are arranged from greatest specificity at left (response to 1 odorant) to lowest specificity at right (response to all 8 odorants). [Reproduced with permission from Takagi, 1986.]

tial patterns in the amplitude of fast oscillatory field potentials, and in the activity-related uptake of 2-deoxyglucose (2-DG). In studies of 2-DG uptake, odor-specific spatial patterns have been consistently demonstrated in the olfactory bulb (Chap. 5), but uptake in piriform cortex has been reported to be uniform in the horizontal dimension (Sharp et al., 1977; Cattarelli et al., 1988), indicating a lack of spatial segregation of cells with similar response properties. When animals were trained with a simple detection task, 2-DG uptake was increased in the anterior olfactory nucleus, but not significantly altered in the piriform cortex (Hamrick et al., 1993).

    In studies with large arrays of recording electrodes, it has been demonstrated that the amplitude of the fast oscillation evoked by odors varies in a complex but consistent way across the surface of the rostral portion of olfactory cortex. Although no differences have been detected between the spatial patterns evoked by different odors (Freeman, 1978), the complex statistical analysis that was required to reveal such patterns in the olfactory bulb (Freeman and Grajski, 1987) has not been applied to the cortex. Aversive conditioning induces a change in a measure of average amplitude of the odor-evoked fast oscillation in the olfactory cortex relative to that in the olfactory bulb that is specific to the reinforced odor (Bressler, 1988), but effects of learning on spatial patterns in fast oscillations have not been investigated in olfactory cortex.

    Taken together, the results of single-unit, oscillatory field potential, and 2-DG uptake studies suggest that there is an *ensemble code* for odor quality where the coding for individual odors is spatially distributed and involves a very large number of different neurons. Furthermore, the studies of Bressler (1988) and McCollum and co-workers (1991) indicate that changes in response properties occur in the piriform cortex during the acquisition of new olfactory discriminations, which is consistent with the participation of this system in the learning of odor-related behaviors.

In addition to recording responses associated with the presentation of odors, Shoen-baum and Eichenbaum (1995) also examined unit activity in the piriform cortex and prefrontal cortex (orbitofrontal area and agranular insula) during other aspects of a complex discrimination task (Fig. 10.21). These included the onset of a light that signaled an impending discrimination trial ("light on" in Fig. 10.21), insertion of the animal's snout into odor delivery and water reinforcement ports ("odor poke" and "water poke" in Fig. 10.21), and the delivery of water reinforcement. The results demonstrated that firing rates of units in the prefrontal cortex change during all of these task components as might be expected from previous studies in the monkey (Fuster, 1985; Goldman-Rakic, 1987), but surprisingly, the activity of units in piriform cortex was indistinguishable from that in prefrontal cortex. This suggests that the role of the piriform cortex in olfactory discrimination and its capacity for associative processing are much greater than previously believed.

FUNCTIONAL CLUES FROM NEURONAL CIRCUITRY

Perhaps the most intriguing feature of the neuronal circuitry in the olfactory cortex is the presence of afferent and association fiber systems that project in a highly divergent fashion to broad areas with no apparent systematic topographical order. Based on cell numbers (see Cell Populations, above) and the highly branched form of both afferent and association axons (Haberly and Bower, 1982; Ojima et al., 1984), it would appear that each cell of origin for afferent or association fibers provides synaptic input to a large number of pyramidal cells and, conversely, that each pyramidal cell receives input from a large number of different cells. Unfortunately, the available evidence provides no insight into the degree to which these connections are established on the basis of specific, functionally relevant pre- and postsynaptic markers that appear to play a key role in the olfactory bulb (Chap. 5).

As discussed previously (Haberly, 1985; Haberly and Bower, 1989), the presence of spatially distributed afferent and association fiber systems, together with the apparent ensemble code for odor quality and a mechanism for activity-dependent synaptic plasticity, are reminiscent of *associative* or *content-addressable* memory models (e.g., Anderson, 1970, 1972; Kohonen et al., 1977; Hopfield, 1982). These models have demonstrated that a large matrix of "neurons" that receives a spatially distributed input, has distributed positive feedback, and is subject to "synaptic" reinforcement triggered by coincident activation (Hebb, 1949; T.H. Brown et al., 1990) has the potential to perform learning, retrieval, and associative functions that would be required for the central processing of odor information. In these network models, "memory traces" are distributed across the entire network and addressed by content rather than location. When delay elements are introduced, temporal as well as spatial patterns can be processed (Tank and Hopfield, 1987; Kleinfeld, 1986). Because the olfactory cortex appears to have the requisite features, is only one synapse removed from its sensory receptors, and has a structure that facilitates circuitry analysis, it would appear to be an ideal system in which to test the applicability of these models to the nervous system. Initial steps have been taken toward the development of models for the olfactory cortex based on this theoretical framework (Granger et al., 1988; Wilson and Bower, 1988; Lynch and Granger, 1991; Hasselmo et al., 1992; Barkai et al., 1994), although simplifying

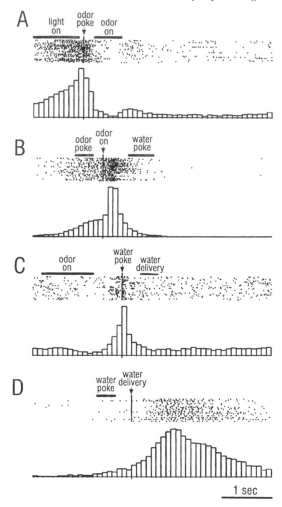

Fig. 10.21. Single-unit activity in piriform cortex and prefrontal cortex of the rat during performance of a previously learned odor discrimination task. Results from the two cortical areas were indistinguishable. **A–D:** Each panel includes a raster display of spikes during each trial (top) and a histogram from pooled data (bottom). After onset of a light ("light on" in A), the rat was required to poke its nose into an odor delivery port ("odor poke") where one of 7 odorants was presented. A "water poke" into a different port was required to receive reinforcement for correct responses. Responses of the 4 single units illustrated in A–D are aligned to the task component during which firing rate was maximal (indicated by vertical line and arrow). Note that firing rate was related to many different task components, not just the delivery of odorants. [Modified from Schoenbaum and Eichenbaum, 1995, with permission.]

assumptions and speculations concerning key features of the circuitry and its operation are still required. Continued development of these models in parallel with circuitry analysis may elucidate the process of olfactory discrimination as well as perhaps provide clues concerning the operation of higher-order "association areas" of the neocortex that, like the olfactory cortex, has strong spatially distributed connections.

11

HIPPOCAMPUS

DANIEL JOHNSTON AND DAVID G. AMARAL

The hippocampus is one of the most thoroughly studied areas of the mammalian central nervous system. There are two main reasons for this. First, it has a distinctive and readily identifiable structure at both the gross and histological levels. The unusual shape of the human hippocampus resembles that of a sea horse, which is what led to its most common name (in Greek *hippo* means "horse" and *kampos* means "sea monster"). The hippocampus is also sometimes called Ammon's horn due to its resemblance to a ram's horn (the Egyptian god Ammon had ram's horns). But it is the histology of the hippocampus that makes it so seductive to neuroscientists. The hippocampus is beautifully laminated; both the neuronal cell bodies and the zones of connectivity are arranged in orderly layers. The hippocampus is one of a group of structures within the limbic system typically called the *hippocampal formation* that includes the dentate gyrus, the hippocampus, the subiculum, presubiculum and parasubiculum, and the entorhinal cortex. The dentate gyrus, hippocampus, and subiculum have a single cell layer with less cellular or acellular layers located above and below it. The other parts of the hippocampal formation have several cellular layers. The highly laminar nature of the dentate gyrus and hippocampus lends them to neuroanatomical and electrophysiological studies.

A second reason for the interest in the hippocampus is that since the early 1950s, it has been recognized to play a fundamental role in some forms of learning and memory. In a landmark paper by Scoville and Milner (1957), the neuropsychological findings from a patient known by his initials, H.M., who underwent bilateral hippocampal removal for the treatment of intractable epilepsy, were reported. HM, probably the most thoroughly studied neuropsychological subject in memory research, suffered a permanent loss of the ability to encode new information into long-term memory. This anterograde memory impairment has been seen in other patients with bilateral damage restricted to the hippocampus (Zola-Morgan et al., 1986). The intense interest in understanding the brain mechanisms involved in learning and memory have helped foster research at the neuroanatomical, physiological, and behavior levels of analysis in the hippocampus. These studies have forged a strong theoretical link between the hippocampus and certain forms of memory (see Functional Synthesis below). The hippocampus is also of interest because of its high seizure susceptibility. It has the lowest seizure threshold of any brain region (Green, 1964). Most patients with epilepsy have seizures that involve the hippocampus, and these seizures are often the most difficult to control medically. Portions of the hippocampal formation, particularly the entorhinal cortex, also appear to be prime targets for the pathology associated with Alzheimer's disease, and the hippocampus is very vulnerable to the effects of ischemia and anoxia.

The anatomical and functional organization of the hippocampus is of particular relevance to this text on the synaptic organization of the brain because in many ways the hippocampus has become a model system for studies of other cortical structures. Much of what is currently known about the physiology and pharmacology of synaptic transmission in the central nervous system has come from studies of the hippocampus. Because the largest portion of the physiological literature on the hippocampal formation deals with either the dentate gyrus or the hippocampus, we will devote most of our coverage to these structures and will focus mainly on the organization of the rat hippocampus.

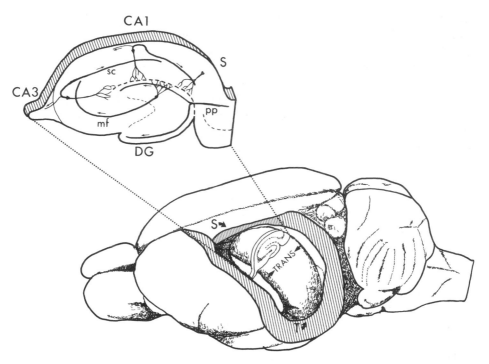

Fig. 11.1. Line drawing of a lateral cutaway view of the rat brain showing the location of the hippocampal formation (rostral is to the left and caudal is to the right). The hippocampus is a banana-shaped structure that extends from the septal nuclei rostrally to the temporal cortex, caudally. The long axis is called the *septotemporal axis* (indicated by S–T) and the orthogonal axis is the *transverse axis* (TRANS). A slice cut perpendicular to the long axis of the hippocampus (above left) shows several fields of the hippocampal formation and several of the intrinsic connections. Slices of this type are typically used for in vitro electrophysiological analyses of the hippocampus. Abbreviations: DG, dentate gyrus; CA3, CA1, fields of the hippocampus; S, subiculum; pp, perforant path fibers from the entorhinal cortex; mf, mossy fibers from the granule cells; sc, Schaffer collateral connections from CA3 to CA1. [From Amaral and Witter, 1989, with permission.]

NEURONAL ELEMENTS

THREE-DIMENSIONAL POSITION AND LAYERS OF THE RAT HIPPOCAMPUS

The three-dimensional position of the rat hippocampal formation in the brain is shown in Figure 11.1. It appears grossly as an elongated structure with its long axis extending in a C-shaped fashion from the septal nuclei rostrally, over and behind the diencephalon, into the temporal lobe caudally and ventrally. The long axis of the hippocampus is referred to as the *septotemporal axis* and the orthogonal axis is referred to as the *transverse axis.*

The various layers of the hippocampal formation are shown in Fig. 11.2. The dentate gyrus consists of three layers: the principal, or granule cell layer, the largely acellular molecular layer that is located above the granule cell layer, and the diffusely cellular polymorphic cell layer (also called the hilus) that is located below the granule cell layer. The hippocampus also has a principal cell layer called the *pyramidal cell layer*. The regions above and below the pyramidal cell layer are divided into a number of strata that we will describe in due course.

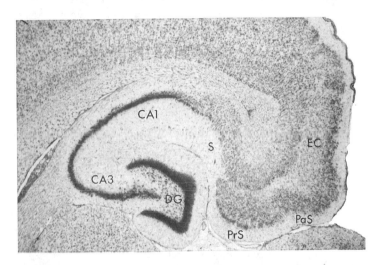

Fig. 11.2. A Nissl-stained horizontal section through the rat hippocampal formation showing all of its cytoarchitectonic divisions. (Caudal is to the right, rostral is to the left, and lateral is to the top.) The dark layers contain stained cell bodies. The acellular regions contain dendrites of the hippocampal neurons and axons from intrinsic and extrinsic sources. The dentate gyrus (DG) has three layers: the molecular layer (m); the granule cell layer (g) and the polymorphic cell layer (pl). The hippocampus is divided into CA3, CA2, and CA1 regions (CA2 not shown). In all hippocampal fields, the surface is formed by the alveus, a thin sheet of outgoing and incoming fibers. The layer occupied by basal dendrites of the pyramidal cells is stratum oriens (o) followed by the pyramidal cell layer (p) where the cell bodies of the pyramidal cells are located. Superficial to the pyramidal cell layer is stratum radiatum (r) and stratum lacunosum-moleculare (l-m) where the apical dendrites of the pyramidal cells are located. The subiculum (S), presubiculum (PrS), parasubiculum (PaS) and entorhinal cortex (EC) are also illustrated. A major input–output fiber bundle is the fimbria (f). The angular bundle (ab) is a fiber region in which the perforant path fibers travel from the entorhinal cortex to the other fields of the hippocampal formation.

PRINCIPAL NEURONS

The principal neurons in the dentate gyrus are the *granule cells*, and in the hippocampus they are the *pyramidal neurons*. The pyramidal cell layer of the hippocampus has been divided into three regions designated *CA1–CA3* (Lorente de Nó, 1934) based on the size and appearance of the neurons.

   The granule cells have small (about 10 μm in diameter), spherically shaped cell bodies that are arranged 4–6 cells thick in the *granule cell layer*. In rodents, the granule cell layer is shaped like the letter "V" or "U," depending on the septotemporal level (see Fig. 11.3). The granule cell dendrites extend perpendicularly to the *granule cell layer*, into the overlying *molecular layer* where they receive synaptic connections from several sources. Because the dendrites emerge only from the top or apical portion of the cell body, granule cells are considered to be monopolar neurons. The axons of the granule cells are called *mossy fibers* because of the peculiar appearance of their synaptic terminals. They typically originate from the basal portion of the cell body, i.e., opposite to where the dendrites originate, and extend into the *polymorphic cell layer* (also called the *hilus*). The mossy fibers synapse onto some of the neurons, such as mossy cells, in the polymorphic cell layer before coalescing into a bundle of fibers that exits the hilus and enters stratum lucidum of CA3. The polymorphic cells are, as the name implies, of various types but they only project to other parts of the dentate gyrus.

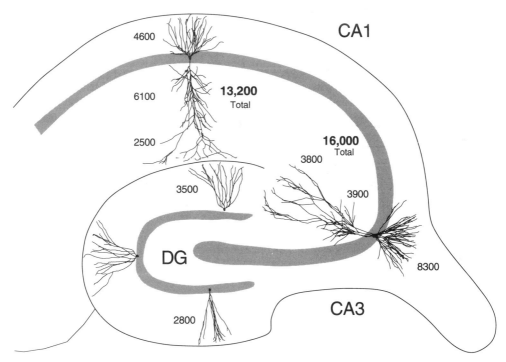

Fig. 11.3. Line drawing showing the shape and size of the principal neurons in the dentate gyrus (DG) and hippocampus (CA3 and CA1). Numbers indicate the total dendritic length of granule cells and of the portions of the dendritic trees located in stratum lacunosum-moleculare, radiatum, and oriens of the hippocampus. For the hippocampal cells, the total dendritic lengths are also given.

The cell bodies of the hippocampal pyramidal neurons are arranged, 3–6 cells deep, in an orderly layer called the *pyramidal cell layer*. These neurons have elaborate dendritic trees extending perpendicularly to the cell layer in both directions and are thus considered to be multipolar neurons but more typically called *pyramidal cells*. The apical dendrites are longer than the basal and extend from the apex of the pyramidal cell body toward the center of the hippocampus, i.e., towards the dentate gyrus (Fig. 11.3). The apical dendrites of CA3 pyramidal cells traverse three strata: stratum lucidum, strata radiatum, and stratum lacunosum-moleculare. The dendrites receive different types of synaptic contacts in each one of these strata. The basal dendrites extend from the base of the pyramidal cell body into stratum oriens.

The hippocampus can clearly be divided into two major regions, a large-celled region closer to the dentate gyrus and a smaller-celled distal region. Ramon y Cajal (1911) called these two regions *regio inferior* and *regio superior*, respectively. However, as noted above, Lorente de Nó (1934), divided the hippocampus into three fields (CA3, CA2, and CA1). He also used the term *CA4*, although this referred to the region occupied by the polymorphic layer of the dentate gyrus; CA4 is typically no longer used. His CA3 and CA2 fields are equivalent to the large-celled regio inferior of Ramon y Cajal and his CA1 is equivalent to regio superior. In addition to differences in the size of the pyramidal cells in CA3 and CA1, there is a clear-cut connectional difference. The CA3 pyramidal cells receive a mossy fiber input from the dentate gyrus and the CA1 pyramidal cells do not.

The CA2 field has been a matter of some controversy. As originally defined by Lorente de Nó, it was a narrow zone of cells interposed between CA3 and CA1, which had large cell bodies like CA3 but did not receive mossy fiber innervation like CA1 cells. The bulk of available evidence indicates that there is, indeed, a narrow CA2 which has both connectional and perhaps even functional differences with the other hippocampal fields. CA2, for example, appears to be more resistant to epileptic cell death than CA3 or CA1 and is sometimes referred to as the *resistant sector* Corsellis and Bruton (1983).

The dendrites of the pyramidal neurons are covered with spines onto which most excitatory synapses terminate. Some of the largest spines in the nervous system are the thorny excrescences, which are located on the proximal dendrites of CA3 and receive the synapses of the mossy fibers. The thorny excrescences are complex branched spines engulfed by a single mossy-fiber bouton (Hamlyn, 1962; see below). The remainder of the dendritic tree of CA3 pyramidal cells and the entire CA1 pyramidal cell dendritic tree have standard "cortical-like" spines on which excitatory, asymmetric synapses are formed.

INTERNEURONS

Intrinsic neurons, or interneurons, have traditionally been defined as neurons with a locally restricted axon plexus that lack spines and release γ-amino butyric acid (GABA). Recently, with advances in cell labeling, staining, and recording, interneurons have been found to be much more diverse than previously thought, and exceptions to all of these traditional views have been described (Buckmaster and Soltesz, 1996).

The vast majority of interneurons in the dentate gyrus and hippocampus (Fig. 11.4) do indeed have locally restricted target regions, lack spines, and are GABAergic

Hippocampus

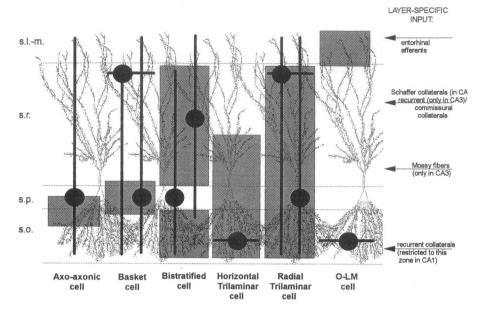

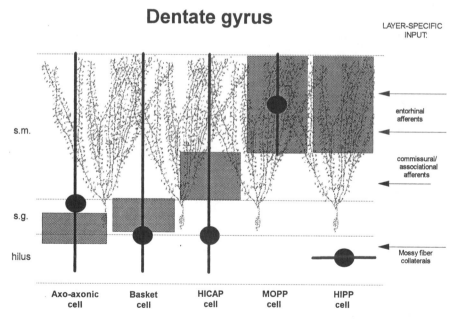

Fig. 11.4. A summary diagram of the various interneurons in the hippocampus and dentate gyrus. Most of the interneurons use GABA as their transmitter. Light profiles in the background show pyramidal cells (in the hippocampus) and granule cells (in the dentate gyrus). The interneurons innervate different portions of these principal neurons. For the interneurons, the locations of the cell bodies are marked with circles. The dark lines emanating from the circles represent the orientation and the laminar location of the major dendrites. The hatched area marks the regions where the axons from each interneuron typically arborizes. The laminar distribution of several of the excitatory inputs to these fields are indicated at right. [From Freund and Buzsaki, 1996, with permission.]

(Freund and Buzsaki, 1996.) In the dentate gyrus, the most prominent class of interneurons is called the *pyramidal basket cell* and the cell bodies of these neurons are typically located at the border between the granule cell layer and the polymorphic cell layer. Axons from these neurons innervate the cell bodies of granule cells. There are at least five different types of these basket cells (Ribak and Seress, 1983). There are also interneurons in the molecular layer. Perhaps the most interesting of these is an axo-axonic cell that terminates on the axon initial segments of granule cells (Kosaka, 1983; Freund and Buzsaki, 1996). There is also a variety of interneurons located in the polymorphic cell layer. Some of these have axons that remain within the polymorphic cell layer while others innervate the granule and molecular layers (Freund and Buzsaki, 1996). There is a class of neurons in the polymorphic layer that are called *mossy cells* (Amaral, 1978). These are excitatory neurons that nonetheless project only to the molecular layer of the dentate gyrus both ipsilaterally and contralaterally. Whereas some investigators have called these *excitatory interneurons*, the fact that they project their axons for long distances on both sides of the hippocampus would seem to preclude the use of the term interneuron. In fact, these neurons tend not to project locally but rather to distant septotemporal levels of the dentate gyrus. These types of neurons would then form an exception to the traditional definitions of interneurons and principal neurons.

Hippocampal interneurons with cell bodies in or near the pyramidal cell layer can be classified into three groups on the basis of their synaptic targets: axo-axonic cells, basket cells, and bistratified cells. As the name implies, *axo-axonic cells* synapse onto the initial segments of pyramidal neurons and thus exert a strong control over action potential initiation. *Basket cells* synapse onto the somata of pyramidal neurons. Each basket cell can make multiple contacts onto a pyramidal neuron, forming what looks like a "basket" into which the soma sits. Finally, *bistratified cells* make synaptic contacts onto apical and basal dendrites of pyramidal neurons. Although there is very little overlap among their target regions, the dendrites of all three cell types project into stratum radiatum and stratum oriens and thus may receive excitatory inputs from Schaffer collaterals, commissural-associational fibers, and feedback synapses from pyramidal neurons in the local region of the interneurons (Buhl et al., 1996; Halasy et al., 1996). There are also mutual inhibitory connections among these interneurons. The mutual inhibitory connections are thought to synchronize the interneurons producing oscillations at various frequencies, including theta (5 Hz) and gamma (40 Hz) frequencies (Jefferys et al., 1996). Many GABAergic interneurons also contain and release neuroactive peptides (see Freund and Buzsaki, 1996, for review).

There are also GABAergic interneurons in stratum radiatum and stratum lacunosum-moleculare which receive excitatory inputs from Schaffer collaterals and perforant path fibers, respectively, and synapse onto pyramidal neuron dendrites in various regions. Among interneurons whose properties and connections are less well known are putative excitatory interneurons in stratum lucidum that receive input from mossy fibers and synapse onto CA3 pyramidal neurons (Soriano and Frotscher, 1993), and interneurons whose postsynaptic targets are exclusively other interneurons (Freund and Buzsaki, 1996).

BASIC CIRCUITS

The basic circuitry of the hippocampal formation has been known since the time of Ramon y Cajal (1911), although details worked out by modern neuroanatomists have contributed to our current understanding, which is illustrated schematically in Fig. 11.5. Andersen and colleagues (1971) emphasized the unique unidirectional progression of excitatory pathways that linked each region of the hippocampal formation and coined the term *trisynaptic circuit*. For simplicity, the entorhinal cortex is considered to be the starting point of the circuit since much of the sensory information that reaches the hippocampus enters through the entorhinal cortex.

Neurons located in layer II of the entorhinal cortex give rise to a pathway, the *perforant path*, that projects through (perforates) the subiculum and terminates both in the dentate gyrus and in the CA3 field of the hippocampus. Cells in the medial entorhinal cortex contribute axons that terminate in a highly restricted fashion within the middle portion of the molecular layer of the dentate gyrus and those from the lateral entorhinal cortex terminate in the outer third of the molecular layer. These two components of the perforant path also end in a laminar pattern in the stratum lacunosum-moleculare of CA3 and CA2. Neurons located in layer III of the entorhinal cortex do not project to the dentate gyrus or CA3 but do project to CA1 and the subiculum. In this case, the projection is not organized in a laminar fashion but rather in a topographic fashion. Axons originating from neurons in the lateral entorhinal cortex terminate in that portion of stratum lacunosum-moleculare located at the border of CA1 with the subiculum. Projections arising from the medial entorhinal cortex terminate in that portion of stratum lacunosum-moleculare of CA1 that is located close to CA3 and in the molecular layer of the subiculum located close to the presubiculum.

The dentate gyrus is the next step in the progression of connections, and it gives rise to the mossy fibers that terminate on the proximal dendrites of the CA3 pyramidal cells. The granule cells also synapse on cells of the polymorphic layer, which provides associ-

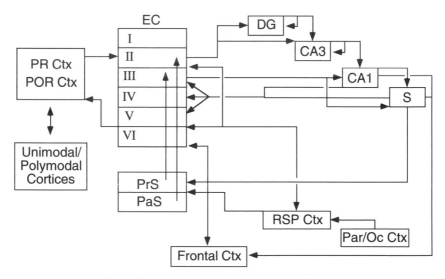

Fig. 11.5. Summary diagram of the major intrinsic connections of the rat hippocampal formation and several of the extrinsic cortical inputs. This diagram emphasizes the serial and parallel aspects of the intrinsic hippocampal circuitry. See text. Abbreviations: DG, dentate gyrus; CA3, CA1 fields of the hippocampus; EC, entorhinal cortex; PR, perirhinal; POR, postrhinal; PrS, presubiculum; PaS, parasubiculum; Par/Oc Ctx, parietal occipital cortices; RSP Ctx, retrosplenial cortex.

ational connections to other levels of the dentate gyrus.The CA3 pyramidal cells, in turn, project heavily to other levels of CA3 as well as to CA1. The projection to CA1 is typically called the *Schaffer collateral projection*. CA1 pyramidal cells give rise to connections both to the subiculum and to the deep layers of the entorhinal cortex. The subiculum also originates a projection to the deep layers of the entorhinal cortex. The deep layers of the entorhinal cortex, in turn, originate projections to many of the same cortical areas that originally projected to the entorhinal cortex. Thus, information entering the entorhinal cortex from a particular cortical area can traverse the entire hippocampal circuit through the excitatory pathways just described and ultimately be returned to the cortical area from which it originated. The transformations that take place through this traversal are presumably essential for enabling the information to be stored as long-term memories.

Now that the basic framework of the connectivity of the hippocampal formation has been layed out, we will delve more deeply into the synaptic organization of the dentate gyrus and hippocampus.

SYNAPTIC CONNECTIONS OF THE DENTATE GYRUS

The dentate granule cells give rise to the distinctive unmyelinated axons called *mossy fibers* (Fig. 11.6). Each mossy fiber gives rise to about seven thinner collaterals within the polymorphic layer before entering the CA3 field of the hippocampus (Claiborne et al., 1986). Within the polymorphic layer, the mossy fiber collaterals have two types of synaptic varicosities. There are about 160 small (0.5–2 μm) varicosities that form contacts on spines and dendritic shafts of polymorphic layer neurons (Claiborne et al.,

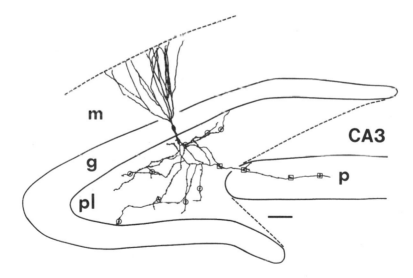

Fig. 11.6. Line drawing of a dentate granule cell and its mossy fiber axonal plexus. The axon originates from the cell body and descends into the polymorphic layer (pl) where it collateralizes. Each collateral has many small synaptic varicosities (small dots) and usually one larger presynaptic terminal (circles) that resemble the mossy fiber expansions found in stratum lucidum. The main mossy fiber axon enters CA3 and demonstrates several en passant and very large (3–8 μm) expansions (boxes) as it traverses the entire CA3 field before entering stratum lucidum. m, molecular layer; g, granule cell layer; p, pyramidal cell layer, pl, polymorphic layer.

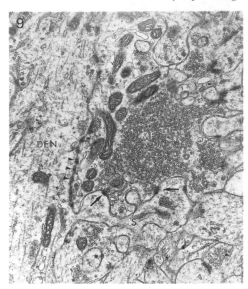

Fig. 11.7. Electron micrograph of a mossy fiber expansion (MF) that makes contact with a pyramidal cell dendrite (DEN). A large, complex thorny excrescence (S) is shown penetrating the expansion. There are several symmetrical contacts between the dendritic shaft and the expansion (arrowheads) which are nonsynaptic puncta adhearentia. There are also several asymmetric synapses between the expansions and the complex spine (arrows). Note that the small, round synaptic vesicles are only associated with the spine specializations. [From Amaral and Dent, 1981, with permission.]

1986). At the ends of each of the collateral branches there are usually single, larger (3–5 μm), irregularly shaped varicosities that resemble the mossy fiber terminals found in the CA3 field. These large mossy fiber terminals in the polymorphic layer establish contacts with the proximal dendrites of the mossy cells, the basal dendrites of the pyramidal basket cells, and other polymorphic layer cells (Ribak and Seress, 1983; Ribak et al., 1985; Scharfman et al., 1990a).

As noted previously, there is a variety of basket cells located close to the granule cell layer. These all appear to contribute to the very dense terminal plexus that is confined to the granule cell layer. The terminals in this basket plexus are GABAergic and form symmetric, presumably inhibitory contacts primarily on the cell bodies and shafts of apical dendrites of the granule cells (Kosaka et al., 1984). GABAergic neurons in the polymorphic layer are themselves innervated by GABAergic terminals (Misgeld and Frotscher, 1986). How widespread is the influence of a single basket cell? Analysis of Golgi-stained axonal plexuses from single basket cells (Struble et al., 1978) indicates that they extend on average 400 μm in the transverse axis and at least 1.1 mm in the septotemporal axis. It is conceivable, therefore, that a single basket cell has influence over a very large number of granule cells.

A second inhibitory input to granule cells originates from the axo-axonic or "chandelier-type" cells located in the molecular layer (Kosaka, 1983; Soriano and Frotscher, 1989). These form symmetric contacts exclusively with the axon initial segment of granule cells. Another intrinsic projection within the dentate gyrus arises from a population of somatostatin immunoreactive neurons scattered throughout the polymorphic layer (Morrison et al., 1982; Bakst et al., 1986). These somatostatin cells, located in the polymorphic layer, colocalize GABA and contribute a plexus of fibers and terminals to the outer portions of the molecular layer. This system of fibers, which forms contacts on the distal dendrites of the granule cells, provides a third means for inhibitory control over granule cell activity (Freund and Buzsaki, 1996).

The inner third of the molecular layer of the dentate gyrus receives a projection that originates exclusively from cells in the polymorphic layer (Blackstad, 1956; Laurberg and Sorensen, 1981). Since this projection originates both on the ipsilateral and contralateral sides, it has been called the *ipsilateral associational/commissural projection*. The ipsilateral associational and commissural projections appear to originate as collaterals from axons of the mossy cells of the hilus (Laurberg and Sorensen, 1981). Most terminals of this pathway form asymmetric, presumably excitatory synaptic terminals on spines of the granule cell dendrites (Laatsch and Cowan, 1967; Kishi et al., 1980). Since the mossy cells are immunoreactive for glutamate (Soriano and Frotscher, 1993), it is likely that they release this excitatory transmitter substance at their terminals within the ipsilateral associational/commissural zone of the molecular layer.

Since the mossy cells are densely innervated by the granule cells, they provide the substrate for a potential feedback loop via their axons to the proximal dendrites of the granule cells. However, a few facts temper the way we think about this feedback loop. The granule cells innervate mossy cells at the same septotemporal level at which their cell bodies are located. However, the mossy cells project not to the same level that their cell bodies are located but to distant levels located both septally and temporally from the level of the cell body. Thus, it would appear that the mossy cells pass on the collective output of granule cells from one septotemporal level to granule cells located at distant levels of the dentate gyrus. The functional significance of the longitudinal distribution of the associational projection cannot be fully appreciated without one further piece of information. In addition to contacting the spines of dentate granule cells, the associational fibers also contact the dendritic shafts of GABAergic basket cells (Frotscher and Zimmer, 1983; Seress and Ribak, 1984). Thus, the associational and commissural projections may function both as a feedforward excitatory pathway and as a disynaptic feedforward inhibitory pathway. A final fact that contributes to this discussion is that the somatostatin/GABA pathway described above (which originates from cells in the polymorphic layer) has a more local and limited terminal distribution. Thus, mossy fiber collaterals terminating on GABA/somatostatin cells in the polymorphic layer may lead predominantly to direct inhibition of granule cells at the same septotemporal level and to either inhibition or excitation (via the ipsilateral associational connection) at more distant levels of the dentate gyrus. The fact that the ipsilateral associational connection appears to be organized primarily to influence cells some distance away from the cell bodies of origin is a significant contradiction to the notion that the hippocampus processes information exclusively in a lamellar fashion, i.e., within slices of the hippocampal banana (Amaral and Witter, 1989).

Synaptic Connections from the Entorhinal Cortex. The major input to the dentate gyrus is from the entorhinal cortex. The major organizational features of this projection have already been described. The projection to the dentate gyrus arises mainly from layer II of the entorhinal cortex (Steward and Scoville, 1976; Schwartz and Coleman, 1981; Ruth et al., 1982, 1988). A minor component of the projection also comes from the deep layers (IV–VI) of the entorhinal cortex (Köhler, 1985). In the molecular layer of the dentate gyrus, the terminals of the perforant path fibers are strictly confined to the outer or superficial two-thirds, where they form asymmetric synapses (Nafstad, 1967). These occur most frequently on the dendritic spines of dentate granule cells, although a small proportion of perforant path fibers terminate on the basket pyramidal interneurons (Zipp et al., 1989). Within the outer two-thirds of the molecular layer, perforant path synapses make up at least 85% of the total synaptic population (Nafstad, 1967). The perforant path is most likely glutamatergic (Fonnum et al., 1979). At least for the projection to the dentate gyrus, the terminals of the lateral perforant pathway are enkephalin immunoreactive, whereas those of the medial pathway are immunoreactive for CCK (Fredens et al., 1984).

Extrinsic Inputs to the Dentate Gyrus. The remainder of this section will deal with the subcortical inputs to the dentate gyrus, which originate mainly from the septal nuclei, supramamillary region of the posterior hypothalamus, and several monoaminergic nuclei in the brainstem, especially the locus coeruleus and raphe nuclei.

The septal projection arises from cells of the medial septal nucleus and the nucleus of the diagonal band of Broca and travels to the hippocampal formation via four routes: the fimbria, dorsal fornix, supracallosal stria, and via a ventral route through and around the amygdaloid complex (Mosko et al., 1973; Swanson, 1978; Amaral and Kurz, 1985). Septal fibers heavily innervate the polymorphic layer, particularly in a narrow band just below the granule cell layer, and terminate more lightly in the molecular layer. Thirty to fifty percent of the cells in the medial septal nucleus and 50–75% of the cells in the nucleus of the diagonal band that project to the hippocampal formation are cholinergic (Amaral and Kurz, 1985; Wainer et al., 1985). Many of the other septal cells that project to the dentate gyrus, however, contain glutamic acid decarboxylase and are presumably GABAergic (Köhler et al., 1984); they terminate in the dentate gyrus and have an apparent preference for terminating on the GABAergic nonpyramidal cells (Freund and Antal, 1988). The septal GABAergic projection provides a striking example of long, projection neurons (not interneurons) that use GABA as their transmitter.

There is only one major hypothalamic projection to the dentate gyrus and this arises from the supramammillary area (Wyss et al., 1979a,b; Dent et al., 1983; Haglund et al., 1984). The supramamillary projection terminates heavily in a narrow zone of the molecular layer located just superficial to the granule cell layer; there is only light innervation of the polymorphic or molecular layers.

The dentate gyrus receives a particularly prominent noradrenergic input primarily from the locus coeruleus (Pickel et al., 1974; Swanson and Hartman, 1975), and the noradrenergic fibers terminate mainly in the polymorphic layer of the dentate gyrus. The serotonergic projection, which originates from the raphe nuclei, also terminates most heavily in the polymorphic layer, but the projection tends to be limited to an immediately subgranular portion of the layer (Conrad et al., 1974). Freund and colleagues

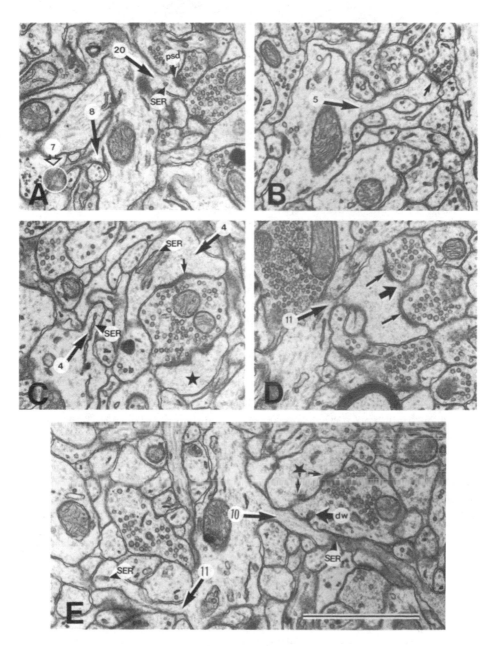

Fig. 11.8. Electron micrographs of axospinous synapses in the CA1 region of the rat hippocampus. **A:** A stubby spine (20) is identified and shows a postsynaptic density (psd). A cistern of smooth endoplasmic reticulum (ser) is in the spine. **B:** A typical thin spine with asymmetrical synapse on its head. **C:** Spine with large spine head making contact with axonal terminal. **D:** Perforated synapse. The spinule (large arrow) perforates the postsynaptic density which forms two patches (small arrows). **E:** Two very thin spine necks (10 and 11). [From Harris and Stevens, 1989, with permission.]

(Halasy et al., 1991) have shown that the serotonergic fibers preferentially terminate on a class of interneurons in the dentate gyrus that primarily innervate the distal dendrites of the granule cells. As with the cholinergic projection, many of the cells in the raphe nuclei that project to the hippocampal formation appear to be nonserotonergic (Köhler and Steinbusch, 1982). The dentate gyrus receives a lighter and diffusely distributed dopaminergic projection that arises mainly from cells located in the ventral tegmental area (Swanson, 1982).

Outputs of the Dentate Gyrus. The dentate gyrus does not project to other brain regions. Within the hippocampal formation, it only projects to CA3 via the mossy fibers. Once the mossy fibers leave the hilus and enter the CA3 region, they have few collaterals. The mossy fibers tend to fasciculate as they extend in stratum lucidum throughout the CA3 field, where they demonstrate the large (3–6 μm in diameter), presynaptic varicosities characteristic of mossy fiber–CA3 pyramidal cell contacts (Claiborne et al., 1986). These large, presynaptic expansions are distributed at approximately 140-μm intervals along the course of the mossy fiber axons. In the part of CA3 located closest to the dentate gyrus, some mossy fibers extend deep to the pyramidal cell layer in what has been called the *infrapyramidal bundle*. In this region, the mossy fibers terminate on large thorny excrescences that are located both on the proximal apical and basal dendrites of the pyramidal cells.

The mossy-fiber presynaptic expansion forms a unique synaptic complex with an equally intricate postsynaptic process called the *thorny excrescence* (Fig. 11.7). These spine-like processes are large, multilobulated entities (with as many as 16 branches) that are surrounded by a single mossy-fiber expansion. A single mossy-fiber expansion can make as many as 37 synaptic contacts with a single CA3 pyramidal-cell dendrite (Chicurel and Harris, 1992). Because of the large size and proximal dendritic location of the mossy fiber synapse, the granule cells are in a unique position to influence the activity of hippocampal pyramidal cells. However, mossy fibers contact relatively few pyramidal cells, perhaps no more than 14 throughout their entire trajectory (Claiborne et al., 1986). Each pyramidal cell receives contacts from approximately 50 dentate granule cells.

The mossy fibers remain at approximately the same septotemporal level as their cells of origin (Gaarskjaer, 1978a,b; Swanson et al., 1978; Claiborne et al., 1986). In this respect, they are different from the organization of the ipsilateral associational connection in the dentate gyrus and the connections of the hippocampus, which tend to have much more extensive septotemporal distributions. Near the CA3–CA2 border, however, the mossy fibers make an abrupt turn temporally and extend for 1 mm or more towards the temporal pole of the hippocampus. The functional significance of this component of the mossy fibers has never been understood.

The mossy fibers are thought to use glutamate (Storm-Mathisen and Fonnum, 1972) as their primary transmitter substance. But some mossy fibers harbor opiate peptides such as dynorphin and enkephalin (Gall et al., 1981; Gall, 1984; van Daal et al., 1989). More recently, mossy fibers have also been shown to be immunoreactive for GABA (Sloviter et al., 1996). However, it is not clear whether this is involved in synaptic transmission or has a more general metabolic role.

SYNAPTIC CONNECTIONS OF CA3

The CA3 pyramidal cells give rise to highly collateralized axons that distribute fibers both within the hippocampus (to CA3, CA2, and CA1), to the same fields in the contralateral hippocampus (the commissural projections), and subcortically to the lateral septal nucleus. CA3 cells, especially those located proximally in the field, and CA2 cells contribute a small number of collaterals that innervate the polymorphic layer of the dentate gyrus.

All of the CA3 and CA2 pyramidal cells give rise to highly divergent projections to all portions of the hippocampus (Ishizuka et al., 1990). The projections to CA3 and CA2 are typically called the *associational connections* and the CA3 projections to the CA1 field are called the *Schaffer collaterals*. There is a highly ordered and spatially distributed pattern of projections from CA3 to CA3 and from CA3 to CA1 (Ishizuka et al., 1990). The essential elements of the organization of these connections include the following.

All portions of CA3 and CA2 project to CA1 but the distribution of terminations in CA1 depends on the transverse location of the CA3/CA2 cells of origin. The older notion that a typical CA3 pyramidal cell sends a single axon to CA1 that extend linearly through the field with equal contact probability at all regions within CA1 is clearly incorrect. The topographic organization of projections from CA3 to CA1 determines a network in which certain CA3 cells are more likely to contact certain CA1 cells. CA3 cells located close to the dentate gyrus, while projecting both septally and temporally for substantial distances, tend to project more heavily to levels of CA1 located septal to their location. CA3 cells located closer to CA1, in contrast, project more heavily to levels of CA1 located temporally. At or close to the septotemporal level of the cells of origin, those cells located proximally in CA3 give rise to collaterals that tend to terminate superficially in stratum radiatum. Conversely, cells of origin located more distally in CA3 give rise to projections that terminate deeper in stratum radiatum and in stratum oriens. At or close to the septotemporal level of origin, CA3 pyramidal cells located near the dentate gyrus tend to project somewhat more heavily to distal portions of CA1 (near the subicular border), whereas CA3 projections arising from cells located distally in CA3 terminate more heavily in portions of CA1 located closer to the CA2 border.

Regardless of the septotemporal or transverse origin of a projection, the highest density of terminal and fiber labeling in CA1 shifts to deeper parts of stratum radiatum and stratum oriens at levels septal to the cells of origin and shifts out of stratum oriens and into superficial parts of stratum radiatum at levels temporal to the origin. Moreover, the highest density of fiber and terminal labeling in CA1 shifts proximally (towards CA3) at levels septal to the origin and distally (towards the subiculum) at levels temporal to the origin. While Schaffer collaterals are often illustrated as extending only through stratum radiatum, it should be emphasized that both stratum radiatum and stratum oriens of CA1 are heavily innervated by CA3 axons. Thus, the Schaffer collaterals are as highly associated with the apical dendrites of CA1 cells in stratum radiatum as they are with the basal dendrites in stratum oriens. Moreover, some Schaffer collaterals that are initially in stratum radiatum ultimately extend into stratum oriens, and thus these axons may terminate on the apical dendrites of some pyramidal cells and the basal dendrites of other pyramidal cells. Although it has been implicit in our discussion of these connections, it should be emphasized that each CA3 neuron makes contacts with many CA1 pyramidal cells. It has been estimated, for example, that a single CA1 neuron may be innervated by more than 5,000 ipsilateral CA3 pyramidal cells (Amaral et al., 1990). The projections from CA3 to CA1 terminate as asymmetric, axospinous synapses located on the apical and basal dendrites of the CA1 pyramidal cells (Fig. 11.8). The sizes and shapes of the spines and presynaptic profiles in this region are quite variable and may be related to the physiological efficacy of the synapses in CA1.

The associational projections from CA3 to CA3 are also organized in a highly systematic fashion and again terminate throughout stratum radiatum and oriens. One somewhat idiosyncratic facet of this projection is that cells located proximally in CA3 only communicate with other cells in the proximal portion of CA3 of the same and adjacent septotemporal levels. Associational projections arising from mid- and distal portions of CA3, however, project throughout much of the transverse extent of CA3 and also project much more extensively along the septotemporal axis.

An important feature of the CA3-to-CA3 associational and CA3-to-CA1 Schaffer collateral projections is that they are both divergently distributed along the septotemporal axis. Single CA3 and CA2 pyramidal cells give rise to highly arborized axonal plexuses that distribute to as much as 75% of the septotemporal extent of the ipsilateral and contralateral CA1 fields (Tamamaki et al., 1984, 1988). Using intracellular techniques, Li et al. (1994) have found that the total length of the axonal plexus from single CA3 neurons can be as long as 150–300 mm and that a single CA3 cell may contact as many as 30,000 to 60,000 neurons in the ipsilateral hippocampus!

In the rat, but not in the monkey (Amaral et al., 1984; Demeter et al., 1985), the CA3 pyramidal cells give rise to commissural projections to the CA3, CA2 and CA1 regions of the contralateral hippocampal formation (Swanson et al., 1978). The same CA3 cells give rise both to ipsilateral and commissural projections (Swanson et al., 1980). Although the commissural projections roughly follow the same topographic organization and generally terminate in homologous regions on both sides, there are minor differences in the distribution of terminals. If a projection is heavier to stratum oriens on the ipsilateral side, for example, it may be heavier in stratum radiatum on the contralateral side (Swanson et al., 1978). As with the commissural projections from the dentate gyrus, CA3 fibers to the contralateral hippocampus form asymmetric synapses on the spines of pyramidal cells in CA3 and CA1 (Gottlieb and Cowan, 1972) but also terminate on the smooth dendrites of interneurons (Frotscher and Zimmer, 1983).

Projections to Other Brain Regions. Until the mid 1970s, it was commonly assumed that the hippocampal fields (CA1–CA3) gave rise to all of the subcortical connections to the basal forebrain and diencephalon. But Swanson and Cowan (1975) demonstrated that most of these projections actually originate from the subiculum. The only sizable subcortical projection from CA3 is to the lateral septal nucleus (Swanson and Cowan, 1977). The CA3 projection to the septal complex is distinct from other hippocampal projections to the septal region in that it is bilateral. Some CA3 fibers cross in the ventral hippocampal commissure to innervate the homologous region of the contralateral lateral septal nucleus. Interestingly, essentially all of the CA3 cells give rise to projections both to CA1 and to the lateral septal nucleus (Swanson et al., 1980). It should be noted that at least some of the hippocampal neurons that project to the septal region are GABAergic (Toth and Freund 1992).

The septal nucleus also provides the major subcortical input to CA3. As with the dentate gyrus, the septal projection originates mainly in the medial septal nucleus and nucleus of the diagonal band of Broca. The projection appears to terminate most heavily in stratum oriens and to a lesser extent in stratum radiatum (Nyakas et al., 1987; Gaykema et al., 1990). As in the dentate gyrus, the GABAergic component of the septal projection to the CA3 field terminates mainly on GABAergic interneurons (Freund and Antal, 1988; Gulyas et al., 1990).

The CA3 field also receives inputs from the noradrenergic nucleus locus coeruleus. Noradrenergic fibers and terminals are most densely distributed in the stratum lucidum and in the most superficial portion of stratum lacunosum-moleculare. A much thinner plexus of noradrenergic axons is distributed throughout the other layers of CA3. Serotonergic fibers are diffusely and sparsely distributed in CA3 and there are few, if any, dopaminergic fibers in this field (Swanson et al., 1987). As in the dentate gyrus, the serotonergic fibers, though diffusely distributed, nonetheless appear to terminate preferentially on interneurons (Freund et al., 1990) with axons that innervate the distal dendrites of pyramidal cells.

SYNAPTIC CONNECTIONS OF CA2

The CA2 field is relatively narrow and is located distal to the end of the mossy fiber projection; it is typically no wider than approximately 250 μm. It is made up of large, darkly staining pyramidal cells, like those of CA3. However, the CA2 pyramidal cells lack the thorny excrescences that are characteristic of CA3 pyramidal cells (Lorente de Nó, 1934; Tamamaki et al., 1988). A number of immunohistochemical studies have also demonstrated differential labeling of CA2. This region demonstrates denser acetylcholinesterase staining and much denser labeling for the calcium-binding protein parvalbumin than adjacent regions of CA3 or CA1 (Bainbridge and Miller, 1982). This is of interest since the calcium-binding proteins are considered to be protective of ischemic or excitotoxic cell death and the CA2 region is purported to be the "resistant sector" described in the human epilepsy literature (Corsellis and Bruton, 1983).

The intrahippocampal connections of CA2 resemble, in part, those of the distal portions of CA3, but there are also some distinguishing characteristics. Like CA3, the CA2 cells give rise to a projection to CA1 (Ishizuka et al., 1990). The projection is rather sparse and diffuse, however, and does not clearly follow the gradient rules established by the CA3 to CA1 projection. Interestingly, more collaterals from CA2 are distributed to the polymorphic layer of the dentate gyrus than from any portion of CA3.

There has been little work dealing specifically with the extrinsic inputs and outputs of CA2. In general, CA2 appears to share the connections of CA3. However, CA2 appears to receive a particularly prominent innervation from the supramammillary area (Haglund et al., 1984) and from the tuberomammillary nucleus (Köhler et al., 1985).

SYNAPTIC CONNECTIONS OF CA1

Unlike the CA3 field, pyramidal cells in CA1 do not appear to give rise to a major set of collaterals that distribute within CA1 (Amaral et al., 1991; Tamamaki et al., 1987), i.e. they have few associational connections. As the CA1 axons extend in the alveus or in stratum oriens towards the subiculum, occasional collaterals do arise and appear to enter stratum oriens and the pyramidal cell layer. It is likely that these collaterals terminate on the basal dendrites of other CA1 cells (Deuchars and Thomson, 1996). What is clear, however, is that the massive associational network which is so apparent in CA3 is largely missing in CA1. Whereas it was thought that the CA1 field gave rise to no commissural connections (Swanson et al., 1978), it now appears that a small number of CA1 neurons may project to the contralateral CA1 (Van Groen and Wyss, 1990).

The CA1 field receives a similar but substantially lighter septal projection than CA3 (Nyakas et al., 1987). As with CA3, the CA1 field receives light noradrenergic and serotonergic projections. The distal portion of CA1 receives a fairly substantial input from the amygdaloid complex (Krettek and Price, 1977b). Fibers originating in the basolateral nucleus terminate in stratum lacunosum-moleculare of the CA1 field; this input from the amygdala appears to be restricted to the temporal third of CA1.

The thalamic inputs to the hippocampal formation have received relatively little attention. It has been known for some time that the anterior thalamic complex is intimately interconnected with the subiculum and the presubiculum. Herkenham (1978) demonstrated fairly prominent projections from midline (or nonspecific) regions of thalamus to several fields of the hippocampal formation. In particular, the small midline nucleus reuniens gives rise to a prominent projection to the stratum lacunosum-moleculare of CA1. Wouterlood and colleagues (1990; Dolleman-Van der Weel and Witter, 1992) found that the nucleus reuniens projections travel to the CA1 field via the internal capsule and cingulum bundle rather than through the fimbria/fornix. The nucleus reuniens projection terminates massively in stratum lacunosum-moleculare and innervates all septotemporal fields. Electronmicroscopic analysis indicates that the nucleus reuniens fibers terminate with asymmetric synapses on spines and thin dendritic shafts in stratum lacunosum-moleculare.

The CA1 field gives rise to two intrahippocampal projections. The first is a topographically organized projection to the adjacent subiculum (Amaral et al., 1991). The second is to the deep layers of the entorhinal cortex.

Axons of CA1 pyramidal cells descend into stratum oriens or the alveus and bend sharply towards the subiculum (Finch et al., 1983; Tamamaki et al., 1988; Amaral et al., 1991). The fibers re-enter the pyramidal cell layer of the subiculum and ramify profusely in the pyramidal cell layer and in the deep portion of the molecular layer. Unlike the CA3 to CA1 projection, which distributes throughout CA1 in a gradient fashion, the CA1 projection ends in a columnar fashion in the subiculum. CA1 cells located proximally in the field project to the distal third of the subiculum, whereas CA1 cells located distally in the field project just across the border into the proximal portion of the subiculum; the mid-portion of CA1 projects to the mid-portion of the subiculum (Amaral et al., 1991). Tamamaki et al. (1988) injected single CA1 pyramidal cells with horseradish peroxidase and demonstrated that individual axonal plexuses distribute to about one-third the width of the subicular pyramidal cell layer. Thus, the CA1 to subiculum projection segments these structures roughly into thirds.

CA1 is the first hippocampal field that originates a return projection to the entorhinal cortex and is thus different from the dentate gyrus and fields CA3/CA2 in this respect. Projections from CA1 to the entorhinal cortex originate from the full septotemporal and transverse extent of CA1 and appear to terminate most densely in the medial entorhinal cortex, although projections also reach the lateral entorhinal cortex. The CA1 projections to the entorhinal cortex terminate predominantly in layer V (Swanson and Cowan, 1977; Finch and Babb, 1980, 1981; Van Groen and Wyss, 1990).

PHYSIOLOGICAL AND PHARMACOLOGICAL PROPERTIES

GENERAL PROPERTIES

Basic Response. As mentioned in previous sections, the highly structured and organized arrangement of synaptic pathways makes the hippocampus ideal for studying synaptic actions in vivo or in vitro (Andersen et al., 1971). Single-shock electrical stimulations to the perforant path, mossy fibers, or Schaffer collaterals result in a characteristic sequence of excitation followed by inhibition in the appropriate target neurons. The excitation typically precedes the inhibition by a few milliseconds but otherwise they overlap in time (Barrionuevo et al., 1986). The inhibition arises from the feedforward and feedback (recurrent) connections described above and often has two phases, a fast and a slow phase (see below). Some of the first recordings of synaptic actions in the hippocampus were made by Andersen and colleagues using electrical field recordings in vivo (see Langmoen and Andersen, 1981).

Extracellular Responses. Electrical field recordings represent the summed responses from a number of neurons in the vicinity of the recording electrode. Because of the orderly arrangement of pyramidal neurons and their dendrites, the electrical fields generated by active neurons have symmetry along the septal-temporal and cell-layer dimensions and asymmetry along the dendritic-somatic axis. This two-dimensional symmetry and one-dimensional assymetry makes electrical field recordings in hippocampus quite informative. For example, it can be shown that under appropriate conditions, the time course of the field potential is approximately equal to the time course of the underlying synaptic current (see Johnston and Wu, 1995). Furthermore, if multiple recordings are made at different sites along the dendritic axis, it is possible to localize the approximate site of generation of the electrical response using a technique called *current-source density analysis* (Haberly and Shepherd, 1973; Richardson et al., 1987).

Because current flows into the dendrites during excitatory synaptic activity, a field-recording electrode in stratum radiatum records first a brief negative-going transient that results from the volley of action potentials in the presynaptic fibers (called the *fiber volley*) followed by a slower negative-going potential with a time course similar to that of the underlying excitatory synaptic currents (refer to Fig. 11.9). This latter waveform is called a *population excitatory postsynaptic potential*, or *pEPSP*, to signify that the measured potential results from the summed activity across a population of neurons. The current flowing into the dendrites during this pEPSP will exit the neurons near the cell body layer so that a field electrode in *stratum pyramidale* will record a positive-going potential during this same synaptic event. If the intensity of the synaptic input is sufficient to evoke action potentials in the neurons, then the field electrode in *stratum pyramidale* will also record a negative-going potential (called a *pspike*) resulting from the inward current during the postsynaptic action potentials. Measurements of the initial slope of the pEPSP measured in either *stratum radiatum* or *stratum pyramidale* provide a reliable estimate of the intensity of synaptic activity, whereas

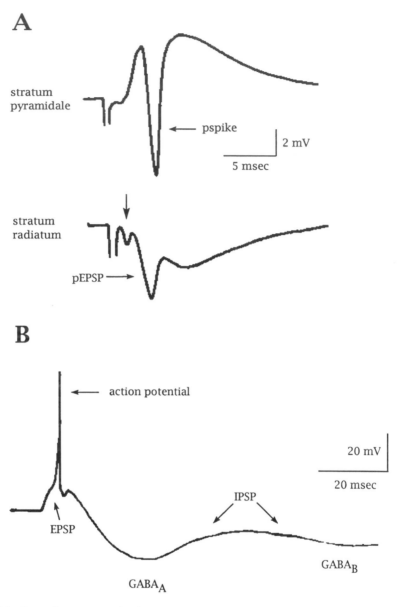

Fig. 11.9. Synaptic responses in hippocampus. **A:** Extracellular recordings from stratum pyramidale (SP) and stratum radiatum (SR) of CA1 in response to stimulation of Schaffer collaterals. The initial positivity from stratum pyramidale corresponds to the large negativity in stratum radiatum and results from synaptic current into the dendrites. This is the pEPSP and can be measured in either stratum pyramidale or stratum radiatum. The large negativity in stratum pyramidale is the pspike. It can be seen as a small positivity in stratum radiatum. The arrow in the stratum radiatum recording indicates the fiber volley (see text). (Modified from Alger et al., 1984, with permission). **B:** Intracellular response in a CA1 neuron to Schaffer collateral stimulation. The initial EPSP triggers an action potential. The EPSP is followed by an IPSP with fast (GABA$_A$) and slow (GABA$_B$) phases. [Modified from Schwartzkroin, 1986, with permission.]

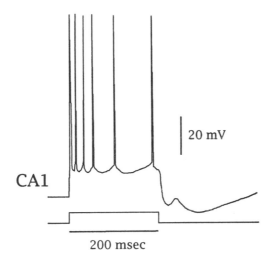

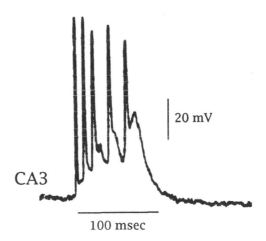

Fig. 11.10. Firing properties of CA1 and CA3 pyramidal neurons. CA1 neurons fire repetitively but show accomodation and fast and slow afterhyperpolarizations. CA3 neurons tend to fire in bursts of action potentials with declining amplitudes. (From Johnston and Wu, 1995, and Johnston and Brown, 1984b.)

a measure of the amplitude of the pspike provides an estimate of the number of neurons reaching threshold from this synaptic input. The amplitude of the fiber volley is proportional to the number of presynaptic axons being activated by the electrical stimulus. These field potentials can be easily recorded from in vitro preparations for many hours and have provided a wealth of information about the physiology and pharmacology of synaptic transmission in hippocampus.

Intracellular Responses. The electrophysiological behavior of the different neurons in the hippocampus is variable. Dentate granule and CA1 pyramidal neurons can fire repetitively at up to several hundred Hz (Schwartzkroin, 1975, 1977), whereas CA3 pyramidal neurons tend to fire in short bursts of 5–10 action potentials (Wong and Prince, 1978; Hablitz and Johnston, 1981; Fig. 11.10). The bursting properties of CA3 were first noticed by Kandel and Spencer (1961a) in their landmark study of hippocampal neurons in vivo and are thought to be important for explaining the seizure susceptibility of the hippocampus (Kandel and Spencer, 1961b; Traub and Llinas, 1979; Traub and Wong, 1981). Another prominent feature of hippocampal neurons firing repetitively is that the frequency of action potentials declines or accomodates during the train and there is a slow afterhyperpolarization (AHP) at the end of the train. Both the frequency accomodation and the slow AHP result in part from the activation of potassium channels by the influx of calcium ions during the train.

Intracellular recordings during electrical stimulation of an afferent pathway reveal the excitation–inhibition (EPSP–IPSP) sequence illustrated in Fig. 11.9B. These recordings can be made with sharp microelectrodes or with whole-cell patch electrodes. Because of recent advances in the visualization of single neurons in brain slices using infrared videomicroscopy (Stuart et al., 1993), the whole-cell patch method has become the technique of choice for most studies. The amplitudes of the electrically evoked EPSPs can range from less than 1 mV to several tens of mV, while the IPSPs, if present, are in the range of 1 to 10 mV. The EPSP rise times (usually measured from 10 to 90% of the peak) are on the order of 5–20 ms and, if not accompanied by an IPSP, decay exponentially according to the membrane time constant, which is about 50 ms (Spruston and Johnston, 1992). IPSPs evoked by stimulation of afferent pathways are typically much slower than EPSPs and are characterized by two components. The fast component peaks in about 20–50 ms from the stimulus and decays nonexponentially in 100–500 ms. The slow component peaks in about 100 ms and can take more than 1 sec to decay. Dendritic IPSPs are slower than somatic IPSPs and more closely follow the time course of NMDA receptor–mediated responses (see below; Pearce, 1993).

If the afferent stimulation is of sufficient intensity, the EPSP will evoke one or more action potentials. These action potentials are usually initiated first in the axon and then propagate into the soma and dendrites as well as down the axon to the synaptic terminals. The threshold for initiating an action potential in the soma of CA1 pyramidal cells is about 10–15 mV depolarized from the usual resting potential of −65 mV. Threshold is 5 to 10 mV higher in CA3 neurons.

In addition to evoked synaptic activity, there is also a high rate of spontaneous synaptic potentials that can be recorded from hippocampal neurons both in vivo and in vitro. These spontaneous synaptic potentials result from random firings of presynaptic neurons and from the quantal release of neurotransmitter from synaptic terminals (Brown et al., 1979; Brown and Johnston, 1984a).

Physiology and Biophysics of Synaptic Actions. Many of the basic hypotheses for synaptic transmission that were first derived from studies of invertebrate preparations have been tested in hippocampal neurons. Presynaptic mechanisms, including the quantal hypothesis for transmitter release and the role of presynaptic calcium, have been studied directly at both mossy fiber and Schaffer collateral synapses (Jonas et al., 1993; Stevens and Wang, 1994; Xiang et al., 1994; Bekkers and Stevens, 1995; see also Johnston and Wu, 1995). As for postsynaptic mechanisms, the properties of conductance-increase and conductance-decrease PSPs have been explored in hippocampal neurons (Barrionuevo et al., 1986). Because excitatory synapses and some inhibitory synapses terminate on the dendrites, the study of the physiology and biophysics of synaptic transmission is complicated by the properties of dendrites, and thus an entire section is devoted below to dendritic properties.

The basic sequence of synaptic transmission begins with an action potential in the presynaptic axon that elicits Ca^{2+} influx into the bouton, and through a number of poorly understood steps, neurotransmitter is released into the cleft from transmitter-containing vesicles in the presynaptic terminal (see Chap. 1). The transmitter molecules diffuse across the synaptic cleft and bind to specific receptors on the postsynaptic neuron opening ion channels. The unit response from a single vesicle is called a *quantum*. Single boutons may have as few as 1 active zone in some Schaffer collateral boutons to as many as 37 active zones on some of the largest mossy fiber terminals (Chicurel and Harris, 1992). A prominent theory is that one vesicle per action potential is released at each active zone with a mean probability of about 1 release every fourth action potential (Korn and Faber, 1991; Allen and Stevens, 1994; Stevens and Wang, 1994). Furthermore, these vesicles can sometimes release their transmitter spontaneously in the absence of a presynaptic action potential (Brown et al., 1979).

Fewer specific details are known about transmission at inhibitory synapses, but they are presumed to function in a similar manner (see Miles and Wong, 1984; Miles, 1990; Ropert et al., 1990). One important difference, however, is that inhibitory neurons can fire repetitively at rates much higher than is typical for excitatory neurons (Schwartzkroin and Mathers, 1978). This means that excitatory input to inhibitory interneurons may trigger a high-frequency train of action potentials in the interneurons, leading to longer-lasting transmitter release and a longer-lasting inhibition of the postsynaptic neuron than from the excitatory response.

NEUROTRANSMITTERS

EXCITATORY NEUROTRANSMITTERS

The major excitatory neurotransmitter in the hippocampus is glutamate (Roberts et al., 1981; Storm-Mathison, 1977). Glutamate is released from the perforant path, mossy fibers, commissural-associational fibers, and Schaffer collaterals, and from the several types of excitatory interneurons described elsewhere. The action of glutamate is on two main types of receptors, ionotropic and metabotropic (Hicks et al., 1987). The ionotropic receptors directly gate ion channels that are part of the receptor–molecule complex, whereas the metabotropic receptors mediate their actions through intermediary G-proteins that either gate ion channels or activate second messenger molecules. There are large families of receptor molecules within each of these classes (Hollmann and Heineman, 1994; see Chap. 2).

The ionotropic glutamate receptors consist primarily of AMPA, kainate, and NMDA receptors, all named for the particular ligand used to characterize them. AMPA and kainate receptors mediate fast EPSPs whereas NMDA receptors mediate slower-rising and slower-decaying EPSPs. Various combinations of AMPA, kainate, and NMDA receptors are present at all of the excitatory pathways of the hippocampus although there may be variations at individual synapses. For example, there are fewer NMDA receptors at mossy fiber synapses (Monaghan et al., 1983). Also, it has been proposed that some Schaffer collateral synapses contain only NMDA receptors (Isaac et al, 1995; Liao et al., 1995). The metabotropic glutamate receptors are also present at glutamatergic synapses, both at the pre- and postsynaptic side of the synapse. They coexist in different combinations with ionotropic receptors postsynaptically and modulate transmitter release presynaptically (Schoepp and Conn, 1993).

All of the ionotropic glutamate receptors open channels that are nonselective for the monovalent cations Na^+ and K^+ (Mayer and Westbrook, 1987). Some of the AMPA and kainate receptors and all of the NMDA receptors are also permeable to Ca^{2+} (MacDermott et al., 1986). In addition to Ca^{2+} permeability, the NMDA receptors have a unique voltage dependency. At membrane potentials near rest, the channel is blocked by Mg^{2+} from the extracellular side, but becomes unblocked at more depolarized potentials (Mayer et al., 1984). The NMDA receptor plays an important role in the induction of certain forms of long-term plasticity (Collingridge and Watkins, 1994; see below).

The AMPA-mediated response to glutamate is fast in comparison to that for NMDA (see Fig. 11.11). Synapses containing both AMPA and NMDA receptors will have a mixture of fast and slow responses, depending on the membrane potential and whether the NMDA receptors are blocked by Mg^{2+}.

Another prominent excitatory transmitter in the hippocampus is acetylcholine (ACh). As with glutamate, ACh acts on both ionotropic and metabotropic receptors. The ionotropic receptors are the nicotinic receptors whereas the metabotropic receptors are muscarinic. Nicotinic receptors are present presynaptically and can modulate glutamate release from excitatory synapses (Gray et al., 1996). They are also on inhibitory interneurons and can modulate inhibition. Muscarinic receptors have been described at both pre- and postsynaptic sites in the hippocampus (Williams and Johnston, 1993). Their presynaptic effects are to decrease glutamate release and thus could be considered inhibitory. Their postsynaptic effects are to decrease a potassium conductance (Brown and Adams, 1980; Brown et al., 1990; Storm, 1990), which in turn produces a depolarization of the postsynaptic neuron, making it more likely to fire an action potential (Halliwell and Adams, 1982). This action is decidedly excitatory because not only is the neuron depolarized by the action of ACh on muscarinic receptors but the decrease in a potassium conductance increases the input resistance, making other concomitant excitatory inputs more likely to fire the neuron.

There are also many other putative excitatory neurotransmitters (see Frotscher et al., 1988), but so far most are believed to be metabotropic and act indirectly through G-proteins. These include norepinephrine, dopamine, serotonin, and a number of neuroactive peptides. With their indirect actions through G-proteins, it is sometimes difficult to classify them as excitatory or inhibitory because their actions often depend on the state of the neuron. They may thus be more accurately described as *neuromodulatory* (Kaczmarek and Levitan, 1987).

INHIBITORY NEUROTRANSMITTERS

The major inhibitory neurotransmitter in the hippocampus is GABA (Roberts et al., 1976). Although glycine is a prominent inhibitory neurotransmitter in the spinal cord and in some brain regions (see olfactory bulb, Chap. 5), it plays little role as a classical neurotransmitter in the hippocampus. Once again, GABA receptors can be divided

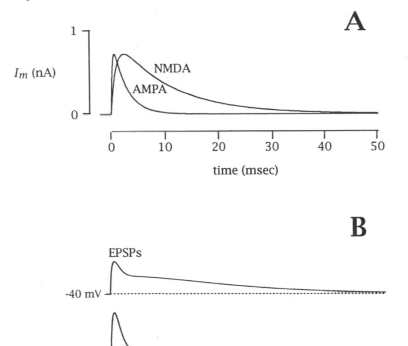

Fig. 11.11. AMPA and NMDA components of synaptic responses. **A:** The time courses of individual AMPA and NMDA currents are indicated and compared. The AMPA current has relatively fast rise and decay times compared with those of the NMDA current. **B:** Mixed AMPA/NMDA EPSPs. The EPSPs recorded at -40 mV is composed of a fast-rising AMPA component and a slow-decaying NMDA component. At -80 mV the NMDA component is much smaller so the EPSP is primarily due to the AMPA component. [Modified from Johnston and Wu, 1995, with permission.]

into ionotropic and metabotropic. The ionotropic receptors ($GABA_A$) open channels permeable to Cl^- and are blocked by picrotoxin and bicuculline. Since the Nernst potential for Cl^- in most adult hippocampal neurons is negative to the resting potential, the opening of these channels results in a hyperpolarization. The opening of these GABA-gated channels also decreases the input resistance of the postsynaptic neurons and can thus reduce the effectiveness of concomitant excitatory inputs. The action of GABA on ionotropic receptors is therefore both a hyperpolarization and a reduction of excitation, each of which can be considered inhibitory.

The metabotropic GABA receptor is called the *$GABA_B$ receptor*, and its action is mediated through G-proteins that open K^+ channels on both the pre- and postsynaptic sides of the synapse (Dutar and Nicoll, 1988a,b; Thalmann, 1988). In the postsynaptic cell this also leads to a hyperpolarization of the membrane potential, but the hyperpolarization has a slower onset and slower decay than the $GABA_A$ response (see Fig. 11.9B). In the presynaptic terminal, activation of $GABA_B$ receptors reduces transmitter release at both glutamatergic and GABAergic synapses.

It was once believed that inhibitory synapses were primarily on the cell bodies of pyramidal neurons (Andersen et al., 1964). There is now much evidence that GABAergic synapses occur both on the cell bodies as well as throughout the dendritic tree. The GABA$_B$ responses are dendritic in origin (Miles et al., 1996), but the GABA$_A$ responses are distributed throughout the neuron. Whether GABA$_A$ and GABA$_B$ receptors coexist at the same synapses is not clear, and some have proposed that the responses are mediated through different interneurons.

Another ionotropic neurotransmitter in the hippocampus is serotonin acting through 5-HT$_3$ receptors (Jackson and Yakel, 1995). These receptors directly gate nonselective cation channels and produce a depolarization. They often occur on inhibitory neurons, however, so that their overall effect is mostly inhibitory. There are also neuromodulatory neurotransmitters acting pre- and/or postsynaptically that under some conditions can be considered inhibitory. These include norepinephrine, serotonin (through non 5-HT$_3$ receptors), dopamine, and neuroactive peptides.

SPECIFIC PATHWAYS

Perforant Pathway. As described previously, the perforant pathway can be separated into two groups of fibers, the lateral and medial perforant paths, depending on the neurons of origin in the entorhinal cortex and the termination zone in the different target regions (Steward, 1976; Yeckel and Berger, 1990, 1995). Both pathways produce glutamatergic EPSPs in the dendrites, although the lateral perforant path also co-releases opioid peptides when there is high-frequency activity of the presynaptic neurons (Gall et al., 1981). It has been reported that opioid peptides influence the induction of long-term potentiation (see below) in the lateral perforant path (Bramham et al., 1988; Breindl et al., 1994; Xie and Lewis, 1995).

Hilar Pathways. The physiology of the hilar region is poorly understood, compared with the rest of the hippocampus. As with other regions, there are inhibitory interneurons or basket cells forming feedforward and feedback inhibition to dentate granule cells. The mossy cells (Scharfman and Schwartzkroin, 1988) receive excitatory inputs from the mossy fibers (see below) and send feedback excitation via glutamatergic synapses to the granule cells (Scharfman, 1995; Jackson and Scharfman, 1996). The functional significance of this pathway is not clear, although it seems to be prominently involved in certain seizure models (Scharfman, 1994).

Mossy Fibers. Mossy fiber boutons are among the largest synapses of the mammalian central nervous system, surpassed only by certain synapses in the cochlear nucleus (see Chap. 4). At each bouton there are multiple active zones (up to 37) resulting in multiple release sites for neurotransmitter (Chicurel and Harris, 1992). The boutons contain large amounts of Zn^{2+} and opioid peptides that are co-released with the main neurotransmitter glutamate (Stengaard-Pedersen et al., 1981; Howell et al., 1984; Aniksztejn et al., 1987). As with most peptides, the opioids are generally only co-released with high-frequency stimulation (McGinty et al., 1983; Hökfelt et al., 1989). As summarized previously, the mossy fibers terminate on the proximal dendrites of CA3 pyramidal cells. This proximal termination site has important practical and functional significance.

Despite these idiosyncratic features, the physiology of mossy-fiber synaptic transmission is nonetheless conventional in many respects. Mossy fiber activity produces fast glutamatergic EPSPs in CA3 neurons. Because of the multiple release sites, however, the EPSPs produced by a single mossy fiber are larger than, for example, those from a single Schaffer collateral. Furthermore, because of the proximal location of the synapses on the dendrites, the EPSPs are less attenuated by the dendrites (see Dendritic Properties). It thus takes fewer active mossy fibers to fire a CA3 neuron than for other types of synapses. The function of the coreleased Zn^{2+} and opioid peptides is not clear, but in part the opioids may play a role in the induction of long-term potentiation at mossy fiber synapses (Williams and Johnston, 1996; Derrick et al., 1992).

One of the practical advantages for the proximal location of the mossy fibers is that better voltage control of the subsynaptic membrane can be achieved from a voltage clamp applied to the soma than for synapses more distally located on the dendritic tree (Johnston and Brown, 1983). Rather detailed studies of synaptic currents and the underlying conductances have been made for mossy fiber synapses (Brown and Johnston, 1983; Jonas et al., 1993). These studies reveal unitary synaptic conductances of around 1 nS and quantal conductances of 100–200 nS. This suggests that each bouton normally releases about 5–10 quanta. The quantal events, when measured with a voltage clamp, have rise times of <1 ms and decay time constants of about 5 ms. These values are close to those derived from the kinetics of the underlying glutamate channels, which suggests that the voltage-clamp measurements are fairly accurate.

In addition to the mossy fibers, statum lucidum also contains recently discovered interneurons (Spruston et al., 1997) that run parallel to stratum lucidum and perpendicular to the dendritic axis of the pyramidal neurons. These interneurons receive input from the mossy fibers and come in two varieties, spiny and aspiny. The aspiny neurons are believed to be GABAergic and mediate feedforward inhibition to the pyramidal neurons. In contrast, the spiny neurons are thought to be glutamatergic and mediate feedforward excitation to pyramidal neurons and thus represent another type of excitatory interneuron. The function of these neurons is not known.

Recurrent Pathways. One of the hallmarks of the CA3 region is the prominent, recurrent excitatory connections among the pyramidal neurons (MacVicar and Dudek, 1980; Miles and Wong, 1986). This recurrent pathway is glutamatergic, and excitatory, and represents a form of positive feedback that makes the CA3 region inherently unstable. In combination with the intrinsic bursting properties of CA3 neurons, subtle increases in the ratio of excitation/inhibition in this region can result in epileptiform activity, which is characterized by spontaneous and synchronous, rhythmic firing among large numbers of neurons (Traub and Miles, 1991). The epileptiform activity in the CA3 region can then spread into CA1 and beyond. Many forms of epilepsy are believed to develop in this manner—that is, from subtle alterations in the balance between excitation and inhibition in areas like CA3 where there is strong, positive synaptic feedback among neurons.

The recurrent connections are also responsible for the so-called "sharp wave" activity (see Functional Synthesis), which is probally the result of a synchronous burst of a small group of CA3 neurons. These sharp waves occur during quiet wakefulness and slow-wave sleep and may be associated with memory formation (Buzsaki, 1989). In fact, the feedback nature of the recurrent pathways has been suggested to provide the substrate for autoassociative memories (see Kohonen, 1978).

Schaffer Collaterals. The Schaffer collaterals are probably the best-studied synaptic pathway in the hippocampus. Each Schaffer collateral axon synapses onto thousands of CA1 pyramidal neurons, but usually with only one or two synaptic contacts per neuron (Sorra and Harris, 1993). The Schaffer collateral pathway has been studied extensively because of interest in the various forms of synaptic plasticity occurring at this synapse. Electrical stimulation of the Schaffer collaterals in stratum radiatum results in the sequence of excitation–inhibition described above. The axons of the CA1 pyramidal neurons also form a recurrent excitatory pathway that synapses back onto other CA1 neurons (Radpour and Thomson, 1991), although it is much sparser and weaker than that in CA3.

SYNAPTIC PLASTICITY

Most of the excitatory synapses in the hippocampus exhibit various forms of use- or activity-dependent synaptic plasticity. These are generally defined as changes in the amplitudes of synaptic potentials that are dependent on the prior activity of the synapse. The different forms are generally distinguished on the basis of their duration or time course and will be briefly described below.

SHORT-TERM PLASTICITIES

The short-term plasticities are facilitation, post-tetanic potentiation, and depression. They range in duration from hundreds of milliseconds to several minutes. Facilitation was first described at the frog neuromuscular junction by Bernard Katz and colleagues (del Castillo and Katz, 1954), but has also been studied in some detail in hippocampus (McNaughton 1982). It is more commonly referred to as *paired-pulse facilitation* (PPF), because it is usually studied by giving a pair of pulses (stimuli) to a synaptic pathway and comparing the amplitude of the second EPSP in the pair to that of the first (Schulz et al., 1994). The amount of PPF depends on the interval between stimuli. At intervals of about 50 ms, PPF can produce several hundred percent increase in the EPSP. PPF decreases with increasing intervals between stimuli. This decay in PPF with time between the pair of pulses is roughly exponential, with a time constant of 100–200 ms.

Post-tetanic potentiation (PTP) represents a transient increase in the amplitude of a synaptic response after a brief train of stimuli. The increase in amplitude can again be several hundred percent immediately following the train and decay over the time course of several minutes after the train. PTP often has two components—a component with a decay time of 5–10 sec, called *augmentation*, and a slower-decaying component, called PTP (see Johnston and Wu 1995). PPF and both phases of PTP result from increases in the probability of transmitter release from the presynaptic terminal triggered by an increase in intraterminal Ca^{2+}. They represent important forms of synaptic plasticity and are highly reproducible from trial to trial and preparation to preparation.

Depression of a synaptic response can have many forms. After repetitive activity of a synapse there can be a short-term depression due to depletion of readily releasable transmitter from the presynaptic terminal. The duration of this depression can be quite variable depending on the amount of transmitter released, but it can range from hundreds of milliseconds to a few minutes. Depression can also occur on a very short time scale (tens of ms), but this is due to desensitization of the postsynaptic transmitter receptor molecules after repeatedly binding neurotransmitter (Stevens and Wang, 1995; Wang and Kelly, 1996).

LONG-TERM PLASTICITIES

There are several forms of synaptic plasticities at glutamatergic, excitatory synapses in hippocampus that have durations of from 30 min to hours, days, or weeks. They typically occur after repetitive trains of synaptic activity and are thought to contribute to the learning and memory functions of the hippocampus (see below). They are called *short-term potentiation and depression* (STP and STD) and *long-term potentiation and depression* (LTP and LTD).

LTP was first described by Bliss and colleagues (Bliss and Lomo, 1973; Bliss and Gardner-Medwin, 1973) and is probably the most intensely studied of all the synaptic plasticities because of its presumed role in learning and memory (Bliss and Collingridge, 1993). Although details of the mechanisms underlying LTP are hotly debated and are far from certain, there are a number of general features of LTP that can be described. LTP is typically induced by giving one or more high-frequency (25–200 Hz) stimulus trains to a synaptic pathway, such as the perforant path, mossy fibers, or Schaffer collaterals. This period of high-frequency stimulation trains is called the *induction phase*. Following the induction phase is the *expression phase*, and during this period the amplitude of the EPSP from a test stimulus is increased some 50–100% above control. One of the characteristics of LTP is that the expression phase lasts much longer than the induction phase. For example, the induction phase can be a few seconds to 1 min in duration whereas the expression phase may last up to several days. The maximum duration of expression is difficult to study, but LTP in hippocampus is unlikely to be permanent.

Another important feature of LTP (and all of the long-term plasticities described in this section) is that it is synapse-specific. In other words, the changes in the synaptic response are generally confined to the synapses receiving the high-frequency stimulation. LTP also has so-called associative properties, in that synapses may exhibit LTP only when they are active at the same time as other synapses. These and other properties (see reviews by Bliss and Lynch, 1988; Madison et al., 1991; Teyler et al., 1994) make LTP an attractive candidate mnemonic device.

The flip side of LTP is LTD. LTD represents a long-term depression of a synaptic response (Christie et al., 1994; Christie et al., 1996; Bear and Abraham, 1996; Goda and Stevens, 1996). It is induced by giving low-frequency stimulation (1–5 Hz) to a synaptic pathway, and the expression of LTD can last from 30 min to an hour or more. A similar phenomenon called *depotentiation* occurs when low-frequency stimulation is given to a synaptic pathway that has already been potentiated and is expressing LTP (Levy and Steward, 1979). Most theories for learning involve strengthening of specific synaptic pathways at the expense of others, and thus the existence of an LTD-like phenomenon has long been theorized.

At many synapses LTP and LTD are dependent on the activation of NMDA receptors. A requirement for the induction of LTP is that there must be a sufficient increase in the intracellular Ca^{2+} concentration near the stimulated synapses. This occurs by the influx of Ca^{2+} ions through NMDA receptors and/or voltage-gated Ca^{2+} channels

(Johnston et al., 1992). At mossy fiber synapses and perhaps at lateral perforant-path synapses, LTP is facilitated by the release of opioid peptides (see above).

STP and STD occur when the stimulation during induction is of insufficient intensity or duration to induce LTP and LTD. In other words, STP and STD have lower induction thresholds than their longer-term counterparts. It is not clear whether STP and STD are just shorter-term versions of LTP and LTD or if they have separate mechanisms (see Schulz and Fitzgibbons, 1997, regarding STP). Nonetheless, they share characteristics, such as a dependence on a rise in intracellular Ca^{2+} concentration in the postsynaptic neuron, and at some synapses, a requirement for NMDA receptor activation.

DENDRITIC PROPERTIES

Hippocampal dendrites are beautiful, tree-like structures that receive all the excitatory and much of the inhibitory synaptic input to the neuron. Approximately 90–95% of the total surface area of a neuron (excluding the axon) is made up of dendrites. A neuron therefore expends a tremendous amount of energy growing and maintaining its dendritic tree. Nevertheless, the function of dendrites has always been somewhat of an enigma. The size and complexity of the dendritic arbor appears to increase during development (Rihn and Claiborne, 1990) and, in particular, when animals are reared in complex sensory environments (Greenough, 1975). These data suggest that dendritic size and branching patterns are important features of normal development and normal function. This conclusion is further supported by data in which dendritic structure was found to be altered in specific ways in patients with certain neurological and psychiatric disorders (Scheibel and Scheibel, 1973; Purpura, 1974; Mehraein et al., 1975; Abede et al., 1991; Scheibel and Conrad, 1993).

A typical CA3 hippocampal pyramidal neuron has a total dendritic length of approximately 16 mm (Fig. 11.3) and receives approximately 25,000 excitatory synapses and fewer inhibitory synapses (Ishizuka et al., 1995). Most of these synapses terminate on dendrites, and it is assumed that dendrites somehow integrate (that is, coordinate and blend into a unified whole) these myriad inputs to produce an output of the neuron in a process called *synaptic integration*. The output of the neuron is usually, but not always, in the form of an action potential. The properties of dendrites that provide this integrative function, as well as the nature of the integration itself, are poorly understood. For many years there have been two somewhat conflicting opinions about dendritic properties: dendrites were considered to be either passive or active.

This distinction concerns the manner in which electrical potentials spread from one point to another in the dendrites. Passive propagation of electrical potentials means that there is no involvement of voltage-gated ion channels and that electrical potentials decrement as they spread because of the so-called cable or electrotonic properties of the neuron (reviewed in Jack et al., 1975; Johnston and Wu, 1995). The active propagation of signals involves the opening of voltage-gated channels to help propel potentials from one point to another with little or no attenuation. For example, the action potential traveling down an axon results from the active properties of the axon. Hippocampal dendrites function in a combined way that includes both passive and active spread of potentials. Some of the functional consequences of this will be presented in the sections below (see also Spruston et al., 1994; Johnston and Wu, 1995; Johnston et al., 1996; Yuste and Tauk, 1996; Stuart et al., 1997; Magee et al., 1998).

PASSIVE PROPERTIES

A number of studies have explored the passive electrotonic properties of hippocampal neurons, including dentate granule cells, CA1 and CA3 pyramidal neurons, and interneurons (Brown et al., 1981; Spruston and Johnston, 1992; Thurbon et al., 1994). The overall conclusions from these studies is that the length constants are quite long (~2 mm) and the membrane time constants are slow (~50 ms). The long length constant suggests that there is very little decay of steady-state potentials through the dendrites, while the time constants determine the rate of decay of synaptic potentials with time and the amount of attenuation of the peak amplitude of synaptic potentials with distance. For example, EPSPs at their site of origin decay approximately monoexponentially with a time constant of about 50 ms. At sites distant from the synapse, however, the EPSP has a much longer total duration and the peak amplitude is less. In other words, the EPSP gets "filtered" by the dendrites in accordance with the membrane time constant and geometrical factors associated with the shape and branching of the dendritic tree. In fact, an EPSP spreading to the soma from the distal half of the dendritic tree may attenuate to 1/5 or less of its original peak amplitude.

Action potentials are also "filtered" by the passive properties of dendrites to an even greater extent than EPSPs. Action potentials spreading into dendrites that do not have active properties decay in amplitude very quickly with distance. One of the functions of active properties (see below) may be to reduce the filtering of EPSPs and to permit active propagation of action potentials in dendrites.

An excellent way of illustrating the filtering properties of dendrites due to passive cable properties is given by the electrotonic transformation (Carnevale et al., 1997). In this transformation, anatomical space is remapped into electrotonic space so that the amount of attenuation of electrical potentials as they spread throughout the dendrites is easily recognized. Attenuation is graphically represented by rescaling the size of a neuron so that larger size means more attenuation. A transformation for a CA1 pyramidal neuron is shown in Fig. 11.12. The difference in the amount of filtering for different frequencies and for signals spreading from the dendrites toward the soma and from the soma out into the dendrites can be estimated from this illustration.

ACTIVE PROPERTIES

It has been known for some time that action potentials can propagate at least part way into the dendrites of hippocampal neurons and perhaps, under certain conditions, even be initiated in the dendrites (Wong et al., 1979; see Johnston et al., 1996). Dendrites therefore must contain certain voltage-gated ion channels such as Na^+ and K^+ channels. The types, distribution, and function of these channels in dendrites, however, has only recently been explored, and in so doing, the full complexity of dendritic integration of synaptic potentials is just beginning to be appreciated.

Voltage-gated Na^+ channels have been recorded in the axon, soma, and distal dendrites of CA1 pyramidal neurons (Magee and Johnston, 1995a). (see Fig. 11.13). The density of these channels is approximately the same throughout the dendrites, soma, and the first 30 μm of the axon (see Fig. 11.14). Beyond this point in the axon, per-

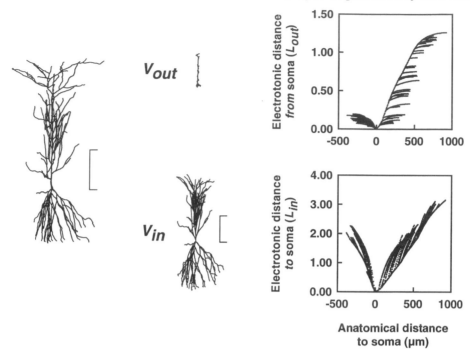

Fig. 11.12. Left: Side view of a detailed morphometric reconstruction of a CA1 pyramidal neuron (scale bar = 200 microns). This cell was mapped from anatomical to electrotonic space using the electrotonic transformation, which computes the logarithm of attenuation for signals spreading along each of its branches. These direction-dependent numeric values are the lengths of the branches in electrotonic space. Center: "Neuromorphic renderings" of the electrotonic transformation at DC (0 Hz). The cell has been redrawn using the electrotonic length of each branch for voltage spreading toward (Vin, bottom) or away from (Vout, top) the soma. The scale bar represents an e-fold attenuation, which is 1 unit of electrotonic distance. Neuromorphic renderings convey an intuitive overview of the electrical signaling properties of the cell by emphasizing regions where attenuation is large and shrinking structures that are nearly isopotential. Right: "L vs. distance plots" of the electrotonic transformation at DC. These give a more quantitative portrait of electrical signaling. Taken together, these figures show that: (1) This CA1 pyramidal cell is electrically more compact for Vout than for Vin; (2) in the Vin transforms, the primary apical dendrite is the site of most attenuation, while the higher order branches and the basilar dendrites are nearly isopotential; (3) Vin voltage gradients are steeper in the higher order branches and basilar dendrites than in the primary apical; (4) Regardless of the direction of signal spread, the spatial profiles of attenuation in the higher order branches and the basil dendrites are very similar to each other; (5) although the cell is not an infinite cylinder, voltage decay along the primary apical dendrite increases nearly exponentially with distance. The rate of decay is greater for Vin than for Vout; (6) in the Vin direction, attenuation along the basilar dendrites is also nearly an exponential function of distance; and (7) while the basil dendrites are physically much shorter than the apical dendritic tree, the electrotonic extents of these two dendritic fields are similar for Vin. (From Carnevale et al., 1997.)

haps at the first node of ranvier, there is a high density of Na$^+$ channels, and it is believed that the action potential is normally initiated here (Colbert and Johnston, 1996; see Fig. 11.15). Once initiated, however, it actively propagates into the soma and at least part way into the dendrites by way of these Na$^+$ channels. This is an extremely important difference from the classical view, which stated that action potentials propagate only in the orthograde (from soma to synapse) direction. In fact, we now know that action potentials, once initiated in the axon, also propagate in the retrograde direction through the soma and into the dendrites (see Fig. 11.16). This has been called *back-propagation*, and is an important new concept for the functioning of hippocampal neurons (Stuart et al., 1997; see Chap. 1).

This back-propagating action potential is not "all or none," like an action potential in an axon. The amplitude of the action potential decrements as it propagates into the dendrites (Turner et al., 1991; Magee and Johnston, 1997). This decrease in amplitude appears to be due to an increasing density of transient K^+ channels so that the action potential is not able to reach its full height in the dendrites (Hoffman et al., 1997). Also, the amplitudes of back-propagating action potentials decrease successively during a train (Spruston et al., 1995; Callaway and Ross, 1995). For example, in the middle of stratum radiatum a single action potential may be 60 mV in amplitude compared with 100 mV in the soma (Fig. 11.16). For a train of about 10 action potentials, however, the last one in the train might be 30 mV compared with 60 mV for the first. This decline in amplitude during a train is both frequency and distance-from-the-soma dependent and is due, in part, to a slow inactivation of Na^+ channels (Colbert et al., 1997). At dendritic branch points, action potentials may fail to invade one or the other of the branches. This is particularly true for the more distal locations where the action potential at the branch point is small (Spruston et al., 1995; Magee and Johnston, 1997).

EPSPs that are too small to trigger a full action potential in the axon may also open some Na^+ channels in the dendrites (Magee and Johnston, 1995b). The opening of

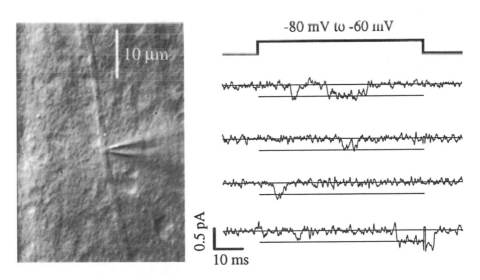

Fig. 11.13. Examples of single-channel recordings from a dendrite of a CA1 pyramidal neuron. On the left is an image of a portion of the apical dendrite approximately 250 μm from the cell body. The image was made using infrared illumination and differential interference optics from a living slice. A patch pipette making a cell-attached patch recording is visible in the picture. On the right are recordings of single T-type Ca^{2+} channels made from this patch (Magee and Johnston, unpublished).

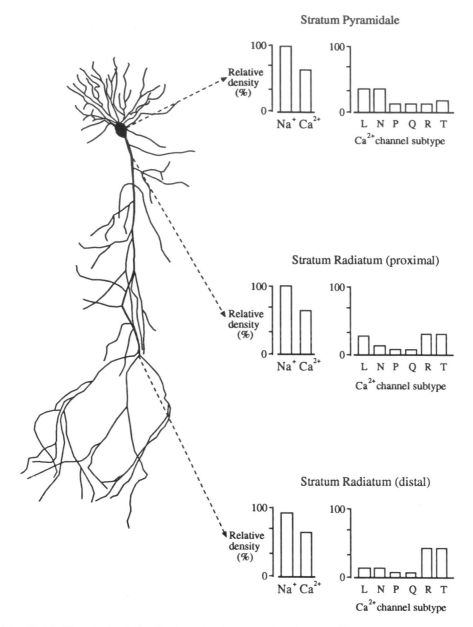

Fig. 11.14. Hypothesized distribution of voltage-gated Na^+ and Ca^{2+} channels in CA1 pyramidal neurons. The bar graphs represent the approximate relative density of the channels in the soma and proximal and distal apical dendrites based on fluorescence imaging and dendritic patch clamping. L, N, P, Q, R, and T represent the different types of Ca^{2+} channels that occur in these neurons [From Johnston et al., 1996, with permission.]

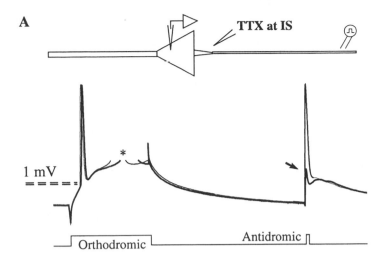

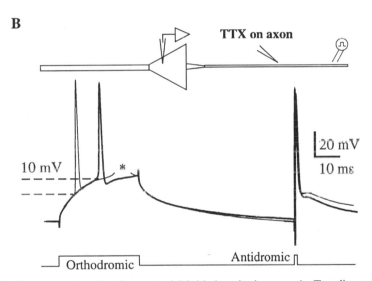

Fig. 11.15. Demonstration of action potential initiation site in axon. **A:** Top diagram indicates a whole-cell recording from the cell body of a subicular pyramidal neuron with TTX applied to the axon initial segment (up to 20 μm from the cell body). Antidromic stimulation is also indicated. Bottom left diagram shows the orthodromic initiation of the action potential with depolarizing current injection to the soma. The threshold voltage is indicated by the dashed lines before and after applying TTX to the initial segment. The threshold is shifted by only 1 mV, suggesting that the initial segment is not the initiation site for the orthodromic action potential. The TTX application, however, does block the somatic invasion of the antidromic action potential as indicated on the right (arrow). **B:** TTX applied in the axon near the beginning of myelination 50 μm from the soma raises threshold by 10 mV, but does not affect antidromic invasion of the action potential. These results and the fact that there is not a high density of Na$^+$ channels in the axon hillock–initial segment of the axon have led to the conclusion that the orthodromic action potential is normally initiated in the axon near the first node of Ranvier. (Modified from Colbert and Johnston, 1996, with permission.]

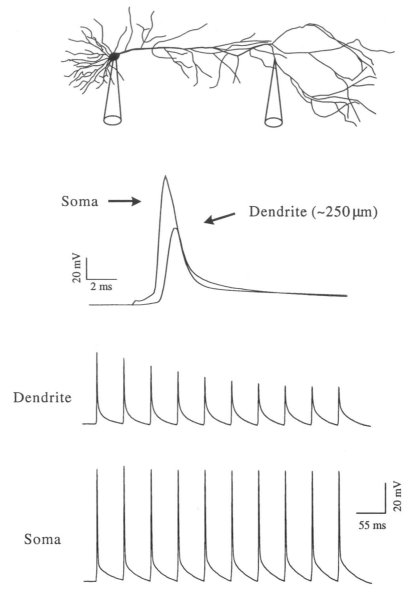

Fig. 11.16. Back-propagation of action potentials. At the top is a diagram of a CA1 neuron with two whole-cell recordings, one in the soma and one in the dendrites about 250 μm from the soma. An action potential is initiated by current injection in the soma. It begins in the axon (Colbert and Johnston, 1996) and then propagates into the soma and later into the dendrites. The action potential in the dendrites is smaller than in the soma because of a high density of A-type K^+ channels. It is delayed from that in the soma because of the conduction time (the conduction velocity of back-propagation is about 0.3 m/sec). The bottom part of the diagram shows the response in the soma and dendrites to a train of action potentials. The action potentials in the soma are all approximately the same amplitude whereas those in the dendrites undergo a frequency-dependent decline in amplitude because of slow inactivation of Na^+ channels and the high density of K^+ channels (Colbert et al., 1997).

these channels provides additional inward current that helps overcome the normal filtering of EPSPs by the passive properties. In this way, EPSPs originating on distal branches may be amplified or boosted by Na^+ channels during their spread to the soma.

In addition to Na^+ channels, voltage-gated Ca^{2+} channels have also been described in hippocampal dendrites (Magee and Johnston, 1995a; Christie et al., 1995). There are many different types of Ca^{2+} channels, some that open with small depolarizations from rest and others that require large depolarizations before opening (Tsien et al., 1988). The distribution of these different Ca^{2+} channels is not homogeneous throughout the neuron (Westenbroek et al., 1990; see Fig. 11.14). There are different channels in dendrites from the soma. For example, the Ca^{2+} channels that open near the resting potential appear to have a higher density in dendrites than in the cell body.

When a back-propagating action potential invades the dendrites, many of these voltage-gated Ca^{2+} channels are activated and produce a significant rise in the concentration of intracellular Ca^{2+} (Jaffe et al., 1992; Miyakawa et al., 1992; Regehr and Tank, 1992; Christie et al., 1995). The change in $[Ca^{2+}]_i$ contributes to the induction of some of the long-term forms of synaptic plasticity discussed above. Furthermore, changes in $[Ca^{2+}]_i$ can activate a number of second-messenger systems that can have myriad effects on the neuron (Kennedy, 1989). Increases in $[Ca^{2+}]_i$ also occur with EPSPs that are too small to trigger action potentials (Magee et al., 1995, 1996). These subthreshold EPSPs activate the Ca^{2+} channels that are opened near the resting potential. This rise in $[Ca^{2+}]_i$ from small EPSPs may also contribute to various forms of synaptic plasticity.

DENDRITIC INTEGRATION OF SYNAPTIC AND ACTION POTENTIALS

The active properties of dendrites can produce highly nonlinear interactions among EPSPs, IPSPs, and action potentials and have powerful influences over neuronal function. The two principal functions of neurons are, first, to decode incoming synaptic input and produce an appropriate output, and, second, to alter the weights or strengths of specific synaptic connections so that certain inputs will, in the future, have more, or less, control over the neuron's output.

As mentioned above, the opening of Na^+ and Ca^{2+} channels by EPSPs may, under certain conditions, lead to an amplification or boosting of distal synaptic events. This would reduce the location–dependent variability among inputs spread across the dendrites in terms of their ability to influence neuronal firing (Cook and Johnston, 1997). This has important consequences for increasing the memory storage ability of the hippocampus and is an example of how active dendrites may play a role in processing synaptic information.

In 1949 neuropsychologist Donald Hebb proposed what has become Hebb's postulate for learning (Stent, 1973). It states that "when an axon of cell A is near enough to excite cell B or repeatedly or consistently takes part in firing it, some growth process or metabolic changes take place in one or both cells such that A's efficiency, as one of the cells firing B, is increased." Hebb's postulate is really a synaptic modification rule relating strengthening of a synaptic connection to some type of correlated firing of pre- and postsynaptic elements (see Brown et al., 1990). It is one of the most influential learning theories in all of neuroscience.

Long-term potentiation (see above) is considered to be the synaptic implementation of Hebb's postulate. A number of studies have shown that simultaneous presynaptic activity and postsynaptic depolarization are required for the induction of LTP (Kelso et al., 1986; Malinow and Miller, 1986; Wigstrom et al., 1986). Under physiological conditions the postsynaptic depolarization may be the back-propagating action potential (Magee and Johnston, 1997; Markram et al., 1997; see Fig. 11.17). It thus can provide the feedback signal from the axon to the synaptic input region than an output of the neuron has occurred. The signal may be the amplitude of the action potential that unblocks NMDA receptors or opens Ca^{2+} channels. Either way, an increase in $[Ca^{2+}]_i$ in the spine and dendrites occurs and leads to LTP of the active synapses. The amplitude of the back-propagating action potential is controlled by local IPSPs and EPSPs (Tsubokawa and Ross, 1996). IPSPs on specific dendritic branches will either reduce the amplitude of the action potential or prevent it from fully propagating into that dendrites. On the other hand, EPSPs will increase the amplitude of back-propagating action potentials and facilitate the propagation of the action potential into specific branches (Magee and Johnston, 1997; Hoffman et al., 1997). In this way, local EPSPs and IPSPs can control and guide the back-propagating action potential into different regions of the dendrites and thus control Hebbian learning. None of this would be possible without the active properties of dendrites.

FUNCTIONAL SYNTHESIS

LEARNING AND MEMORY

Perhaps the most widely accepted and long-lived proposal about hippocampal function relates to its role in memory (Eichenbaum, 1994). It has been known for nearly a century that damage to certain brain regions can result in an enduring amnesic syndrome that is characterized by a complete, or near complete, anterograde amnesia. Affected patients are incapable of recreating a record of day-to-day events. It is now clear that damage isolated to the human hippocampal formation is sufficient to produce this form of memory impairment. The most famous example of this is the patient with the initials H.M. As a young man, H.M. suffered from epilepsy that was so severe that it was life threatening. In 1953, H.M. underwent a neurosurgical procedure in which the hippocampal formation and surrounding brain tissue on both sides of his brain were removed. Although this surgery substantially reduced his seizures, there was a dramatic side effect. From the time of his surgery until the present day, H.M. has not been able to store any new information into long-term memory. In all other respects, however, H.M.'s cognitive functions appear normal. More recently, a number of other patients with bilateral damage confined to the hippocampus have been described. Patient R.B. was reported by Zola-Morgan and colleagues (1986). R.B. became ischemic following coronary bypass surgery and was neuropsychologically evaluated for 5 years after the incident. Like H.M., R.B. demonstrated a substantial anterograde memory impairment with little or no loss of memories formed before his surgery. R.B.'s brain was subjected to postmortem analysis and the only pathology that could be associated with his memory defect was a bilateral, complete loss of the CA1 field of the hippocampus. Since his amnesia was less severe than H.M.'s, it has been proposed that the severity of the memory impairment may depend on the amount of the hippocampal formation

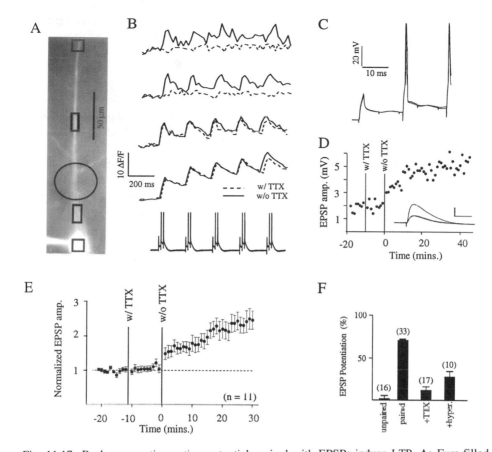

Fig. 11.17. Back-propagating action potentials paired with EPSPs induce LTP. **A:** Fura-filled CA1 pyramidal neuron with somatic electrode. Approximate area of TTX application shown by oval. **B:** Superimposed optical recordings of changes in fura-2 fluorescence from regions of the neuron delimited by the boxes in A. An increase in $[Ca^{2+}]_i$ is represented by an increase in $\triangle F/F$. Traces are from progressively more proximal regions moving down the column in B. Dashed lines are average $\triangle F/F$ during pairing protocol given along with a transient application of 10 μM TTX to dendrite. Solid lines are average $\triangle F/F$ during pairing protocol given without TTX application (approximately 11 min later). The rise in $[Ca^{2+}]_i$ is similar in regions of the neuron proximal to the TTX application and significantly reduced in those regions distal to TTX application site. Lower trace is somatic voltage during paired train. **C:** Expanded somatic voltage recordings during the first burst of paired stimuli for trains with the TTX application and without it. No appreciable differences are observable. First current injection was subthreshold in all traces, so only two action potentials were evoked during each individual burst. **D:** Plot of EPSP amplitude for the same neuron showing that paired stimuli without back-propagating action potentials do not modify EPSP amplitude, whereas subsequent paired stimuli with back propagating action potentials do result in a long-term, large magnitude increase in EPSP amplitude. Average EPSPs for last 2 min of each period shown in inset (control, +TTX, −TTX). **E:** Grouped data showing normalized EPSP amplitude after paired stimulation with and without TTX application. **F:** Summary of mean LTP amplitude under various experimental conditions. Plot shows the amount of EPSP potentiation, plotted as percent of control, for all cells under each condition. Potentiation was calculated by dividing the average EPSP amplitude at 10–15 min post-stimulation by the average control EPSP amplitude. [From Magee and Johnston, 1997, with permission.]

or adjacent cortex that is included in the lesion. It is clear, however, that damage confined to the human hippocampus is sufficient to produce a clinically significant amnesic syndrome.

Although the types of tasks that are used to assess memory in animal models are typically quite different from those used in humans, like humans, damage confined to the hippocampal formation of rats produces a severe memory impairment. One standard task of spatial memory is called the *Morris water maze*. In this task, rats are placed to swim in a small pool of milky water. Somewhere in the pool is a submerged platform that the animals can't see but which provides a means for them to get out of the water. The rat ultimately learns the location of the platform through its position relative to spatial cues that exist in the testing room and exhibits rapid swimming from the starting point to the platform. Animals with lesions of the hippocampus are dramatically impaired in this task and never really learn the position of the platform.

Electrophysiological studies also conducted primarily in rodents have demonstrated that neurons in the hippocampus are preferentially activated by certain stimuli located in the environment. If one records the neural activity of single hippocampal cells while a rat is running around in a maze, for example, the cell might be activated when the rat travels through a certain location of the maze (called *place cells*). Data of this type have prompted the suggestion that the hippocampus can form a "cognitive map" of the outside world (Okeefe, 1979). In a more general sense, it might be thought that the neurons of the hippocampal formation, acting as an assembly of differentially activated units, can form a representation of ongoing experience. Perhaps the interaction of this hippocampal representation of experience with the more detailed information of the experience located in the neocortex is the route through which long-term memories are formed (Wilson and McNaughton, 1993, 1994; McHugh et al., 1996). One implication of the electrophysiological data is that neurons in the hippocampal formation are not uniquely sensitive to certain types of information. Rather, neurons in the hippocampal formation may act more like random-access memory (RAM) in a computer and are therefore potentially activated by all types of information. Since it would be difficult for evolution to anticipate all the various forms of information that might need to be stored as memory, a generalized memory buffer system would be highly adaptive.

The hippocampus displays very characteristic brain-wave activity that may be associated with learning and memory. When animals are exploring their environment, electroencephalographic (EEG) activity of 5–10 Hz frequencies (theta) are recorded (Okeefe, 1979; Buzsaki, 1989). When the animal stops exploring and is in a period of quiet wakefulness, the theta frequencies cease and are replaced by sharp-wave activity consisting of large amplitude, irregularly occurring waveforms. These two types of EEG patterns are mutually exclusive. One theory holds that during theta (exploratory) activity the hippocampus is acquiring a new representation of its environment while during sharp-wave (quiet) activity (and also during slow-wave sleep) the hippocampus is facilitating the consolidation of this information in the form of long-term memories elsewhere in the cortex (Buzsaki, 1989; Skaggs and McNaughton, 1996).

DISEASES OF THE HIPPOCAMPUS

The hippocampus has been implicated in a number of neurological and psychiatric disorders, including epilepsy, Alzheimer's disease, and schizophrenia. As mentioned at the beginning of this chapter, the hippocampus has the lowest seizure threshold in the brain. In animal models of epilepsy, much of the electrical activity associated with seizures can be recorded from the hippocampus either in vivo or in vitro (Traub et al., 1989; see Fig. 11.18). The epileptiform activity so recorded is characterized by large, synchronous discharges that occur rhythmically and are often initiated in the CA2 or CA3 regions (Johnston and Brown, 1981, 1984, 1986). The propensity for the hippocampus to exhibit this epileptiform activity has been attributed to the recurrent excitatory connections among pyramidal neurons and the tendency for CA3 neurons to fire in bursts of action potentials. Under normal conditions the strong inhibition mediated by the various GABAergic interneurons described above prevents this abnormal activity from manifesting itself. Subtle changes in the firing properties of neurons or in the balance between excitation and inhibition, however, can permit a breakthrough of this hyperexcitable state leading to seizures.

An early and devastating feature of the onset of Alzheimer's disease is the inability to form new memories. Ultimately, even old memories weaken and fail. Because of the important role of the hippocampus in learning and memory, it is not surprising that the hippocampus is heavily damaged in Alzheimer's disease. In fact, it has been suggested that the hippocampus is functionally disconnected from the rest of the brain in this disease (Hyman et al., 1984). Moreover, there is suggestive evidence that the en-

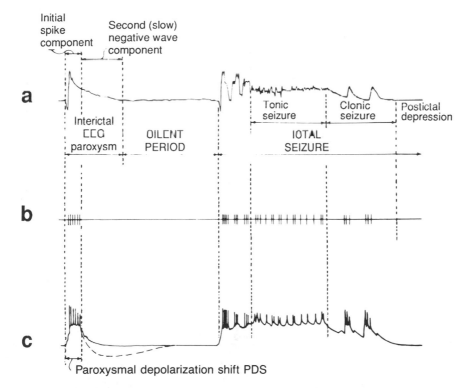

Fig. 11.18. Relationship between (a) cortical EEG and (b) extracellular and (c) intracellular discharges from a feline, penicillin-induced, spontaneous epileptiform discharge. [From Ayala et al., 1970, with permission.]

torhinal cortex may be one of the first brain regions in which Alzheimer's pathology becomes apparent. Although other parts of the brain are also affected, the ability of the hippocampus to process new information is seriously impaired in Alzheimer's disease. The hippocampus is also particularly vulnerable to ischemia and anoxia. In many patients who sustain these conditions, the hippocampus is one of only a few brain regions in which neuronal loss is observed. It appears that this loss is due to an excitotoxicity that may be mediated through the NMDA receptor. Some have proposed that the price the hippocampus pays for being able to rapidly encode new information is that it is inherently unstable and thus prone to a number of metabolic stressors. Finally, the link between schizophrenia and the hippocampus is not so clear. The principal finding is that the hippocampus is significantly smaller and has altered morphology in patients with schizophrenia (Luchins, 1990). Why these alterations should lead to the hallucinations and other altered mentation associated with schizophrenia is not known.

12

NEOCORTEX

RODNEY DOUGLAS AND KEVAN MARTIN

Many of the brain regions discussed in this volume are examples of cortical ("bark-like") structures. Taking its place alongside the archicortex (hippocampus) and paleo-cortex (olfactory bulb) is the neocortex, which is the most recent arrival in evolution-ary history and is arguably the most impressive example of the genre. It has certainly impressed paleontologists whose research on the fossil record of hominids has demon-strated that the size of the hominid brain has trebled over the past 3 million years. En-docasts of the fossil hominid skulls indicate that this increase in size is largely due to the expansion of the neocortex and its connections. The massive and rapid changes in the size of the neocortex are paralleled in the phylogenetic differences we see in con-temporary mammalian brains (Fig. 12.1). Of land mammals, the primates have the largest brains in proportion to their body weight. However, the human brain is three times as large as might be expected for a primate of equivalent weight (Passingham, 1982). Furthermore, the human brain is not simply a scaled-up version of our closest primate relative, i.e., the Bonobo chimpanzee. The greatest expansion is in the corti-cal structures, particularly the cerebellum and neocortex. Within the neocortex itself, the expansion is uneven. In comparison with nonhuman primates of equivalent body weight, the association and premotor areas have expanded relative to the sensory ar-eas. When added together, the neocortex and its connections form a massive 80% by volume of the human brain (Passingham, 1982).

In all mammals the neocortex consists of a sheet of cells, about 2 mm thick. Con-ventionally it is divided into 6 layers, but in many regions more than 6 laminae are in evidence (Fig. 12.2). Each cubic millimeter contains approximately 50,000 neurons. The study of the laminar organization of these cells in the neocortex began in the early part of the 20th century and became known as *cytoarchitectonics*. In conjunction with studies of the organization of myelinated fibers, called *myeloarchitectonics*, cytoar-chitectonics was applied by Campbell in England and by Vogt and Brodmann in Ger-many, to divide the neocortex into about 20 different regions. Although many more areas have since been identified, there are three major cytoarchitectural divisions of the neocortex. The *koniocortex*, or granular cortex of the sensory areas, contains small, densely packed neurons in the middle layers. These small neurons are large absent in the *agranular* cortex of the motor and premotor cortical areas. The third type of cor-tex has varying populations of granule cells and is called *eulaminate* or *homotypical*

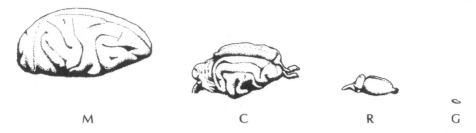

Fig. 12.1. Brains of modern vertebrates: goldfish (G), rat (R), cat (C), and Old World monkey (M). Scaled to body weight, the neocortex and its connections form an increasingly greater proportion of the brain volume. The neocortex in monkey completely envelops all other brain structures.

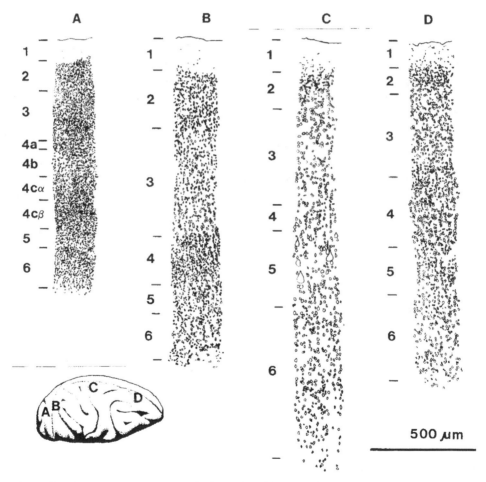

Fig. 12.2. The laminar organization of neurons in different cortical areas of the macaque monkey cortex (inset). **A:** Area 17 (striate visual cortex). **B:** Area 18 (extrastriate cortex). **C:** Area 4 (motor cortex). **D:** Area 9 (frontal cortex). A basic six-layered structure can be identified in all areas. The pia covers layer 1; the white matter is below layer 6. Note the marked difference in cell size and density among the different areas, but additional layers are apparent in some areas (e.g., Area 17). The giant neurons in layer 5 of area 4 are the Betz cells. (Celloidin-embedded brain, cut in 40 μm thick parasagittal sections, stained for Nissl substance, uncorrected for shrinkage.)

460

cortex. It includes much of "*association cortex*," which is a convenient description for cortex whose function has yet to be discovered (Fig. 12.2). Within each of these areas there are many subdivisions, both functional and anatomical. Some are clearly delimited by their cytoarchitectonic structure, as in the case of area 17, the primary visual cortex, or by myeloarchitectonics, as in the case of the middle temporal visual area (MT). Other areas, such as area 18 in the monkey, can only be subdivided by more elaborate immunochemical, histological, or physiological methods.

In a planar view the map of these architectonically defined areas looks like a patchwork quilt. The functional properties and subdivisions of these have been mapped most extensively in the monkey cortical areas concerned with vision. The exponential growth of functional imaging studies in humans means that more and more is becoming known about the equivalent subdivisions of the human brain. In addition to the basic sensory and motor functions, the human cortex appears to be particularly involved in high-level functions, such as speech production and comprehension. Indeed, the concept of cortical localization of function derives from studies in the last century that correlated damage of specific areas of human cortex with specific deficits in speech production. Similar modern case studies of aphasias have become celebrated in the popular culture of books, television, and films. With the advent of functional imaging studies with positron emission tomography (PET), functional magnetic resonance imaging (fMRI), and electroencephalography (EEG), there has been a rapid increase in our knowledge of the functional and anatomical map of human cortex. These techniques, however, do not attempt to identify the the mechanisms or neuronal circuits responsible for these functions. Thus, the challenge is to discover what is actually happening when different regions of the cortex are activated under different sensory or behavioral tasks. Fundamental to this central endeavor is an understanding of the structure and function of the microcircuits of the neocortex and their components.

NEURONAL ELEMENTS

Nearly 100 years ago, Ramon y Cajal outlined the basic approach to studying the elementary pattern of cortical organization (Cajal, 1911). The method is to reveal the complete structure of neurons, including their axons, and then piece together these components in a jigsaw-puzzle fashion to produce circuits. He, and many since, studied the morphology and circuitry of the neocortex with the silver impregnation technique discovered by Golgi. Although this techniques has been superseded by much more sophisticated modern techniques, the basic classes of neurons revealed by the Golgi technique used by Ramon y Cajal have remained largely unaltered. All three cytoarchitectural divisions of the neocortex contain the same two basic types of neurons: those whose dendrites bear spines (the stellate and pyramidal cells, Fig. 12.3) and those whose dendrites are smooth (smooth cells, Fig. 12.4). Occasionally, *sparsely spiny cells* have been described, but these neurons form a very small subclass of cortical neurons.

Modern electron microscopic and immunochemical techniques have been used to determine the proportion of the different types in the different regions of cortex. These studies have shown that while the different types may be differentially distributed between laminae within a single cortical area, the overall proportions of a given neuronal type remain approximately constant between different areas. The pyramidal cells form

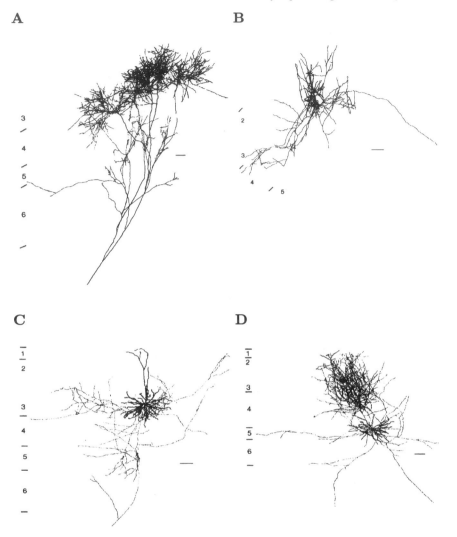

Fig. 12.3. Thalamic afferent and several spiny neurons from cat visual cortex. **A:** Y-type thalamic afferent. Note extensive but patchy arbor in layer 4. This axon formed over 8000 boutons. **B:** Spiny stellate neuron of layer 4. **C:** Pyramidal neuron of layer 3. Note characteristic apical dendrite extending to layer 1. Many collateral branches arise from the main axon before it leaves the cortex (below). **D:** Pyramidal neuron of layer 5. Note the very rich axon collateral arbor in the superficial layers. This neuron did not project out of area 17. The thalamic afferent and neurons were filled intracellularly in vivo with horseradish peroxidase. Cortical layers are as indicated. Bars = 100 μm.

about 70% of the neurons (Sloper et al., 1979; Powell, 1981) and the smooth cells form about 20% of the neurons (Peters, 1987) in all cortical areas examined. These morphological differences in the dendritic structure are only one of many differences between these two basic types. For example, the spiny cells are excitatory, whereas the smooth neurons are inhibitory. Spiny neurons use quite different neurotransmitters from

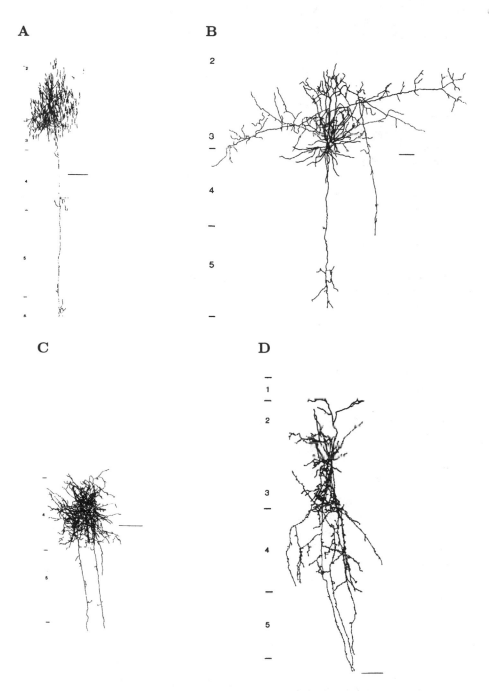

Fig. 12.4. Smooth neurons from cat visual cortex. **A:** Chandelier cell. **B:** Large basket cell of layer 3. Note lateral axon collaterals. **C:** Small basket cell of layer 4. The major portion of the axon arbor is confined to layer 4. **D:** Double bouquet cell. The axon collaterals run vertically. Cortical layers are as indicated. Bars = 100 μm.

smooth neurons; their respective synapses are associated with a quite different set of receptors and this is reflected in the morphology of the synapses.

SPINY NEURONS

Spiny neurons are called this because their dendrites bear small processes called spines. Spines are usually club shaped, with a head of about 1 μm diameter and a shaft, or *neck*, of about 0.1 μm diameter. The length of the neck varies greatly, from virtually nothing as in "stubby" spines, in which the head attaches directly to the dendritic shaft, to necks that are several micrometers long (Jones and Powell, 1969c). At the high magnifications achieved with the electron microscope, spines can be distinguished from other dendritic elements in the neuropil by the presence of a characteristic *spine apparatus*, which is composed of a calcium-binding protein, and this has been an important marker for spines in quantitative electron microscopic studies (cf. Chap. 7, Fig. 7.6A) although similar structural elements are found in dendritic shafts.

Pyramidal Neurons. The major subtype of spiny neurons are the pyramidal cells (Fig. 12.3C,D), which constitute about two-thirds of the neurons in the neocortex. Pyramidal neurons are found in all cortical layers except layer 1. Their most prominent feature is an apical dendrite that may extend through all the layers of the cortex above the soma. Pyramidal cells are the major output neurons of the neocortex. They participate both in connections between the different cortical areas and to subcortical structures such as the thalamus and superior colliculus. However, they also are a major provider of excitatory input to the area in which they are found: each pyramidal neuron has a rich collateral network that forms part of the local cortical circuitry.

The proximal shafts of the dendrites of the spiny cell types are nearly devoid of spines. The spine density varies considerably between different types of neurons. At one extreme is the sparsely spiny neuron, which may bear fewer than 100 spines over the entire dendritic tree. These neurons form a small subclass of the inhibitory neuron population. At another extreme are neurons such as the *Betz cell*, a large pyramidal cell that is found in the motor cortex (area 4) and bears about 10,000 spines. Each spine forms a type 1 synapse with a presynaptic bouton. Thus, simply counting spines gives a lower limit on the number of type 1 synapses. However, because not all type 1 synapses are formed on spines, the degree of underestimation can only be determined by quantitative electron microscopy of the dendrites of identified neurons. Due to this methodological bottleneck, accurate estimates of the number and positions of synapses onto particular neuronal types are unfortunately extremely rare.

Relatively little attempt has been made to divide up the spiny neurons into different classes and they are usually defined according to the lamina in which their soma is located. However, many types can be distinguished on the basis of their dendritic morphology. The clearest distinction is that some spiny neurons have an apical dendrite (*pyramidal cells*) and some do not (*spiny stellate cells*). Many subgroups of the pyramidal cells can be distinguished on the basis of their morphology or functional characteristics and in each layer pyramidal cells can be found whose morphology and axonal projections are exclusive to that layer. For example, in layer 4, Lorente de Nó identified "star" pyramids, which got their name because of their symmetric and radially orientated basal dendrites. The most prominent pyramidal cells in the neocortex are the Betz cells of area 4, the *motor* cortex. The Betz cells are very large pyramidal cells located in layer 5 (see Fig. 12.3D). Their axons form part of the pyramidal tract that descends to the spinal cord. The primary visual cortex also has a distinct set of exceptionally large pyramidal neurons, called the *solitary cells of Meynert.* These pyramidal cells, which are found in the deep layers (5 or 6, depending on species), project to other cortical areas and down to the midbrain structures such as the superior colliculus and the pons. Within layer 5 in the visual cortex two distinct types of pyramidal cells have now been distinguished on the basis of a correlated structure–function relationship. One type has a thick apical dendrite that ascends to layer 1 where it forms a terminal tuft. These neurons have a bursting discharge of action potentials in response to a depolarizing current. The other type has a regular discharge and their apical dendrite is thin and terminates without branching in layer 2 (Chagnac-Amitai et al., 1990; Mason and Larkman, 1990). This observation has led to theoretical work suggesting that the shape of the dendritic tree itself is a major factor in controlling the pattern of spike output from the neurons (Mainen and Sejnowski, 1996).

Spiny Stellate Neurons. A second group of spiny neurons, the spiny stellate neurons, are found exclusively in layer 4 of the granular cortex (Cajal, 1911). These also have spiny dendrites, but do not have the apical dendrite that is the characteristic of the pyramidal cells. Instead, dendrites of approximately equal length radiate out from the soma and give these neurons a star-like appearance, hence their name. Occasionally these neurons do project to other areas, but most have axonal projections confined to the area in which they occur. It has been proposed that these neurons are simply pyramidal neurons without an apical dendrite. However, they differ in a number of important respects from pyramidal cells, e.g., they have much lower spine densities and many more excitatory synapses on their dendritic tree (Anderson et al., 1994). They should be considered as a distinct cell type confined to layer 4 of sensory cortex. Previously the spiny stellate cells were thought to be the sole recipients of the thalamic input to the sensory cortices, but it is clear that although they probably are the major recipient, thalamic neurons also connect to the pyramidal cells and smooth cells (Hersch and White, 1981; Hornung and Garey, 1981; Freund et al., 1985; Ahmed et al., 1994).

SMOOTH NEURONS

The class of neurons with spine-free dendrites is frequently referred to as smooth stellates, but since their dendritic morphology is rarely stellate, a more accurate term is simply *smooth neurons*. They tend to have elongated dendritic trees, both in the radial and the tangential dimension. Their dendritic morphologies have been described as multipolar, bipolar, bitufted and stellate, but the most useful discriminator of the different types has been the axonal arbor. At least 19 different types of smooth neurons have been described (Szentágothai, 1978; Peters and Regidor, 1981) but the basket cell, first described by Ramón y Cajal, appears to be the most common. These smooth neurons do not just have morphologically distinct axonal arbors, they also form quite specific synaptic connections, as will be described below.

The most prominent smooth neuron is the cortical *basket cell.* As with basket cells in the cerebellum (Chap. 7) and hippocampus (Chap. 11), the axons of the basket cells form nests or baskets around the somata of their targets, usually pyramidal cells. However, modern studies have shown that basket cell boutons form most of their synapses on the dendrites and spines of pyramidal cells. In superficial and deep layers, the main feature of the basket cell axonal arborization is the lateral extension of the axon (Fig. 12.4B). In the middle layers, the basket cells have much more compact axonal arbors (Fig. 12.4C). As with the well-studied patterns of thalamic afferents to the visual cortex (see below), which underlie the functional ocular dominance columns, these differences in the axonal arborizations most probably relate to the functional architecture of the piece of cortex in which they are located.

As with the spiny cells, some morphological types of smooth neurons are found only in particular layers. Layer 1, for example, has two types that are not found in other layers: the *Retzius-Cajal neuron*, which has a horizontally elongated dendritic tree, and the *small neuron of layer 1*, which has highly localized dendritic and axonal arbors. Many of the smooth types have descending or ascending axon collaterals in addition to their lateral extensions. Most notable of these is the *double bouquet cell* of Ramón y Cajal (Fig. 12.4D), which is characterized by elongated dendrites extending radially above and below the somata, and an axon that forms a cascade of vertically orientated collaterals. Another neuron with a vertical organization is the Martinnoti cell, whose soma is located in layer 6, but whose axon processes span all layers. Perhaps the most evocative description of a smooth cell was given by *Szentágothai* to the *chandelier cell*, so named because its axonal boutons are arranged in a series of vertical "candles" which give the whole axonal arborization the appearance of a chandelier (Fig. 12.4A).

Histochemical methods have revealed the existence of a further smooth neuronal type, which is sparse in the gray matter, but which forms a distinct layer at the border of the gray and white matter. These neurons stain positively for the enzyme NADPH-diaphorase, which is a synthetic enzyme for nitric oxide gas. Although they are few in number, their axonal ramifications are immense and provide a rich plexus of axons throughout the gray matter.

AFFERENTS

Thalamus. The thalamus projects to all cortical areas and provides input to most layers of the cortex. The densest projections are to the middle layers, where they form about 5–10% of the synapses in those layers (LeVay and Gilbert, 1976; White, 1989; Ahmed et al., 1994). The main feature of this input is that it is highly ordered. The sensory inputs are represented centrally in a way that their topographic arrangement in the periphery is preserved. This mapping is achieved by preserving the nearest-neighbor relationships of the arrangements of the sensory or motor elements in the periphery. Such topographic projections are a ubiquitous feature of the cortex. The precision of the mapping does vary between areas, however. The primary sensory and motor areas usually preserve the highest detail of the topography, which degrades progressively through secondary and tertiary and higher order areas of cortex.

An important transform in the topography from the periphery to the center is that the regions of highest receptor density have the largest representation in the cortex. This transformation is described as the *magnification factor* of the projection (Daniel and Whitteridge, 1961). In the visual system of the primate, the fovea of the retina contains the highest density of photoreceptors and the primary visual cortex represents this by devoting cortex in the ratio of 30 mm per degree of visual field to this representation. In the far periphery of the visual field the ratio falls off to about 0.01 mm/degree of visual field. In the somatosensory system the hand and face have high densities of touch receptors and these parts have a magnified representation in the primary somatosensory cortex. One of the most remarkable cortical representations is that of the whiskers of rats and mice. Each whisker has a separate representation in the cortex, which appears as a barrel when looked at in a tangential section of the cortex (Woolsey and Van der Loos, 1970). The centers of the barrels are formed by clusters of thalamic afferents that convey impulses from each whisker. The cortical map of the whiskers forms a representation that is topologically equivalent to the arrangement of whiskers on the face of the rat or mouse. This whisker map dominates the representation of the somatosensory surface of the rodent.

In the cat visual cortex, the terminal arbors of each individual thalamic afferent may extend over 1–5 mm of the cortical surface so that each point in layer 4 is covered by the arbors of at least 1000 separate thalamic relay cells (Freund et al., 1985). Thus, the dendritic tree of an average layer 4 neuron, which extends for 200–300 μm, could receive input from many more thalamic afferents. However, the connections are not made randomly between the geniculate afferents and the cortical neurons. Selectivity is revealed in several ways. For example, there is a high degree of precision in the visuotopic map recorded in the first-order cortical neurons in the input layer, i.e., those receiving monosynaptic activation by the thalamic afferents. This clustering is made according to the eye preference of the arbors. Those thalamic relay neurons that are driven by the right eye cluster together in regions about 0.5 mm in diameter and are partially segregated from the afferents that are driven by the left eye. This segregation forms the basis of ocular dominance columns. In addition there is some clustering of the afferents according to whether they are ON or OFF center. This clustering of inputs forms the basis of the ON and OFF subfields of the simple cells. In the somatosensory pathway there are segregations according to the modality of the sensory information, e.g., light touch is segregated from deep pressure and so on (Powell and Mountcastle, 1959).

Other Subcortical Regions. Although the thalamus is a major source of input to the neocortex, it is not the only one. More than 20 different subcortical structures projecting to the neocortex have been identified (Tigges and Tigges, 1985). These structures include the claustrum, locus coeruleus, basal forebrain, the dorsal and median raphe, and the pontine reticular system. As has been pointed out in many earlier chapters, these pathways have distinct neurochemical signatures, which has made the analysis of their cortical targets more tractable. The contributions of these different pathways vary from one cortical area to the next and among species for a homologous cortical area. There are also wide differences in the laminar projections of the terminals of these neurons between areas and in very few cases have the synaptic targets of these projections been identified. Thus, it is as yet not possible to offer a simple schematic of these pathways, but there are a few whose role in plasticity and development have been examined.

Because of their relative ease of identification, the monoaminergic innervation of the cerebral cortex has been studied most intensively. These systems are generally thought to be diffuse and nonspecific, both in terms of the information they carry and in terms of their lack of spatial specificity and anatomical organization. Physiological examinations of these neurons are rare, but closer examinations of the anatomy have generally revealed a higher degree of specificity (Parnevelas and Papadopoulos, 1989). Three main types of monoamine-containing cortical afferents have been described: the dopamine-positive fibers arising from the rostral mesencephalon, the noradrenaline-containing axons originating from the locus coeruleus, and the serotonin (5-HT) fibers that originate from the mesencephalic raphé nuclei. There has been some doubt as to the mode of release of the transmitter, because early studies failed to find clear ultra-structural evidence of synapses. This was consistent with an older concept of the brain as a complex neuroendocrine organ where neurosecretion was the means by which brain activity was modulated. However, it is now clear that monoaminergic fibers in the neocortex do form conventional synapses and can show a high degree of anatomical specificity, both for particular cortical areas and for particular laminae within a single cortical area.

The projections of the locus coeruleus, which lies in the dorsal pons, have been relatively well studied. The nucleus is small, but projects to most of the neocortex in a roughly topographic arrangement (Waterhouse et al., 1983). Neurons in the dorsal portion project to posterior regions of the neocortex, such as the visual regions, whereas neurons in the ventral portion project to frontal cortical areas. In primates, the strongest projections are to the primary motor and somatosensory cortices and their related association areas in frontal and parietal lobes (Tigges and Tigges, 1985). The fine, unmyelinated, axons ramify horizontally, most prominently in layer 6, and form synapses with spine shafts and somata (Papadopoulos et al., 1987). The neurons synthesize norepinephrine, which is thought to be involved in the development and plasticity of thalamocortical projections in the visual cortex. These fibers develop early and their removal by neurotoxins prevents plasticity of the columns formed by the thalamic afferents arbors driven by the left and right eye (Daw et al., 1983; Pettigrew, 1982). Activity in locus coeruleus neurons correlates with changes in the EEG, which suggests that it is involved in the arousal response induced by sensory stimuli.

The raphé nuclei and pontine reticular formation are a complex of nuclei that contain the highest density of neurons that synthesize serotonin. These neurons project to all cortical areas with varying degrees of laminar specificity (Tigges and Tigges, 1985; Mulligan and Tork, 1988). There are clear differences between projections to the homologous areas in different species that make generalizations impossible, e.g., the strongest projections in the monkey are to the thalamorecipient layers of area 17, whereas these layers are relatively poorly innervated in the adult cat. In the kitten, however, there is a transient surge of serotonergic innervation of the thalamorecipient layer 4, which may indicate a relationship to the critical period (Gu et al., 1990).

The third monoamine projection to cortex is the dopaminergic pathway. It has been suggested that a dysfunction of the dopaminergic innervation of the prefrontal cortex is one of the factors in the pathogenesis of schizophrenia. The dopaminergic projection to the frontal cortex originates from the ventral tegmental area, the rostral mesencephalic groups, and the nucleus linearis. They form symmetric synapses with the dendrites of pyramidal cells and with GABAergic smooth neurons (van Eden et al., 1987; Verney et al., 1990; Smiley and Goldman-Rakic, 1993). All layers except layer 4 receive dopaminergic input. Dopaminergic projections are strongest to the rostral cortical areas, especially the prefrontal cortex. Here they target pyramidal cells, particularly spines, which they share with an excitatory synapse.

Although there are intrinsic sources of acetylcholine from neurons within the cortex, the major sources of the acetylcholinergic fibers in the cortex are extrinsic. These fibers originate from the nucleus basalis of Meynert and the diagonal band of Broca, which constitute the nuclei of the basal forebrain. These cholinergic projections to the neocortex have been of particular interest because of their possible involvement in the pathology of Alzheimer's disease. The terminals of the acetylcholinergic fibers distribute through all cortical layers, with the densest innervation in layer 1 and relatively sparse innervation of the deep layers (de Lima and Singer, 1986; Aoki and Kabak, 1992). They form synapses with dendritic shaft and spines but show some bias for the GABAergic neurons.

Although it was previously thought that all GABAergic synapses were derived from intrinsic sources in the cortex, it has now been demonstrated that there are GABAergic projections from subcortical nuclei to the cortex. These afferents arise from the basal forebrain, the ventral tegmental area, and the zona incerta. The GABAergic neurons of the zona incerta project to sensory and motor cortex, but not to the frontal cortex. As with the acetylcholinergic fibers from the same source, the GABAergic neurons of the visual cortex are a major target of the GABAergic afferents of the basal forebrain (Beaulieu and Somogyi, 1991).

The claustrum is also a nucleus of the basal forebrain. It connects reciprocally and topographically with the cerebral cortex (LeVay and Sherk, 1981; Tigges and Tigges, 1985). However, the reciprocal connections do not form a single continuous map, but are segregated into function specific divisions. Thus, the claustrum is not strictly multimodal, although it contains representations of visual, auditory, somatosensory, limbic and perhaps motor functions. These functions are represented separately in the nuclear mass of the claustrum and there is no evidence of integration of the different modalities. In this respect, the claustrum follows the principle of separate representation of these modalities adopted by the neocortex and thalamus. In the case of the visual system it is clear that many, perhaps all, of the retinotopically organized visual areas converge on the claustrum and it in turn projects divergently back to them. In the primary visual cortex the projection to the claustrum arises from a subset of the layer 6 pyramidal cells. The claustrum sends a sparse projection back to all layers of visual cortex where it forms excitatory connections mainly with the spines of excitatory neurons, except in layer 4 where synapses with dendritic shafts form about half the targets (LeVay and Sherk, 1981).

Cortico-Cortical Connections. Although anatomists have emphasized the long fiber tracts between the neocortex and their subcortical targets and suppliers, the major input to any cortical area is from other cortical areas. Braitenberg and Schüz (1991) have calculated that only 1 in 100 or even 1 in 1000 fibers in the white matter is involved in subcortical projection. Most of the fibers in the white matter are involved in the intrahemispheric connections and interhemispheric connections. Over the past 20 years these connections have been intensively studied, particularly in the primate visual cortex. The pattern that has emerged is that the pyramidal cells of the superficial layers project to the middle layers (principally layer 4) of their target area, whereas the deep layer pyramidals project outside the middle layers to superficial and deep layers. These patterns have been used to classify patterns as *feedforward* (projecting to layer 4), or *feedback* (projecting outside layer 4) (Felleman and Van Essen, 1991; Kennedy et al., 1991). All cortical areas are reciprocally connected by these feedforward and feedback pathways. In the face of multiple parallel pathways projecting to and from cortical and subcortical areas such simple classifications of feedforward and feedback may not translate into functional significance. However, it is clear that the substantial majority of the neuronal targets of these corticocortical connections are pyramidal neurons.

One of the most important principles in cortical circuitry is the need to save "wire," i.e., reduce the length of the axons that interconnect neurons (Mead, 1990; Mitchison, 1992). The dimensions of this problem are evident in the statistics of the amount of wire involved. Each cubic millimeter of white matter contains about 9 m of axon, and an equal volume of gray matter contains about 3 km of axon. The volume occupied by axons would be greatly increased if each neuron had to connect to every other neuron in a given area, or if every neuron were involved in long-distant connections between cortical areas. Instead, the design principles of cortex are that neurons are sparsely connected, that most connections are local, and only restricted subsets of neurons are involved in long-distance connections.

The constraint on volume can also lead to multiple cortical areas. If separate areas are fused into a single area that preserves the total cortical thickness of 2 mm, then the components of the original areas must spread over a larger area (Mitchison, 1992). The original connections between neurons now have to span larger distances and so contribute to a larger volume for the same number of neurons. Mitchison has shown that fusing 100 cortical areas leads to a 10-fold increase in the cortical volume. Of course, if all the cortical areas are fused into one area, then much of the white matter can be eliminated. However, the increase in the volume of the *intra*areal axons far exceeds the reduction of the *inter*areal axons. Similar arguments can be raised for the patchiness of connections within a cortical area that are a cardinal feature of cortical organization. A given cluster of neurons projects to a number of sites within a given cortical area. These clusters tend to link areas of common functional properties. The size of the clusters—about 400 μm—is remarkably uniform between cortical areas. This size is similar to the spread of the dendritic arbor. Malach (1992) has shown theoretically that such an organization increases the diversity of sampling across a cortical area that has a nonuniform distribution of functional properties.

SYNAPTIC CONNECTIONS

TYPES

Gray used the electron microscope to make the fundamental observation that there are two basic types of synapses in the neocortex, which he called *types 1 and 2* (Gray, 1959). The synapses made by the vast majority of the cortical spiny neurons and by some of the subcortical projections, such as the thalamic and claustral afferents, are type 1. Type 2 synapses are made by smooth neurons and some of the subcortical projections, such as the noradrenergic fibers. His classification was based on the appearance of the electron-dense staining adjacent to the pre- and postsynaptic membranes. The type 1 synapses have a thicker postsynaptic than presynaptic density, giving them an *asymmetrical* appearance. The type 2 synapses have equally thick pre- and postsynaptic densities, which given them a more *symmetrical* appearance. There are additional morphological criteria that have been used to classify the synapses (see Chap. 1). The synaptic cleft of the type 1 synapses is wider than that of type 2 synapses; the vesicles associated with type 1 synapses tend to be round, while the type 2 synapses are pleomorphic (Colonnier, 1968). Significantly, these morphological distinctions correlate with the physiological divisions, excitatory in most cases being type 1 and inhibitory, type 2 synapses.

Both types of synapses are found throughout the cortex in approximately constant proportions. In each cubic millimeter of neocortex there are 2.78×10^8 synapses, 84% of which are type 1 synapses and 16% are type 2 (Beaulieu and Colonnier, 1985). Both types are found on all cortical neurons, but their locations on the dendritic trees of the different types differ (Fig. 12.5; Gray, 1959; Szentágothai, 1978; White and Rock,

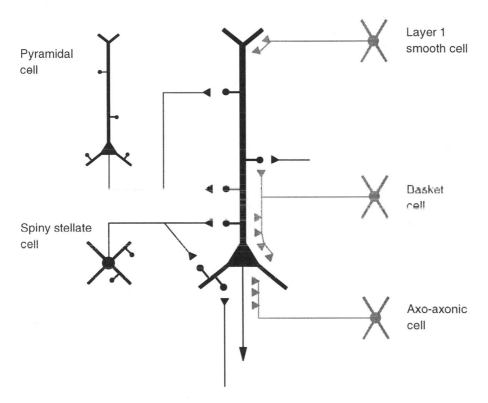

Fig. 12.5. Synaptic connections in neocortex. Configurations of excitatory and inhibitory connections made onto a typical pyramidal neuron (center). The excitatory (spiny) cells (black, left) and thalamic afferents (black, bottom) form synapses with the spines of the target pyramidal cell. Layer 6 pyramidal cell (not shown) are the exception to this rule. They form synapses mainly with the dendritic shafts of target spiny cells. There are a number of different classes of inhibitory (smooth) cells (gray, right), each with a characteristic pattern of connection to the pyramidal cell. Three classes are shown here. Each smooth cell makes multiple synapses with its target. The superficial smooth cell synapses with the apical tuft. The basket cell synapses with the soma, dendritic trunk, and dendritic spines. The chandelier cell synapses with the initial segment of the axon.

1980; Beaulieu and Colonnier, 1985; White, 1989). Pyramidal cells receive few type 1 synapses on their dendritic shafts and none at all on their somata or initial segment of the axon. Conversely, type 2 synapses are found on the proximal dendritic shafts, on the somata, and on the axon initial segment of pyramidal cells. Nearly every spine of pyramidal cells forms a type 1 synapse, but only about 7% of spines form an additional type 2 synapse. Similar distributions have been reported for the spiny stellate cells of the mouse somatosensory cortex, but the pattern for the spiny stellate cells in layer 4 of the primary visual cortex is different. About 60% of the type 1 synapses are formed with the proximal and distal dendritic shafts, the remainder are formed on the heads of the dendritic spines (Ahmed et al., 1994; Anderson et al., 1994). Type 2 synapses are found on the somata, but synapses are rarely found on the axon initial segment. Although the type 2 synapses are clustered in higher density on the proximal dendrites, about 40% of the type 2 synapses are on distal portions of the dendrites (i.e., more than 50 μm from the soma).

The smooth neurons by definition do not bear spines, so both type 1 and type 2 synapses are formed on the beaded dendrites that are a characteristic feature of smooth neurons. The beads themselves are the sites of clusters of synaptic inputs. The pattern of input to the smooth neurons is quite different from that of the spiny neurons: both types of synapses cluster on the proximal dendrites and somata at about 2–3 times the density found for spiny dendrites. The type 2 synapses are rarely found on the distal regions of the dendritic tree and the density of type 1 synapses on the distal dendrites is less than on the proximal dendrites. The initial segment of the axon of smooth neurons does not form synapses.

SPINY NEURONS

The axons of the spiny neurons form the vast majority of the synapses in the cortex. The synapses they form are type 1 in morphology and almost all are on spines (80–90% of targets) (Sloper and Powell, 1979a; Martin, 1988). One type of spiny neuron, a layer 6 pyramidal neuron, is the exception to this general rule: it forms most of its synapses preferentially with the shafts of spiny neurons in layer 4 (see White, 1989). Some synapses of the spiny stellate or pyramidal neurons are formed with dendrites or somata of smooth neurons, but these constitute only about 10% of their output. A feature of the output of the spiny neurons is that they contribute only a few synapses to any individual postsynaptic target. Conversely, any single neuron receives its excitatory input from the convergence of many thousands of neurons, most of which are in the same cortical area. The thalamic afferents, which provide the principle sensory input to cortex, form about 10% or less of the synapses in layer 4, the main thalamorecipient layer (White, 1989; Ahmed et al., 1994; Fig. 12.6).

SMOOTH NEURONS

The synaptic connections of the smooth neurons differ in a number of significant respects from the spiny neurons. Their axons are less extensive than those of the spiny neurons and they make multiple synapses on their targets. This means they contact many fewer targets on average than spiny neurons. Whereas the spiny neurons generally form synapses with dendritic spines, the smooth neurons target a variety of sites. In addition, different smooth neuron types form synapses specifically with different

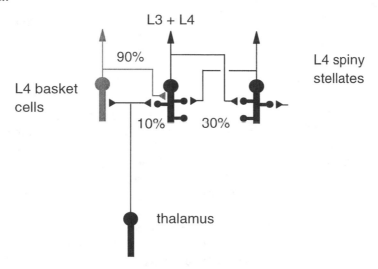

Fig. 12.6. Fractions of synaptic connections onto spiny stellate neurons in layer 4 of cat striate cortex (Ahmed et al., 1994). Only about 10% of the excitatory synapses are derived from the lateral geniculate nucleus. Thirty percent arise from other spiny stellate neurons in layer 4, and a further 40% from the layer 6 pyramidal cells (not shown). Ninety percent of the inhibitory inputs arise from layer 4 basket cells.

portions of the neuron (Fig. 12.5). The major output of the smooth neurons, however, is to spiny neurons. The smooth neurons form no more than 15% of the targets of the spiny neurons.

Basket cells (Fig. 12.4B) are the most frequently encountered smooth neuron in Golgi preparations and in intracellular physiological studies. Kisvárday (1992) has estimated that they form at least 20% of all GABAergic neurons. They have a very characteristic axon that forms the most extensive lateral connections of any of the smooth cell types. The basket cells of the superficial and deep layers have axons that radiate from the soma up to distances of 1–2 mm. In layer 4 the small basket cell (also called a *clutch cell*, in this context; see Fig. 12.4C) axon is more localized and extends about 0.5 mm laterally in most cases (Mates and Lund, 1983; Kisvárday et al., 1985). Each basket cell forms multiple synapses with about 300–500 target neurons and makes about 10 synapses on average with each target. Ramón y Cajal originally provided the descriptive name "basket" cells because in the Golgi preparations the axons of the basket cells form pericellular "nests," or baskets, around the soma of the pyramidal cells (Cajal, 1911). Modern light and electron microscopic studies on the axonal boutons of intracellularly labeled basket cells have revealed, as noted above, that the major targets of the basket cell axons are the dendritic shafts and spines of pyramidal and spiny stellate cells (Somogyi et al., 1983; Kisvárday, 1992). The "basket" seen by Ramón y Cajal is formed by the convergence of about 10–30 basket cells each contributing a twiglet to the perisomatic nest. Superficial and deep basket cells and clutch cells make about 20–40% of their synapses with spines, 20–40% with dendritic shafts, and the remainder with the somata.

The chandelier cell (Fig. 12.4A) is rarely encountered in Golgi preparations and in intracellular recordings in vitro and in vivo. However, they have been a focus of interest because their sole output is to the initial segment of the axons of pyramidal cells. Such specificity is not seen with any other neocortical cell although it is common elsewhere in the brain (see earlier chapters). The chandelier cells seem to be found only in the superficial layers and layer 4, but some have a descending axon collateral that innervates the deep layer pyramidal cells. Correspondingly, electron microscopic examination of the initial segments of the pyramidal cells has indicated that there are about three times as many synapses along the initial segment of the axon of superficial layer pyramidal cells as compared with deep layer pyramidal cells (Somogyi, 1977; Sloper et al., 1979; Peters, 1984). In the superficial layers, the axon initial segment forms about 40 type 2 synapses with the boutons of the chandelier cell. Each pyramidal cell receives input from 3 to 5 chandelier cells and each chandelier cell forms synapses with about 300 pyramidal cells over a surface area about 200–400 μm across (Somogyi et al., 1982; Peters, 1984).

Double bouquet neurons (Fig. 12.4D) are smooth neurons found in the superficial layers and having a bitufted axonal system that spans several layers (Cajal, 1911; Somogyi and Cowey, 1981). In contrast to the laterally directed axons of the basket cell, the predominant orientation of the double bouquet cell's axon is vertical. For this reason, it was originally thought that the vertically oriented apical dendrites of the pyramidal cells were the major target of multiple synapses from the pallisades of double bouquet axons. There is no clear evidence of multiple synapses between double bouque axons and apical dendrites, but the pyramidal cells are nevertheless major targets. About 40% of the type 2 synapses of double bouquet cells are formed with dendritic shafts and most of the remainder are formed with dendritic spines (Somogyi and Cowey, 1981).

The synaptic connections formed by the axons of layer 1 neurons have been studied rarely. The small neurons of layer 1 have as their major target the spines and dendritic shafts of pyramidal cell apical dendritic tufts that form most of the neuropil of layer 1. The connections made by the Cajal-Retzius cells are unknown. Similarly, the connections made by other smooth neurons of the neocortex have yet to be determined.

BASIC CIRCUIT

An article of faith among neuroanatomists from the beginning of the study of the cortical circuits was that there was an elementary pattern of cortical organizations. Anatomists studying Golgi stained material were generally convinced that there were structural details that remained constant despite variations in cell number, form, size, and type of neurons. This constant, according to Lorente de Nó, was the "arrangement of the plexuses of dendrites and axonal branches," by which he meant the synaptic connections between cortical neurons. However, subsequent examination of the details of cortical circuitry still leaves considerable leeway in interpretation of the pattern of connections. Any attempt to suggest a common basic pattern of connections necessarily will be open to the criticism that such models are based on the intensive study of a very small number of areas, mainly primary sensory areas at that (White, 1989). Nevertheless, the great advantage of having some hypothetical circuit is that it focuses ideas and gives form to otherwise simply descriptive accounts of cells and connections within a given area that have been the standard works in the anatomical field.

Most modern models of cortical circuits are derived from functional studies. In contradistinction to the great diversity of cell types and interconnections that characterize the anatomical descriptions, the circuits derived from physiological experiments strip off all the embellishment and detail: simple circuits of excitatory cells make up the core of these models. The Hubel-Wiesel models of the local circuits of visual cortex are the best-known examples (Hubel and Wiesel, 1977). In these circuits, the inhibitory neurons are added as a means of providing the lateral inhibition that is such a feature of sensory processing at all levels. Two basic designs have emerged. In the dominant model, the processing is strictly serial: input arrives in the cortical circuit, it is fed forward through a short chain of two or three neurons within the local area, and then it is transmitted to other areas by the output neurons. This feedforward model follows from the simple idea that sensory input must pass through several processing stages in the neocortex before it arrives at a motor output.

An alternative view was first given form by Lorente de Nó. He supposed that the rich interconnections between the different cortical layers made the cortical circuit a unitary system, with no clear basis for a distinction between input, association, and output layers. In his view, impulses circulate through these recurrent circuits and the activity in the cortical circuit is modified by the action of the association fibers arriving at critical points within the circuit. In turn, the effect of the incoming input depends on the activity in the circuit at that point in time.

Both the feedforward and the recurrent recurrent model agree, however, that the processing that occurs in the neocortex is essentially local and vertical. In this arrangement, the anatomy and the physiology agree. In most cortical areas the function being represented is laid out topographically, as in the retinotopic maps of the visual cortex or the motor maps in the motor cortex. For example, portions of the sensory surface that will receive related input are nearest neighbors in their cortical representation. The vertical connectivity within the cortex is similarly local. The axons of cortical neurons do not extend more than a few millimeters laterally in any area. Thus the monosynaptic connections at least are local. This corresponds with the physiological findings of Mountcastle, Hubel and Wiesel, and others who discovered that neurons with similar functional properties are organized in "columns" that extend from the cortical surface to the white matter (Powell and Mountcastle, 1959; Hubel and Wiesel, 1977; Fig. 12.7).

In fact, with few exceptions, most arrangements of neurons are only strictly columnar when viewed with the one-dimensional tool of the microelectrode. The clearest view arises from optical imaging in which the activity of large numbers of nerve cells can be viewed indirectly by measuring the changes in the oxygenation of hemoglobin that occur during the increased oxygen demand of neural activity. Such imaging techniques have been used to show that in the lateral dimension, the different functional maps take the form of slabs or pinwheels. The widths of the slabs vary according to the particular property being mapped, but are of the order of 0.5 mm in the case of the best-studied system—the ocular dominance system of the primary visual cortex. In this system, the afferents of the lateral geniculate nucleus representing left and right eye map into a series parallel slabs that look like a zebra's stripes when viewed from the surface. Such segregation and patchiness are seen at the level of single axonal arbors and appear to be the means by which the cortex maps multiple processes into a single area. In the few cases in which it has been examined, the rule of connectivity between patches is that "like" connects to "like." For example, a number of different functional dimensions are represented within the retinotopic map of the primary visual cortex of primates. These dimensions are seen physically in the ocular dominance and orientation slabs and the cytochrome oxidase columns, which are called "blobs" because of their appearance when viewed in tangentially cut sections of the cortex (Hendrickson et al., 1981; Horton and Hubel, 1981; Wong-Riley and Carroll, 1984; Fig. 12.7). In each of these systems, neurons of like function interconnect.

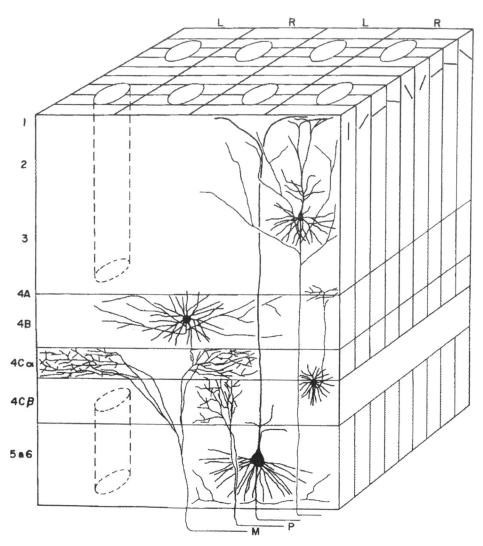

Fig. 12.7. "Ice cube" model of visual cortex in the macaque monkey devised by Hubel and Wiesel. L and R indicate ocular dominance "columns" or "slabs." The narrower orientation columns run orthogonally. The cytochrome oxidase rich "blobs" appear as cylinders in the center of ocular dominance columns. M, P: Thalamic afferents originating from the magno and parvocellular layers of the lateral geniculate nucleus, respectively, and terminating in separate subdivisions of layer 4, within appropriate ocular dominance slabs.

CORTICAL OUTPUT

All projection neurons have recurrent collaterals that participate in local cortical circuits, so there are no layers that have exclusively output functions. The output neurons from the cortex are generally pyramidal cells. These same cells, however, may also be *input* neurons in that they may receive direct input from the thalamus. There is a laminar-specific organization of the output according to the location of their targets. A simplified view of the laminar organization is provided in the summary figure Fig. 12.8. The general rule-of-thumb is that cortico-cortical connections arise mainly from the superficial cortical layers and the subcortical projections arise from the deep layers. Within the deep layers, there is an output to regions that have a motor-related function, e.g., the superior colliculus, basal ganglia, brainstem nuclei, and spinal cord. These regions receive their cortical output from a relatively small number of layer 5 pyramidal cells. There is also an output to the subcortical relay nuclei in the thalamus, which are the source of the primary sensory input to the cortex. This cortico-thalamic projection generally arises from the layer 6 pyramidal cells. However, there are clear exceptions to this rule of thumb. In area 4, the projections into the pyramidal tract, which supplies the spinal cord and cerebellum, arise from both layer 5 and from layer 3 pyramidal cells. The cortico-cortical connections may also arise from neurons in the deep layers. However, the simplifications are not extreme and offer a useful constraint on the connections that can be made within the basic circuits. For example, if a circuit in cat visual cortex requires an output to the eye-movement maps of the superior colliculus, then it necessarily will have to connect to the output pyramidal cells of layer 5. Although particular laminae are the source of the outputs to these different cortical and subcortical regions, the set of output neurons within a given lamina may not be uniform. Thus, within layer 6, the pyramidal cells that give rise to the cortico-thalamic projection are morphologically different from those that give rise to the cortico-

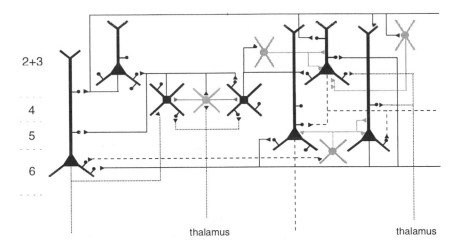

Fig. 12.8. Basic circuit for visual cortex. Smooth, GABAergic, neurons and their connections are indicated in gray. Spiny neurons and their connections are indicated in black. Cortical layers as indicated.

claustral projection (Katz, 1987). These two groups of pyramidal cells also have different local projection patterns: the cortico-thalamic pyramidal cells have a rich projection to layer 4, whereas the cortico-claustral cells project within layer 6 itself. The receptive fields of the cortico-thalamic neurons are significantly smaller than those of the cortico-claustral neurons (Grieve and Sillito, 1995).

As with the local intra-areal connectivity, the output neurons that project to other cortical areas also appear to be organized in patchy systems. One of the most elaborate discovered so far is the output from primary (V1) to the secondary visual area (V2), which arises from at least three specific subgroups of neurons in V1. These neurons project to another stripe system in area V2 in the monkey. These pathways may be visualized by the pattern of cytochrome oxidase staining (Gilbert and Kelly, 1975; Gilbert and Wiesel, 1979). Neurons located in the cytochrome oxidase blobs in V1 project to a series of thin cytochrome oxidase blobs in V2. The neurons in layer 3 outside the blobs project to pale stripe (interstripes) in V2, while the third group of projection neurons located in layer 4B of V1 project to a series of thick cytochrome stripes in V2. The stripes formed by these projections themselves reveal the organization of output from V2 to other cortical areas: the thin cytochrome stripes project to visual area 4 (V4), the interstripes to V3 and V4, and the thick stripes to area MT.

SYNAPTIC ACTIONS

Release of neurotransmitter at synapses is triggered by the membrane depolarization associated with the arrival of an action potential. Consequently, the pattern of arrival of APs at the end terminal is one of the fundamental factors governing the interaction of pre- and postsynaptic neuron. It is usually assumed that the pattern of action potentials seen by the presynaptic terminal is exactly the pattern that was generated at the beginning of the presynaptic axon. That is, we assume that the axon acts as a simple transmission line for action potentials, and that there are no factors that selectively alter its transmission characteristics over moderate time intervals. The presynaptic axon begins at the initial segment, which is also the site at which the axonal action potential transmission begins. The initial segment is electrotonically close to the soma, and therefore we assume the electrical events of the initial segment can be recorded from the soma, which is the most probable site of impalement by intracellular electrodes. Most of our knowledge about interneuronal communication rests on interpretations of electrical events in the soma, and in particular, on the assumption that the action potentials that we observe in the soma will ultimately affect postsynaptic targets.

NEURONAL EXCITABILITY

In considering the action of synapses, there are two key issues. One is the effect of the synapses on the neuron at the site of the synapses; the other, the response of the whole neuron to the local synaptic actions. The latter issue includes the attributes of the neuron, such as its membrane properties, the ionic currents involved, and the shape and cable properties of the neuron.

Sodium Currents. Action potential generation entails regenerative depolarization followed by a restorative repolarization. In cortical neurons, as in most other neurons, these two phases are mediated by a fast, voltage-dependent, inactivating sodium current (Connors et al., 1982), and a delayed, voltage-dependent potassium current (Prince and Huguenard, 1988), respectively. In addition to the inactivating sodium current, cortical neurons also exhibit a non-inactivating, voltage-dependent sodium current (Stafstrom et al., 1982, 1984) similar to that observed in cerebellar Purkinje cells (Llinás and Sugimori 1980a,b; see Chap. 7) and hippocampal pyramidal cells (Hotson et al., 1979; Connors et al., 1982; see Chap. 11), and analogous to the slow inward calcium current (I_i) seen in spinal motoneurons (Schwindt and Crill, 1980; see Chap. 4). In cortical neurons this "persistent" sodium current (I_{NaP}) is activated about 10–20 mV positive to the resting potential and attains steady-state conductance within about 4 ms. It remains persistent and large up to at least 50 mV above resting potential (Stafstrom et al., 1984). These properties suggest that I_{NaP} can be activated by EPSPs, and that I_{NaP} acts as a current amplifier for depolarizing inputs. Indeed, I_{NaP} can itself provide regenerative depolarization that is able to drive the membrane to the level where the larger spike generating sodium current is activated (Stafstrom et al., 1982). The difference in kinetics between these two regenerative sodium currents is probably responsible for the indistinct transition between the subthreshold rise of membrane potential and the rapid initial rise of the action potential (Stafstrom et al., 1984).

By recording directly from the apical dendrites of the pyramidal cells (Stuart and Sakmann, 1994), it has been shown that the dendrites contain active sodium conductances. However, they appear to be at a much lower density than at the soma or axon initial segment, which has the highest density and is the main site of initiation of the action potential, as was originally proposed from recordings from the motoneuron (Fuortes et al., 1957; Eccles 1957).

Potassium Currents. The inward sodium currents that accompany spike depolarization are opposed by an increase in outward potassium currents, and these currents ultimately restore the neuronal membrane to its resting level. The classical action potential mechanism provides a restorative outward current by just one delayed voltage-dependent potassium conductance, but the restorative outward current of cortical neurons is enhanced by several additional potassium currents. These currents affect the dynamics of membrane during postspike recovery and also during the subthreshold response to depolarizing inputs. Consequently, they affect the neuron's repetitive discharge behavior.

In the simplest case, a suprathreshold sustained depolarizing input current will evoke a train of action potentials. Each action potential ends with a repolarization that drives the membrane potential below threshold. The subsequent interspike interval will depend on the rate of postspike depolarization, since this will determine the interval to the next threshold crossing. If the time constants of the membrane currents are all short (i.e., of the order of an action potential duration), then the interspike intervals will be of equal duration and the neuron will exhibit sustained regular discharge. But some of the potassium conductances have much longer time constants and so their outward currents can be active throughout successive interspike intervals. Since these outward potassium currents oppose the depolarizing input currents, they retard threshold crossing and so increase the interspike interval. These interactions are the basis of adaptation, often referred to as *spike-frequency adaptation*, the progressive lengthening of interspike interval that occurs during a sustained depolarizing input to some cortical neurons. The process of adaptation in cortical cells is interesting because it imposes an intrinsic restriction on their discharge. It is calcium-dependent, it can be modified by neurotransmission, and adaptation characteristics correlate with morphological cell type.

The outward potassium currents that underly the impulse afterhyperpolarizations (AHP) are seen in cortical neurons both in vivo and in vitro (Connors et al., 1982). Three separate AHPs have been identified in layer 5 neurons of sensorimotor cortex: a fast, medium, and slow AHP (Schwindt et al., 1988b). The fast AHP has a duration of milliseconds, and follows spike repolarization. It is often followed by a transient delayed afterdepolarization (ADP). The medium AHP follows a brief train of spikes. It has a duration of tens of milliseconds, and its amplitude and duration are increased by the frequency and number of spikes in the train. The slow AHP (sAHP) is evoked by sustained discharge, and has a duration of seconds. All three hyperpolarizations are sensitive to extracellular potassium concentration, but they have different sensitivities to divalent ion substitutions and pharmacological manipulations (Schwindt et al. 1988a,b). This suggests that they are mediated by at least three distinct potassium conductances. However, the individual potassium conductances have not been identified completely. This is partly because of the difficulty in comparing the characteristics of the many potassium conductance types found in various excitable cells, the many different regimes of investigation, and inconsistent nomenclature.

There is evidence that neocortical cells have at least four potassium conductances: a delayed rectifier, a fast, transient, voltage-dependent (A-like) current; a slow, calcium-mediated (AHP-like) current; and a slow, receptor-modulated, voltage-dependent (M-like, mAHP) current (Connors et al., 1982; Schwindt et al., 1988a,b). Thus, the potassium currents of neocortical neurons appear qualitatively similar to those reported in hippocampal neurons of archicortex (see Chap. 11). But the situation is rather more complicated than this, as the following examples illustrate. The transient fast current of cortex is TEA sensitive (Schwindt et al., 1988a). The mAHP current is due to a calcium-mediated potassium conductance and so is superficially similar to AHP currents seen in hippocampal neurons. But the cortical conductance mechanism is not sensitive to TEA whereas the hippocampal current is. The cortical conductance is sensitive to apamin, whereas the hippocampal current is not (Schwindt, 1992). Muscarine and beta-adrenergic agonists abolish the sAHP but have no effect on the mAHP (Schwindt et al., 1988), whereas in hippocampus acetylcholine affects both the M and AHP currents (Madison and Nicoll 1984). These and other conductance differences may be due to important functional constraints on the discharge of neocortical neurons that are different from the discharge requirements of hippocampal neurons. An alternative view is that the differences have less to do with unique discharge requirements than with the variations of parallel evolution.

Some outward current conductances can be modulated by neurotransmitters. The outward potassium M current of cortical pyramids is reduced by activation of muscarinic receptors (Brown, 1988; McCormick and Prince, 1985). Since the outward current is reduced, the effect of depolarizing currents is enhanced. The slow Ca^{2+}-activated potassium (AHP) current of cortical pyramids is also decreased by acetylcholine (McCormick and Prince, 1986b). These modulations of slow outward currents are the means whereby acetylcholine enhances discharge frequency and decreases adaptation. Similar effects have been noted in hippocampal neurons (Benardo and Prince, 1982; Cole and Nicoll, 1984; Madison and Nicoll, 1984). Neurotransmitters may also modulate currents that interact with the slow hyperpolarizing potassium currents. Schwindt et al. (1988b) have shown that low concentrations of muscarine abolish the sAHP, but at higher concentrations the sAHP is replaced by a slow after-depolarization (sADP) that is not potassium sensitive, nor is it sensitive to the sodium channel blocker TTX. The mechanism of the sADP is unknown.

In addition to the above effects, acetylcholine also evokes a transient early inhibition of pyramidal neurons. However, two findings indicate that this inhibition is probably an indirect effect of the excitation of inhibitory interneurons. First, the inhibition is mediated by a chloride conductance similar to that activated by GABA. Second, ACh has a rapid excitatory effect on the fast-spiking (presumably GABA-ergic) cortical neurons (McCormick and Prince, 1985, 1986b), and smooth cells are known to have cholinergic afferents (Houser et al., 1985).

Calcium Conductances. Calcium currents also contribute to the dynamics of cortical neurons. Somatic recordings from antidromically activated pyramidal tract neurons in vivo indicated the existence of fast prepotentials (Deschênes, 1981). Blocking the sodium channel blocker with QX-314 left these prepotentials intact, suggesting they were mediated by calcium channels in the dendrites (Hirsch et al., 1995).

These currents may affect the dynamics directly by contributing to the electrical behavior of the membrane, or indirectly by changing the internal calcium concentration, which in turn affects potassium conductance (described above). Where calcium currents are voltage-dependent, they operate as sodium currents do and so could contribute to spike generation. However, the calcium currents appear to be relatively small in cortical neurons, and must be unmasked by both blocking the sodium currents and depressing the potassium currents. Under these conditions, a Ca^{2+} spike can be elicited from some cortical neurons (Connors et al., 1982; Stafstrom et al., 1985). The threshold for this spike is about 30–40 mV positive to the resting potential, and therefore well above the activation thresholds for the sodium currents, I_{NaP} and I_{Na}.

Calcium spikes have been observed in hippocampal pyramidal cells (see Chap. 11) and elsewhere, and in these cases, they can be evoked after blockade of the sodium currents alone (Schwartzkroin and Slawsky, 1977; Wong et al., 1979). In order to initiate a calcium spike the conductance for calcium must be much larger than that for potassium. Presumably, g_K is large in cortical cells, and must be depressed in order to obtain a conductance ratio favorable for calcium spike initiation. Therefore, the need to depress the potassium conductance in cortical cells implies either that g_K is larger in cortical neurons than other calcium-spiking cells, or that the calcium conductance is smaller. An alternative explanation is that the site of the calcium conductance is located in the dendrites, electrotonically distant from the soma. In this case, a depolarization large enough to drive the distant site to the activation threshold of the calcium conductance would also strongly activate the more proximal voltage dependent potassium conductances. The resulting increase in potassium conductance would shunt depolarizing current injected into the soma, and so prevent the dendritic membrane from reaching the threshold for calcium current activation.

Stafstrom et al. (1985) suggest that there are two calcium conductances in cortical neurons, and that these are distributed along the soma-dendrite. The somatic calcium conductance is slow and small and has a high threshold. The dendritic conductance is both faster and larger than its somatic counterpart. Its threshold is also high, but this may be partly due to electrotonic distance from the soma, which makes it relatively difficult to activate from an electrode in the soma. Both somatic and dendritic currents contribute to the calcium spike. Somatic depolarization activates the somatic calcium current and that in turn activates the more distal dendritic calcium conductance that powers the calcium spike. Both currents are probably persistent and so they require activation of an outward current to effect the recovery phase of the spike. This outward current is provided by the slow potassium (AHP) current that is activated by the influx of calcium in cortical (Hotson and Prince, 1980) and hippocampal (Madison and Nicoll, 1984; Lancaster and Adams, 1986) neurons.

Direct evidence for the existence of dendritic voltage-sensitive calcium channels has come from membrane patches of apical dendrites (Huguenard et al., 1989) and by calcium imaging of the dendrites (Yuste et al., 1994). The imaging studies showed that the dendritic accumulation of calcium took place immediately after calcium spikes were triggered, followed by a slower diffusion of intracellular calcium. Confocal and two-photon microscopic imaging of calcium has revealed the sites of calcium channels in the dendritic shaft (Markram and Sakmann, 1994) and in spine heads (Yuste and Denk, 1995). It appears that calcium channels are distributed over the whole dendritic tree. The in vivo study of Hirsch et al. (1995) indicated that calcium spikes may be initiated in cat visual cortex in the absence of sodium spikes. However, Svoboda et al. (1997) found that sodium spikes were required to activate calcium spikes in rat barrel cortex.

The issue of the role of spines in the compartmentalization of calcium has also been addressed by a number of studies, unfortunately none as yet in neocortical pyramidal cells. The first studies that used optical methods to image the spines in hippocampal pyramidal cells indicated that individual spines could have quite different calcium dynamics from their parent dendrites (Muller and Connor, 1991; Guthrie et al., 1991). However, further studies in the hippocampal pyramids in which two-photon microscopy was used to image the spines of hippocampal pyramidal cells loaded with a Ca-sensitive dye indicate that individual spines are only activated under subthreshold conditions. If the neuron fires an action potential, then calcium enters the spines (Denk et al., 1996). Neocortical pyramidal cells have similar dimensions to those of the hippocampal pyramidal cells and it is likely that similar phenomena will be observed. Theoretically, the restriction of calcium in the spine during subthreshold synaptic activation could serve to segregate the potential that occurs on spines during coactivation of pre- and postsynaptic neuron (Rall, 1974a).

Repetitive Discharge. The repetitive discharge properties of neocortical cells has been investigated both in vivo (e.g., Calvin and Sypert, 1976) and in vitro (e.g., Ogawa et al., 1981). McCormick et al. (1985) originally reported three electrophysiological cell types in neocortex: fast-spiking, regular spiking, and bursting cells. The fast-spiking cells were sparsely spiny or aspiny neurons. These "smooth cells" are the GABA-containing, inhibitory neurons of cortex. The regular and bursting cells were both pyramidal neurons. "Regular firing" which is somewhat of a misnomer, refers to the adapting pattern of discharge in response to an injection of constant current into the soma. This was the predominant behavior of most pyramidal cells. Only a small percentage of these pyramidal cells exhibited a bursting discharge and they were located mainly in the deep cortical layers (Connors and Gutnick, 1990). However, it is now clear that there are exceptions to the general function–structure relationships described and smooth neurons are found that have the adapting pattern that was thought to be a characteristic of pyramidal cells. Kawaguchi (1995), for example, has found chandelier cells, double bouquet cells, and neurogliaform cells with adapting patterns of discharge that are more commonly associated with spiny neurons.

The discharge of regular spiking neurons showed various degrees of adaptation, and the presence of both AHP and M currents could be demonstrated in these cells. A transient, fast voltage-dependent (A) current is present in pyramids and this may contribute to their adaptation (Schwindt et al., 1988a). The structure–function correlations of the burst/nonburst firing pyramidal cells of layer 5 have been determined (Chagnac-Amitai et al., 1990; Connors and Gutnick, 1990; Mason and Larkman, 1990; Kim and Connors, 1993). The regular firing pyramids have thin apical dendrites that do not branch extensively in layer 1. The burst-firing pyramids by contrast have thick apical dendrites and an extensive tuft in layer 1. Multipolar and bitufted neurons with bursting patterns have been described by Kawaguchi (1995) who called them *low-threshold spike cells*. These neurons would respond with a burst of action potentials when the neuron was depolarized from a hyperpolarized potential. Their dendrites had few spines.

Bursting neurons (Connors et al., 1982; McCormick et al., 1985; Kawaguchi, 1995) respond to depolarization by generating a short burst of about three spikes. McCormick and Gray (1996) have reported another class of bursting cell, which they called a *chattering cell*. This cell produces a series of bursts during sustained depolarization. The exact mechanism of bursting in cortical neurons is unknown, but it has been explained by various mechanisms, including the activation of low- and high-threshold calcium currents (McCormick et al., 1985; Jahnsen, 1986a; McCormick and Gray, 1996), by a calcium-dependent potassium current (Berman et al., 1989), and most recently by the distribution of sodium channels in the dendritic tree (Mainen and Sejnowski, 1996). In theory, it is possible to achieve a short burst in a neuron that has limited fast outward current and a dominant AHP current (Berman et al., 1989). The reduced fast-outward current encourages a short interspike interval and consequently a rapid discharge. The discharge would be terminated by the growing AHP current. Thus, variations in the parameters of the same outward current conductances could determine whether a pyramidal neuron discharges in regular or burst mode. In the model of Mainen and Sejnowski (1996), the dendritic sodium conductances promote propagation of the somatic action potential back into the dendrites. When the soma has repolarized, current returns from the dendrites to produce a late depolarization and some maintained action-potential discharge. This effect was enhanced by high-threshold, voltage-gated Ca^{2+} channels. Schwindt et al. (1988a) have shown that reduction of the transient fast potassium conductance converts normal firing into burst firing, whereas specific reduction of mAHP increases the instantaneous discharge rate but does not affect adaptation (Schwindt, 1992).

The fast-spiking cells encompass a variety of smooth neuron types (Kawaguchi 1995). The action potentials of fast-spiking cells are brief by comparison with pyramidal neurons. The repolarization phase of the action potential is rapid and followed by a significant undershoot. This indicates the presence of an unusually large and fast repolarizing potassium current. Indeed, Hamill et al. (1991) were able to demonstrate that fast-spiking cells have a higher density of "delayed rectifier" potassium currents than do pyramidal cells. The spike repolarization is followed by a transient afterhyperpolarization. These cells showed little or no adaptation. The initial slopes of their current-discharge relation were steeper and their maximum discharge frequencies were higher than those of pyramidal neurons. There was no evidence of either the AHP or M potassium currents in these neurons; the absence of these longer time-constant outward currents in fast-spiking cells would explain their lack of adaptation.

Long-Term Potentiation. Brief tetanic stimulation of a set of input fibers potentiates synapses in hippocampal excitatory synapses for many hours (Bliss and Lömo, 1973). The mechanisms of this process have been extensively studied in the brain (see Chaps. 10 and 11) and the same processes are found in neocortical neurons. Homosynaptic (specific to the stimulated pathway) long-term potentiation (LTP) was first seen in neocortex in vivo, along with the converse phenomenon of heterosynaptic (affecting nonstimulated pathways) long-term depression (LTD), in which the synapses become weaker (Tsumoto and Suda, 1979). Subsequent investigation in vitro confirmed the presence of both LTP and LTD in neocortical neurons of young rats and kittens (Komatsu et al., 1981; Artola and Singer, 1987; Bindman et al., 1988; Artola et al., 1990; Aroniadou and Teyler, 1992). However, while LTP could be readily induced in neocortical neurons that showed bursting behavior (Artola and Singer, 1987), LTP was only induced in other cortical neurons in the presence of bicuculline, the GABAa antagonist (Artola and Singer, 1987).

LTP of inhibitory synapses has also been observed in visual cortex of developing rat (Komatsu and Iwakiri, 1993). Tetanic stimulation of an inhibitory pathway onto layer 5 pyramidal cells leads to a long (more than 1 hr) potentiation of the IPSPs. Weaker stimuli led to a short-term potentiation. The effects were specific to the stimulated pathway.

Artola et al. (1990) provided evidence that identical stimulation could produce either LTD or LTP, depending on the level of depolarization of the postsynaptic neurons. They suggested that if the EPSPs produced a depolarization that exceeds a certain level but remains below the threshold for activation of the NMDA receptor, then LTD results. If, however, the threshold for the NMDA receptor is reached, then LTP results. This is essentially the theoretical model of Bienenstock et al. (1982). Kimura et al. (1990) found that tetanic stimulation that would otherwise produce LTP will produce LTD if postsynaptic calcium ions are chelated. This indicates that the prevailing calcium concentration may be important for the production of LTP or LTD. Kirkwood et al. (1993) showed that one of the most effective means of producing LTD is by low-frequency (1 Hz) stimulation and that the induction of LTD was dependent on NMDA receptors. This suggests that the actual level of calcium might be critical for determining whether LTP (high postsynaptic calcium) or LTD (low postsynaptic calcium) is induced. However, a recent study (Neveu and Zucker, 1996) indicates that this is not the simple solution.

The precise roles of LTP and LTD in the neocortex remain a matter of speculation; the widely held belief that they have something to do with memory remains the central dogma. However, the existence of a clear *critical period* of development in the sensory cortex, in particular, has led to the obvious hypothesis that these synaptic processes are part of the cascade that leads to the formation and modification by experience of nerve connections. Investigations of mouse barrel cortex and rat visual cortex of the rat have indicated that LTP, induced without the aid of GABA antagonists, has a critical period. For example, in barrel cortex, it was possible to potentiate the thalamo-cortical synapses during the first week of life, but not the second (Crair and Malenka, 1995). This matches approximately the time course of structural plasticity of the thalamocortical afferents (Schlaggar et al., 1993). The LTP was dependent on NMDA-receptor activation and on increases in postsynaptic calcium.

In rat visual cortex, Kirkwood et al. (1995) also demonstrated that there is a critical period for LTP that corresponds to the falling phase for the plasticity of left and right eye inputs to cortex (ocular dominance plasticity). LTP was evoked in layer 3 by tetanic stimulation in the white matter. Unlike in adult rat cortex (described above), the LTP could be induced without blocking the GABA receptors. LTP could, however, be preserved beyond the normal end of the critical period by dark-rearing the pups. This procedure is known to delay the critical period in cats (Cynader and Mitchel, 1980) and appears to have some effect in rats. This dark-rearing paradigm has also been used to study the model of Bienenstock et al. (1982), which predicts that synapses that are used a lot will be more prone to LTD, while synapses that are used less will potentiate more readily. The history of synapse use therefore is an important factor in deciding whether a particular stimulation will lead to LTD or LTP. Kirkwood et al. (1996) found that in dark-reared rats, LTP was enhanced, whereas LTD was hard to evoke. The effect was reversed after dark-reared rats were exposed to light after just two days.

The processes of LTP and LTD have been studied in a number of different cortical areas. In the motor cortex (area 5a) of young adult cats, brief tetanic stimulation of the same area or area 1 and 2 could evoke LTP (Keller et al., 1990). This study was one of few to examine the phenomenon in vivo and to identify the neurons being recorded. They found that LTP could be evoked in both spiny (pyramidal cells) and smooth neurons. However, LTP was induced only in those neurons that produced monosynaptic EPSPs in response to stimulation. Thalamic input to the motor cortex could also be potentiated in vivo by coactivation with the cortico-cortical pathway (Iriki et al., 1991). Tetanic stimulation of the ventrobasal thalamus alone did not product LTP.

There are, however, some differences in the plasticity seen in rat sensory (granular) cortex and motor (agranular) cortex in vitro (Castro-Alamancos et al., 1995). Although both cortical areas could reliably generate homosynaptic LTD, LTP was more reliably generated in sensory cortex than in motor cortex, unless inhibition was reduced by application of GABA receptor antagonists. In both areas, the application of NMDA antagonists blocked the induction of both LTP and LTD. However, the kainate/AMPA receptor-mediated responses are also potentiated (Aroniadou and Keller, 1995) in rat motor cortex in vitro.

EXCITATORY SYNAPSES

In the neocortex the main excitatory neurotransmitter is the amino acid glutamate. The postsynaptic membrane of glutamate synapses contains a collection of different receptor types. The amino acid sequences of many of these receptor proteins have now been identified and specific antibodies have been raised that recognize subunits of the receptors (see Chap. 2). Although additional species of glutamate receptor may well be identified, the immediate goal is to discover the role of these different receptor subtypes in the different cortical circuits.

The glutamate receptors have been divided into three major types on the basis of their amino acid sequences and agonists. These three are the AMPA/kianate receptor, the NMDA receptor, and a more recently discovered class of metabotropic receptor. Of these, the ionotropic NMDA and AMPA/kianate receptors have been best studied. The AMPA receptor is ligand gated and unlike the NMDA receptor, is not voltage-dependent. Both receptors are involved in fast synaptic transmission, although the activation of the NMDA receptor is relatively slow compared with the AMPA receptor and contributes minimally to the peak amplitude of unitary EPSPs (see Chap. 2).

Activation of the AMPA receptor in cortical neurons evokes a short-duration conductance change to sodium and to a lesser extent, potassium (Hablitz and Langmoen, 1982; Crunelli et al., 1984). The permeability of the AMPA receptors to calcium is low. Activation of the NMDA receptor evokes a long-duration conductance change (tens of milliseconds), during which cations flow through the channel. Although a significant flux of calcium can occur through the NMDA channels, they are much less conductive to calcium than the voltage-sensitive calcium channels. Consequently, most of the current is carried by sodium and potassium ions. However, the entry of calcium through the NMDA receptor appears to be important for the activation of the CaM kinase II and protein phosphorylation of the AMPA receptors that is important for potentiation.

Although the current–voltage relationships for the NMDA channel have been studied in vitro, they have yet to be done in vivo. In vitro, the resting potential of the membrane is sufficiently negative that the channel is probably blocked by magnesium, thus endowing the channel with its voltage sensitivity. However, because neurons are spontaneously active in vivo, it is likely that they are much closer to the firing threshold. Thus, in vivo the NMDA receptors may be released from their magnesium block under resting conditions and their current–voltage behaviour may resemble more that of conventional AMPA receptors. Thus, the notion derived from experiments in hippocampal slices in vitro (e.g., Collingridge et al., 1983a,b) that NMDA receptors only contribute to synaptic excitation during high-frequency stimulation, or after a reduction in inhibition, is probably not true for neocortex. In vivo evidence from visual cortex (Fox et al., 1990) and rat barrel cortex (Armstrong-James et al., 1993) suggests that, although there may be laminar differences in the involvement of NMDA receptors, they are clearly involved in synaptic responses to natural stimuli.

As with the ionotropic glutamate receptors, the metabotropic glutamate receptors (mGluR) are widely distributed through the brain. They are found on pre- and postsynaptic sites. They are coupled to G-proteins and their action is slower than that of the slow ionotropic receptor, NMDA. The time course of the metabotropic receptors depends on the particular set of subunits involved in a given receptor. The slowly developing depolarization of Purkinje cells induced by low-frequency stimulation of the parallel fibers can be blocked by RS-α-methyl-4-carboxyphenylglycine (MCPG) the competitive antagonist of the group I and II mGluRs.

In the neocortex, studies of the action of metabotropic receptors in the neocortex are in their infancy and have mainly addressed issues of development and plasticity. Few have considered their functional roles. The direct action of the mGluR on pyramidal cells, after blocking AMPA and NMDA receptors, was to produce a slow depolarization after evoked spikes (Greene et al., 1994). In burst-firing neurons that project to the superior colliculus or pons, application of mGluR agonists inhibited the burst firing and changed the neurons to a tonic mode of firing (McCormick et al., 1993; Wang and McCormick, 1993). This effect is mediated by a decrease in a potassium conductance. In isolated neocortical neurons, Sayer et al. (1992) found that mGluR activation reduced the high-threshold Ca^{2+} current mediated by L-type calcium channels.

In slices of frontal cortex of immature rats, Burke and Hablitz (1995) provided evidence that mGlu receptors are located on both pre- and postsynaptic terminals. It appeared from their pharmacological dissection that different receptor subtypes were localized at the pre- and postsynaptic sites. When $GABA_A$ receptors were blocked, mGluR agonists increased epileptiform discharges, whereas the antagonist MCPG suppressed epileptiform activity. Ionophoretic application of mGluR agonists in rat barrel cortex in vivo produced disinhibition in response to natural stimulation of the vibrissae, whereas application of the antagonists reversed these disinhibitory effects (Wan and Cahusac, 1995). The effect might be mediated by a presynaptic receptor that depresses the release of GABA.

Locations of Excitatory Synapses. The major fraction (65–85%) of excitatory synapses made on pyramidal cells are on their spines, the remainder being on dendritic shafts. No excitatory synapses are made on the somata of pyramidal cells. It was previously supposed that spiny stellate cells followed the pattern of innervation of pyramidal cells. This is true for spiny stellate cells of the mouse barrel cortex (White, 1989), but it is not true for spiny stellates of layer 4a in area 17 of the cat (Ahmed et al., 1994; Anderson et al., 1994). It also may not be true for monkey spiny stellates. In the cat, about 60% of the excitatory input arrives on shafts of dendrites. The excitatory inputs to smooth neurons are onto both the dendritic shafts and the soma. In the case of the cat, at least some of the layer 4 smooth neurons form somatic synapses with the thalamic afferents (see Synaptic Connections, above).

The strength of the excitatory synaptic coupling between excitatory neurons has been studied in a variety of cortical areas in rat and cat. Mason et al. (1991) made the first recordings from pairs of pyramidal neurons in the superficial layers of the rat visual cortex. They reported that the synapses produced small-amplitude EPSPs, about 0.1–0.4 mV as recorded in the soma. Thomson et al. (1993) studied the connections between pyramidal cells in the deep layers of the rat's motor cortex. They found that synaptic transmission was mediated by both NMDA and non-NMDA glutamate receptors. These synapses produce an EPSP with an amplitude of 1–2 mV, recorded in the soma, which was depressed by repetitive stimulation. Similar findings have been made by Markram and Tsodyks (1996) recording from pairs of neighboring layer 5 pyramidal cells in rat somatosensory cortex.

Stratford et al. (1996) examined the excitatory input to spiny stellate neurons in layer 4 of cat visual cortex. The advantage of the spiny stellate neuron for these studies is that its dendritic tree is symmetrical and electrotonically compact. Thus variations in amplitude and time course of the EPSPs are more due to synaptic properties than to the cable properties of the dendrites. The intracortical sources of excitation were spiny stellate neurons similar to the target, and also layer 6 pyramidal cells. These two types of cortical neuron had very different synaptic physiologies. The spiny stellate to spiny stellate synapse produced EPSPs with an amplitude recorded in the soma of about 1.5 mV, which depressed slightly with repetitive stimulation. The layer 6 pyramid synapses produced comparatively small-amplitude EPSPs (0.4 mV), which showed strong facilitation with repetitive stimulation. In addition they were able to demonstrate large-amplitude (2.0 mV) EPSPs from putative single thalamic fiber inputs to these same spiny stellate cells. Unlike the EPSPs of cortical origin, these putative thalamic EPSPs showed remarkably little variance in amplitude from trial to trial, and only slight depression with repetitive stimulation. Thus, the excitatory synapses formed with a single type of neuron can show a variety of static and dynamic properties, according to their source.

INHIBITORY SYNAPSES

The existence of inhibition in the cortex has been demonstrated repeatedly using intracellular recording. The first recodings were made in the Betz cells of the cat motor cortex in vivo (Phillips 1959). By antidromically activating the pyramidal tract neurons, Phillips demonstrated the presence of a recurrent inhibitory pathway in the cortex. Later studies were made in visual cortex (Li et al., 1960; Pollen and Lux, 1966; Creutzfeldt et al., 1966; Krnjević and Schwartz, 1967; Toyama et al., 1974). These confirmed Phillips's (1959) observation that every neuron received an inhibitory input. Electrical stimulation of either the subcortical thalamic nuclei or local cortical stimulation produced a long-lasting (100–200 msec) IPSP. The role and mode of operation of inhibition in generating the stimulus-specific responses of neurons in the visual cortex remain questions of intense interest (Somers et al., 1995; Douglas et al., 1995; Ferster et al., 1996).

A number of chemical substances have inhibitory effects on cortical neurons, but the most dominant inhibitor appears to be GABA. Krnjević and Schwartz (1967) performed a direct comparison between the membranc cffccts of GABA and naturally occurring IPSPs in mammalian cortex. They used surface stimulation to evoke IPSPs in neurons of pericruciate cortex, and recorded IPSPs that reached peaks at about 20–30 ms, had durations of 200–300 ms, and amplitudes of about −10 mV at the resting membrane potential. These IPSPs could be reversed by current injection or intracellular Cl injection (Krnjević and Schwartz, 1967; Dreifuss et al., 1969). Application of GABA usually hyperpolarized the cells and reduced the amplitude of the IPSPs (Krnjević and Schwartz, 1967). The reduction in IPSP amplitude was dependent on the GABA ejection current. The highest ejection currents flattened the IPSP (Krnjević and Schwartz, 1967), and sometimes slightly inverted them (Dreifuss et al., 1969). The applied GABA increased the input conductance, whose time course was similar to that of the IPSP voltage response, and decayed with a time-constant of about 50 ms. Direct application of GABA also gave a marked increase in input conductance, together with hyperpolarization in most instances. The reversal potentials for the direct GABA effect and the IPSP were similar. Dreifuss et al. (1969) therefore concluded that GABA was the source of the cortical IPSP. The development of a specific GABA receptor antagonist, bicuculline, allowed confirmation that cortical inhibitory processes were GABA mediated and had an important functional role in shaping cortical responses

(Sillito, 1975; Tsumoto et al., 1979). Subsequent identification of the structure of the GABA receptor (Barnard et al., 1987) has allowed specific antibodies to be developed for the GABA receptor subunits and so enabled the regional distribution of GABA receptor subunits to be mapped (Fritschy and Mohler, 1995).

Receptor Types. In their original paper on the heterogeneity of hippocampal responses to GABA, Alger and Nicoll (1982) proposed that there were two different mechanisms mediating GABA inhibition and that these two mechanisms were activated by two different GABA receptor types. However, the details of their hypothesis differed considerably from current models of GABA action in hippocampus. Alger and Nicoll (1982) suggested that there was only one hyperpolarizing mechanism, and that it was distributed throughout both soma and dendrites. This hyperpolarization was Cl-dependent. Their second mechanism was depolarizing. They were uncertain of the ion conductance involved, but it was slightly sensitive to chloride. However, the presence of both hyperpolarizing and depolarizing responses on the dendrite, and both sensitive to chloride, did not seem attractive! They proposed two species of GABA receptor, a single receptor type mediating hyperpolarization, and a second mediating depolarization. The hyperpolarizing receptor was seen as being the true (subsynaptic) receptor, whereas the depolarizing variety was extrasynaptic. They began on the assumption that both ought to be blocked by bicuculline. Thus, they ascribed their failure to block the hyperpolarizing response in dendrites to the subsynaptic location of the GABA receptors that activated the (putative chloride) hyperpolarizing conductance. In their view, the subsynaptic receptors would be relatively protected from the bicuculline and so the (chloride) depolarizing response would be more effectively blocked. They argued that this arrangement would explain why the application of bicuculline to the dendrites would sometimes unmask a hyperpolarizing response. The residual hyperpolarization arose from the subsynaptic GABA conductance, which was unopposed by the blocked extrasynaptic (depolarizing) mechanism. Thus the two receptors of Ager and Nicoll (1982) are very different from the two receptors now thought to mediate $GABA_{A/B}$, unless we interpret the depolarizing response to be $GABA_B$. But this interpretation does not fit, because they were able to show that the depolarizing response was blocked by bicuculline.

$GABA_A$. In early studies it was found that the conductance changes, reversal potential, and sensitivity to chloride of GABA ionophoresis and IPSPs were similar (Eccles, 1964), suggesting that they were both mediated by chloride channels. The GABA receptor associated with the chloride conductance is now known as the $GABA_A$ receptor. It is the receptor that also binds benzodiazepine and barbiturate (see Matsumoto, 1989). The $GABA_A$ receptor is selectively blocked by bicuculline. There are 16 known $GABA_A$ receptor subunits that may assemble in various combinations of 5 (pentamers) that form the functional chloride channels (Barnard et al., 1987; Nayeem et al., 1994). The β subunit contains the $GABA_A$ receptor site, whereas the α subunit contains the benzodiazepine receptor site. Benzodiazepines increase the effect of GABA by increasing the frequency of channel opening in the presence of GABA. Picrotoxin acts by interference with the chloride ionophore (Barker et al., 1983). At low concentrations, barbiturates prolong the duration of $GABA_A$ channel opening without affecting

conductance (Study and Barker 1981) and at concentrations of the order 50 μM they directly activate chloride channels (?). Alphaxalone has similar effects (Cottrell et al., 1987). The GABA$_A$ receptor sensitivity is reduced in the presence of the raised intracellular calcium associated with the calcium spike (Inoue et al., 1986).

GABA$_B$. The failure of the specific GABA$_A$-receptor antagonist, bicuculline, to block the long-duration IPSP in cortex (Curtis et al., 1970; Godfraind et al., 1970; Curtis and Felix, 1971) indicated the presence of another GABA-mediated response. Bowery and colleagues (Hill and Bowery, 1981; Bowery et al., 1987) discovered a second class of GABA receptor, which was not sensitive to barbiturates or benzodazipines (Alger and Nicoll, 1982; Blaxter et al., 1986; Bormann, 1988). These GABA$_B$ receptors are activated by the antispastic drug, baclofen, which is ineffective at GABA$_A$ receptors (Bowery et al., 1984). The GABA$_B$ receptor has now been cloned (Kaupmann et al., 1997). It forms part of the G-protein-coupled receptor superfamily (Bowery, 1993). The GABA$_B$ receptor is indirectly coupled to calcium and potassium channels via GTP-binding proteins and perhaps protein kinase C (Dutar and Nicoll, 1988b; Dolphin and Scott, 1986). In frontal cortex, G proteins are involved in the postsynaptic response, and the short latency of the GABA$_B$ IPSPs suggests a close coupling between receptor and ionophore (Hablitz and Thalmann, 1987). The GABA$_B$ receptors are also found presynaptically, where they activate potassium channels or inhibit calcium conductances. This may reduce the GABA released and reduce the overall level of GABA-mediated inhibition. On excitatory terminals, the GABA$_B$ receptors may also reduce the release of excitatory neurotransmitter (Thomson et al., 1993). Connors et al. (1988) showed in cortical slices that baclofen, the GABA$_B$ agonist, activated a long time-course hyperpolarization with a reversal potential around the potassium reversal potential, and similar observations were made in cat visual cortex in vivo (Douglas et al., 1988; Douglas and Martin, 1991).

Two low-potency GABA$_B$ antagonists, phaclofen and saclophen, have been used as GABA$_B$ receptor blockers (Kerr et al., 1987, 1988). They block the long-duration late component of the IPSPS in vitro in frontal cortex (Karlsson et al., 1988) and in visual cortex (Connors et al., 1988; Hirsch and Gilbert, 1991). Due to the low potency of phaclofen, its effects on orientation and direction selectivity of visual cortical neurons in vivo has proved inconclusive (Baumfalk and Albus, 1988), whereas blocking GABA$_A$ receptors with n-m-bicuculline produces a marked reduction in the selectivity of visual cortical neurons to visual stimuli (Sillito, 1975).

In addition to their role in postsynaptic inhibitory process, GABA$_B$ receptors also inhibit transmitter release in neocortical neurons via a presynaptic mechanism (Deisz and Prince, 1989). The mechanism is probably by reducing the entry of calcium into the presynaptic terminal and thus lowering the probability of transmitter release. Phaclophen is ineffective at the presynaptic GABA$_B$ sites (Dutar and Nicoll, 1988b).

ELECTRICAL PROPERTIES OF THE IPSP

Responses to GABA. There are at least three distinct responses to direct GABA applications to cortical neurons in vitro (Scharfman and Sarvey, 1987). The first response is a fast hyperpolarization; this predominated when the GABA was ejected close to the soma. It produced a large increase in the input conductance. The second was a longer-lasting depolarization, which was evoked most readily by application of GABA to the distal dendrites. It was associated with a moderate increase in the input conductance. The third was a slow hyperpolarization that appeared on the trailing edge of the depolarization. It was a prolonged response that decayed over many seconds and was associated with a moderate increase in the input conductance. The three compounds are often mixed. For example, ejection in the vicinity of soma may show early somatic hyperpolarizing response followed by a relatively late depolarization (as GABA diffuses onto dendrites and evokes a dendritic response). GABA ejected in the vicinity of proximal dendrites evokes both a somatic and a dendritic response.

The somatic response had a reversal potential of -65 mV, was chloride-dependent, and was blocked by bicuculline (Scharfman and Sarvey, 1987; Connors et al., 1988). The dendritic depolarization is probably also mediated by GABA$_A$ receptors since it is blocked by bicuculline and picrotoxin and is potentiated by benzodiazepines (Blaxter and Cottrell, 1985). The differences in the response between somatic and dendritic activation of the same receptor have been explained by possible differences in the chloride concentrations in dendrites and soma (Thomson et al., 1988). Lambert et al. (1991) have proposed that the GABA$_A$ receptors in the hippocampus mediate their dendritic responses via a different ionophore. By contrast the dendritic hyperpolarization evoked by GABA is mimicked by baclofen, the specific GABA$_B$ agonist. This hyperpolarization reverses at -90 mV (Ogawa et al., 1986; Scharfman and Sarvey, 1987; Connors et al., 1988). The GABA hyperpolarization is potassium-dependent and can be evoked alone by small doses of GABA applied to the dendrites (Wong and Watkins, 1982) or by blocking the depolarizing component with bicuculline (Inoue et al., 1985a,b). This dendritic hyperpolarization is blocked by phaclofen and thus is probably mediated by the GABA$_B$ receptor (Dutar and Nicoll, 1988b).

In neocortical slices, long and short IPSPs have been observed (Ogawa et al., 1981; Connors et al., 1982). The stimulus threshold for the late, long IPSPs mediated by the GABA$_B$ receptor is higher than for the early, short IPSPs, which are mediated by the GABA$_A$ receptors (Connors et al., 1982). In most neurons the early IPSPs were depolarizing because the resting potential of the cortical neurons was more negative than the reversal potential of chloride (Connors et al., 1982; McCormick et al., 1985).

Sites of Action of Inhibitory Synapses. Fatt and Katz (1953) found that the main effect of inhibitory input to crustacean muscle fiber was to attenuate the amplitude of end-plate potentials. The membrane potential of the muscle fiber was hardly affected by the inhibitory input, unless the membrane was polarized away from resting, in which case the effect of the inhibitory input was to drive the membrane towards the original resting membrane potential. The inhibitory input was associated with a 20–50% increase in membrane conductance. They estimated this increase in conductance from the change in the membrane time-constant as reflected in the rate of decay of the end-plate potential. Fatt and Katz did not use the term *shunting inhibition*, nor did they place particular emphasis on the interaction between the end-plate potential amplitude and the increase in conductance evoked by the inhibitory input. They were more concerned to point out that hyperpolarizing inhibition was not a sufficient explanation for the decrement in EPSP amplitude observed (it could account for only about 5%, whereas an 80% reduction was observed). They emphasized the possible interaction between the excitatory and inhibitory neurotransmitter at the receptor, rather than analyzing the interaction of postsynaptic potentials.

The soma or the proximal dendrites are the regions where anatomical and immuno-cytochemical studies have revealed the major concentration of symmetric (Gray's type II), GABA-ergic synapses (LeVay, 1973; Ribak, 1978; White and Rock, 1980; Freund et al., 1983; Peters, 1987). In brain slice preparations large conductance changes occur only transiently at the onset of an electrically evoked IPSP and last for 15–25 msec. The long phase of the IPSP is associated with a small conductance change (Ogawa et al., 1981). Intracellular recordings from visual cortical neurons in vivo revealed hyperpolarization during a long period of visually evoked inhibition (Douglas et al., 1988; Ferster, 1988; Ferster and Jagadeesh, 1992) but they did not show large conductance changes that would have been expected on the basis of the in vitro studies.

It is possible that the large conductance inhibitory synapses are located more distally on the dendritic tree and would thus be more difficult to detect. Indeed, a more distal location would enhance the shunting effect of the synapse since the input conductance of the trunk dendrite decreases relative to the active conductance of the inhibitory synapse. In these peripheral sites, the degree of conductance increase could be masked by the impedance properties of the intervening dendritic tree. While this is a suitable theoretical explanation for the absence of large changes in somatic input conductance, the current neuroanatomical data (LeVay, 1973; Ribak, 1978; White and Rock, 1980; Freund et al., 1983; Peters, 1987) do not support the existence of a large population of putative inhibitory synapses located distally on the dendrites of cortical neurons.

An extreme example would have the shunting inhibitory synapse located on the spine head, or distally on the neck. Under these circumstances, a large increase in conductance evoked in the spine head would provide very specific shunting of an excitatory synapse on the spine head, but the conductance change would be masked from the soma by the high axial resistance of the spine neck. However, the present neuroanatomical data suggest that relatively few excitatory synapses could be influenced in this way: only 7% of spines have both synaptic types (Beaulieu and Colonnier, 1985). Even if this figure is an underestimate by 100%, there remain a large number of spines without inhibitory input. Since the major excitatory input to pyramidal cells is thought to arrive on spines (LeVay, 1973; Peters, 1987; Colonnier, 1968; Szentágothai, 1973); most of this input could not be selectively inhibited.

NEUROTRANSMITTERS

AMINO ACID TRANSMITTERS

The establishment of the identity of cortical neurotransmitters has been one of the most tortuous activities of the last 40 years. Hayashi (1954) first proposed the amino acids L-glutamate and L-aspartate as candidates for the excitatory neurotransmitters in the cerebral cortex. This was supported by Krnjévic and Phillis (1963) and by the super-fusion studies of Jasper et al. (1965), who found that glutamate, aspartate, glycine and taurine were released during activation of the cortex. Clark and Collins (1976) showed that the release of glutamate, aspartate, and GABA were calcium-dependent. However, resistance to accepting glutamate as a neurotransmitter was strong because glutamate is distributed throughout the brain in high concentrations, a quite different picture from the restricted location and lower concentrations of acknowledged neurotransmitters, such as acetylcholine and catecholamines.

Other acidic amino acids also exert an excitatory effect of neurons. Some of these are more potent than the endogenous amino acids. The D-isomer of *N*-methyl aspartate is much more potent than L-glutamate (Curtis and Watkins 1963). The extraction of kainate and quisqualate from plants provided more agents that had stronger excitatory effects on neurons than L-glutamate (Shinozaki and Konishi, 1970). An antagonist, L-glutamic acid diethylester (GDEE), proved to be more effective against L-glutamate than other excitatory amino acids and indicated that there may be more than one type of excitatory amino acid receptor (Haldeman et al., 1972; Haldeman and McLennan, 1972). With the recent effort devoted to the characterization of receptor subunits, L-glutamate has emerged as the major excitatory amino acid transmitter of the cerebral cortex.

The acceptance of the amino acid GABA as the major inhibitory neurotransmitter has been as slow as that for glutamate. This occurs, despite the demonstration by Krnjévic and Schwartz (1967) that ionophoretically applied GABA profoundly inhibited cortical neurons and the evidence that GABA was released from active cortical synapses (Iversen et al., 1971). Application of n-m-bicuculline, the GABA$_A$ receptor antagonist, has a marked effect on the receptive field structure of visual cortical cells (Sillito, 1975; Tsumoto et al., 1979) and on the shape of the electrically evoked IPSP (Connors et al., 1988; Douglas et al., 1989). Antibodies directed against the synthetic enzyme for GABA, glutamate decarboxylase, or against the amino acid itself, indicate that about 20% of the neocortical neurons synthesize and contain GABA (Naegele and Barnstable, 1989).

Acetylcholine. Ionophoretic application of acetylcholine modifies the response to visual stimulation of most neurons in the cat visual cortex (Sillito and Kemp, 1983). The effect is usually facilitatory and seems to enhance the signal-to-noise ratio, rather than being generally excitatory. In deep layer pyramidal neurons, ACh induces a depolarization accompanied by an increase in resistance. The reversal potential is above that for potassium, suggesting that the action of ACh is to decrease the conductance for potassium (Krnjévic et al., 1971) by modulation of the slow outward potassium M current. The ACh response is mediated by a muscarinic receptor. The slow depolarization is preceded by a short latency hyperpolarization and a decrease in resistance that is probably due to the rapid muscarinic excitation of the inhibitory neurons (McCormick and Prince, 1985, 1986a). The inhibitory neurons are innervated by cholinergic afferents (Houser et al., 1985).

The onset of the depolarizing muscarinic excitation is slow and the response is sustained for many seconds. Some of the effects of ACh are mediated by second messengers (Stone and Taylor, 1977). Low concentrations of muscarine abolish the slow AHP (sAHP), but at higher concentrations the sAHP is replaced by a slow after depolarization (sADP) that is not mediated by potassium or sodium (Schwindt et al., 1988b; Schwindt, 1992). ACh-induced excitation can be enhanced selectively by somatostatin, although somatostatin itself inhibits spontaneous firing (Mancillas et al., 1986).

Biogenic Amines. Norepinephrine depresses the spontaneous extracellular activity of most cortical neurons (Reader et al., 1979; Armstrong-James and Fox, 1983). Some cortical cells in the deep layers are excited by low concentration of norepinephrine but inhibited by higher concentrations (Armstrong-James and Fox, 1983). Waterhouse et al. (1990) found that visual cortical cells in the rat showed enhanced responses to visual stimuli during ionophoresis of norepinephrine but depressed responses during serotonin ionophoresis.

Neuropeptides. The GABAergic neurons of the neocortex colocalize various peptides, including somatostatin (SSt), cholecystokinin, neuropeptide Y, vasoactive intestinal polypeptide (VIP), and substance P (Hendry et al., 1984; Schmechel et al., 1984; Somogyi et al., 1984; Demeulemeester et al., 1988). VIP and substance P are also associated with cholinergic axons (Vincent et al., 1983a; Eckenstein and Baughman, 1984).

The physiological role of neuropeptides remains obscure. Salt and Sillito (1984) showed that SSt could inhibit or excite cortical neurons. They were unable to demonstrate a modulatory effect on either GABAergic or cholinergic transmission. Mancillas et al. (1986) found that SSt inhibited rat cortical neurons. Cholecystokinin and VIP (Grieve et al., 1985a,b) produce mild excitation in some neurons. The difficulty in detecting effects, and the variety of effects produced, suggests that the role of these peptides is not primarily fast neurotransmission. Possibly, they are part of some cascade of effects acting over time courses of many hours or days, rather than the hour or so for conventional experiments that require receptive field mapping.

DENDRITES

The surface area of the dendrites is one to two orders of magnitude larger than that of the soma and the dendrites receive the vast majority of the synaptic inputs to the neuron. This arrangement suggests that the role of the dendrites is to integrate synaptic input, the result of which the neuron then expresses as the discharge activity of the soma. Unfortunately, in most cases the diameters of the dendrites of typical cortical neurons are too small to obtain stable recordings using available electrophysiological techniques and so most of our understanding of their electrical behaviour is derived indirectly, from recordings made from the somata and apical dendrites (Stuart and Sakmann, 1994). These methods are now being supplemented by sophisticated imaging techniques such as calcium imaging and two-photon microscopy (Denk et al., 1995).

The simplest electrical model of a dendrite is the passive electrotonic structure (Rall, 1977, 1989; Segev, 1995; Johnston and Wu, 1995). In this *cable model*, the dendrites are composed of cylindrical segments of membrane that are linked in a tree-like structure. The membranous wall of the cylinders has capacitance and linear conductance and the interior of the cylinders presents a linear axial conductance to the longitudinal passage of current. Such cylinders are electrically distributed (nonisopotential) structures and an input current injected at a point will establish voltage gradients along the dendrite. For simple cylindrical dendrites, the voltages at any point along their length is specified by the cable equation. The solution of this equation, and so the voltage profile, depends on the boundary conditions at the ends of the dendritic cylinder. These boundaries are usually approximated as either an infinite cable, a cut (short circuit) end, or sealed (open circuit) end. Rall (1959a,b) showed that the cable equation could also be solved for branching cylindrical dendrites, provided that there was a 3/2 power relationship between the parent and daughter branch diameters. When this relationship and a few other restrictions hold, then the entire dendrite can be reduced to a single equivalent cable of constant diameter.

In real neurons the synaptic voltages attenuate more rapidly toward the soma than toward the dendritic terminations. The electrical asymmetry of the dendritic tree arises because the terminations are sealed ends and little synaptic current is lost from them, whereas the somatic end has many other dendrites attached and so presents a large conductance load to the source synapse located on one of the dendrites. The voltage attenuation from dendrites to soma may be as much as a few hundred-fold. This implies that a number of EPSPs must occur within a membrane time-constant in order to displace the somatic potential across a 10–20 mV threshold. If the effect of a synapse depended only on its peak voltage, then the response of the neuron would be very sensitive to the displacement along the dendrite of the synapse. But, if the entire EPSP is considered, the situation is different. The passive dendrite behaves as a low-pass filter, and so the temporal form of the synaptic potentials becomes significantly broader as they spread from distal synaptic sites towards the soma. Although the peak synaptic voltages are attenuated, the attenuation of the time integral of the EPSP at the soma is smaller and not much affected by synaptic location. This is also true of the integral of the synaptic current at the soma (synaptic charge delivery). Since the synapses exert their effect collectively, by sustained depolarization of the somatic membrane, it is the charge delivery to the soma that best expresses synaptic efficacy (Bernander et al., 1994).

The broadening of the EPSP as it spreads centripetally has the effect of delaying the signal, and makes the response at the soma sensitive to the temporal order of synaptic events applied in the dendrites. This means that the dendrite can usefully compute functions such as direction of motion (Rall, 1964; Koch et al., 1982). Passive dendrites can also act on different time scales. For example, extensively branched distal dendrites provide a large area for charge equilibration, and so the time constant for synaptic integration is much shorter (about $0.1 \, \tau_m$) there than closer to the soma. The briefer synaptic events in the distal arbors interact as coincidence detectors, whereas the longer events closer to the soma integrate (Agmon-Snir and Segev, 1992).

The morphology of the dendritic tree is important, at least in so far as it affects the passive spread of currents from the synapses to the initial segment (Mainen and Sejnowski, 1996). Most cortical neurons are electrotonically compact, whether measured electrophysiologically (Stafstrom et al., 1985) or anatomically (Douglas and Martin, 1993). However, the apical dendrite of the pyramidal cells is a special case. The electrotonic length of the apical dendrite is about 2–3 times greater than that of the basal dendrites, and the synaptic inputs injected into the apical tuft at the distal end of the apical dendrite are greatly attenuated en route to the soma (Bernander et al., 1994). This apparent ineffectiveness of the distal apical input is counterintuitive. Important interareal projections make their synapses there, and there has been no phylogenetic trend to dispense with apical dendrites (with the possible exception of layer 4 spiny neurons). One possibility is that the apical dendrite makes use of active currents to enhance selectively signal transmission to the soma (Bernander et al., 1994). Where the dendrites are long and narrow, and so electrotonically short, the dendrite can decompose into electrotonically separate subunits, each of which can compute a relatively independent function (Koch et al., 1982). It is unlikely that such conditions exist in cortical neurons, except possibly in the apical tufts.

ACTIVE PROPERTIES

The cable model has been extremely useful in obtaining qualitative insights into the behavior of quiescent dendrites. However, it has two significant failings that limit its application to cortical neurons. First, the approximation to a cable across the branches in a dendrite requires that a particular relationship of diameters hold between the parent and daughter segments of the branch. This relationship is only rarely true across the dendritic branches of cortical neurons. Second, it is clear that the majority of cortical neurons have many active conductances in their dendrites (Stuart and Sakmann, 1994), and so the linear cable approximation is only useful under very restricted conditions. Active dendritic conductances include voltage-dependent sodium, potassium, and calcium currents (Markram and Sakmann, 1994; Stuart and Sakmann, 1994; Magee and Johnston, 1995b). When the nonlinearities due to the active conductances are included, the dendritic models have mathematic descriptions that cannot be solved analytically. The models must then be investigated by numerical simulations of compartmental approximations to the dendrites. In these compartmental models, the dendritic segments are considered to be electrotonically short (isopotential) compartments linked by axial resistors according to the topology of the dendrite. When the dendritic quantization is sufficiently small, the compartmental description with only passive components converges to the continuous description of the cable equation. However, the important interest in the compartmental approach is not the passive cable behavior, but the effects of active conductances.

The active conductances are able to generate a variety of subthreshold nonlinearities and may cross the thresholds for calcium or sodium action potentials. The exact roles of the active dendritic conductances are unknown, but they could support a number of interesting functions. Sodium spikes are able to propagate retrogradely into the dendritic tree (Stuart et al., 1997). The action potential propagates more reliably centrifugally than it does centripetally, because in the latter case the branching dendritic tree presents a large impedance load to the small action potential currents generated in the narrow peripheral dendrites. The retrograde spikes could provide a signal to hebbian synapses that the postsynaptic cell is active. For example, Yuste and Denk (1995) have used two-photon microscopy of hippocampal pyramidal cells to show that the centrifugal action potential invades the dendritic spines and leads to a local rise in their calcium ion concentration.

The introduction of active conductances in the apical dendrite could provide amplification and linearization of synaptic inputs to the apical tuft (Bernander et al., 1994), or decompose the dendritic tree into a number of distant multiplicative subunits (Mel, 1993). The active conductances could also amplify selective combinations of input by nonlinear multiplicative interactions (Mel, 1993). Since these effects are usually associated with increases in conductance, increasing stimulation will cause the multiplicative and subregion effects to become more localized in space and time (Mel, 1993).

Dendrites with slow active currents that are partly decoupled from the fast spike generating currents at the soma can produce a wide repertoire of temporal patterns of output spikes, including bursting (Pinsky and Rinzel, 1994; Mainen and Sejnowski, 1996). Activation of dendritic potassium conductances could also offset large dendritic input currents, thus providing an adaptive mechanism to keep the dendrite in a favorable operating range (Bernander et al., 1991, 1994).

SPINES

One of the most prominent features of cortical neurons is their dendritic spines (Cajal, 1911). They are the major recipients of excitatory input, and play an important role in activity-dependent modification of synaptic efficacy such as LTD and LTP (for a review see Shepherd, 1996). Although these structures have been extensively examined by light and electron microscopy, physiological data has been more difficult to obtain because of their tiny dimensions, and so their functional role is still not entirely understood. Fortunately, recent advances in imaging techniques are making it possible to measure calcium dynamics in individual spines with high time resolution (Denk et al., 1996).

The simplest views of spine function were mechanical. They were thought to be convenient physical connections whereby *en passant* axonal boutons could more easily connect to dendrites (Peters and Kaiserman-Abramof, 1970; Swindale, 1981). More elaborate views have considered the electrical and chemical properties of the spinous connection (see Chap. 1).

ELECTRICAL MODELS

The membrane area of the spine neck is very small and consequently, little synaptic current flows through the neck membrane. Therefore most of the synaptic current injected into the spine head reaches the trunk dendrite via the spine neck. Nevertheless, the resistance to current flow through the neck is high, on the order of $100 \, M\Omega$ or more (Segev and Rall, 1988). This is roughly the input resistance of a typical spiny dendrite about half a length-constant from the soma. So the spine neck will attenuate by about half the voltage applied at the spine head. Thus the neck resistance could be used to control the efficacy of the synapse (Rall, 1962) and so provide a basis for synaptic plasticity (Fifkova and Anderson, 1981). The resistance could be changed by modifying the neck diameter or length (Rall, 1974a,b), or by partial occlusion of the neck by the spine apparatus (Rall and Segev, 1987). However, attempts to correlate changes in spine dimensions in relation to, for example, LTP induction have been unconvincing (Fifkova and van Harreveld, 1977; Andersen et al., 1987; Desmond and Levy, 1990).

The *twitching spine* hypothesis of Crick (1982) proposed that a change in spine length could be achieved quickly, by calcium activation of myosin and actin localized in the spine neck (Fifkova and Delay, 1982; Markham and Fifkova, 1986). In theory, a burst discharge of the excitatory afferent could raise the free calcium concentration in a spine to the level required to activate the actin (Gamble and Koch, 1987). The twitching spine hypothesis is one of the interesting suggestions that could soon be tested by the new imaging techniques.

Saturating Spines. The flow of synaptic current through the spine input resistance will shift the spine head potential toward the EPSP reversal potential and reduce the driving potential for the synaptic current. For small synaptic conductances the synaptic current saturates. This interdependence gives rise to a sigmoidal relationship between synaptic conductance and synaptic current (Fig. 12.9). We do not know exactly where on this relationship the operating range of the neocortical synapse lies.

That spines generally receive only one excitatory synapse can be interpreted in two opposing ways, in this context. It may reflect the need to avoid saturating the synapse, or it may indicate that a single synapse on a spine always saturates the synapse, so that additional inputs would be redundant. If the synapse is driven into saturation, then the spine potential will be relatively insensitive to the exact amount of neurotransmitter delivered to the synapse. The spine head will simply turn on to a repeatable voltage level. Moreover, because the spine neck resistance is at least as large as that of the parent dendritic trunk, the spine approximates a constant current source attached to the dendrite. The synapse on the spine head is less susceptible to changes in the dendritic input resistance than is a synapse located on the dendritic trunk.

Spine Action Potentials. A special case of saturation behavior arises if the spine head membrane contains active conductances that could amplify the synaptic signal (Jack et al., 1975; Perkel and Perkel, 1985; Miller et al., 1985; Rall and Segev, 1987; Segev and Rall, 1988). Shepherd et al. (1985) and others (Rall and Segev, 1987; Baer and

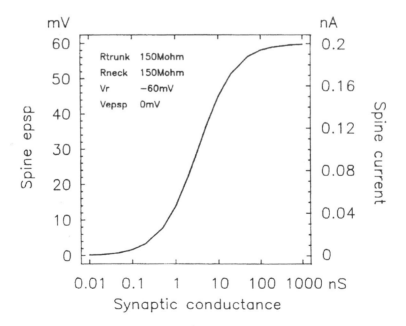

Fig. 12.9. Simulation of steady-state activation of synapse on the spine head. Effect of synaptic conductance on the amplitude of EPSP in the spine head, and the magnitude of the current delivered through the spine neck resistance (R_{neck}) to the trunk dendrite resistance (R_{trunk}) for a simulated spine and dendrite. V_r, resting potential; V_{EPSP}, reversal potential of EPSP.

Rinzel, 1991) have suggested that this amplification could lead to spinous action potentials. The saltatory transmission of these action potentials from spine to spine, conditional on their synaptic input, could form the basis of Boolean algebraic-like processing along the dendrite. Although these notions are attractive, the experimental evidence consistent with spiking spines has been obtained only in cerebellar Purkinje neurons (Denk et al., 1995).

Nonsaturating Spines. If the synapse on the spine is not driven into saturation, but operates instead within the linear range of Fig. 12.9, then the synapse will be particularly susceptible to nonlinear interactions with other spines. Because the resistance of the spine head membrane is much greater than the axial resistance of the neck, the dendritic potential is transferred to the spine head with little attenuation. Consequently, a depolarization of the dendritic trunk will reduce the driving potential of the spine synapse and mediate nonlinear interactions between neighboring spines. These interactions are only possible if the spines operate in their linear range. If the spines operate in saturation, then their synapse will be insensitive to modulations of local driving potential.

Inhibition on Spines. A small proportion (about 10%) of neocortical spines receive input from a type 2 (GABA-ergic) synapse in addition to the type 1 (excitatory) synapse (Jones and Powell, 1969c; Peters and Kaiserman-Abramof, 1970; Sloper and Powell, 1979b; Somogyi et al., 1983; Beaulieu and Colonnier, 1985; Dehay et al., 1991). This arrangement raises the possibility that some excitatory inputs receive selective inhibition. Nonlinear inhibition of excitatory inputs on the same spine can be large and is essentially limited to the affected spine (Koch and Poggio, 1983). The large series resistance of the spine neck masks changes that occur in the head from the trunk dendrite and so may effectively restrict the inhibitory control to the affected spine. This specific effect has attracted much theoretical interest (Koch and Poggio, 1983; Segev and Rall, 1988) because of its computational possibilities, but only a small percentage of the excitatory input onto a single neuron could be gated in this way. It is possible that the spines that are controlled by an inhibitory synapse all receive input from a strategically important class of afferents, such as the thalamocortical inputs for example. However, Dehay et al. (1991) have shown that this selective inhibition does not occur.

Less selective locations of inhibitory synapses may also permit strong nonlinear effects. For example, inhibitory synapses on the trunk dendrite would reduce interspine communication and could control saltatory conduction between spines (Shepherd and Brayton, 1987). This raises the possibility of enabling or disabling selected branches of dendrites. However, logical computations in spines do not necessitate inhibitory inputs. Triggering an action potential could also be conditioned by activation of the spine-head synapse (e.g., the NMDA receptor is voltage-dependent only if gated by neurotransmitter). If saltatory conduction were conditional on excitatory input, then this arrangement would provide an elegant means of signal gating that depends on the coincidence of excitatory inputs, rather than the interaction of excitatory and inhibitory inputs.

BIOCHEMICAL COMPARTMENTS

The strong role of calcium in synaptic plasticity and the need to localize plasticity to the activated synapse have led to the suggestion that the spines provide the necessary isolated biochemical compartment (Gamble and Koch, 1987; Zador et al., 1990). The notion is that the spine neck limits the diffusion of calcium between the head and the dendrite. It is proposed that restriction in calcium movement through the neck arises from the calcium sink created by the calcium pumps in the neck membrane. Their activity has the effect of shortening the calcium space constant in the neck, leading to significant calcium attenuation across the neck.

Calcium could enter the head through NMDA channels, voltage-dependent calcium channels, and second-messenger channels. Studies in hippocampal neurons have provided evidence that calcium levels in the spine head are to some extent uncoupled from those in the parent dendrite (Guthrie et al., 1991; Muller and Connor, 1991; Yuste and Denk, 1995). Similar experiments in neocortical neurons are awaited.

FUNCTIONAL OPERATIONS

SINGLE NEURONS OR NEURAL NETWORKS

The history of ideas of cortical function makes a fascinating account of the interplay of hypothesis and experiment (Martin, 1988). In particular, the experimental results from microelectrode recordings from single cortical units (neurons) have had a deep influence on our ideas of cortical function. Much of fhe motivation for studying the functional properties of single units in the cortex in such detail arises from the fact that the activities of cortical neurons are thought to describe the world and so to reflect our subjective experiences. However, the nature of the encoding used by the neurons to represent the world is still a matter of intense and interesting debate.

The encoding problem is important because it determines to a large extent the success with which the nervous system can interact with the world. It is clear that the attributes of the world must be encoded in the variables of the nervous system. If the neural encoding is suitable, then the nervous system will be able to represent the world well, and the efficiency interactions with the physical world will be enhanced. For example, in artificial neural networks, learning and generalization improve with the quality of data representation.

One central question is whether the nervous system uses a data representation in which the encoding of objects is distributed across many neurons, or whether the representation is localized. This debate is usually couched in the domain of perception. There the question is whether the discharge of a combination of neurons, or the discharge of just one neuron, reflects the experience of a percept. These opposing views of the operation of cortex have a long and distinguished history. Sherrington (1941), for example, contrasted the notion of "one ultimate pontifical nerve-cell . . . [as] the climax of the whole system of integration [with the concept of mind as] a million-fold democracy, whose each unit is a cell."

The case for localized encoding has been formalized in the *neuron doctrine* proposed by Barlow (1972). He proposed five dogmas that encapsulate the powerful idea that percepts are the product of the activity of certain individual cortical neurons, rather than by some more complex (and obscure) properties of the combinatorial rules of the usage of nerve cells. The force of Barlow's thesis in molding our ideas is evident in most textbooks of psychology and neurobiology, which are well stocked with illustrations showing how the specificity of neurons arises from a hierarchical sequence of processing through the cortical circuits.

Recently, the pendulum has begun to swing back. The antithetical proposition that perceptual processing occurs through the collective properties of parallel cortical networks rather than through the activity of single units has been receiving close attention from theoreticians working on *neural networks* or *connectionist* models of cortical function. Results obtained from computer simulations of these hypothetical nerve circuits have led to a model of cortical function that is quite different from that proposed in the neuron doctrine.

The dialectic of the one versus many neurons is best considered in the context of the visual system, where the physiology and anatomy are known in greatest detail, and where the behavioral performance is well established.

SINGLE NEURONS OR NEURAL NETWORKS?

It is evident that visual perception is a complex task. We need only to only not determine the form, movement, and position in space of the objects we encounter, but also to recognize them as being particular objects. Solving this key problem was central to Barlow's development of the neuron doctrine. He proposed that the primary visual cortex dealt only with the elemental building blocks of perception, the detection of orientated line segments, or the local motion of these segments, for example. In order to build these responses into neurons that were selective for, e.g., a cat, chair, or grandmother, he proposed a hierarchical sequence of processing within single cortical areas and through the many visual areas. Thus, the *grandmother cell* scheme is essentially a classification network in which the input is classified according to which output neuron is activated. In nervous systems, the classification occurs in a hierarchical network. The neurons at each stage of the hierarchy become progressively more selective to the attributes of the stimulus, so that while the neurons in the primary visual cortex would respond to many objects, neurons at the highest level of the hierarchy would respond only to particular objects. Barlow (1972) suggested that the activity of about 1000 of these high-level *cardinal* neurons would be sufficient to represent a single visual scene. Because the number of possible percepts is very large, however, the total number of cardinal cells would have to be a substantial fraction of the 10^{10} cells of the human neocortex (Barlow, 1972).

The single neuron representation faces two major difficulties: poor generalization, and limited encoding capacity. If individual objects are very specifically encoded by single neurons, then it is difficult for the neurons to generalize their classification to novel intermediate cases. For example, given only a "red apple" neuron and a "green apple" neuron, how does the nervous system respond to a yellow apple? Either it must quickly recruit a new neuron with very similar connections and assign it to yellow apples, or else the yellow apple percept must arise from some combination of the activity of the red and green neurons, in which case the single-cell encoding hypothesis is weakened. Moreover, if new neurons must be recruited for each new feature (such as yellow) that is added to the classification scheme, then the number of neurons required to encode selectively the various combinations of features increases explosively and soon exceeds the number of neurons available.

Despite these difficulties, selective encoding representation has remained a popular implicit hypothesis in experimental neuroscience. Since 1972 many of the visual areas beyond area 17 have been explored in some detail. Efforts to discover whether cardinal cells reside in these visual areas have met with mixed success. In most areas, the stimulus requirements for activating neurons are not very different in quality from those for area 17. If anything, the requirements are less restrictive, in that only a single property of the stimulus might be important, such as its direction of motion, or color, or depth in visual space. Only in the primate inferotemporal region of cortex have neurons with higher-order properties been found (Gross et al., 1972). These neurons respond preferentially to parts of the body, especially faces, although they respond to other visual stimuli as well (Gross et al., 1972; Bruce et al., 1981; Richmond et al., 1983; Young and Yamane, 1992). Other cells in the inferotemporal region have large receptive fields that respond quite specifically to complex shapes, but close neighbors tend to respond to similar features (Tanaka et al., 1991; Fujita et al., 1992; Miyashita, 1988; Miyashita and Chang 1988). Neurons in these areas appear to "learn" specific complex stimuli.

Direct examination of neuronal responses involved in the perceptual foundation of a decision process (Salzman and Newsome, 1994; Shadlen and Newsome, 1996) have also brought some support for the cardinal cell view. It appears that in the motion discrimination task, the reliability of the animal's decision is not much better than that of a single observed neuron, which argues against the view that the animal bases its decision on an average across many neurons.

Nevertheless, the general conclusion from the many studies that have examined encoding is that individual neurons do not respond completely selectively to single *trigger features*. Instead, each neuron is sensitive to a number of different stimulus characteristics, such as contrast, dimension, depth, and orientation. Single cortical neurons appear unable to signal unambiguously the presence of a particular stimulus, and therefore cannot act as cardinal cells. An important reason why such cardinal cells are not found may lie in the basic organization of the cortical circuitry, which expresses much stronger lateral and recurrent interactions between neurons than is expected of a feed-forward classification network.

NEW DESIGNS FOR THE VISUAL CIRCUITS

When Barlow proposed his neuron doctrine in 1972, the modern study of cortical microcircuitry was in its infancy. Anatomical studies had emphasized the vertical, columnar structure of cortex. This view was reinforced by many electrophysiological studies, which showed vertical functional columns. Technical advances since the late 1970s have resulted in a wealth of new information about the cortical microcircuitry. The technique of intracellular labeling of neurons (e.g., Figs 12.3 and 12.4) has revealed an extensive system of horizontal connections within the cortex. Certain markers, such as horseradish peroxidase or biocytin, fill the entire axonal arborization, including the boutons, and so estimates of the number and spatial distribution of the synapses made by a single neuron are now available for the first time. The horizontal spread of connections means that each point in cortex is covered by axons of a very large number of neurons. For example, estimates for the number of geniculate X cells (see Chap. 8) that provide input to any point in cat area 17 range from 400 to 800 (Freund et al., 1985), whereas the figure for Y cells may be even higher. The geniculate axons form less than 10% of the excitatory synapses on spiny stellate neurons in layer 4 (Ahmed et al., 1994; see Synaptic Connections, above), so the number of cortical neurons providing the input to a single point must be considerably higher. Because one cortical neuron supplies only a few synapses to any other cortical neuron, each neuron can potentially be activated by hundreds of other neurons. It is this highly divergent and convergent connectivity that is the feature of neocortex, and that differs considerably from that of the lateral geniculate nucleus (Chap. 8), where there is a much tighter coupling between neurons.

The widespread and rich connections of the thalamic afferents ensure that even the smallest detectable disturbance of the retinal receptor layer—for example, that induced by a dim flash of light—alters the probability of firing of thousands of cortical neurons in the primary visual cortex. The signal is then amplified by the divergent axonal arbors of the cortical neurons, which ensure that many thousands more neurons are activated both within area 17 and in the other cortical areas to which these neurons project. Thus, although there certainly is the convergence of many inputs that is required to create the cardinal cells, the considerable divergence of the connections of each neuron ensures the simultaneous activation of many neurons. In such a context it is difficult to see that the activity of any single neuron can be completely isolated from that of its companions in order to signal a unique percept. Instead, the combined activity of large numbers of cortical neurons seems more likely to be the basis of our perceptual experience. However, distributed representations have problems of their own, such as the ambiguity of interpretation when a particular neuron is permitted to respond in more than a single context. For example, many neurons may implement the distributed encoding of apples, and some common fraction of these will be activated by particular red, yellow, and green apples. If this common fraction is activated in a number of different contexts, what is the unique neural object that defines a particular apple? Von der Malsburg (1981) has proposed that the population of neurons activated by the stimuli of a particular physical object is bound together transiently by a common physiological process. One possibility is that the 40 Hz oscillation of discharge observed in cortical neurons reflects such a binding process (Gray and Singer, 1989; Crick and Koch, 1992; Singer, 1994).

PARALLEL PROCESSING IN NEURAL NETWORKS

It is evident from the above discussion that normal vision involves the activity of very large numbers of cortical neurons. These large numbers do not simply reflect redundancy, which an efficient coding must avoid, but are a necessary part of perception. This is evident in the example of color vision, where both behavioral and theoretical studies show that the relative stability of the perceived color of objects in the face of changing illumination (e.g., moving from indoors to outdoors) requires the comparison of the reflected wavelengths over a large region of the visual field (Jameson and Hurvich, 1959; Land, 1959a,b, 1983). This phenomenon of color constancy necessarily involves the coordinated activity of large numbers of cortical neurons. Similar considerations apply in the case of binocular vision, where two slightly different views of the same complex scene must be fused to produce a single vision and stereopsis. Attempts to replicate this performance have shown that it is a difficult task (Marr and Poggio, 1979; Mahowald, 1994). Yet we fuse the image and extract the exact three-dimensional information effortlessly and far more rapidly than any computer yet can. One reason for this difference is that the strict hierarchy of serial processing used by computers with von Neumann architecture is slow. In the cerebral cortex, by contrast, the higher degree of divergence in the connections makes it likely that much of the processing occurs simultaneously through parallel pathways. Of course, computers have transistors that can generate digital impulses at very high rates and transmit them at light speeds to perform their computations. By comparison, neurons generate impulses at very low rates and transmit them at meters/second. However, the neocortex makes many connections to and from each neuron, whereas the limitations of size and thickness mean that silicon components have limited connectivity. Thus advantages of speed are offset against limited connectivity.

The increase in speed offered by parallel processing has been exploited in a number of models of visual processing based on feedforward artificial neural networks. The most common form of feedforward network is composed of three layers of highly abstract neurons whose activity typically varies between 0 and 1. A first layer, or *input layer*, connects extensively to units of a second, *hidden layer*, which in turn sends its output to the third, *output layer*. The sensory input is applied via the input layer. The responses of units in the hidden and output layers are determined by summing activities of all the units in the previous layer. The effect of each of the inputs is governed by a synaptic *weight*, which may be positive (excitatory) or negative (inhibitory). The values of these weights determine what functions of the input the network can compute, and so what overall task the network performs. These weights may be specified directly, but more often they are organized by a learning algorithm, for example, *back-propagation* (Rumelhart and McClelland, 1986; Hertz et al., 1991; Anderson, 1995). Such networks turn out to be powerful and are capable of solving some of the perceptual problems of depth, form, and motion perception (Lehky and Sejnowski, 1988; Zipser and Andersen, 1988).

ARE NEURAL NETWORKS LIKE CORTICAL CIRCUITS?

The neural network models, besides being functionally successful, have a strong appeal because of their superficial resemblance to the structure of the cortex: they are layered and have highly interconnected units. However, this superficial resemblance should be examined more critically in the light of our knowledge of the structure of area 17. The basic circuit of Fig. 12.10 illustrates some of the main neuronal components and their connections within area 17. Comparing this figure with the feedforward neural network of Fig. 12.11 shows a number of similarities. The first layer in the neural network corresponds to the map of the geniculate terminals, the second layer units, to the neurons in layer 4 that project to the superficial layers, and the third, to the pyramidal neurons projecting from cortical layers 2 and 3. In respect of this laminar organization, the pattern of the model corresponds to that of cortex in that very few neurons of layer 4 provide an output to other cortical areas, whereas a large proportion (70%) of the pyramidal neurons in layers 2 and 3 do project to other areas. However, it is evident at a glance that the organization of cortex shown

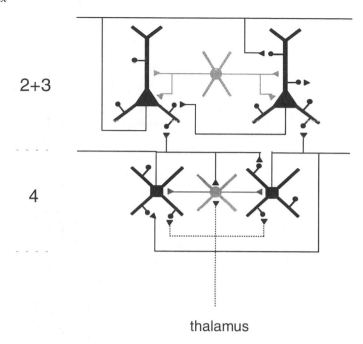

2+3

4

thalamus

Fig. 12.10. Possible recurrent connections in neocortex. This figure is an elaboration of Figs. 12.8 and 12.6. The feedforward thalamic inputs synapse with spiny stellate neurons and a small basket cell in layer 4. Some of the spiny stellate connections are recurrent to other spiny stellates. They also synapse onto superficial pyramidal cells that in turn have recurrent connections with one another.

in Fig. 12.10 is in many important respects different from the neural network circuit of Fig. 12.11.

Unlike the neural network, the primate visual cortex receives at least two physiologically and anatomically distinct inputs from the thalamus, which are laminar specific. The cortex has twice as many or more layers, particularly if the subdivisions of the six basic layers are taken into account. This may be a requirement of the cortex to divide its output destinations ("addresses") into laminar-specific zones. However, the internal connectivity and physiology differ in different layers, indicating that there may be important differences in the processing within layers. In contrast to the units within a single layer of the neural network, there are extensive lateral connections within a single lamina or sublamina of cortex. Thus, the local connectivity of cortical neurons resembles that of the recurrent neural networks (Hopfield, 1982, 1984). However, unlike typical recurrent artificial neural networks, the cortical ones are not fully connected. Instead, they are quite sparsely connected. Similarly, the interconnections between cortical laminae are highly specific and do not simply connect adjacent layers as in the units of the neural network. Both the vertical and the lateral connections in the cortex are clustered, focusing on discrete zones. This columnar structure is a feature of cortical organization, but it is the exception rather than the rule to incorporate such horizontal organization within network models.

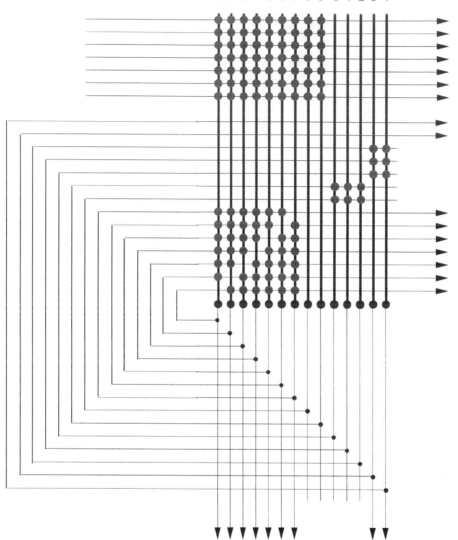

Fig. 12.11. A hypothetical cortical neuronal network composed of two subnetworks; one feedforward, and the other feedback. Neurons of the network (black) receive input synapses (gray circles) onto their dendrites (thick black vertical lines). The effects of these neurons are integrated into the neuronal somata (black circles) and their outputs are transmitted along their axons (thin black lines). Branch points of the axons are indicated as small black dots on the axons. The neurons are numbered from 1 to 14. Feedforward inputs enter via the 7 horizontal axons above. **Feedforward network:** The feedforward inputs synapse with the first layer of cortical neurons (8 and 9), which project to the second layer (10, 11, and 12), and from there to the final layer (13 and 14), whose outputs project out of this region of cortex. The intermediate computations of this entirely feedforward network are unaffected by connections between cells in the same layer, or by backward projections from later layers. **Feedback network:** The feedforward inputs synapse with the distal dendrites of the recurrently connected population of neurons (1 through 7). Their axons synapse with all other members of their population (but not with

It is somewhat surprising, given the activity in this area, that the rules of connectivity for neocortex have still to be discovered. At this stage, we know that the different types of neurons connect with some degree of specificity to particular regions of other neurons, e.g., dendritic shafts or spines, but whether single neuron to single neuron connections are specified is still quite unclear. At this stage it seems likely that neurons do not connect on a point-to-point basis, but on a point-to-zone basis, targeting particular subsets of neurons within a zone.

The point is readily made that these and other differences show that the artificial neural networks are different in important respects from the cerebral cortex. Finally, artificial *neural* networks are not really very neural. They are just networks operating according to a specific algorithm, and it would be rash to press their analogy to cortical circuits too far. Nevertheless, the potential usefulness of network models that are biologically based cannot be overestimated. The major problem lies in trying to bridge the gap between experimental data and theory. Our knowledge of the structure of the cortical microcircuitry outstrips our understanding of the function of these circuits. This disparity, together with the sheer complexity of the cortical circuits, is a significant barrier to moving from networks that are simply *neurally inspired* to those that actually incorporate basic features of the biology. To achieve this step, the cortical connections shown in Fig. 12.8, and their associated physiology, have to be simplified. Given the outline of the preceding sections, one such simplification can now be suggested (Fig. 12.12). The form of this "canonical" circuit was arrived at from an analysis of the structure and function of local circuits in the visual cortex (Douglas et al., 1989, 1995; Douglas and Martin, 1991). However, an analysis of the circuits of other cortical structures such as the olfactory cortex (paleocortex) and hippocampus (archicortex) reveals that they, too, bear many resemblances to the circuits of the neocortex (Shepherd, 1988a,b; see Chap. 1). Thus, it is tempting to suppose that there may be some common basic principles that underly the organization and operation of all cortical circuits.

A CANONICAL CORTICAL CIRCUIT

From the anatomy, several components and connections seem to dominate in most cortical areas (Fig. 12.12). Any realistic model must separate inhibitory (GABAergic) and excitatory neurons into distinct populations. The excitatory group (80% of the cortical neurons) can be subdivided into two major pools, one being found in the granular and supragranular layers (layers 2–4), and the other in the deep layers (layers 5 and 6). Although these groups are extensively interconnected, this division is made because their outputs are distinct, and because inhibition appears to be stronger in the deep layers (Douglas et al., 1989). The different types of GABAergic smooth neurons cannot yet be distinguished on functional grounds; they are therefore represented in the diagram of Fig. 12.12 by a single population.

---

themselves). In this case, the evolving response of each neuron comes to influence the computations of its fellows. The overall computation is iterative in quality, and converges on a solution which is, in some sense, a consensus amongst the cooperating neurons. The state of the population is transmitted out of this region of cortex.

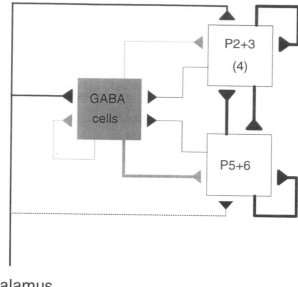

thalamus

Fig. 12.12. The canonical microcircuit for striate cortex. Three populations of neurons interact
with one another: One population is inhibitory (GABAergic cells, gray synapses), and two are
excitatory (solid synapses) representing superficial (P2 + 3) and deep (P5 + 6) pyramidal neurons. The properties of layer 4 stellates (4), which contribute 10% of neurons in granular cortex, less elsewhere, are similar to those of the superficial pyramids. The thickness of the connecting lines indicates the functional strength of the input. Note that the dominant connection is
between excitatory neurons, so that a relatively weak thalamic input can be greatly amplified by
the recurrent excitation of the spiny neurons.

   Neurons within each division form connections with other members of that division.
The dominant interlaminar connections are between the superficial and deep layer
groups of spiny neurons, whereas the inhibitory neurons connect across the laminae to
both groups of spiny neurons. All three groups receive direct activation from the thalamic afferents, but because the thalamic input provides only about 10% of the excitatory input, 90% of the excitation is provided here by intracortical connections between
pyramidal neurons. This recurrent excitation may provide selective amplification of
geniculate input (Douglas et al., 1989, 1995). Such intracortical amplification provides
the basis for a number of recent models of cortical computation (Mahowald, 1994;
Ben-Yishai et al., 1995; Douglas et al., 1995; Somers et al., 1995; Suarez et al., 1995).
Inhibition acts by modulating the recurrent excitation, and so is effective even though
it may be relatively weak (Douglas et al., 1995).
   The excitatory neurotransmitters act on two major receptor types, the NMDA and
non-NMDA receptors. The inhibitory neurotransmitter GABA acts via the GABA$_A$ and
the GABA$_B$ receptors. These distinctions are made because the receptor types have
distinctly different kinetics. The biophysical characteristics of the cortical neurons, as
outlined in the previous sections, also need to be incorporated to give the appropriate
response characteristics.

This recurrent excitation model provides the minimum specifications that seem necessary for basic cortical circuits, based on our present level of knowledge. The form of this simplified model is sufficiently general that it can be applied equally well to visual cortex as to motor cortex, and as such, has the properties of a canonical circuit. This circuit forms only a basic building block. Obviously, each cortical area has individual features that need to be incorporated. However, simplicity encourages the convergence of theory and biology through common models, and such convergence is imperative if we are to understand how the synaptic organization of the neocortex produces the complexity of cortical function.

REFERENCES

Abbott, L.F., Varela, J.A., Sen, K., and Nelson, S.B. 1997. Synaptic depression and cortical gain control. Science 275: 220–224.

Ache, B.W. 1994. Towards a common strategy for transducing olfactory information. Semin. Cell Biol. 5: 55–64.

Adams, J.C. 1976. Single unit studies on the dorsal and intermediate acoustic striae. J. Comp. Neurol. 170: 97–106.

Adams, J.C. 1983. Multipolar cells in the ventral cochlear nucleus project to the dorsal cochlear nucleus and the inferior colliculus. Neurosci. Lett. 37: 205–208.

Adams, J.C. and Mugnaini, E. 1987. Patterns of glutamate decarboxylase immunostaining in the feline cochlear nuclear complex studied with silver enhancement and electron microscopy. J. Comp. Neurol. 262: 375–401.

Adams, P. 1982. Voltage-dependent conductances of vertebrate neurones. Trends Neurosci. 2: 116–119.

Adams, P.R. and Galvan, M. 1986. Voltage-dependent currents of vertebrate neurons and their role in membrane excitability. Adv. Neurol. 44: 137–170.

Adrian, E.D. 1942. Olfactory reactions in the brain of the hedgehog. J. Physiol. (Lond.) 100: 459–473.

Adrian, E.D. 1950. The electrical activity of the mammalian olfactory bulb. Electroencephalogr. Clin. Neurophysiol. 2: 377–388.

Adrian, E.D. 1953. Sensory messages and sensation. The response of the olfactory organ to different smells. Acta Physiol. Scand. 29: 5–14.

Aghajnian, G.K. 1985. Modulation of a transient outward current in serotonergic neurones by alpha1-adrenoceptors. Nature 315: 501–503.

Agmon-Snir, H. and Segev, I. 1992. Signal delay and propagation velocity in passive dendritic structures. J. Neurophysiol. 70: 2066–2085.

Ahlsén, G., Lindström, S., and Lo, F.-S. 1984. Inhibition from the brainstem of inhibitory interneurones of the cat's dorsal lateral geniculate nucleus. J. Physiol. (Lond.) 347: 539–609.

Ahmed, B., Anderson, J., Douglas, R., Martin, K., and Nelson, C. 1994. Polyneuronal innervation of spiny stellate neurons in cat visual cortex. J. Comp. Neurol. 341: 39–49.

Ahnelt, P., Keri, C., and Kolb. H. 1990. Identification of pedicles of putative blue-sensitive cones in the human retina. J. Comp. Neurol. 293: 39–53.

Albuquerque, E.X., Peieira, E.F., Castro, N.G., and Alkondon, M. 1995. Nicotinic receptor function in the mammalian central nervous system. Ann. N.Y. Acad. Sci. 757: 48–72.

Albus, J.S. 1971. A theory of cerebellar function. Math. Biosci. 10: 25–61.

Alger, B.E., Dhanjal, S.S., Dingledine, R., Garthwaite, J., Henderson, G., King, G.L., Lipton, P., North, A., Schwartzkroin, P.A., Sears, T.A., Segal, M., Whittingham, T.S., and Williams, J. 1984. Brain slice methods. In: Brain Slices. (Dingledine, R., eds.) New York: Plenum Press, pp. 381–437.

Alger, B.E. and Nicoll, R. 1982. Feed-forward dendritic inhibition in rat hippocampal pyramidal cells studied in vitro. J. Physiol. (Lond.) 328: 105–123.

Allen, C. and Stevens, C.F. 1994. An evaluation of causes for unreliability of synaptic transmission. Proc. Natl. Acad. Sci. U.S.A. 91: 10380–10383.

Allison, A.C. 1953. The morphology of the olfactory system in the vertebrates. Biol. Rev. 28: 195–244.

Altschuler, R.A., Betz, H., Parakkal, M.H., Reeks, K.A., and Wenthold, R.J. 1986. Identification of glycinergic synapses in the cochlear nucleus through immunocytochemical localization of the postsynaptic receptor. Brain Res. 369: 316–320.

Amaral, D.G. 1978. A Golgi study of the cell types in the hilar region of the hippocampus in the rat. J. Comp. Neurol. 182: 851–914.

Amaral, D.G. 1979. Synaptic extensions from mossy fibers of fascia dentata. Anat. Embryol. 155: 241–251.

Amaral, D.G. 1993. Emerging principles of intrinsic hippocampal organization. Curr. Opin. Neurobiol. 3: 225–229.

Amaral, D.G. and Dent, J.A. 1981. Development of the mossy fibers of the dentate gyrus: I. A light and electron microscopic study of the mossy fibers and their expansions. J. Comp. Neurol. 195: 51–86.

Amaral, D.G., Dolorfo, C., and Alvarez-Royo, P. 1991. Organization of CA1 projections to the subiculum: A PHA-L analysis in the rat. Hippocampus 1: 415–436.

Amaral, D.G., Insausti, R., and Cowan, W.M. 1984. The commissural connections of the monkey hippocampal formation. J. Comp. Neurol. 224: 307–336.

Amaral, D.G., Ishizuka, N., and Claiborne, B. 1990. Neurons, numbers and the hippocampal network. In: Progress in Brain Research, Understanding the Brain Through the Hippocampus: The Hippocampal Region as a Model for Studying Structure and Function (Storm-Mathisen, J., Zimmer, J., and Ottersen, O.P., eds.) Amsterdam: Elsevier, pp. 1–11.

Amaral, D.G. and Kurz, J. 1985. An analysis of the origins of the cholinergic and noncholinergic septal projections to the hippocampal formation of the rat. J. Comp. Neurol. 240: 37–59.

Amaral, D.G. and Witter, M.P. 1989. The three dimensional organization of the hippocampal formation: A review of anatomical data. Neuroscience 31: 571–591.

Amaral, D.G. and Witter, M. 1995. Hippocampal formation. In: The Rat Nervous System (G. Paxinos, eds.). San Diego: Academic Press, pp. 443–493.

Amthor, F.R. and Grzywacz, N.M. 1993. Directional selectivity in vertebrate retinal ganglion cells. Rev. Oculomot. Res. 5: 79–100.

Amthor, F.R., Takahashi, E.S., and Oyster, C.W. 1989. Morphologies of rabbit retinal ganglion cells with complex receptive fields. J. Comp. Neurol. 280:97–121.

Andersen, P., Blackstad, T., Hulleberg, G., and Al, E. 1987. Changes in spine morphology associated with ltp in rat dentate granule cells. Proc. Physiol. Soc. 50: 288.

Andersen, P., Bliss, T.V.P., and Skrede, K. 1971. Lamellar organization of hippocampal excitatory pathways. Exp. Brain Res. 13: 222–238.

Andersen, P., Eccles, J.C., and Loyning, Y. 1964a. Location of postsynaptic inhibitory synapses on hippocampal pyramids. J. Neurophysiol. 27: 592–607.

Andersen, P., Eccles, J.C., and Voorhoeve, P.E. 1964b. Postsynaptic inhibition of cerebellar Purkinje cells. J. Neurophysiol. 27: 1139–1153.

Anderson, J.A. 1970. Two models for memory organization using interacting traces. Math. Biosci. 8: 137–160.

Anderson, J.A. 1972. A simple network generating an interactive memory. Math. Biosci. 14: 197–220.

Anderson, J.A. 1995. An Introduction to Neural Networks. Cambridge, MA: Bradford Books.

Anderson, J.C., Douglas, R., Martin, K.A.C., Nelson, C., and Whitteridge, D. 1994. Synaptic output of physiologically identified spiny neurons in cat visual cortex. J. Comp. Neurol. 341: 16–24.

Anderson, O.S. and Koeppe, R.E.I. 1992. Molecular determinants of channel function. Physiol. Rev. 72(Suppl.): S89–S158.

Andres, K. 1965. Der Feinbau des Bulbus Olfactorius der Ratte unter besonderer Berüksichtgung der Synaptischen Verbindungen. Z. Zellforsch. Mikrosk. Anat. 65: 530–561.

Aniksztejn, L., Charton, G., and Ben-Ari, Y. 1987. Selective release of endogenous zinc from the hippocampal mossy fibers in situ. Brain Res. 404: 58–64.

Aoki, C. and Kabak, S. 1992. Cholinergic terminals in the cat visual cortex: Ultrastructural basis for interaction with glutamate-immunoreactive neurons and other cells. Vis. Neurosci. 8: 177–191.

Arcelli, P., Frassoni, C., Regondi, M.C., De Biasi, S., and Spreafico, R. 1997. GABAergic neurons in mammalian thalamus: A marker of thalamic complexity? Brain Res. Bull. 42: 27–37.

Arle, J.E. and Kim, D.O. 1991. Neural modeling of intrinsic and spike-discharge properties of cochlear nucleus neurons. Biol. Cybern. 64: 273–283.

Armstrong, D.M. 1974. Functional significance of connections of the inferior olive. Physiol. Rev. 54: 358–417.

Armstrong-James, M. and Fox, K. 1983. Effects of iontophoresed noradrenaline on the spontaneous activity of neurons in rat primary somatosensory cortex. J. Physiol. (Lond.) 335: 427–447.

Armstrong-James, M., Welker, I., and Callahan, C. 1993. The contribution of NMDA and non-NMDA receptors to fast and slow transmission of sensory information in the rat SI barrel cortex. J. Neurosci. 13: 2149–2160.

Aroniadou, V. and Keller, A. 1995. Mechanisms of long term potentiation induction in rat motor cortex in vitro. Cereb. Cortex 5: 353–362.

Aroniadou, V. and Teyler, T. 1992. Induction of NMDA receptor independent long-term potentiation of LTP in visual cortex of adult rats. Brain Res. 584: 169–173.

Artola, A., Brocher, S., and Singer, W. 1990. Different voltage-dependent thresholds for inducing long-term depression and long-term potentiation in slices of rat visual cortex. Nature 347: 69–72.

Artola, A. and Singer, W. 1987. Long-term potentiation and NMDA receptors in rat visual cortex. Nature 330: 649–652.

Arvidsson, U., Cullheim, S., Ulfhake, B., Bennett, G.W., Fone, K.C.F., Cuello, A.C., Verhofstad, A.A.J., Visser, T.J., and Hökfelt, T. 1990. 5-Hydroxytryptamine, substance P, and thyrotropin-releasing hormone in the adult spinal cord segment L7: Immunohistochemical and chemical studies. Synapse 6: 231–270.

Ascher, P. and Nowak, L. 1987. Electrophysiological studies of NMDA receptors. Trends Neurosci. 10: 284–287.

Atick, J.J. and Redlich, A.N. 1992. What does the retina know about natural scenes? Neural Comp. 4: 196–210.

Attwell, D. 1986. Ion channels and signal processing in the outer retina. Q. J. Exp. Physiol. 71: 497–536.

Ayala, G.F., Matsumoto, H., and Gumnit, R.J. 1970. Excitability changes and inhibitory mechanisms in neocortical neurons during seizures. J. Neurophysiol. 33: 73–85.

Ayoub, G.S., Korenbrot, J.I., and Copenhagen, D.R. 1989. The release of endogenous glutamate from isolated cone photoreceptors of the lizard. Neurosci. Res. (Suppl.) 10: 547–556.

Azzopardi, P. and Cowey, A. 1993. Preferential representation of the fovea in the primary visual cortex. Nature 361: 719–721.

Baer, S. and Rinzel, J. 1991. Propagation of dendritic spikes mediated by excitable spines: A continuum theory. J. Neurophysiol. 65: 874–890.

Bainbridge, K.G. and Miller, J.J. 1982. Immunohistochemical localization of calcium-binding protein in the cerebellum, hippocampal formation and olfactory bulb of the rat. Brain Res. 245: 223–229.

Baker, F.H. and Malpeli, J.G. 1977. Effects of cryogenic blockade of visual cortex on the responses of lateral geniculate neurons in the monkey. Exp. Brain. Res. 29: 433–444.

Baker, H. 1988. Neurotransmitter plasticity in the juxtaglomerular cells of the olfactory bulb. In: Molecular Neurobiology of the Olfactory System (F.L. Margolis and T.V. Getchell, eds.). New York: Plenum Press, pp. 185–216.

Baker, H., Kwano, T., Margolis, F.L., and Joh, T.H. 1983. Transneural regulation of tyrosine hydroxylase expression in olfactory bulb of mouse and rat. J. Neurosci. 3: 69–78.

Bakst, I., Avendano, C., Morrison, J.H., and Amaral, D.G. 1986. An experimental analysis of the origins of somatostatin-like immunoreactivity in the dentate gyrus of the rat. J. Neurosci. 6: 1452–1462.

Baldissera, F. and Gustafsson, B. 1974. Firing behavior of a neurone model based on the afterhyperpolarization conductance time course. First interval firing. Acta Physiol. Scand. 91: 528–544.

Baldissera, F., Hultborn, H., and Illert, M. 1981. Integration in spinal neuronal systems. In: Handbook of Physiology, Section 1: The Nervous System, Vol. III: Motor Control, Part 1 (Brooks, V.B., eds.). Bethesda: American Physiological Society, pp. 509–595.

Banks, M.I., Haberly, L.B., and Jackson, M.B. 1996. Layer-specific properties of the transient K current (I_A) in piriform cortex. J. Neurosci. 16: 3862–3876.

Banks, M.I. and Sachs, M.B. 1991. Regularity analysis in a compartmental model of chopper units in the anteroventral cochlear nucleus. J. Neurophysiol. 65: 606–629.

Barber, P.C. and Lindsay, R.M. 1982. Schwann cells of the olfactory nerves contain glial fibrillary acidic protein and resemble astrocytes. Neuroscience 7: 2687–2695.

Bargas, J., Galarraga, E., and Aceves, J. 1988. Electrotonic properties of neostriatal neurons are modulated by extracellular potassium. Exp. Brain Res. 72: 390–398.

Barkai, E., Bergman, R.E., Horwitz, G., and Hasselmo, M.E. 1994. Modulation of associative memory function in a biophysical simulation of rat piriform cortex. J. Neurophysiol. 72: 659–677.

Barkai, E. and Hasselmo, M.E. 1994. Modulation of the input/output function of rat piriform cortex pyramidal cells. J. Neurophysiol. 72: 664–658.

Barker, J., McBurney, R., and Mathers, D. 1983. Convulsant induced depression of amino acid responses in cultured mouse spinal neurons studied under voltage clamp. Br. J. Pharmacol. 80: 619–629.

Barlow, H.B. 1953. Summation and inhibition in the frog's retina. J. Physiol. (Lond.) 119: 69–88.

Barlow, H.B. 1972. Single units and sensation: A neuron doctrine for perceptual psychology. Perception 1: 371–394.

Barlow, H.B. 1982. General principles: The senses considered as physical instruments. In: The Senses (Barlow, H.B. and Mollon, J.D., eds.). Cambridge: Cambridge University Press, pp. 1–33.

Barlow, H.B., Fitzhugh, B.R., and Kuffler, S.W. 1957. Change of organization in the receptive fields of the cat's retina during dark adaptation. J. Physiol. (Lond.) 137: 338–354.

Barlow, H.B., Levick, W.R., and Yoon, M. 1971. Responses to single quanta of light in retinal ganglion cells of the cat. Vision Res. S3: 87–101.

Barnard, E., Darlison, M., and Seeburg, P. 1987. Molecular biology of the receptor: The receptor/channel superfamily. Trends Neurosci. 10: 502–509.

Barnes, J.M. and Henley, J.M. 1992. Molecular characteristics of excitatory amino acid receptors. Prog. Neurobiol. 39: 113–133.

Barrett, E.F. and Barrett, J.N. 1976. Separation of two voltage-sensitive potassium currents, and demonstration of a tetrodotoxin-resistant calcium current in frog motoneurones. J. Physiol. (Lond.) 255: 737–774.

Barrett, E.F., Barrett, J.N., and Crill, W.E. 1980. Voltage-sensitive outward currents in cat motoneurones. J. Physiol. (Lond.) 304: 251–276.

Barrett, E.F. and Magleby, K.L. 1976. Physiology of cholinergic transmission. In: Biology of Cholinergic Function (Goldberg, A.M. and Hanin, E., eds.). New York: Raven Press, pp. 29–100.

Barrett, J.N. and Crill, W.E. 1974. Specific membrane properties of cat motoneurones. J. Physiol. (Lond.) 239: 301–324.

Barrionuevo, G. and Brown, T.H. 1983. Associative long-term potentiation in hippocampal slices. Proc. Natl. Acad. Sci. USA 80: 7347–7351.

Barrionuevo, G., Kelso, S.R., Johnston, D., and Brown, T.H. 1986. Conductance mechanism responsible for long-term potentiation in monosynaptic and isolated excitatory synaptic inputs to hippocampus. J. Neurophysiol. 55: 540–550.

Bartlett, J.R., Doty, R.W., Sr., Lee, B.B., and Sakakura, H. 1976. Influence of saccadic eye movements on geniculostriate excitability in normal monkeys. Exp. Brain Res. 25: 487–509.

Bassett, J.L., Shipley, M.T., and Foote, S.L. 1992. Localization of corticotropin-releasing factor-like immunoreactivity in monkey olfactory bulb and secondary olfactory areas. J. Comp. Neurol. 316: 348–362.

Baumfalk, U. and Albus, K. 1988. Phaclofen antagonizes baclofen-induced suppression of visually evoked responses in the cats striate cortex. Brain Res. 463: 398–402.

Baylor, D.A., Fuortes, M.G.F., and O'Bryan, P.M. 1971. Receptive fields of cones in the retina of the turtle. J. Physiol. (Lond.) 214: 265–294.

Baylor, D.A., Nunn, B.J., and Schnapf, J.L. 1984. The photocurrent, noise and spectral sensitivity of rods of the monkey *Macaca fascicularis*. J. Physiol. (Lond.) 357: 575–607.

Bean, B.P. 1989. Classes of calcium channels in vertebrate cells. Annu. Rev. Physiol. 51: 367–384.

Bear, M.F. and Abraham, W.C. 1996. Long-term depression in hippocampus. Annu. Rev. Neurosci. 19: 437–462.

Beaulieu, C. and Colonnier, M. 1983. The number of neurons in the different laminae of the binocular and monocular regions of area 17 in the cat. J. Comp. Neurol. 217: 337–344.

Beaulieu, C. and Collonier, M. 1985. A laminar analysis of the number of round-asymmetrical and flat-symmetrical synapses on spines, dendritic trunks, cell bodies in area 17 of the cat. J. Comp. Neurol. 231: 180–189.

Beaulieu, C. and Somogyi, P. 1991. Enrichment of cholinergic synaptic terminals on GABAergic neurons and coexistence of immunoreactive GABA and choline acetyltransferase in the same synaptic terminals in the striate cortex of the cat. J. Comp. Neurol. 304: 666–680.

Beckstead, R.M. 1979. An autoradiographic examination of corticocortical and subcortical projections of the mediodorsal-projection (prefrontal) cortex in the rat. J. Comp. Neurol. 184: 43–62.

Behan, M., Johnson, D.M.G., Feig, S.L., and Haberly, L.B. 1995. A new anatomically and physiologically distinct subdivision of the piriform (olfactory) cortex. Soc. Neurosci. Abstr. 21: 1186.

Bekkers, J.M. and Stevens, C.F. 1995. Quantal analysis of EPSPs recorded from small numbers of synapses in hippocampal cultures. J. Neurophysiol. 73: 1145–1156.

Benardo, L. and Prince, D. 1982. Cholinergic excitation of hippocampal pyramidal cells. Brain Res. 249: 315–333.

Bender, D.B. 1983. Visual activation of neurons in the primate pulvinar depends on cortex but not colliculus. Brain Res. 279: 258–261.

Bennett, B.D. and Bolam, J.P. 1993. Characterization of calretinin-immunoreactive structures in the striatum of the rat. Brain Res. 609: 137–148.

Bennett, B.D. and Bolam, J.P. 1994. Synaptic input and output of parvalbumin-immunoreactive neurons in the neostriatum of the rat. Neuroscience 62: 707–719.

Bennett, M.V.L. 1977. Electrical transmission: A functional analysis and comparison to chemical transmission. In: Handbook of Physiology, Section 1: The Nervous System, Vol. I: Cellular Biology of Neurons, Part 1 (Kandel, E.R., eds.). Washington, DC: American Physiological Society, pp. 357–416.

Benson, T.E. and Brown, M.C. 1990. Synapses formed by olivocochlear axon branches in the mouse cochlear nucleus. J. Comp. Neurol. 294: 52–70.

Benson, T.E., Burd, G.D., Greer, C.A., Landis, D.M., and Shepherd, G.M. 1985. High-resolution 2-deoxyglucose autoradiography in quick-frozen slabs of neonatal rat olfactory bulb. Brain Res. 339: 67–78.

Benson, T.E., Ryugo, D., and Hinds, J. 1984. Effects of sensory deprivation on developing mouse olfactory system. J. Neurosci. 4: 638–653.

Ben-Yishai, R., Lev Bar-Or, R., and Sompolinsky, H. 1995. Theory of orientation tuning in visual cortex. Proc. Natl. Acad. Sci. USA 92: 3844–3848.

Berg, H.C. 1993. Random Walks in Biology. Princeton: Princeton University Press.

Berkowicz, D.A., Trombley, P.Q., and Shepherd, G.M. 1994. Evidence for glutamate as the olfactory receptor cell neurotransmitter. J. Neurophysiol. 71: 2557–2561.

Berman, N., Bush, P., and Douglas, R. 1989. Adaptation and bursting may be controlled by a single fast potassium current. Q. J. Exp. Physiol. 74: 223–226.

Bernander, O., Douglas, R., and Koch, C. 1994. Amplification and linearization of synaptic input to the apical dendrites of cortical pyramidal neurons. J. Neurophysiol. 72: 2743–2753.

Bernander, O., Douglas, R., Martin, K.A.C., and Koch, C. 1991. Synaptic background activity influences spatiotemporal integration in single pyramidal cells. Proc. Natl. Acad. Sci. U.S.A. 88: 11569–11573.

Berrebi, A.S., Morgan, J.I., and Mugnaini, E. 1990. The Purkinje cell class may extend beyond the cerebellum. J. Neurocytol. 19: 643–654.

Berrebi, A.S. and Mugnaini, E. 1991. Distribution and targets of the cartwheel cell axon in the dorsal cochlear nucleus of the guinea pig. Anat. Embryol. 183: 427–454.

Berson, D.M. and Graybiel, A.M. 1983. Organization of the striate-recipient zone of the cat's lateralis posterior-pulvinar complex and its relations with the geniculostriate system. Neuroscience 9: 337–372.

Berson, D.M., Pu, M., and Famiglietti, E.V. 1996. The zeta cell: A new ganglion cell type in cat retina. Invest. Ophthalmol. Vis. Sci. Abstr. 37: S631.

Berson, D.M., Pu, M., and Isayama, T. 1997. The eta cell: a new ganglion cell type in cat retina. Invest. Ophthalmol. Vis. Sci. Abstr. 38: S51.

Betz, H. 1991. Glycine receptors: Heterogeneous and widespread in the mammalian brain. Trends. Neurosci. 14: 458–461.

Bhalla, U.S. and Bower, J.M. 1993. Exploring parameter space in detailed single neuron models: Simulations of the mitral and granule cells of the olfactory bulb. J. Neurophysiol. 69: 1948–1965.

Bickford, M.E., Günlük, A.E., Guido, W., and Sherman, S.M. 1993. Evidence that cholinergic axons from the parabrachial region of the brainstem are the exclusive source of nitric oxide in the lateral geniculate nucleus of the cat. J. Comp. Neurol. 334: 410–430.

Bickford, M.E., Günlük, A.E., Van Horn, S.C., and Sherman, S.M. 1994. GABAergic projection from the basal forebrain to the visual sector of the thalamic reticular nucleus in the cat. J. Comp. Neurol. 348: 481–510.

Biedenbach, M.A. and Stevens, C.F. 1969. Synaptic organization of the cat olfactory cortex as revealed by intracellular recording. J. Neurophysiol. 32: 204–214.

Biella, G. and de Curtis, M. 1995. Associative synaptic potentials in the piriform cortex of the isolated guinea-pig brain in vitro. Eur. J. Neurosci. 7: 54–64.

Bienenstock, E.L., Cooper, L.N., and Munro, P.W. 1982. Theory for the development of neuron selectivity: Orientation specificty and binocular interaction in visual cortex. J. Neurosci. 2: 32–48.

Binder, M.D., Heckman, C.J., and Powers, R.K. 1993. How different inputs control motoneuron discharge and the output of the motoneuron pool. Curr. Opin. Neurobiol. 3: 1028–1034.

Bindman, L., Meyer, T., and Prince, C. 1988. Comparison of the electrical properties of neocortical neurones in slices in vitro and in the anaesthetized rat. Brain Res. 68: 489–496.

Birnbaumer, L., Campbell, K.P., Catterall, W.A., Harpold, M.M., Hofmann, F., Horne, W.A., Mori, Y., Schwartz, A., Snutch, T.P., Tanabe, T., and Tsien, R.W. 1994. The naming of voltage-gated calcium channels. Neuron 13: 505–506.

Bishop, G.A., Chang, H.T., and Kitai. 1982. Morphological and physiological properties of neostriatal neurons: An intracellular horseradish peroxidase study in the rat. Neuroscience 7: 179–191.

Bisti, S., Iosif, G., Marchesi, G.F., and Strata, P. 1971. Pharmacological properties of inhibitions in the cerebellar cortex. Exp. Brain Res. 14: 24–37.

Björklund, A. and Lindvall, O. 1984. Dopamine-containing systems in the CNS. In: Handbook of Chemical Neuroanatomy, Vol. 2: Classical Transmitters in the CNS, Part I. (Björklund A. and Hökfelt, T., eds.). Amsterdam: Elsevier, pp. 55–122.

Blackburn, C.C. and Sachs, M.B. 1989. Classification of unit types in the anteroventral cochlear nucleus: PST histograms and regularity analysis. J. Neurophysiol. 62: 1303–1329.

Blackburn, C.C. and Sachs, M.B. 1990. The representation of the steady-state vowel sound /ɛ/ in the discharge patterns of cat anteroventral cochlear nucleus neurons. J. Neurophysiol. 63: 1191–1212.

Blackstad, T.W. 1956. Commissural connections of the hippocampal region in the rat, with special reference to their mode of termination. J. Comp. Neurol. 105: 417–537.

Blackstad, T.W. and Kjaerheim, A. 1961. Special axo-dendritic synapses in the hippocampal cortex electron and light microscopic studies on the layer of mossy fibers. J. Comp. Neurol. 117: 133–159.

Blackstad, T.W., Osen, K.K., and Mugnaini, E. 1984. Pyramidal neurones of the dorsal cochlear nucleus: A Golgi and computer reconstruction study in cat. Neuroscience 13: 827–854.

Blaxter, T., Carlen, P., Davies, M., and Kujitan, P. 1986. γ-aminobutyric acid hyperpolarizes rat hippocampal pyramidal cells through a calcium-dependent potassium conductance. J. Physiol. (Lond.) 373: 181–194.

Blaxter, T. and Cottrell, G. 1985. Actions of gaba and ethylenediamine on CA1 pyramidal neurones in the rat hippocampus. Q. J. Exp. Physiol. 70: 75–93.

Bliss, T.V.P. and Collingridge, G.L. 1993. A synaptic model of memory long-term potentiation in the hippocampus. Nature 361: 31–39.

Bliss, T.V.P. and Gardner-Medwin, A.R. 1973. Long-lasting potentiation of synaptic transmission in the dentate area of the unanaesthetized rabbit following stimulation of the perforant path. J. Physiol. (Lond.) 232: 357–374.

Bliss, T.V.P. and Lomo, T. 1973. Long-lasting potentiation of synaptic transmission in the dentate area of the unanaesthetized rabbit following stimulation of the perforant path. J. Physiol. (Lond.) 232: 331–356.

Bliss, T.V.P. and Lynch, M.A. 1988. Long-term potentiation of synaptic transmission in the hippocampus: properties and mechanisms. In: Long-Term Potentiation. From Biophysics to Behavior (Landfield, P.W. and Deadwyle, S.A., eds.). New York: Alan R. Liss, pp. 3–72.

Bliss, T.V.P. and Rosenberg, M. 1979. Activity-dependent changes on conduction velocity in the olfactory nerve of the tortoise. Pflugers Arch. 381: 209–216.

Bloedel, J.R. and Courville, J. 1981. Cerebellar afferent systems. In: Handbook of Physiology, Section I: The Nervous System, Vol. II: Motor Control, Part 2 (Brooks, V.B., eds.). Bethesda, MD: American Physiological Society, pp. 735–829.

Bloom, F.E., Hoffer, B.J., and Siggins, G.R. 1971. Studies on norepinephrine-containing afferents to Purkinje cells of rat cerebellum. I. Localization of the fibers and their synapses. Brain Res. 25: 501–521.

Bloomfield, S.A. 1992. Relationship between receptive and dendritic field size of amacrine cells in the rabbit retina. J. Neurophysiol. 68: 711–725.

Bloomfield, S.A., Hamos, J.E., and Sherman, S.M. 1987. Passive cable properties and morphological correlates of neurones in the lateral geniculate nucleus of the cat. J. Physiol. (Lond.) 383: 653–692.

Bloomfield, S.A. and Sherman, S.M. 1989. Dendritic current flow in relay cells and interneurons of the cat's lateral geniculate nucleus. Proc. Natl. Acad. Sci. USA 86: 3911–3914.

Boahen, K.A. 1996. Retinomorphic vision systems: Reverse engineering the vertebrate retina. Ph.D. Thesis, California Institute of Technology.

Bodnarenko, S.R., Jeyarasasingam, G., and Chalupa, L. 1995. Development and regulation of dendritic stratification in retinal ganglion cells by glutamate-mediated afferent activity. J. Neurosci. 15: 7037–7045.

Bogan, N., Brecha, N., Gall, C., and Karten, H.J. 1982. Distribution of enkephalin-like immunoreactivity in the rat main olfactory bulb. Neuroscience 7: 895–906.

Bolam, J.P., Clarke, D.J., Smith, A.D., and Somogyi, P. 1983. A type of aspiny neuron in the rat neostriatum accumulates [^{3}H]gamma-aminobutyric acid: Combination of Golgi-staining, autoradiography, and electron microscopy. J. Comp. Neurol. 213: 121–134.

Bolam, J.P., Ingham, C.A., Izzo, P.N., Levey, A.I., Rye, D.B., Smith, A.D., and Wainer, B.H. 1986. Substance P-containing terminals in synaptic contact with cholinergic neurons in the neostriatum and basal forebrain: A double immunocytochemical study in the rat. Brain Res. 397: 279–289.

Bolam, J.P., Somogyi, P., Totterdell, S., and Smith, A.D. 1981. A second-type of striatonigral neuron: A comparison between retrogradely labelled and Golgi-stained neurons at the light and electron microscopic levels. Neuroscience 6: 2141–2157.

Bolam, J.P., Wainer, B.H., and Smith, A.D. 1984. Characterization of cholinergic neurons in the rat neostriatum. A combination of choline acetyltransferase immunocytochemistry, Golgi-impregnation and electron microscopy. Neuroscience 12: 711–718.

Bolz, J., Thier, P., Voight, T., and Wässle, H. 1985. Action and localization of glycine and taurine in the cat retina. J. Physiol. (Lond.) 362: 395–413.

Boos, R., Schneider, H., and Wässle, H. 1993. Voltage- and transmitter-gated currents of AII-amacrine cells in a slice preparation of the rat retina. J. Neurosci. 13: 2874–2888.

Borges, S., Gleason, E., Turelli, M., and Wilson, M. 1995. The kinetics of quantal transmitter release from retinal amacrine cells. Proc. Natl. Acad. Sci. USA 92: 6896–6900.

Bormann, J. 1988. Electrophysiology of GABA$_A$ and GABA$_B$ receptor subtypes. Trends Neurosci. 11: 112–116.

Bormann, J. and Feigenspan, A. 1995. GABA$_C$ receptors. Trends Pharmacol. Sci. 18: 515–519.

Boudreau, J.C. and Tsuchitani, C. 1970. Cat superior olive S-segment cell discharge to tonal stimulation. Contrib. Sens. Physiol. 4: 143–213.

Bourassa, J., Pinault, D., and Deschênes, M. 1995. Corticothalamic projections from the cortical barrel field to the somatosensory thalamus in rats: A single-fibre study using biocytin as an anterograde tracer. J. Neurosci. 7: 19–30.

Bourk, T.R. 1976. Electrical Responses of Neural Units in the Anteroventral Cochlear Nucleus of the Cat. Ph.D. thesis, Massachusetts Institute of Technology, Cambridge, MA.

Bourk, T.R., Mielcarz, J.P., and Norris, B.E. 1981. Tonotopic organization of the anteroventral cochlear nucleus of the cat. Hear. Res. 4: 215–241.

Bowery, N. 1993. GABA$_B$ receptor pharmacology. Annu. Rev. Pharmacol. Toxicol. 33: 109–147.

Bowery, N., Price, G., Hudson, A., Hill, D., Wilkin, G., and Turnbull, M. 1984. GABA receptor multiplicity: Visualization of different receptor types in the mammalian CNS. Neuropharmacology 23: 219–231.

Bowery, N.G., Hudson, A.L., and Price, G.W. 1987. GABA-A and GABA-B receptor site distribution in the rat central nervous system. Neuroscience 20: 365–383.

Bowling, D.B. and Michael, C.R. 1984. Terminal patterns of single, physiologically characterized optic tract fibers in the cat's lateral geniculate nucleus. J. Neurosci. 4: 198–216.

Bowmaker, J.K., Govardovskii, V.I., Shukolyukov, S.A., Zueva, L.V., Hunt, D.M., Sideleva, V.G., and Smirnova, O.G. 1994. Visual pigments and the photic environment: The cottoid fish of Lake Baikal. Vision Res. 34: 591–605.

Boycott, B.B. and Dowling, J.E. 1969. Organization of the primate retina. Light microscopy. Phil. Trans. R. Soc. (Lond.) B 255: 109–184.

Boycott, B.B. and Kolb, H. 1973. The connections between bipolar cells and photoreceptors in the retina of the domestic cat. J. Comp. Neurol. 148: 91–114.

Boycott, B.B. and Wassle, H. 1974. The morphological types of ganglion cells of the domestic cat's retina. J. Physiol. (Lond.) 240: 397–419.

Boycott, B.B. and Wässle, H. 1991. Morphological classification of bipolar cells of the primate retina. Eur. J. Neurosci. 3: 1069–1088.

Boyd, I.A. and Davey, M.R. 1968. Composition of Peripheral Nerves. Edinburgh: E. & S. Livingstone.

Braitenberg, V. and Atwood, R.P. 1958. Morphological observations in the cerebellar cortex. J. Comp. Neurol. 109: 1–34.

Braitenberg, V. and Schüz, A. 1991. Anatomy of the Cortex: Statistics and Geometry. New York: Springer-Verlag.

Bramham, C.R., Errington, M.L., and Bliss, T.V.P. 1988. Naloxone blocks the induction of long-term potentiation in the lateral but not in the medial perforant pathway in the anesthetized rat. Brain Res. 449: 352–356.

Brandstätter, J.H., Koulen, P., Kuhn, R., van der Putten, H., and Wässle, H. 1996. Compartmental localization of a metabotropic glutamate receptor (mGluR7): Two different active sites at a retinal synapse. J. Neurosci. 16: 4749–4756.

Brännström, T. 1993. Quantitative synaptology of functionally different types of cat medial gastrocnemius alpha-motoneurons. J. Comp. Neurol. 330: 439–454.

Brawer, J.R., Morest, D.K., and Kane, E.C. 1974. The neuronal architecture of the cochlear nucleus of the cat. J. Comp. Neurol. 155: 251–300.

Brazier, M.A.B. 1960. The historical development of neurophysiology. In: Handbook of Physiology, Section 1: Neurophysiology, Vol. I (Magoun, H.W., ed.). Bethesda: American Physiological Society, pp. 1–58.

Brecha, N., Johnson, D., Peichl, L., and Wässle, H. 1988. Cholinergic amacrine cells of the rabbit retina contain glutamate decarboxylse and gamma-aminobutyrate immunoreactivity. Proc. Natl. Acad. Sci. USA 85: 6187–6191.

Bredt, D.S., Glatt, C.E., Hwang, P.M., Fotuhi, M., Dawson, T.M., and Snyder, S.H. 1991. Nitric oxide synthase protein and mRNA are discretely localized in neuronal populations of the mammalian CNS together with NADPH diaphorase. Neuron 7: 615–624.

Bredt, D.S., Hwang, P.M., and Snyder, S.H. 1990. Localization of nitric oxide synthase indicating a neural role for nitric oxide. Nature 347: 768–770.

Bredt, D.S. and Snyder, S.H. 1992. Nitric oxide, a novel neuronal messenger. Neuron 8: 3–11.

Breer, H. 1994. Odor recognition and second messenger signaling in olfactory receptor neurons. Semin. Cell Biol. 5: 25–32.

Breer, H. and Shepherd, G.M. 1993. Implications of the NO/cGMP system for olfaction. Trends Neurosci. 16: 5–9.

Breindl, A., Derrick, B.E., Rodriguez, S.B., and Martinez, J.L.J. 1994. Opioid receptor-dependent long-term potentiation at the lateral perforant path-CA3 synapse in rat hippocampus. Brain Res. Bull. 33: 17–24.

Bressler, S.L. 1988. Changes in electrical activity of rabbit olfactory bulb and cortex to conditioned odor stimulation. Behav. Neurosci. 102: 740–747.

Brock, L.G., Coombs, J.S., and Eccles, J.C. 1952. The recording of potentials from motoneurones with an intracellular electrode. J. Physiol. (Lond.) 117: 431–460.

Brodal, A. 1981. Neurological Anatomy. Oxford: Oxford University Press.

Brown, A.G. 1981. Organization in the Spinal Cord: The Anatomy and Physiology of Identified Neurones. Berlin: Springer-Verlag.

Brown, A.G. and Fyffe, R.E.W. 1981. Direct observations on the contacts made between Ia afferents and α-motoneurones in the cat's lumbosacral spinal cord. J. Physiol. (Lond.) 313: 121–140.

Brown, A.G., Rose, P.K., and Snow, P.J. 1977. The morphology of spinocervical tract neurones revealed by intracellular injection of horseradish peroxidase. J. Physiol. (Lond.) 270: 747–764.

Brown, D.A. 1988. M-currents: An update. Trends Neurosci. 44: 294–299.

Brown, D.A. and Adams, P.R. 1980. Muscarinic suppression of a novel voltage-sensitive K^+ current in a vertebrate neurone. Nature 283: 673–676.

Brown, D.A., Gahwiler, B.H., Griffith, W.H., and Halliwell, J.V. 1990a. Membrane currents in hippocampal neurons. Prog. Brain Res. 83: 141–160.

Brown, D.A. and Kukulka, C.G. 1993. Human flexor reflex modulation during cycling. J. Neurophysiol. 69: 1212–1224.

Brown, M.C., Berglund, A.M., Kiang, N.Y.S., and Ryugo, D.K. 1988. Central trajectories of type II spiral ganglion neurons. J. Comp. Neurol. 278: 581–590.

Brown, T.H., Fricke, R.A., and Perkel, D.H. 1981. Passive electrical constants in three classes of hippocampal neurons. J. Neurophysiol. 46: 812–827.

Brown, T.H. and Johnston, D. 1983. Voltage-clamp analysis of mossy fiber synaptic input to hippocampal neurons. J. Neurophysiol. 50: 487–507.

Brown, T.H., Kairiss, E.W., and Keenan, C.L. 1990b. Hebbian synapses: Biophysical mechanisms and algorithms. Annu. Rev. Neurosci. 13: 475–511.

Brown, T.H., Wong, R.K.S., and Prince, D.A. 1979. Spontaneous miniature synaptic potentials in hippocampal neurons. Brain Res. 177: 194–199.

Brownstone, R.M., Gossard, J.P., and Hultborn, H. 1994. Voltage-dependent excitation of motoneurons from spinal locomoter centers in the cat. Exp. Brain Res. 102: 34–44.

Bruce, C., Desimone, R., and Gross, C. 1981. Visual properties of neurons in a polysensory area in superior temporal sulcus of the macaque. J. Neurophysiol. 46: 369–384.

Bruce, H.M. 1959. An exteroceptive block to pregnancy in the mouse. Nature 184: 105.

Brughera, A.R., Stutman, E.R., Carney, L.H., and Colburn, H.S. 1996. A model with excitation and inhibition for cells in the medial superior olive. Auditory Neurosci. 2: 219–233.

Brunjes, P.C. 1994. Unilateral naris closure and olfactory system development. Brain Res. Revs. 19: 146–160.

Buchsbaum, G. and Gottschalk, A. 1983. Trichromacy, opponent colours coding and optimum colour information transmission in the retina. Proc. R. Soc. (Lond) B 220: 89–113.

Buck, L.D. and Axel, R. 1991. A novel multigene family may encode odorant receptors: A molecular basis for odorant recognition. Cell 65: 175–187.

Buckmaster, P.S. and Soltesz, I. 1996. Neurobiology of hippocampal interneurons: A workshop review. Hippocampus 6: 330–339.

Buckmaster, P.S., Wenzel, J.H., Kunkel, D.D., and Schwartzkroin, P.A. 1996. Axon arbors and synaptic connections of hippocampal mossy cells in the rat in vivo. J. Comp. Neurol. 366: 270–292.

Bufler, J., Zufall, F., Franke, C., and Hatt, H. 1992. Patch-clamp recordings of spiking and nonspiking interneurons from rabbit olfactory bulb slices: GABA- and other transmitter receptors. J. Comp. Physiol. A 170:153–159.

Buhl, E.H., Szilagyi, T., Halasy, K., and Somogyi, P. 1996. Physiological properties of anatomically identified basket and bistratified cells in the CA1 area of the rat hippocampus in vitro. Hippocampus 6: 294–305.

Bührle, C.P. and Sonnhof, U. 1985. The ionic basis of postsynaptic inhibition of motoneurons of the frog spinal cord. Neuroscience 14:581–592.

Buonviso, N. and Chaput, M.A. 1990. Response similarity to odors in olfactory bulb output cells presumed to be connected to the same glomerulus: Electrophysiological study using simultaneous single unit recordings. J. Neurophysiol. 63: 447–454.

Buonviso, N., Revial, M.F., and Jourdan, F. 1991. The projections of mitral cells from small local regions of the olfactory bulb: An anterograde tracing study using PHA-L (Phaseolus vulgaris leucoagglutinin). Eur. J. Neurosci. 3: 493–500.

Burd, G. 1980. Myelinated dendrites and neuronal perikarya in the olfactory bulb of the mouse. Brain Res. 181: 450–454.

Burgi, P.-Y. and Grzywacz, N.M. 1994. Model for the pharmacological basis of spontaneous synchronous activity in developing retinas. J. Neurosci. 14: 7426–7439.

Burian, M. and Gestoettner, W. 1988. Projection of primary vestibular afferent fibres to the cochlear nucleus in the guinea pig. Neurosci. Lett. 84: 13–17.

Burke, J. and Hablitz, J. 1995. Modulation of epileptiform activity by metabotropic glutamate receptors in immature rat neocortex. J. Neurophysiol. 73: 205–217.

Burke, R.E. 1967. The composite nature of the monosynaptic excitatory postsynaptic potential. J. Neurophysiol. 30: 1114–1137.

Burke, R.E. 1968. Firing patterns of gastrocnemius motor units in the decerebrate cat. J. Physiol. (Lond.) 196: 631–645.

Burke, R.E. 1981. Motor units: Anatomy, physiology and functional organization. In: Handbook of Physiology, Section 1: The Nervous System, Vol. II: Motor Control, Part 1 (Brooks, V.B., eds.). Bethesda: American Physiological Society, pp. 345–422.

Burke, R.E. 1991. Selective recruitment of motor units. In: Motor Control: Concepts and Issues (Humphrey, D.R. and Freund, H.-J., eds.). Chichester: John Wiley & Sons, pp. 5–21.

Burke, R.E., Dum, R.P., Fleshman, J.W., Glenn, L.L., Lev-Tov, A., O'Donovan, M.J., and Pinter, M.J. 1982. An HRP study of the relation between cell size and motor unit type in cat ankle extensor motoneurons. J. Comp. Neurol 209: 17–28.

Burke, R.E., Fedina, L., and Lundberg, A. 1971. Spatial synaptic distribution of recurrent and group Ia inhibitory systems in cat spinal motoneurones. J. Physiol. (Lond.) 214: 305–326.

Burke, R.E., Fyffe, R.E.W., and Moschovakis, A.K. 1994. Electrotonic architecture of cat gamma motoneurons. J. Neurophysiol. 72. 2302–2316.

Burke, R.E. and Glenn, L.L. 1996. Horseradish peroxidase study of the spatial and electrotonic distribution of group Ia synapses on type-identified ankle extensor motoneurons of the cat. J. Comp. Neurol. 372: 465–485.

Burke, R.E., Jankowska, E., and ten Bruggencate, G. 1970. A comparison of peripheral and rubrospinal synaptic input to slow and fast twitch motor units of triceps surae. J. Physiol. (Lond.) 207: 709–732.

Burke, R.E., Levine, D.N., Tsairis, P., and Zajac, F.E. 1973. Physiological types and histochemical profiles in motor units of the cat gastrocnemius. J. Physiol. (Lond.) 234: 723–748.

Burke, R.E. and Nelson, P.G. 1971. Accommodation to current ramps in motoneurons of fast and slow twitch motor units. Int. J. Neurosci. 1: 347–356.

Burke, R.E. and Rudomin, P. 1977. Spinal neurons and synapses. In: Handbook of Physiology, Section 1: The Nervous System, Vol. I: The Cellular Biology of Neurons, Part 2 (Kandel, E.R., ed.). Bethesda: American Physiological Society, pp. 877–944.

Burke, R.E., Rudomin, P., and Zajac, F.E. 1976a. The effect of activation history on tension production by individual muscle units. Brain Res. 109: 515–529.

Burke, R.E., Rymer, W.Z., and Walsh, J.V. 1976b. Relative strength of synaptic input from short latency pathways to motor units of defined type in cat medial gastrocnemius. J. Neurophysiol. 39: 447–458.

Burke, R.E., Strick, P.L., Kanda, K., Kim, C.C., and Walmsley, B. 1977. Anatomy of medial gastrocnemius and soleus motor nuclei in cat spinal cord. J. Neurophysiol. 40: 667–680.

Burke, R.E. and Tsairis, P. 1977. Histochemical and physiological profile of a skeletofusimotor (beta) unit in cat soleus muscle. Brain Res. 129: 341–345.

Büttner, U. and Fuchs, A.F. 1973. Influence of saccadic eye movements on unit activity in simian lateral geniculate and perigeniculate nuclei. J. Neurophysiol. 36: 127–141.

Buzsaki, G. 1989. Two-stage model of memory trace formation: A role for "noisy" brain states. Neuroscience 31: 551–570.

Caggiano, M., Kauer, J.S., and Hunter, D.D. 1994. Globose basal cells are neuronal progenitors in the olfactory epithelium: A lineage analysis using a replication-incompetent retrovirus. Neuron 13: 339–352.

Caicedo, A. and Herbert, H. 1993. Topography of descending projections from the inferior colliculus to auditory brainstem nuclei in the rat. J. Comp. Neurol. 328: 377–392.

Cajal, S. Ramon y. 1888. Estructura de los centros nerviosos de los aves. Rev. Trimestr. Histol. Normal Patol. 1: 305–315.

Cajal, S. Ramon y. 1904. La Textura del Sistema Nervioso del Hombre y los Vertebrados. Madrid: Moya.

Cajal, S. Ramon y. 1911. Histologie du Système Nerveux de l'Homme et des Vertebres, Vol. II (trans. L. Azoulay). Paris, Maloine.

Cajal, S. Ramon y. 1955. Studies on the Cerebral Cortex (Limbic Structures) (trans., L.M. Kraft). London: Lloyd-Luke.

Cajal, S. Ramon y. 1972. The Structure of the Retina. Springfield, IL: Charles C. Thomas.

Calabresi, P., Lacey, M.G., and North, R.A. 1989. Nicotinic excitation of rat ventral tegmental neurones in vitro studied by intracellular recording. Br. J. Pharmacol. 98: 135–140.

Calabresi, P., Mercuri, N.B., and Bernardi, G. (eds.). 1993. Chemical modulation of synaptic transmission in the striatum. In: Chemical Signalling in the Basal Ganglia (Arbuthnott, G. and Emson, P.C., eds.). Prog. Brain Res. 99: 299–308.

Calabresi, P., Pisani, A., Mercuri, N.B., and Bernardi, G. 1996. The corticostriatal projection: From synaptic plasticity to dysfunctions of the basal ganglia. Trends Neurosci. 19: 19–24.

Calancie, B., Needham-Shropshire, B., Jacobs, P., Willer, K., Zych, G., and Green, B.A. 1994. Involuntary stepping after chronic spinal cord injury. Evidence for a central rhythm generator for locomotion in man. Brain 117: 1143–1159.

Calkins, D.J., Schein, S., Tsukamoto, Y., and Sterling, P. 1994. M and L cones in macaque fovea connect to midget ganglion cells via different numbers of excitatory synapses. Nature 371: 70–72.

Calkins, D.J. and Sterling, P. 1996. Absence of spectrally specific lateral inputs to midget ganglion cells in primate retina. Nature 381: 613–615.

Calkins, D.J. and Sterling, P. 1997a. Microcircuitry of the primate blue/yellow ganglion cell. (Submitted).

Calkins, D.J. and Sterling, P. 1997b. Midget (P) ganglion cells in retina of trichromatic primates are not wired for color opponency. (Submitted).

Calkins, D.J., Tsukamoto, Y., and Sterling, P. 1996. Foveal cones form basal as well as invaginating contacts with diffuse ON bipolar cells. Vision Res. 36: 3373–3381.

Callaway, J.C. and Ross, W.N. 1995. Frequency dependent propagation of sodium action potentials in dendrites of hippocampal CA1 pyramidal neurons. J. Neurophysiol. 74: 1395–1403.

Calleja, C. 1893. La Region Olfactoria del Cerebro. Madrid Moya.

Calvin, W.H. and Schwindt, P.C. 1972. Steps in the production of motoneuron spikes during rhythmic firing. J. Neurophysiol. 35: 297–310.

Calvin, W.H. and Sypert, G. 1976. Fast and slow pyramidal tract neurons: An intracellular analysis of their contrasting repetitive firing properties in the cat. J. Neurophysiol. 39: 420–434.

Cant, N.B. 1981. The fine structure of two types of stellate cells in the anterior division of the anteroventral cochlear nucleus of the cat. Neuroscience 6: 2643–2655.

Cant, N.B. 1982. Identification of cell types in the anteroventral cochlear nucleus that project to the inferior colliculus. Neurosci. Lett. 32: 241–246.

Cant, N.B. 1992. The cochlear nucleus: Neuronal types and their synaptic organization. In: The Mammalian Auditory Pathway: Neuroanatomy (Webster, D.B., Popper, A.N., and Fay, R.R., eds.) Berlin: Springer-Verlag, pp. 66–116.

Cant, N.B. 1993. The synaptic organization of the ventral cochlear nucleus of the cat: The peripheral cap of small cells. In: The Mammalian Cochlear Nuclei (Merchán, M.A., Juiz, J.M., Godfrey, D.A., and Mugnaini, E., eds.). New York: Plenum, pp. 91–105.

Cant, N.B. and Gaston, K.C. 1982. Pathways connecting the right and left cochlear nuclei. J. Comp. Neurol. 212: 313–326.

Cant, N.B. and Morest, D.K. 1979a. Organization of the neurons in the anterior division of the anteroventral cochlear nucleus of the cat. Light-microscopic observations. Neuroscience 4: 1909–1923.

Cant, N.B. and Morest, D.K. 1979b. The bushy cells in the anteroventral cochlear nucleus of the cat. A study with the electron microscope. Neuroscience 4: 1925–1945.

Cant, N.B. and Morest, D.K. 1984. The structural basis for stimulus coding in the cochlear nucleus of the cat. In: Hearing Science, Recent Advances (Berlin C.I., eds.). San Diego: College-Hill Press, pp. 371–421.

Carbonne, E. and Lux, H.D. 1984. A low voltage-activated calcium conductance in embryonic chick sensory neurons. Biophys. J. 46: 413–418.

Carmichael, S.T., Clugnet, M.-C., and Price, J.L. 1994. Central olfactory connections in the macaque monkey. J. Comp. Neurol. 346: 403–434.

Carnevale, N.T., Tsai, K.Y., Claiborne, B.J., and Brown, T.H. 1997. Comparative electronic analysis of 3 classes of rat hippocampal neurons. J. Neurophysiol. 78: (In press).

Carpenter, D.O., Matthews, M.R., Parsons, P.J., and Hori, N. 1994. Long-term potentiation in the piriform cortex is blocked by lead. Cell. Mol. Neurobiol. 14: 723–733.

Casagrande, V.A. and Norton, T.T. 1996. Lateral geniculate nucleus: A review of its physiology and function. In: The Neural Basis of Visual Function (Leventhal A.G., eds.) London: MacMillan, pp. 41–84.

Casini, G. and Brecha, N.C. 1992. Colocalization of vasoactive intestinal polypeptide and GABA immunoreactivities in a population of wide-field amacrine cells in the rabbit retina. Vis. Neurosci. 8: 373–378.

Caspary, D.M., Backoff, P.M., Finlayson, P.G., and Palombi, P.S. 1994. Inhibitory inputs modulate discharge rate within frequency receptive fields of anteroventral cochlear nucleus neurons. J. Neurophysiol. 72: 2124–2133.

Castillo, J.d. and Katz, B. 1954. Statistical factors involved in neuromuscular facilitation and depression. J. Physiol. (Lond.) 124: 574–585.

Castro-Alamancos, M., Donoghue, J., and Connors, B. 1995. Different forms of synaptic plasticity in somatosensory and motor areas of the neocortex. J. Neurosci 15: 5324–5333.

Cattarelli, M., Astic, L., and Kauer, J.S. 1988. Metabolic mapping of 2-deoxyglucose uptake in the rat piriform cortex using computerized image processing. Brain Res. 442: 180–184.

Catterall, W.A. 1988. Structure and function of voltage-sensitive ion channels. Science 242: 50–61.

Catterall, W.A. 1992. Cellular and molecular biology of voltage-gated sodium channels. Physiol. Rev. 72 (Suppl. 4): 515–548.

Catterall, W.A. 1995. Structure and function of voltage-gated ion channels. Annu. Rev. Biochem. 64: 493–531.

Chagnac-Amitai, Y., Luhmann, H., and Prince, D. 1990. Burst-generating and regular spiking layer 5 pyramidal neurons of rat neocortex have different morphological features. J. Comp. Neurol. 296: 598–613.

Chandy, K.G. and Gutman, G.A. 1995. Voltage-gated potassium channel genes. In: Ligand- and Voltage-Gated Channels (North, A., ed.). Boca Raton, FL: CRC Press, pp. 1–71

Chang, H.T. and Kitai, S.T. 1982. Large neostriatal neurons in the rat: An electron microscopic study of gold-toned Golgi-stained cells. Brain Res. Bull. 8: 631–643.

Chang, H.T., Wilson, C.J., and Kitai, S.T. 1981. Single neostriatal efferent axons in the globus pallidus: a light and electron microscopic study. Science 213: 915–918.

Chang, H.T., Wilson, C.J., and Kitai, S.T. 1982. A Golgi study of rat neostriatal neurons: Light microscopic analysis. J. Comp. Neurol. 208: 107–126.

Chan-Palay, V. 1977. Cerbellar Dentate Nucleus. New York: Springer-Verlag.

Chan-Palay, V., Palay, S.L., and Wu, J.Y. 1979. Gamma-aminobutyric acid pathways in the cerebellum studied by retrograde and anterograde transport of glutamic acid decarboxylase antibody after in vivo injections. Anat. Embryol. 157: 1–14.

Charpak, S., Gähwiler, B.H., Do, K.Q., and Knopfel, T. 1990. Potassium conductances in hippocampal neurons blocked by excitatory amino-acid transmitters. Nature 347: 765–767.

Chen, C. and Thompson, R. 1995. Temporal specificity of long-term depression in parallel fiber–Purkinje synapses in rat cerebellar slice. Learn. Memory 2: 185–198.

Chen, W.R., Midtgaard, J., and Shepherd, G.M. 1997a. Forward- and back-propagation of action potentials in mitral cell dendrites. Soc. Neurosci. Abstr. 27 (In press).

Chen, W.R., Midtgaard, J., and Shepherd, G.M. 1997b. Initiation and propagation of action potentials in the mitral cell primary dendrite of the rat olfactory bulb. ISOT Abstr. (In press).

Chesselet, M.F. and Graybiel, A.M. 1986. Striatal neurons expressing somatostatin-like immunoreactivity evidence for a peptidergic interneuronal system in the cat. Neuroscience 17: 547–571.

Chicurel, M.E. and Harris, K.M. 1992. Three-dimensional analysis of the structure and composition of CA3 branched dendritic spines and their synaptic relationships with mossy fiber boutons in the rat hippocampus. J. Comp. Neurol. 325: 169–182.

Chiu, K. and Greer, C.A. 1996. Immunocytochemical analyses of astrocyte development in the olfactory bulb. Dev. Brain Res. 95: 28–37.

Choi, W.S., Kim, M.O., Lee, B.J., Kim, J.H., Sun, W., Seong, J.Y., and Kim, K. 1994. Presence of gonadotropin-releasing hormone mRNA in the rat olfactory piriform cortex. Brain Res. 648: 148–151.

Christensen, T.A., Heinbockel, T., and Hildebrand, J.G. 1996. Olfactory information processing in the brain: Encoding chemical and temporal features of odors. J. Neurobiol. 30: 82–91.

Christensen, T.A. and Hildebrand, J.G. 1987. Male-specific, sex pheromone–selective projection neurons in the antennal lobes of the moth *Manduca sexta*. J. Comp. Physiol. A 160: 553–569.

Christensen, T.A., Waldrop, B.R., Harrow, I.D., and Hildebrand, J.G. 1993. Local interneurons and information processing in the olfactory glomeruli of the moth *Manduca sexta*. J. Comp. Physiol. A 173: 385–99.

Christie, B.R., Eliot, L.S., Ito, K.I., Miyakawa, H., and Johnston, D. 1995. Different Ca^{2+} channels in soma and dendrites of hippocampal pyramidal neurons mediate spike-induced Ca^{2+} influx. J. Neurophysiol. 73: 2553–2557.

Christie, B.R., Kerr, D.S., and Abraham, W.C. 1994. Flip side of synaptic plasticity long-term depression mechanisms in the hippocampus. Hippocampus 4: 127–135.

Christie, B.R., Magee, J.C., and Johnston, D. 1996. The role of dendritic action potentials and Ca^{2+} influx in the induction of homosynaptic long-term depression in hippocampal CA1 pyramidal neurons. Learn. Memory 3: 160–169.

Chujo, T., Yamada, Y., and Yamamoto, C. 1975. Sensitivity of Purkinje cell dendrites to glutamic acid. Exp. Brain Res. 23: 293–300.

Chun, M.-H., Grünert, U., Martin, P.R., and Wässle, H. 1996. The synaptic complex of cones in the fovea and in the periphery of the macaque monkey retina. Vision Res. 36: 3383–3395.

Chun, M.-H. and Wässle, H. 1989. GABA-like immunoreactivity in the cat retina: Electron microscopy. J. Comp. Neurol. 279: 55–67.

Cinelli, A.R. and Kauer, J.S. 1994. Voltage-sensitive dyes and functional activity in the olfactory pathway. Annu. Rev. Neurosci. 15: 321–351.

Claiborne, B.J., Amaral, D.G., and Cowan, W.M. 1986. A light and electron microscopic analysis of the mossy fibers of the rat dentate gyrus. J. Comp. Neurol. 246: 435–458.

Claiborne, B.J., Amaral, D.G., and Cowan, W.M. 1990. A quantitative three-dimensional analysis of granule cell dendrites in the rat dentate gyrus. J. Comp. Neurol. 302: 206–219.

Clark, R. and Collins, G. 1976. The release of endogenous amino acids from the rat visual cortex. J. Physiol. (Lond.) 263: 383–400.

Clark, W.E. le Gros 1957. Inquiries into the anatomical basis of olfactory discrimination. Proc. R. Soc. Lond. B Biol. Sci. 146: 299–319.

Cleland, B.G., Dubin, M.W., and Levick, W.R. 1971. Sustained and transient neurones in the cat's retina and lateral geniculate nucleus. J. Physiol. (Lond.) 217: 473–496.

Cleland, B.G. and Freeman, A.W. 1988. Visual adaptation is highly localized in the cat's retina. J. Physiol. (Lond.) 404: 591–611.

Cleland, B.G. and Levick, W.R. 1974. Properties of rarely encountered types of ganglion cells in the cat's retina and an overall classification. J. Physiol. (Lond.) 240: 457–492.

Cohen, E. and Sterling, P. 1986. Accumulation of [^{3}H] glycine by cone bipolar neurons in the cat retina. J. Comp. Neurol. 250: 1–7.

Cohen, E. and Sterling, P. 1990a. Demonstration of cell types among cone bipolar neurons of cat retina. Phil. Trans. R. Soc. (Lond.) B 330: 305–321.

Cohen, E. and Sterling, P. 1990b. Convergence and divergence of cones onto bipolar cells in the central area of cat retina. Phil. Trans. R. Soc. (Lond.) B 330: 323–328.

Cohen, E. and Sterling, P. 1992. Parallel circuits from cones to the ON-beta ganglion cell. Eur. J. Neurosci. 4: 506–520.

Cohen, E.D., Zhou, Z.J., and Fain, G.L. 1994. Ligand-gated currents of alpha and beta ganglion cells in the cat retinal slice. J. Neurophysiol. 72: 1260–1269.

Colbert, C.M. and Johnston, D. 1996. Axonal action-potential initiation and Na$^+$ channel densities in the soma and axon initial segment of subicular pyramidal neurons. J. Neurosci. 16: 6676–6686.

Colbert, C.M., Magee, J.C., Hoffman, D., and Johnston, D. 1997. Slow recovery from inactivation of Na$^+$ channels underlies the activity-dependent attenuation of dendritic action potentials in hippocampal Ca1 pyramidal neurons. J. Neurosci. (In press).

Cole, A. and Nicoll, R. 1984. Characterization of a slow cholinergic postsynaptic potential recorded in vitro from rat hippocampal pyramidal cells. J. Physiol. (Lond.) 352: 173–188.

Cole, K.S. 1968. Membrane, Ions and Impulses. A Chapter of Classical Biophysics. Berkeley, CA: University of California Press.

Collingridge, G.L. and Bliss, T.V.P. 1987. NMDA receptors—Their role in long-term potentiation. Trends Neurosci. 10: 288–293.

Collingridge, G.L., Herron, C., and Lester, R. 1988b. Synaptic activation of N-methyl-D-aspartate receptors in the Schaffer collateral-commissural pathway of rat hippocampus. J. Physiol. (Lond.) 399: 283–300.

Collingridge, G.L., Herron, C., and Lester, R. 1988a. Frequency-dependent N-methyl-D-aspartate receptor-mediated synaptic transmission in rat hippocampus. J. Physiol. (Lond.) 399: 301–312.

Collingridge, G.L. and Watkins, J.C. (eds.). 1994. The NMDA Receptor. New York: Oxford University Press.

Collins, G.G.S. 1993. Actions of agonists of metabotropic glutamate receptors on synaptic transmission and transmitter release in the olfactory cortex. Br. J. Pharmacol. 108: 422–430.

Collins, G.G.S. 1994. The characteristics and pharmacology of olfactory cortical LTP induced by theta-burst high frequency stimulation and 1S,3R-ACPD. Neuropharmacology 33: 87–95.

Colonnier, M. 1968. Synaptic patterns on different cell types in the different laminae of the cat visual cortex. An electron microscope study. Brain Res. 9: 268–287.

Connor, J.A. and Stevens, C.F. 1971. Voltage clamp studies of a transient outward membrane current in gastropod neural somata. J. Physiol. (Lond.) 213: 21–30.

Connors, B.W. and Gutnick, M.J. 1990. Intrinsic firing patterns of diverse neocortical neurons. Trends Neurosci. 13: 99–104.

Connors, B.W., Gutnick, M.J., and Prince, D.A. 1982. Electrophysiological properties of neocortical neurons in vitro. J. Neurophysiol. 48: 1302–1320.

Connors, B.W., Malenka, R., and Silva, L. 1988. Two inhibitory postsynaptic potentials, and $GABA_a$ and $GABA_b$ receptor-mediated responses in neocortex of rat and cat. J. Physiol. (Lond.) 406: 443–468.

Conrad, L.C.A., Leonard, C.M., and Pfaff, D.W. 1974. Connections of the median and dorsal raphe nuclei in the rat: An autoradiographic and degeneration study. J. Comp. Neurol. 156: 179–206.

Conradi, S., Cullheim, S., Gollnik, L., and Kellerth, J.-O. 1983. Electron microscopic observations on the synaptic contacts of group Ia and muscle spindle afferents in the cat lumbosacral spinal cord. Brain Res. 265: 31–40.

Conradi, S., Kellerth, J.-O., and Berthold, C.-H. 1979. Electron microscopic studies of cat spinal α-motoneurons: II. A method for the description of neuronal architecture and synaptology from serial sections through the cell body and proximal dendritic segments. J. Comp. Neurol. 184: 741–754.

Constanti, A., Bagetta, G., and Libri, V. 1993. Persistent muscarinic excitation in guinea-pig olfactory cortex neurons involvement of a slow post-stimulus afterdepolarizing current. Neuroscience 56: 887–904.

Constanti, A. and Galvan, M. 1983a. Fast inward-rectifying current accounts for anomalous rectification in olfactory cortex neurones. J. Physiol. (Lond.) 335: 153–178.

Constanti, A. and Galvan, M. 1983b. M-current in voltage-clamped olfactory cortex neurones. Neurosci. Lett. 39: 65–70.

Constanti, A., Galvan, M., Franz, P., and Sim, J.A. 1985. Calcium-dependent inward currents in voltage-clamped guinea-pig olfactory cortex neurones. Pflugers Arch. 404: 259–265.

Constanti, A. and Libri, V. 1992. Trans-ACPD induces a slow post-stimulus inward tail current (IADP) in guinea-pig olfactory cortex neurones in vitro. Eur. J. Pharmacol. 216: 463–464.

Constanti, A. and Sim, J.A. 1987a. Muscarinic receptors mediating suppression of the M-current in guinea-pig olfactory cortex neurones may be of the M2-subtype. Br. J. Pharmacol. 90: 3–5.

Constanti, A. and Sim, J.A. 1987b. Calcium-dependent potassium conductance in guinea-pig olfactory cortex neurones in vitro. J. Physiol. (Lond.) 387: 173–194.

Cook, E.P. and Johnston, D. 1997. Active dendrites reduce location-dependent variability of synaptic input trains. J. Neurophysiol. (In press).

Cook, P.B. and Werblin, F.S. 1994. Spike initiation and propagation in wide field transient amacrine cells of the salamander retina. J. Neurosci. 14: 3852–3861.

Coombs, J.S., Eccles, J.C., and Fatt, P. 1955. Excitatory synaptic actions in motoneurons. J. Physiol. (Lond.) 130: 374–395.

Cooper, J.R., Bloom, F.E., and Roth, R.H. 1987. The Biochemical Basis of Neuropharmacology, 5th ed. New York: Oxford University Press.

Copenhagen, D.R. and Jahr, C.E. 1989. Release of endogenous excitatory amino acids from turtle photoreceptors. Nature 341: 536–539.

Corsellis, J.A.N. and Bruton, C.J. 1983. Neuropathology of status epilepticus in humans. Adv. Neurol. 34: 129–139.

Cotman, C.W., Monaghan, D.T., Ottersen, O.P., and Storm-Mathisen, J. 1987. Anatomical organization of excitatory amino acid receptors and their pathways. Trends Neurosci. 10: 273–280.

Cottrell, G., Lambert, J., and Peters, J. 1987. Modulation of $GABA_A$ receptor activity by alophaxalone. Br. J. Pharmacol. 90: 491–500.

Coulter, D.A., Huguenard, J.R., and Prince, D.A. 1990. Differential effects of petit mal anticonvulsants and convulsants on thalamic neurones: calcium current reduction. Br. J. Pharmacol. 100: 800–806.

Cowan, R.L. and Wilson, C.J. 1994. Spontaneous firing patterns and axonal projections of single corticostriatal neurons in the rat medial agranular cortex. J. Neurophysiol. 71: 17–32.

Cowan, R.L., Wilson, C.J., Emson, P.C., and Heizmann, C.W. 1990. Parvalbumin-containing GABAergic interneurons in the rat neostriatum. J. Comp. Neurol. 302: 198–205.

Cox, C.L., Huguenard, J.R., and Prince, D.A. 1996. Heterogeneous axonal arborizations of rat thalamic reticular neurons in the ventrobasal nucleus. J. Comp. Neurol. 366: 416–430.

Cox, J.F. and Rowe, M.H. 1996. Linear and nonlinear contributions to step responses in cat retinal ganglion cells. Vision Res. 36: 2047 2060.

Crair, M. and Malenka, R. 1995. A critical period for long-term potentiation at thalamocortical synapses. Nature 375: 325–328.

Creed, R.S., Denny-Brown, D., Eccles, J.C., Liddell, E.G.T., and Sherrington, C.S. 1932. Reflex Activity of the Spinal Cord. Oxford: Oxford University Press.

Crepel, F., Daniel, H., Hemart, N., and Jaillard, D. 1993. Mechanisms of synaptic plasticity in the cerebellum. In: Long-Term Potentiation: A Debate of Current Issues (Baudry, M. and Davis, J., eds.) Cambridge, MA: MIT Press, pp. 145–150.

Crepel, F., Dhanjal, S.S., and Sears, T. 1982. Effect of glutamate, aspartate and related derivatives on cerebellar Purkinje cell dendrites in the rat: An in vitro study. J. Physiol. (Lond.) 329: 297–317.

Crepel, F. and Jaillaes, D. 1990. Protein kinases, nitric oxide and long-term depression of synapses in the cerebellum. NeuroReport 1: 133–136.

Crepel, F. and Penit-Soria, J. 1986. Inward rectification and low threshold calcium conductance in rat cerebellar Purkinje cells. An in vitro study. J. Physiol. (Lond.) 372: 1–23.

Creutzfeldt, O., Lux, D., and Watanabe, S. 1966. Electrophysiology of cortical cells. In: The Thalamus. (Purpura, D. and Yuhr, Y., eds.). New York: Columbia University Press, pp. 209–235.

Crick, F. 1982. Do dendritic spines twitch? Trends Neurosci. 5: 44–46.

Crick, F. 1984. Function of the thalamic reticular complex: The searchlight hypothesis. Proc. Natl. Acad. Sci. USA 81: 4586–4590.

Crick, F. and Koch, C. 1992. The problem of consciousness. Sci. Am. 267: 152–159.

Crone, C., Hultborn, H., Kiehn, O., Mazieres, L., and Wigström, H. 1988. Maintained changes in motoneuronal excitability by short-lasting synaptic inputs in the decerebrate cat. J. Physiol. (Lond.) 405: 321–343.

Crooks, J. and Kolb, H. 1992. Localization of GABA, glycine, glutamate and tyrosine hydroxylase in the human retina. J. Comp. Neurol. 315: 287–302.

Crowell, J.A. and Banks, M.S. 1988. Physical limits of grating visibility: fovea and periphery. Invest. Ophthalmol. Vis. Sci. 29: 139 (Abstract).

Crunelli, V., Forda, S., and Kelly, J. 1984. The reversal potential of excitatory amino acid action on granule cells of the rat dentate gyrus. J. Physiol. (Lond.) 351: 327–342.

Crunelli, V., Lightowler, S., and Pollard, C.E. 1989. A T-type Ca^{2+} current underlies low-threshold Ca^{2+} potentials in cells of the cat and rat lateral geniculate nucleus. J. Physiol. (Lond.) 413: 543–561.

Cucchiaro, J.B., Bickford, M.E., and Sherman, S.M. 1991. A GABAergic projection from the pretectum to the dorsal lateral geniculate nucleus in the cat. Neuroscience 41: 213–226.

Cucchiaro, J.B., Uhlrich, D.J., and Sherman, S.M. 1993. Ultrastructure of synapses from the pretectum in the A-laminae of the cat's lateral geniculate nucleus. J. Comp. Neurol. 334: 618–630.

Cudeiro, J., Grieve, K.L., Rivadulla, C., Rodríguez, R., Martínez-Conde, S., and Acuña, C. 1994a. The role of nitric oxide in the transformation of visual information within the dorsal lateral geniculate nucleus of the cat. Neuropharmacology 33: 1413–1418.

Cudeiro, J., Rivadulla, C., Rodriguez, R., Martinez-Conde, S., Acuña, C., and Alonso, J.M. 1994b. Modulatory influence of putative inhibitors of nitric oxide synthesis on visual processing in the cat lateral geniculate nucleus. J. Neurophysiol. 71: 146–149.

Cudeiro, J., Rivadulla, C., Rodriguez, R., Martinez-Conde, S., Martinez, L., Grieve, K.L., and Acuña, C. 1996. Further observations on the role of nitric oxide in the feline lateral geniculate nucleus. Eur. J. Neurosci. 8: 144–152.

Cudeiro, J. and Sillito, A.M. 1996. Spatial frequency tuning of orientation-discontinuity-sensitive corticofugal feedback to the cat lateral geniculate nucleus. J. Physiol. (Lond.) 490: 481–492.

Cull-Candy, S.G. and Usowicz, M.M. 1987. Multiple-conductance channels activated by excitatory amino acids in cerebellar neurons. Nature 325: 525–528.

Cullheim, S., Fleshman, J.W., Glenn, L.L., and Burke, R.E. 1987. Membrane area and dendritic structure in type-identified triceps surae alpha-motoneurons. J. Comp. Neurol. 255: 68–81.

Cullheim, S. and Kellerth, J.-O. 1978a. A morphological study of the axons and recurrent axon collaterals of cat α-motoneurones supplying different hind-limb muscles. J. Physiol. (Lond.) 281: 285–299.

Cullheim, S. and Kellerth, J.-O. 1978b. A morphological study of axons and recurrent axon collaterals of cat α-motoneurones supplying different functional types of muscle unit. J. Physiol. (Lond.) 281: 301–313.

Cullheim, S. and Kellerth, J.-O. 1981. Two kinds of recurrent inhibition of cat spinal α-motoneurones as differentiated pharmacologically. J. Physiol. (Lond.) 312: 209–224.

Cullheim, S., Kellerth, J.-O., and Conradi, S. 1977. Evidence for direct synaptic interconnections between cat spinal α-motoneurons via the recurrent axon collaterals: A morphological study using intracellular injection of horseradish peroxidase. Brain Res. 132: 1–10.

Curcio, C.A., Allen, K.A., Sloan, K.R., Lerea, C.L., Hurley, J.B., Klock, I.B., and Milam, A.H. 1991. Distribution and morphology of human cone photoreceptors stained with anti-blue opsin. J. Comp. Neurol. 312: 610–624.

Curcio, C.A., Sloan, K.R., Kalina, R.E., and Hendrickson, A.E. 1990. Human photoreceptor topography. J. Comp. Neurol. 292: 497–523.

Curtis, D.R., Duggan, A., Felix, D., and Johnston, G. 1970. GABA, bicuculline and central inhibition. Nature 226: 1222–1224.

Curtis, D.R. and Eccles, J.C. 1960. Synaptic action during and after repetitive stimulation. J. Physiol. (Lond.) 150: 374–398.

Curtis, D.R. and Felix, D. 1971. The effect of bicuculline upon synaptic inhibition in the cerebral and cerebellar cortices of the cat. Brain Res. 34: 301–321.

Curtis, D.R., Gynther, B.D., Beattie, D.T., and Lacey, G. 1995. An in vivo electrophysiological investigation of group Ia afferents fibres and ventral horn terminations in the cat spinal cord. Exp. Brain Res. 106: 403–417.

Curtis, D.R. and Johnston, G.A.R. 1974. Amino acid transmitters in the mammalian central nervous system. Ergeb. Physiol. 69: 98–188.

Curtis, D.R., Lodge, D., Bornstein, J.C., and Peet, M.J. 1981. Selective effects of (−) baclofen on spinal synaptic transmission in the cat. Exp. Brain Res. 42: 158 170.

Curtis, D.R. and Watkins, J. 1963. Acidic amino acids with strong excitatory actions on mammalian neurones. J. Physiol. (Lond.) 166: 1–14.

Cynader, M. and Mitchell, D. 1980. Prolonged sensitivity to monocular deprivation in dark reared cats. J. Neurophysiol. 43: 1041–1054.

Czarkowska, J., Jankowska, E., and Sybirska, E. 1981. Common interneurones in reflex pathways from group Ia and Ib afferents of knee flexors and extensors in the cat. J. Physiol. (Lond.) 319: 367–380.

Dacey, D.M. 1989a. Axon-bearing amacrine cells of the macaque monkey retina. J. Comp. Neurol. 284: 275–293.

Dacey, D.M. 1989b. Monoamine-accumulating ganglion cell type of the cat's retina. J. Comp. Neurol. 288: 59–80.

Dacey, D.M. 1990. The dopaminergic amacrine cell. J. Comp. Neurol. 301: 461–489.

Dacey, D.M. 1993. The mosaic of midget ganglion cells in the human retina. J. Neurosci. 13: 5334–5355.

Dacey, D.M. 1996. Circuitry for color coding in the primate retina. Proc. Natl. Acad. Sci. USA 93: 582–588.

Dacey, D.M. and Brace, S. 1992. A coupled network for parasol but not midget ganglion cells in the primate retina. Vis. Neurosci. 9: 279–290.

Dacey, D.M., Lee, B.B., Stafford, D.K., Pokorny, J., and Smith, V.C. 1996. Horizontal cells of the primate retina: cone specificity without spectral opponency. Science 271: 656–659.

Dacheux, R.F. and Raviola, E. 1986. The rod pathway in the rabbit retina: A depolarizing bipolar and amacrine cell. J. Neurosci. 6: 331–345.

Dacheux, R.F. and Raviola, E. 1995. Light responses from one type of ON-OFF amacrine cells in the rabbit retina. J. Neurophysiol. 74: 2460 2467.

Dale, H H 1935. Pharmacology and nerve endings. Proc. R. Soo. Med. 28: 319 332.

Daniel, H., Hemart, N., Jaillard, D., and Crepel, F. 1993. Long-term depression requires nitric oxide and guanosine 3′-5′ cyclic monophosphate production in cerebellar Purkinje cells. Eur. J. Neurosci. 5: 1079–1082.

Daniel, P. and Whitteridge, D. 1961. The representation of the visual field on the cerebral cortex in monkeys. J. Physiol. (Lond.) 159: 203–221.

Dann, J.F., Buhl, E.H., and Peichl, L. 1988. Postnatal dendritic maturation of alpha and beta ganglion cells in cat retina. J. Neurosci. 8: 1485–1499.

Darian-Smith, I. 1984. The sense of touch: Performance and peripheral neural processes. In: Handbook of Physiology, Section 1: The Nervous System, Vol. III: Sensory Processes, Part 2 (Darian-Smith, I., ed.). Bethesda: American Physiological Society, pp. 739–788.

Datiche, F., Luppi, P.-H., and Cattarelli, M. 1995. Projection from nucleus reuniens thalami to piriform cortex. A tracing study in the rat. Brain Res. Bull. 38: 87–92.

Datiche, F., Luppi, P.-H., and Cattarelli, M. 1996. Serotonergic and non-serotonergic projections from the raphe nuclei to the piriform cortex in the rat: A cholera toxin B subunit (CTb) and 5-HT immunohistochemical study. Brain Res. 671: 27–37.

Davies, C.H., Starkey, S.J., Pozza, M.F., and Collingridge, G.L. 1991. GABA$_B$ autoreceptors regulate the induction of LTP. Nature 349: 609–611.

Davis, B.J., Burd, G.D., and Macrides, F. 1982. Localization of moetionine-enkephalin, substance P and somatostatin immunoreactivities in the main olfactory bulb of the hamster. J. Comp. Neurol. 204: 377–383.

Davis, K.A., Miller, R.L., and Young, E.D. 1996a. Effects of somatosensory and parallel-fiber stimulation on neurons in dorsal cochlear nucleus. J. Neurophysiol. 76: 3012–3024.

Davis, K.A., Miller, R.L., and Young, E.D. 1996b. Presumed cartwheel cells in the cat dorsal cochlear nucleus (DCN) are excited by somatosensory and parallel fiber stimulation. Abstr. Assoc. Res. Otolaryngol. 19: 171.

Daw, N., Rader, R., Robertson, T., and Ariel, M. 1983. Effects of 6-hydroxydopamine on visual deprivation in the kitten striate cortex. J. Neurosci. 3: 907–914.

Deacon, T.W., Eichenbaum, H., Rosenberg, P., and Eckmann, K.W. 1983. Afferent connections of the perirhinal cortex in the rat. J. Comp. Neurol. 220: 168–190.

Degtyarenko, A.M., Simon, E.S., and Burke, R.E. 1996. Differential modulation of disynaptic cutaneous inhibition and excitation in ankle flexor motoneurons during fictive locomotion. J. Neurophysiol. 76: 2972–2985.

Dehay, C., Douglas, R., Martin, K., and Nelson, C. 1991. Excitation by geniculocortical synapses is not "vetoed" at the level of dendritic spines in cat visual cortex. J. Physiol. (Lond.) 440: 723–734.

Deisz, R. and Prince, D. 1989. Frequency-dependent depression of inhibition in the guinea-pig neocortex in vitro by $GABA_B$ receptor feed-back on GABA release. J. Physiol. (Lond.) 412: 513–542.

de la Villa, P., Kurahashi, T., and Kaneko, A. 1995. L-glutamate-induced responses and cGMP-activated channels in retinal bipolar cells dissociated from the cat. J. Neurosci. 15: 3571–3582.

del Cerro, S., Jung, M., and Lynch, G. 1992. Benzodiazepines block long-term potentiation in slices of hippocampus and piriform cortex. Neuroscience 49: 1–6.

de Lima, A.D., Montero, V.M., and Singer, W. 1985. The cholinergic innervation of the visual thalamus: An EM immunocytochemical study. Exp. Brain Res. 59: 206–212.

de Lima, A.D. and Singer, W. 1986. Cholinergic innervation of the cat striate cortex: A choline acetyltransferase immunocytochemical analysis. J. Comp. Neurol. 250: 324–338.

de Lima, A.D. and Singer, W. 1987. The brainstem projection to the lateral geniculate nucleus in the cat: identification of cholinergic and monoaminergic elements. J. Comp. Neurol. 259: 92–121.

DeLong, M.R. 1973. Putamen: Activity of single units during slow and rapid arm movements. Science 179: 1240–1242.

Dembner, J.M. and Greer, C.A. 1994. Topological distribution of olfactory receptor cell axons in olfactory bulb glomeruli: A confocal microscopic analysis of DiI staining. Assoc. Chemorecep. Sci. Abstr. 16: 333.

Demeter, S., Rosene, D.L., and Van Hoesen, G.W. 1985. Interhemispheric pathways of the hippocampal formation, presubiculum and entorhinal and posterior parahippocampal cortices in the rhesus monkey: The structure and organization of the hippocampal commissures. J. Comp. Neurol. 233: 30–47.

Demeulemeester, H., Vandesande, F., Orban, G., Brandon, C., and Vanderhaegen, J. 1988. Heterogeneity of GABAergic cells in cat visual cortex. J. Neurosci 8: 988–1000.

de Monasterio, F.M. 1978. Properties of concentrically organized X and Y ganglion cells of macaque retina. J. Neurophysiol. 41: 1394–1417.

de Monasterio, F.M., Schein, S.J., and McCrane, E.P. 1981. Staining of blue-sensitive cones of the macaque retina by a fluorescent dye. Science 213: 1278–1281.

de Montigny, C. and Lamarre, Y. 1974. Rhythmic activity induced by harmaline in the olivo-cerebellar-bulbar systems of the cat. Brain Res. 53: 81–95.

Deniau, J.M. and Chevalier, G. 1985. Disinhibition as a basic process in the expression of striatal functions. II. The striato-nigral influence on thalamocortical cells of the ventromedial thalamic nucleus. Brain Res. 334: 227–233.

Denk, W., Sugimori, M., and Llinas, R. 1995. Two types of calcium response limited to single spines in cerebellar Purkinje cells. Proc. Natl. Acad. Sci. USA 92: 8279–8282.

Denk, W., Yuste, R., Svoboda, K., and Tank, D. 1996. Imaging caclium dynamics in dendritic spines. Curr. Opin. Neurobiol. 6: 372–378.

Denny-Brown, D. 1929. On the nature of postural reflexes. Proc. R. Soc. Lond. B Biol. Sci. 104: 252–301.

Denny-Brown, D. 1949. Interpretation of the electromyogram. Arch. Neurol. Psychiatry 61:99–128.

Dent, J.A., Galvin, N.J., Stanfield, B.B., and Cowan, W.M. 1983. The mode of temination of the hypothalamic projection to the dentate gyrus: An EM autoradiographic study. Brain Res. 258: 1–10.

de Olmos, J., Hardy, H., and Heimer, L. 1978. The afferent connections of the main and the accessory olfactory bulb formations in the rat: An experimental HRP-study. J. Comp. Neurol. 181: 213–244.

De Quidt, M.E. and Emson, P.C. 1986. Distribution of neuropeptide Y-like immunoreactivity in the rat central nervous system. II. Immunocytochemical analysis. Neuroscience 18: 545–618.

Derrick, B.E., Rodriguez, S.B., Lieberman, D.N., and Martinez, J. 1992. Mu opioid receptors are associated with the induction of hippocampal mossy fiber long-term potentiation. J. Pharmacol. Exp. Ther. 263: 725–733.

Derrington, A.M. and Lennie, P. 1982. The influence of temporal frequency and adaptation level on receptive field organization of retinal ganglion cells in cat. J. Physiol. (Lond.) 333: 343–366.

Derrington, A.M., Lennie, P., and Wright, M.J. 1979. The mechanism of peripherally evoked responses in retinal ganglion cells. J. Physiol. (Lond.) 289: 299–310.

de Ruyter van Steveninck, R. and Laughlin, S.B. 1996. The rate of information transfer at graded-potential synapses. Nature 379: 642–645.

Deschênes, M. 1981. Dendritic spikes induced in fast pyramidal tract neurons by thalamic stimulation. Exp. Brain Res. 43: 304–308.

Deschênes, M., Bourassa, J., Doan, V.D., and Parent, A. 1996. A single-cell study of the axonal projections arising from the posterior intralaminar thalamic nuclei in the rat. Eur. J. Neurosci. 8: 329–343.

Desmedt, J.E. and Godaux, E. 1977. Ballistic contractions in man: Characteristic recruitment pattern of single motor units of the tibialis anterior muscle. J. Physiol. (Lond.) 264: 673–694.

Desmond, N. and Levy, W. 1990. Morphological correlates of long-term potentiation imply the modification of existing synapses, not synaptogenesis, in the hippocampal dentate gyrus. Synapse 5: 139–143.

Destombes, J., Horcholle-Bossavit, G., and Thiesson, D. 1992. Distribution of glycinergic terminals on lumbar motoneurons of the adult cat—An ultrastructural study. Brain Res. 599: 353–360.

Deuchars, J. and Thomson, A.M. 1996. CA1 pyramid-pyramid connections in rat hippocampus in vitro: Dual intracellular recordings with biocytin filling. Neuroscience 74: 1009–1018.

Devor, M. 1976. Fiber trajectories of olfactory bulb efferents in the hamster. J. Comp. Neurol. 166: 31–48.

DeYoe, E.A., Felleman, D.J., Van Essen, D.C., and McClendon, E. 1994. Multiple processing streams in occipitotemporal visual cortex. Nature 371: 151–154.

Diamond, M.E., Armstrong-James, M., Budway, M.J., and Ebner, F.F. 1992. somatic sensory responses in the rostral sector of the posterior group (POm) and in the ventral posterior medial nucleus (VPM) of the rat thalamus: Dependence on the barrel field cortex. J. Comp. Neurol. 319: 66–84.

DiFiglia, M. and Aronin, N. 1982. Ultrastructural features of immunoreactive somatostatin neurons in the rat caudate nucleus. J. Neurosci. 2: 1267–1274.

DiFiglia, M. and Carey, J. 1986. Large neurons in the primate neostriatum examined with the combined Golgi-electron microscopic method. J. Comp. Neurol. 244: 36–52.

DiFiglia, M., Pasik, P., and Pasik, T. 1976. A Golgi study of neuronal types in the neostriatum of monkeys. Brain Res. 114: 245–256.

DiFiglia, M. and Rafols, J.A. 1988. Synaptic organization of the globus pallidus. J. Electron Microsc. Tech. 10: 247–263.

DiFrancesco, D. 1985. The cardiac hyperpolarization-activated current I_f: Origins and developments. Prog. Biophys. Mol. Biol. 46: 163–183.

Dinerman, J.L., Dawson, t.M., Schell, M.J., Snowman, A., and Snyder, S.H. 1994. Endothelial nitric oxide synthase localized to hippocampal pyramidal cells: Implications for synaptic plasticity. Proc. Natl. Acad. Sci. USA 91:4214–4218.

Dingledine, R. and Kelly, J.S. 1977. Brain stem stimulation and the acetylcholine-evoked inhibition of neurones in the feline nucleus reticularis thalami. J. Physiol. (Lond.) 271: 135–154.

Dodge, F.A. 1979. The nonuniform excitability of central neurons as exemplified by a model of the spinal motoneuron. In The Neurosciences: Fourth Study Program (Schmitt, F.O., eds.). Cambridge: MIT Press, pp. 439–455.

Dodt, H.U. and Misgeld, U. 1986. Muscarinic slow excitation and muscarinic inhibition of synaptic transmission in the rat neostriatum. J. Physiol. (Lond.) 380: 593–608.

Dolleman-Van der Weel, M.J. and Witter, M.P. 1992. Organization of nucleus reuniens thalami projections to the hippocampal region, studied by multiple retrograde tracing in the rat. Eur. J. Neurosci. Suppl. 5: 69.

Dolphin, A.C. and Scott, R.H. 1986. Inhibition of calcium currents in cultured rat dorsal root ganglion neurones by (−)-baclofen. Br. J. Pharmacol. 88: 213–220.

Domroese, M.E. and Haberly, L.B. 1995. NMDA-dependent induction of epileptiform activity in piriform cortex in vitro does not involve kinases that are required for LTP. Soc. Neurosci. Abstr. 21: 982.

Domroese, M.E. and Haberly, L.B. 1996. Dual origin of slow regenerative potentials in the endopiriform nucleus. Soc. Neurosci. Abstr. 22: 2103.

Doucet, J.R., Gillespie, M.B., and Ryugo, D.K. 1996. Ventral cochlear nucleus projections to the dorsal cochlear nucleus. Abstr. Assoc. Res. Otolaryngol. 19: 166.

Doucette, R. 1993. Glial cells in the nerve fiber layer of the main olfactory bulb of embryonic and adult mammals. Microsc. Res. Tech. 24: 113–130.

Douglas, R., Koch, C., Mahowald, M., Martin, K.A.C., and Suarez, H.H. 1995. Recurrent excitation in neocortical circuits. Science 269: 981–985.

Douglas, R. and Martin, K.A.C. 1991. A functional microcircuit for cat visual cortex. J. Physiol. (Lond.) 440: 735–769.

Douglas, R. and Martin, K.A.C. 1993. Exploring cortical microcircuits: A combined anatomical, physiological, computational approach. In: Single Neuron Computation (McKenna, J.D.T. and Zornetzer, S., eds.). Orlando, FL: Academic Press, pp. 381–412.

Douglas, R., Martin, K.A.C., and Whitteridge, D. 1988. Selective responses of visual cortical cells do not depend on shunting inhibition. Nature 332: 642–644.

Douglas, R., Martin, K.A.C., and Whitteridge, D. 1989. A canonical microcircuit for neocortex. Neural Comput. 1: 480–488.

Dowling, J.E. 1986. Dopamine: A retinal neuromodulator? Trends Neurosci. 9: 236–240.

Dowling, J.E. and Boycott, B.B. 1965. Neural connections of the retina: Fine structure of the inner plexiform layer. Cold Spring Harb. Symp. Quant. Biol. 30: 393–402.

Dowling, J.E. and Boycott, B.B. 1966. Organization of the primate retina: Electron microscopy. Proc. R. Soc. Lond. B Biol. Sci. 166: 80–111.

Dowling, J.E. and Cowan, W.M. 1966. An electron microscope study of normal and degenerating centrifugal fiber terminals in the pigeon retina. Z. Zellforsch. Mikrosk. Anat. 71: 14–28.

Dreifuss, J., Kelly, J., and Krnjevic, K. 1969. Cortical inhibition and γ-aminobutyric acid. Exp. Brain Res. 9: 137–154.

Dubé, L., Smith, A.D., and Bolam, J.P. 1988. Identification of synaptic terminals of thalamic or cortical origin in contact with distinct medium-size spiny neurons in the rat neostriatum. J. Comp. Neurol. 267: 455–471.

Dubin, H. 1976. The inner plexiform layer of the vertebrate retina: A quantitative and comparative electron microscopic analysis. J. Comp. Neurol. 140: 479–506.

Dulac, C. and Axel, R. 1995. A novel family of genes encoding putative pheromone receptors in mammals. Cell 83: 195–206.

Dunlap, K. and Fischbach, G.D. 1981. Neurotransmitters decrease the calcium conductance activated by depolarization of embryonic chick sensory neurons. J. Physiol. (Lond.) 317: 519–535.

Dupont, J.L., Crepel, F., and Delhaye-Bouchaud, N. 1979. Influence of bicuculline and picrotoxin on reversal properties of excitatory synaptic potentials in cerebellar Purkinje cells of the rat. Brain Res. 173: 577–580.

Durand, D. 1984. The somatic shunt cable model for neurons. Biophys. J. 46: 645–653.

Dutar, P. and Nicoll, R.A. 1988a. A physiological role for GABA_B receptors in the central nervous system. Nature 332: 156–158.

Dutar, P. and Nicoll, R.A. 1988b. Pre- and postsynaptic GABA_B receptors in the hippocampus have different pharmacological properties. Neuron 1: 585–591.

Dykes, R.W. 1983. Parallel processing of somatosensory information: A theory. Brain Res. Rev. 6: 47–115.

Easter, S.S. and Stuermer, C. 1984. An evaluation of the hypothesis of shifting terminals in goldfish optic tectum. J. Neurosci. 4: 1052–1063.

Eblen, F. and Graybiel, A.M. 1995. Highly restricted origin of prefrontal cortical inputs to striosomes in the macaque monkey. J. Neurosci. 15: 5999–6013.

Eccles, J. 1957. The Physiology of Nerve Cells. Baltimore: Johns Hopkins Press.

Eccles, J.C. 1964. The Physiology of Synapses. New York: Academic Press.

Eccles, J.C., Eccles, R.M., and Lundberg, A. 1957. The convergence of monosynaptic excitatory afferents onto many different species of alpha-motoneurones. J. Physiol. (Lond.) 137: 22–50.

Eccles, J.C., Eccles, R.M., and Lundberg, A. 1960. Types of neurone in and around the intermediate nucleus of the lumbosacral cord. J. Physiol. (Lond.) 154: 89–114.

Eccles, J.C., Fatt, P., and Koketsu, K. 1954. Cholinergic and inhibitory synapses in a pathway from motor-axon collaterals to motoneurones. J. Physiol. (Lond.) 126: 524–562.

Eccles, J.C., Fatt, P., and Landgren, S. 1956. The central pathway for the direct inhibitory action of impulses in the largest afferent fibers to muscle. J. Neurophysiol. 19: 75–98.

Eccles, J.C., Llinàs, R., and Sasaki, K. 1966a. The excitatory synaptic action of climbing fibers on the Purkinje cells of the cerebellum. J. Physiol. (Lond.) 182: 268–296.

Eccles, J.C., Llinàs, R., and Sasaki, K. 1996b. The inhibitory interneurons within the cerebellar cortex. Exp. Brain Res. 1: 1–16.

Eccles, J.C., Llinàs, R., and Sasaki, K. 1966c. Parallel fiber stimulation and the responses induced thereby in the Purkinje cells of the cerebellum. Exp. Brain Res. 1: 17–39.

Eccles, J.C., Llinàs, R., and Sasaki, K. 1966d. The mossy fibre-granule cell relay of the cerebellum and its inhibitory control. Exp. Brain Res. 1: 82–101.

Eccles, R.M. and Lundberg, A. 1958. Integrative pattern of Ia synaptic actions on motoneurones of hip and knee muscles. J. Physiol. (Lond.) 144: 271–298.

Eccles, R.M. and Lundberg, A. 1959. Synaptic action in motoneurones by afferents which may evoke the flexion reflex. Arch. Ital. Biol. 97: 199–221.

Eckenstein, F. and Baughman, R. 1984. Two types of cholinergic innervation in the cortex, one co-localised with vasoactive intestinal polypeptide. Nature 309: 153–155.

Eckert, M.P. and Buchsbaum, G. 1993a. Efficient coding of natural time varying images in the early visual system. Phil. Trans. R. Soc. (Lond.) B 339: 385–395.

Eckert, M.P. and Buchsbaum, G. 1993b. Effect of tracking strategies on the velocity structure of two-dimensional image sequences. J. Opt. Soc. Am. 10: 1582–1585.

Edwards, C. and Ottoson, D. 1958. The site of impulse initiation in a nerve cell of a crustacean stretch receptor. J. Physiol. (Lond.) 143: 138–148.

Edwards, F.R., Redman, S.J., and Walmsley, B. (1976) Statistical fluctuations in charge transfer at Ia synapses on spinal motoneurones. J. Physiol. (Lond.) 259: 665–688.

Eeckman, F.H. and Freeman, W.J. 1990. Correlations between unit firing and EEG in the rat olfactory system. Brain Res. 528: 238–244.

Eichenbaum, H. 1994. The hippocampal system and the declarative memory in humans and animals: Experimental analysis and historical origins. In: Memory Systems (Schacter, D.L. and Tylving, E., eds.). Cambridge, MA: MIT Press, pp. 147–201.

Ekstrand, J.J. and Haberly, L.B. 1995. GABAergic neurons in the molecular layer of piriform (olfactory) cortex have lamina-specific axonal arbors. Soc. Neurosci. Abstr. 21: 1186.

Ekstrand, J.J., Johnson, D.M.G., Feig, S.L., and Haberly, L.B. 1996. Cajal-Retzius cells in anterior piriform cortex mediate fast feedforward inhibition in a large area of the piriform cortex, anterior olfactory nucleus, and olfactory tubercle. Soc. Neurosci. Abstr. 22: 1824.

Emonet-Denand, F., Jami, L., and Laporte, Y. 1975. Skeletofusimotor axons in hind-limb muscles of the cat. J. Physiol. (Lond.) 249: 153–166.

Eng, D.L. and Kocsis, J.D. 1987. Activity dependent changes in extracellular potassium and excitability in turtle olfactory nerve. J. Neurophysiol. 57: 740–754.

Engberg, I. and Marshall, K.C. 1979. Reversal potentials for Ia excitatory post synaptic potentials in spinal motoneurons of cats. Neuroscience 4: 1583–1591.

Ennis, M., Zimmer, L.A. and Shipley, M.T. 1996. Olfactory nerve stimulation activates rat mitral cells via NMDA and non-NMDA receptors in vitro. Neuroreport 7: 989–992.

Enoch, J.M. 1981. Retinal receptor orientation and photoreceptor optics. In: Vertebrate Photoreceptor Optics (Enoch, J.M. and Tobey, F.L.J., eds.). Berlin: Springer-Verlag, pp. 127–168.

Enroth-Cugell, C. and Robson, J.G. 1966. The contrast sensitivity of retinal ganglion cells of the cat. J. Physiol. (Lond.) 187: 517–552.

Enz, R., Brandstätter, J.H., Wässle, H., and Bormann, J. 1996. Immunocytochemical localization of GABA$_C$ receptor rho subunits in the mammalian retina. J. Neurosci. 16: 4479–4490.

Erişir, A., Van Horn, S.C., Bickford, M.E., and Sherman, S.M. 1977a. Immunocytochemistry and distribution of parabrachial terminals in the lateral geniculate nucleus of the cat: A comparison with corticogeniculate terminals. J. Comp. Neurol. 377: 535–549.

Erişir, A., Van Horn, S.C., and Sherman, S.M. 1977b. Relative numbers of cortical and brainstem inputs to the lateral geniculate nucleus. Proc. Natl. Acad. Sci. USA 94: 1517–1520.

Esclapez, M., Tillakaratne, N.J.K., Tobin, A.J., and Houser, C.R. 1993. Comparative localization of mRNAs encoding two forms of glutamic acid decarboxylase with nonradioactive in situ hybridization methods. J. Comp. Neurol. 331: 339–362.

Euler, T., Schneider, H., and Wässle, H. 1996. Glutamate responses of bipolar cells in a slice preparation of the rat retina. J. Neurosci. 16: 2934–2944.

Evans, E.F. and Nelson, P.G. 1973. The responses of single neurons in the cochlear nucleus of the cat as a function of their location and the anaesthetic state. Exp. Brain Res. 17: 402–427.

Ezeh, P.I., Davis, L.M., and Scott, J.W. 1995. Regional distribution of rat electroolfactogram. J. Neurophysiol. 73: 2207–2220.

Fadiga, E. and Brookhart, J.M. 1960. Monosynaptic activation of different portions of the motor neuron membrane. Am. J. Physiol. 198: 693–703.

Fahrenbach, W.H. 1985. Anatomical circuitry of lateral inhibition in the eye of the horseshoe crab, *Limulus polyphemus*. Proc. R. Soc. Lond. [B] Biol. Sci. 225: 219–249.

Fallon, J.H. and Leslie, F.M. 1986. Distribution of dynorphin and enkephalin peptides in the rat brain. J. Comp. Neurol. 249: 293–336.

Famiglietti, E.V. 1991. Synaptic organization of starburst amacrine cells in rabbit retina: Analysis of serial thin sections by electron microscopy and graphic reconstruction. J. Comp. Neurol. 309: 40–70.

Famiglietti, E.V. 1992a. Dendritic co-stratification of ON and ON-OFF directionally selective ganglion cells with starburst amacrine cells in rabbit retina. J. Comp. Neurol. 324: 322–335.

Famiglietti, E.V. 1992b. Polyaxonal amacrine cells of rabbit retina: Size and distribution of PA1 cells. J. Comp. Neurol. 316: 406–421.

Famiglietti, E.V. and Kolb, H. 1976. Structural basis for ON- and OFF-center responses in retinal ganglion cells. Science 194: 193–195.

Famiglietti, E.V., Jr. and Peters, A. 1972. The synaptic glomerulus and the intrinsic neuron in the dorsal lateral geniculate nucleus of the cat. J. Comp. Neurol. 144: 285–334.

Farbman, A.I. 1986. Prenatal development of mammalian olfactory receptor cells. Chem. Senses 11: 3–18.

Farbman, A.I. 1994. Developmental biology of olfactory sensory neurons. Semin. Cell Biol. 5: 3–10.

Fatt, P. 1957. Sequence of events in synaptic activation of a motoneurone. J. Neurophysiol. 20: 61–80.

Fatt, P. and Katz, B. 1953. The effect of inhibitory nerve impulses on a crustacean muscle fibre. J. Physiol. (Lond.) 121: 374–389.

Feldman, A. and Orlovsky, G. 1975. Activity of interneurons mediating reciprocal Ia inhibition during locomotion. Brain Res. 84: 181–194.

Feldman, M.L. 1984. Morphology of the neocortical pyramidal neuron. In: Cerebral Cortex, Vol. 1: Cellular Components of the Cerebral Cortex (Peters, A. and Jones, E.G., eds.). New York: Plenum Press, pp. 123–200.

Feliciano, M., Saldaña, E., and Mugnaini, E. 1995. Direct projections from the rat primary auditory neocortex to nucleus salgulum, paralemniscal regions, superior olivary complex and cochlear nucleus. Auditory Neurosci. 1: 287–308.

Felleman, D.J. and van Essen, D.C. 1991. Distributed hierarchical processing in the primate cerebral cortex. Cereb. Cortex 1: 1–47.

Feller, M.B., Wellis, D.P., Stellwagen, D., Werblin, F.S., and Shatz, C.J. 1996. Requirement of cholinergic synaptic transmission in the propagation if spontaneous retinal waves. Science 272: 1182–1187.

Feng, J.J., Kuwada, S., Ostapoff, E.M., Batra, R., and Morest, D.K. 1994. A physiological and structural study of neuron types in the cochlear nucleus. I. Intracellular responses to acoustic stimulation and current injection. J. Comp. Neurol. 346: 1–18.

Fernandez, C. and Karapas, F. 1967. The course and termination of the striae of Monakow and Held in the cat. J. Comp. Neurol. 131: 371–386.

Ferster, D. 1988. Spatially opponent excitation and inhibition in simple cells of the cat visual cortex. J. Neurosci 8: 1172–1180.

Ferster, D., Chung, S., and Wheat, H. 1996. Orientation selectivity of thalamic input to simple cells of cat visual cortex. Nature 380: 249–252.

Ferster, D. and Jagadeesh, B. 1992. EPSP-IPSP interactions in cat visual cortex studied with in vivo whole-cell patch recording. J. Neurosci 12: 1262–1274.

Ferster, D. and Koch, C. 1987. Neuronal connections underlying orientation selectivity in cat visual cortex. Trends Neurosci. 10: 487–492.

Fetcho, J.R. 1987. A review of the organization and evolution of motoneurons innervating the axial musculature of vertebrates. Brain Res. Rev. 12: 243–280.

Fifkova, E. and Anderson, C. 1981. Stimulation induced changes in the dimensions of stalks of dendritic spines in the dentate molecular layer. Exp. Neurol 74: 621–627.

Fifkova, E. and Delay, R. 1982. Cytoplasmic actin in dendritic spines as possible mediator of synaptic plasticity. J. Cell Biol. 95: 345–350.

Fifkova, E.F. and Harreveld, A.v. 1977. Long-lasting morphological changes in the dendritic spines of dentate granular cells following stimulation of the entorhinal area. J. Neurocytol. 6: 211–230.

Finch, D.M. and Babb, T.L. 1980. Inhibition in subicular and entorhinal principal neurons in response to electrical stimulation of the fornix and hippocampus. Brain Res. 196: 89–98.

Finch, D.M. and Babb, T.L. 1981. Demonstration of caudally directed hippocampal efferents in the rat by intracellular injection of horseradish peroxidase. Brain Res. 214: 405–410.

Finch, D.M., Nowlin, N.L., and Babb, T.L. 1983. Demonstration of axonal projections of neurons in the rat hippocampus and subiculum by intracellular injection of HRP. Brain Res. 271: 201–216.

Finkel, A.S. and Redman, S.J. 1983. The synaptic current evoked in cat spinal motoneurones by impulses in single group Ia axons. J. Physiol. (Lond.) 342: 615–632.

Fisher, S.K. and Boycott, B.B. 1974. Synaptic connexions made by horizontal cells within the outer plexiform layer of the retina of the cat and the rabbit. Proc. R. Soc. (Lond.) B 186: 317–331.

Fitzpatrick, D., Conley, M., Luppino, G., Matelli, M., and Diamond, I.T. 1988. Cholinergic projections from the midbrain reticular formation and the parabigeminal nucleus to the lateral geniculate nucleus in the tree shrew. J. Comp. Neurol. 272: 43–67.

Fitzpatrick, D., Diamond, I.T., and Raczkowski, D. 1989. Cholinergic and monoaminergic innervation of the cat's thalamus: Comparison of the lateral geniculate nucleus with other principal sensory nuclei. J. Comp. Neurol. 288: 647–675.

Fitzpatrick, D., Lund, J.S., Schmechel, D.E., and Towles, A.C. 1987. Distribution of GABAergic neurons and axon terminals in the macaque striate cortex. J. Comp. Neurol. 264: 73–91.

Fitzpatrick, D., Penny, G.R., and Schmechel, D.E. 1984. Glutamic acid decarboxylase-immunoreactive neurons and terminals in the lateral geniculate nucleus of the cat. J. Neurosci. 4: 1809 1829.

Flaherty, A.W. and Graybiel, A.M. 1991. Corticostriatal transformations in the primate somatosensory system. Projections from physiologically mapped body-part representations. J. Neurophysiol. 66: 1249–1263.

Flaherty, A.W. and Graybiel, A.M. 1994. Input-output organization of the sensorimotor striatum in the squirrel monkey. J. Neurosci. 14: 599–610.

Fleshman, J.W., Lev-Tov, A., and Burke, R.E. 1984. Peripheral and central control of flexor digitorum longus and flexor hallucis longus motoneurons: The synaptic basis of functional diversity. Exp. Brain Res. 54: 133–149.

Fleshman, J.W., Munson, J.B., and Sypert, G.W. 1981a. Homonymous projection of individual group Ia-fibers to physiologically characterized medial gastrocnemius motoneurons in the cat. J. Neurophysiol. 46: 1339–1348.

Fleshman, J.W., Munson, J.B., Sypert, G.W., and Friedman, W.A. 1981b. Rheobase, input resistance, and motor-unit type in medial gastrocnemius motoneurons in the cat. J. Neurophysiol. 46: 1326–1338.

Fleshman, J.W., Rudomin, P., and Burke, R.E. 1988a. Supraspinal control of a short-latency cutaneous pathway to hindlimb motoneurons. Exp. Brain Res. 69: 449–459.

Fleshman, J.W., Segev, I., and Burke, R.E. 1988b. Electrotonic architecture of type-identified alpha-motoneurons in the cat spinal cord. J. Neurophysiol. 60: 60–85.

Floris, A., Diño, M., Jacobowitz, D.M., and Mugnaini, E. 1994. The unipolar brush cells of the rat cerebellar cortex and cochlear nucleus are calretinin-positive: A study by light and electron microscopic immunocytochemistry. Anat. Embryol. 189: 495–520.

Fonnum, F., Karlsen, R.L., Malthe Sorenssen, D., Skrede, K.K., and Walaas, I. 1979. Localization of neurotransmitters, particularly glutamate, in hippocampus, septum, nucleus accumbens and superior colliculus. Prog. Brain Res. 51: 167–191.

Fonnum, F., Storm-Mathisen, J., and Walberg, F. 1970. Glutamate decarboxylase in inhibitory neurons. A study of the enzyme in Purkinje cells axons and boutons in the cat. Brain Res. 20: 259–270.

Fonnum, F. and Walberg, F. 1973. An estimation of the concentration of gamma-aminobutyric acid and glutamate decarboxylase in the inhibitory Purkinje axon terminals in the cat. Brain Res. 54: 115–127.

Foote, S.L., Bloom, F.E., and Aston-Jones, G. 1983. Nucleus locus ceruleus: New evidence of anatomical and physiological specificity. Physiol. Rev. 63: 844–914.

Forssberg, H. 1979. Stumbling corrective reaction: A phase-dependent compensatory reaction during locomotion. J. Neurophysiol. 42: 936–953.

Fox, C.A., Andrade, A.N., Hillman, D.E., and Schwyn, R.C. 1971. The spiny neurons in the primate striatum: A Golgi and electron microscopic study. J. Hirnforsch. 13: 181–201.

Fox, C.A., Hillman, D.E., Seigesmund, K.A., and Dutta, C.R. 1967. The primate cerebellar cortex: A Golgi study and electron microscopical study. In: Progress in Brain Research, Vol. 25 (Fox, C.A. and Sneider, R., eds.). Amsterdam: Elsevier, pp. 174–225.

Fox, C.A. and Rafols, J.A. 1976. The striatal efferents in the globus pallidus and in the substantia nigra. In: The Basal Ganglia (Yahr, M.D., ed.). New York: Raven Press, pp. 37–55.

Fox, K., Sato, H., and Daw, N. 1990. The effect of varying stimulus intensity on NMDA-receptor activity in cat visual cortex. J. Neurophysiol. 64: 1413–1429.

Fox, S., Krnjevic, K., Morris, M.E., Puil, E., and Werman, R. 1978. Action of baclofen on mammalian synaptic transmission. Neuroscience 3: 495–515.

Frank, B.D. and Hollyfield, J.G. 1987. Retinal ganglion cell morphology in the frog, *Rana pipiens*. J. Comp. Neurol. 266: 413–434.

Frank, K. 1959. Basic mechanisms of synaptic transmission in the central nervous system. IRE Trans. Med. Electr. ME-6: 85–88.

Frank, K. and Fuortes, M.G.F. 1956. Stimulation of motoneurones with intracellular electrodes. J. Physiol. (Lond.) 134: 451–460.

Frank, K. and Fuortes, M.G.F. 1957. Presynaptic and postsynaptic inhibition of monosynaptic reflexes. Fed. Proc. 16: 39–40.

Frazier-Cierpial, L. and Brunjes, P.C. 1989. Early postnatal cellular proliferation and survival in the olfactory bulb rostral migratory stream of normal and unilateral odor-deprived rats. J. Comp. Neurol. 289: 481–492.

Fredens, K., Steengaard-Pedersen, K., and Larsson, L.I. 1984. Localization of enkephalin and cholecystokinin immunoreactivities in the perforant path terminal fields of the rat hippocampal formation. Brain Res. 304: 255–263.

Frederickson, R.C.A., Neuss, M., Morzorati, S.L., and McBride, W.J. 1978. A comparison of inhibitory effects of taurine and GABA on identified Purkinje cells and other neurons in the cerebellar cortex of the rat. Brain Res. 145: 117–126.

Freed, M.A., Kier, C.K., Buchsbaum, G., Smith, R.G., and Sterling, P. 1997. How the spatio-temporal distribution of transmitter quanta determines beta ganglion cell sensitivity. (Submitted).

Freed, M.A. and Nelson, R. 1994. Conductances evoked by light in the ON-β ganglion cell of the cat retina. Vis. Neurosci. 11: 261–269.

Freed, M.A., Pflug, R., Kolb, H., and Nelson, R. 1996. ON-OFF amacrine cells in cat retina. J. Comp. Neurol. 364: 556–566.

Freed, M.A., Smith, R.G., and Sterling, P. 1987. Rod bipolar array in the cat retina: Pattern of input from rods and GABA-accumulating amacrine cells. J. Comp. Neurol. 266: 445–455.

Freed, M.A., Smith, R.G., and Sterling, P. 1992. Computational model of the ON-alpha ganglion cell receptive field based on bipolar circuitry. Proc. Natl. Acad. Sci. USA 89: 236–240.

Freed, M.A. and Sterling, P. 1988. The ON-alpha ganglion cell of the cat retina and its presynaptic cell types. J. Neurosci. 8: 2303–2320.

Freeman, W.J. 1974. Relation of glomerular neuronal activity to glomerular transmission attenuation. Brain Res. 65: 91–107.

Freeman, W.J. 1975. Mass Action in the Nervous System. New York: Academic Press.

Freeman, W.J. 1978. Spatial properties of an EEG event in the olfactory bulb and cortex. Electroencephalogr. Clin. Neurophysiol. 44: 586–605.

Freeman, W.J. 1983. Dynamics of image formation by nerve cell assemblies. In: Synergetics of the Brain (Basar, E., Flohr, H., and Mandell, A.J., eds.). New York: Springer-Verlag, pp. 102–121.

Freeman, W.J. and Grajski, K.A. 1987. Relation of olfactory EEG to behavior factor analysis. Behav. Neurosci. 101: 766–777.

Frerking, M. and Wilson, M. 1996. Effects of variance in mini amplitude on stimulus-evoked release: A comparison of two models. Biophys. J. 70: 2078–2091.

Freund, T.F. and Antal M., 1988. GABA-containing neurons in the septum control inhibitory interneurons in the hippocampus. Nature 336: 170–173.

Freund, T.F. and Buzsaki, G. 1996b. Interneurons of the hippocampus. Hippocampus 6: 345–470.

Freund, T.F., Gulyás, A.I., Acsády, L., Görcs, T., and Tóth, K. 1990. Serotonergic control of the hippocampus via local inhibitory interneurons. Proc. Natl. Acad. Sci. USA 87: 8501–8505.

Freund, T.F., Martin, K.A.C., Smith, A.D., and Somogyi, P. 1983. Glutamate decarboxylase-immunoreactive terminals of Golgi impregnated axo-axonic neurons and of presumed basket neurons in synaptic contact with pyramidal neurons of the cat's visual cortex. J. Comp. Neurol. 221: 263–278.

Freund, T.F., Martin, K.A.C., Somogyi, P., and Whitteridge, D. 1985. Innervation of cat visual areas 17 and 18 by physiologically identified x- and y-type thalamic afferents. II. Identification of postsynaptic targets by GABA immunocytochemistry and Golgi impregnation. J. Comp. Neurol. 242: 275–291.

Freund, T.F., Powell, J.F., and Smith, A.D. 1984. Tyrosine hydroxylase-immunoreactive boutons in synaptic contact with identified striatonigral neurons, with particular reference to dendritic spines. Neuroscience 13: 1189–1215.

Friedman, B. and Price, J.L. 1984. Fiber systems in the olfactory bulb and cortex. A study in adult and developing rats, using the Timm method with the light and electron microscope. J. Comp. Neurol. 223: 88–109.

Friedman, W.A., Sypert, G.W., Munson, J.B., and Fleshman, J.W. 1981. Recurrent inhibition in type-identified motoneurons. J. Neurophysiol. 46: 1349–1359.

Friedrich, R. and Korsching, S.I. 1996. Representation of odorant information by spatial afferent activity patterns in the zebrafish olfactory bulb. Soc. Nuerosci. Abstr. 22: 1072.

Frisina, R.D., Smith, R.L., and Chamberlain, S.C. 1990. Encoding of amplitude modulation in the gerbil cochlear nucleus: I. A hierarchy of enhancement. Hear. Res. 44: 99–122.

Fritschy, J.-M. and Mohler, H. 1995. GABA$_A$-receptor heterogeneity in the adult rat brain: Differential regional and cellular distribution of seven major subunits. J. Comp. Neurol 359: 154–194.

Frotscher, M., Kugler, P., Misgeld, U., and Zilles, K. 1988. Neurotransmission in the hippocampus. In: Advances in Anatomy, Embryology, and Cell Biology (Beck, F., Hild, W., Kriz, W., Ortmann, R., Pauly, J.E., and Schiebler, T.H., eds.). Berlin: Springer-Verlag, pp.

Frotscher, M. and Leranth, C. 1985. Cholinergic innervation of the rat hippocampus as revealed by choline acetyltransferase immunocytochemistry. J. Comp. Neurol. 239: 237–246.

Frotscher, M. and Zimmer, J. 1983. Commisural fibers terminated on non-pyramidal neurons in the guinea pig hippocampus–A combined Golgi/EM degeneration study. Brain Res. 265: 289–293.

Fujita, I., Tanaka, K., Ito, M., and Cheng, K. 1992. Columns for visual features in monkey inferotemporal cortex. Nature 360: 343–346.

Funke, K., Pape, H.-C., and Eysel, U.T. 1993. Noradrenergic modulation of retinogeniculate transmission in the cat. J Physiol (Lond.) 463: 169–191.

Fuortes, M., Frank, K., and Becker, M. 1957. Steps in the production of motoneuron spikes. J. Gen. Physiol. 40: 735–752.

Fuster, J.M. 1985. The prefrontal cortex and temporal integration. In: Cerebral Cortex (Jones, E.G. and Peters, A., eds.). New York: Plenum, pp. 151–177.

Fyffe, R.E.W. 1984. Afferent fibers. In: Handbook of the Spinal Cord, Vol. 1: Physiology (Davidoff, R.E., ed.). New York: Marcel Dekker, pp. 79–136.

Fyffe, R.E.W. 1990. Evidence for separate morphological classes of Renshaw cells in the cat's spinal cord. Brain Res. 536: 301–304.

Fyffe, R.E.W. 1991a. Glycine-like immunoreactivity in synaptic boutons of identified inhibitory interneurons in the mammalian spinal cord. Brain Res. 547: 175–179.

Fyffe, R.E.W. 1991b. Spatial distribution of recurrent inhibitory synapses on spinal motoneurons in the cat. J. Neurophysiol. 65: 1134–1149.

Fyffe, R.E.W. and Light, A.R. 1984. The ultrastructure of group Ia afferent fiber synapses in the lumbosacral spinal cord of the cat. Brain Res. 300: 201–209.

Gaarskjaer, F.B. 1978a. Organization of the mossy fiber system of the rat studied in extended hippocampi. I. Terminal area related to number of granule and pyramidal cells. J. Comp. Neurol. 178: 49–72.

Gaarskjaer, F.B. 1978b. Organization of the mossy fiber system of the rat studied in extended hippocampi. II. Experimental analysis of fiber distribution with silver impregnation methods. J. Comp. Neurol. 178: 73–88.

Gall, C. 1984. Ontogeny of dynorphin-like immunoreactivity in the hippocampal formation of the rat. Brain Res. 307: 327–331.

Gall, C., Brecha, N., Karten, H.J., and Chang, K.J. 1981. Localization of enkephalin-like immunoreactivity to identified axonal and neuronal populations of the rat hippocampus. J. Comp. Neurol. 198: 335–350.

Galupo, M.P. and Stripling, J.S. 1995. All-or-none threshold for expression of LTP in the olfactory bulb and piriform cortex: Modulation by behavioral state. Soc. Neurosci. Abstr. 21: 1185.

Gamble, E. and Koch, C. 1987. The dynamics of free calcium in dendritic spines in response to repetitive synaptic input. Science 236: 1311–1315.

Gan, L., Xiang, M., Zhou, L., Wagner, D.S., Klein, W.H., and Nathans, J. 1996. POU domain factor Brn-3b is required for the development of a large set of retinal ganglion cells. Proc. Natl. Acad. Sci. USA 93: 3920–3925.

Garnett, R. and Stephens, J.A. 1981. Changes in the recruitment threshold of motor units produced by cutaneous stimulation in man. J. Physiol. (Lond.) 311: 463–473.

Gaykema, R.P.A., Luiten, P.G.M., Nyakas, C., and Traber, J. 1990. Cortical projection patterns of the medical septum-diagonal band complex. J. Comp. Neurol. 293: 103–124.

Geisert, E.E., Langsetmo, A., and Spear, P.D. 1981. Influence of the cortico-geniculate pathway on response properties of cat lateral geniculate neurons. Brain Res. 208: 409–415.

Geisler, W.S. 1989. Sequential ideal-observer analysis of visual discriminations. Psychol. Rev. 96: 267–314.

Gellman, R.L. and Aghajanian, G.K. 1994. 5-HT2-receptor mediated excitation of interneurons in piriform cortex antagonism by atypical antipsychotic drugs. Neuroscience 58: 515–525.

Gellman, R.L. and Aghajanian, G.K. 1993. Pyramidal cells in piriform cortex receive a convergence of inputs from monoamine activated GABAergic interneurons. Brain Res. 600: 63–73.

Gerfen, C.R. 1984. The neostriatal mosaic. Compartmentalization of corticostriatal input and striatonigral output systems. Nature 311: 461–464.

Gerfen, C.R. 1985. The neostriatal mosaic. I. Compartmental organization of projections of the striatonigral system in the rat. J. Comp. Neurol. 236: 454–476.

Gerfen, C.R. 1989. The neostriatal mosaic. Striatal patch-matrix organization is related to cortical lamination. Science 246: 385–388.

Gerfen, C.R., Baimbridge, K.G., and Thibault, J. 1987. The neostriatal mosaic III. Biochemical and developmental dissociation of patch-matrix mesostriatal systems. J. Neurosci. 7: 3935–3944.

Gerfen, C.R., Engber, T.M., Mahan, L.C., Susel, Z., Chase, T.N., Monsma, F.J., and Sibley, D.R. 1990. D1 and D2 dopamine receptor-regulated gene expression of striatonigral and striatopallidal neurons. Science 250: 1492–1432.

Gerfen, C.R. and Young, W.S. 1988. Distribution of striatonigral and striatopallidal peptidergic neurons in both patch and matrix compartments: An in situ hybridization histochemistry and fluorescent retrograde tracing study. Brain Res. 460: 161–167.

Gerschenfeld, H.M., Piccolino, M., Neyton, J. 1980. Feed-back modulation of cone synapses by L-horizontal cells of turtle retina. J. Exp. Biol. 89: 177–192.

Gesteland, R.C. 1986. Speculation on receptor cells as analyzers and filters. Experientia 42: 287–291.

Getchell, T.V. and Shepherd, G.M. 1975a. Short-axon cells in the olfactory bulb: Dendrodendritic synaptic interactions. J. Physiol. (Lond.) 251: 523–548.

Getchell, T.V. and Shepherd, G.M. 1975b. Synaptic actions on mitral and tufted cells elicited by olfactory nerve volleys in the rabbit. J. Physiol. (Lond.) 251: 497–522.

Ghosh, S., Fyffe, R.E.W., and Porter, R. 1988. Morphology of neurons in area 4τ of the cat's cortex studied with intracellular injection of HRP. J. Comp. Neurol. 269: 290–312.

Gilbert, C. and Kelley, J.P. 1975. The projection of cells in the different layers of the cat's visual cortex. J. Comp. Neurol. 163: 81–106.

Gilbert, C. and Wiesel, T. 1979. Morphology and intracortical projections of functionally characterised neurons in the cat visual cortex. Nature 280: 120–125.

Giuffrida, R. and Rustioni, A. 1988. Glutamate and aspartate immunoreactivity in corticothalamic neurons of rats. In: Cellular Thalamic Mechanisms (Bentivoglio, M. and Spreafico, R., eds.). Amsterdam: Elsevier, pp. 311–320.

Gobel, S., Falls, W.M., Bennett, G.J., Abhelmoumene, M., Hayashi, H., and Humphrey, E. 1980. An EM analysis of the synaptic connections of horseradish peroxidase-filled stalked cells and islet cells in the substantia gelatinosa of adult cat spinal cord. J. Comp. Neurol. 194: 781–807.

Goda, Y. and Stevens, C.F. 1996. Long-term depression properties in a simple system. Neuron 16: 103–111.

Godfraind, J., Krnjevic, K., and Pumain, R. 1970. Doubtful value of bicuculline as a specific antagonist of GABA. Nature 228: 675–670.

Godfrey, D.A., Kiang, N.Y.S., and Norris, B.E. 1975a. Single unit activity in the posteroventral cochlear nucleus of the cat. J. Comp. Neurol. 162: 247–268.

Godfrey, D.A., Kiang, N.Y.S., and Norris, B.E. 1975b. Single unit activity in the dorsal cochlear nucleus of the cat. J. Comp. Neurol. 162: 269–284.

Godwin, D.W., Vaughan, J.W., and Sherman, S.M. 1996a. Metabotropic glutamate receptors switch visual response mode of lateral geniculate nucleus cells from burst to tonic. J. Neurophysiol. (in press).

Godwin, D.W., Zhou, Q., and Sherman, S.M. 1996b. Evidence for activation of feedforward GABAergic circuitry in cat LGN via a specific metabotropic glutamate receptor. Soc. Neurosci. Abstr. 22: 1606.

Gogan, P., Gueritaud, J.P., Horchclle-Bossavit, G., and Tyc-Dumont, S. 1977. Direct excitatory interactions between spinal motoneurones of the cat. J. Physiol. (Lond.) 272: 755–767.

Goldberg, J.M. and Brown, P.B. 1969. Response of binaural neurons of dog superior olivary complex to dichotic tonal stimuli: Some physiological mechanisms of sound localization. J. Neurophysiol. 32: 613–636.

Goldberg, J.M. and Brownell, W.E. 1973. Discharge characteristics of neurons in anteroventral and dorsal cochlear nuclei of cat. Brain Res. 64: 35–54.

Golding, N.L. and Oertel, D. 1995. Evidence that cartwheel cells of the dorsal cochlear nucleus excite other cartwheel cells and inhibit principal cells with the same neurotransmitter, glycine. Abstr. Soc. Neurosci. 21: 399.

Golding, N.L. and Oertel, D. 1996. Context-dependent synaptic action of glycinergic and GABAergic inputs in the dorsal cochlear nucleus. J. Neurosci. 16: 2208–2219.

Golding, N.L., Robertson, D., and Oertel, D. 1995. Recordings from slices indicate that octopus cells of the cochlear nucleus detect coincident firing of auditory nerve fibers with temporal precision. J. Neurosci. 15: 3138–3153.

Goldman, D.E. 1943. Potential, impedance, and rectification in membranes. J. Gen. Physiol. 27: 37–60.

Goldman, P.S. and Nauta, W.J.H. 1977. An intricately patterned prefronto-caudate projection in the rhesus monkey. J. Comp. Neurol. 171: 369–385.

Goldman-Rakic, P.S. 1982. Cytoarchitectonic heterogeneity of the primate neostriatum—Subdivision into island and matrix cellular compartments. J. Comp. Neurol. 205: 398–413.

Goldman-Rakic, P.S. 1987. Circuitry of primate prefrontal cortex and regulation of behavior by representational memory. In: Handbook of Physiology, The Nervous System, Higher Functions of the Brain (F. Plum and V.B. Mountcastle, eds.). Bethesda: American Physiology Society, pp. 373–417.

Golgi, C. 1886. Sulla fina Anatomia degli Organi Centrali del Sistema Nervoso. Milano: Hoepli.

Gonzalez, M.L., Malemud, C.J., and Silver, J. 1993. Role of astroglial extracellular matrix in the formation of rat olfactory bulb glomeruli. Exp. Neurol. 123: 91–105.

Goodchild, A.K., Chan, T.L., and Grünert, U. 1996a. Horizontal cell connections with short-wavelength-sensitive cones in macaque monkey retina. Vis. Neurosci. 13: 833–845.

Goodchild, A.K., Ghosh, K.K., and Martin, P.R. 1996b. Comparison of photoreceptor spatial density and ganglion cell morphology in the retina of human, macaque monkey, cat, and the marmoset *Callithrix jacchus*. J. Comp. Neurol. 366: 55–75.

Gossard, J.-P., Floeter, M.K., Kawai, Y., Burke, R.E., Chang, T. and Schiff, S.J. 1994. Fluctuations of excitability in the monosynaptic reflex pathway to lumbar motoneurons in the cat. J. Neurophysiol. 72: 1227–1239.

Gottlieb, D.I. and Cowan, W.M. 1972. On the distribution of axonal terminals containing spheroidal and flattened synaptic vesicles in the hippocampus and dentate gyrus of the rat and cat. Z. Zellforsch. Mikrosk. Anat. 129: 413–429.

Graham, B. and Redman, S. 1994. A simulation of action-potentials in synaptic boutons during presynaptic inhibition. J. Neurophysiol. 71: 538–549.

Granger, R., Ambros-Ingerson, J., and Lynch, G. 1988. Derivation of encoding characteristics of layer II cerebral cortex. J. Cogn. Neurosci. 1: 61–87.

Graveland, G.A. and DiFiglia, M. 1985a. The frequency and distribution of medium-sized neurons with indented nuclei in the primate and rodent neostriatum. Brain Res. 327: 308–311.

Graveland, G.A. and DiFiglia, M. 1985b. A Golgi study of the human neostriatum—Neurons and afferent fibers. J. Comp. Neurol. 234: 317–333.

Gray, C.M. and Singer, W. 1989. Stimulus-specific neuronal oscillations in orientation columns of cat visual cortex. Proc. Natl. Acad. Sci. USA 86: 1698–1702.

Gray, C.M. and Skinner, J.E. 1988. Centrifugal regulation of neuronal activity in the olfactory bulb of the waking rabbit as revealed by reversible cryogenic blockade. Exp. Brain Res. 69: 378–386.

Gray, E.G. 1959. Axo-somatic and axo-dendritic synapses of the cerebral cortex: An electron-microscopic study. J. Anat. 93: 420–433.

Gray, R., Rajan, A.S., Radcliffe, K.A., Yakehiro, M., and Dani, J.A. 1996. Hippocampal synaptic transmission enhanced by low concentrations of nicotine. Nature 383: 713–716.

Graybiel, A.M., Aosaki, T., Flaherty, A.W., and Kimura, M. 1994. The basal ganglia and adaptive motor control. Science 265: 1826–1831.

Graybiel, A.M., Baughman, R.W., and Eckenstein, F. 1986. Cholinergic neuropil of the striatum observes striosomal boundaries. Nature 323: 625–627.

Graybiel, A.M., Ragsdale, C.W., Jr., Yoneoka, E.S., and Elde, R.P. 1981. An immunohistochemical study of enkephalin and other neuropeptides in the striatum of the cat with evidence that opiate peptides are arranged to form mosaic patterns in register with striosomal compartments visible by acetylcholinesterase staining. Neuroscience 6: 377–397.

Graybiel, A.M. and Ragsdale, C.W., Jr. 1983. Biochemical anatomy of the striatum. In: Chemical Neuroanatomy (Emson, P.C., ed.). New York: Raven Press, pp. 427–503.

Graziadei, P.P.C. and Monti-Graziadei, G.A. 1979. Neurogenesis and neuron regeneration in the olfactory system of mammals. I. Morphological aspects of differentiation and structural organization of the olfactory sensory neurons. J. Neurocytol. 8: 1–18.

Green, J.D. 1964. The hippocampus. Physiol. Rev. 44: 561–608.

Greene, C., Schwindt, P., and Crill, W. 1994. Properties and ionic mechanisms of a metabotropic glutamate receptor-mediated slow after depolarization in neocortical neurons. J. Neurophysiol. 72: 693–704.

Greenough, W.T. 1975. Experimental modification of the developing brain. Sci. Am. 63: 37–46.

Greer, C.A. 1984. A Golgi analysis of granule cell development in the neonatal rat olfactory bulb. Soc. Neurosci. Abstr. 10: 531.

Greer, C.A. 1987. Golgi analyses of dendritic organization among denervated olfactory bulb granule cells. J. Comp. Neurol. 257: 442–452.

Greer, C.A. 1988. High voltage electromicroscopic analyses of olfactory bulb granule cell spine geometry. J. Comp. Neurol. 257: 442–452.

Greer, C.A. and Halasz, N. 1987. Plasticity of dendrodendritic microcircuits following mitral cell loss in the olfactory bulb of the murine mutant PCD. J. Comp. Neurol. 256: 284–298.

Greer, C.A., Kaliszewski, C.K., and Cameron, H.A. 1989. Ultrastructural analyses of local circuits in the olfactory system. Proc. EMSA 47: 790–791.

Greer, C.A. and Shepherd, G.M. 1982. Mitral cell degeneration and sensory function in the neurological mutant mouse Purkinje cell degeneration (PCD). Brain Res. 235: 156–161.

Greer, C.A., Stewart, W.B., Teicher, M.H., and Shepherd, G.M. 1982. Functional development of the olfactory bulb and a unique glomerular complex in the neonatal rat. J. Neurosci. 2: 1744–1759.

Grieve, K., Murphy, P., and Sillito, A. 1985a. The actions of VIP and ACh on the visual responses of neurons in the striate cortex. Br. J. Pharmacol. [Suppl.] 85: 253.

Grieve, K., Murphy, P., and Sillito, A. 1985b. An evaluation of the role of CCK and VIP in the cat visual cortex. J. Physiol. (Lond.) 365: 42P.

Grieve, K. and Sillito, A. 1995. Differential properties of cells in the feline primary visual cortex providing the corticofugal feedback to the lateral geniculate nucleus and visual claustrum. J. Neurosci. 15: 4868–4874.

Grillner, S. 1981. Control of locomotion in bipeds, tetrapods and fish. In: Handbook of Physiology, Section 1: The Nervous System, Vol. II: Motor Control, Part 2 (Brooks, V.P., ed.). Bethesda: American Physiological Society, pp. 1179–1236.

Gross, C., Rocha-Miranda, C., and Bender, D. 1972. Visual properties of neurons in inferotemporal cortex of the macaque. J. Neurophysiol. 35: 96–111.

Grünert, U., Martin, P.R., and Wässle, H. 1994. Immunocytochemical analysis of bipolar cells in the macaque monkey retina. J. Comp. Neurol. 348: 607–627.

Grünert, U. and Wässle, H. 1990. GABA-like immunoreactivity in the macaque monkey retina: A light and electron microscopic study. J. Comp. Neurol. 297: 509–524.

Gu, Q., Patel, B., and Singer, W. 1990. The laminar distribution and postnatal development of serotonin-immunoreactive axons in the cat primary visual cortex. Exp. Brain Res. 81: 257–266.

Guido, W., Lu, S.-M., and Sherman, S.M. 1992. Relative contributions of burst and tonic responses to the receptive field properties of lateral geniculate neurons in the cat. J. Neurophysiol. 68: 2199–2211.

Guido, W., Lu, S.-M., Vaughan, J.W., Godwin, D.W., and Sherman, S.M. 1995. Receiver operating characteristic (ROC) analysis of neurons in the cat's lateral geniculate nucleus during tonic and burst response mode. Vis. Neurosci. 12: 723–741.

Guido, W. and Weyand, T. 1995. Burst responses in thalamic relay cells of the awake behaving cat. J. Neurophysiol. 74: 1782–1786.

Guillery, R.W. 1966. A study of Golgi preparations from the dorsal lateral geniculate nucleus of the adult cat. J. Comp. Neurol. 128: 21–50.

Guillery, R.W. 1969a. A quantitative study of synaptic interconnections in the dorsal lateral geniculate nucleus of the cat. Z. Zellforsch. 96: 39–48.

Guillery, R.W. 1969b. The organization of synaptic interconnections in the laminae of the dorsal lateral geniculate nucleus of the cat. Z. Zellforsch. 96: 1–38.

Guillery, R.W. 1995. Anatomical evidence concerning the role of the thalamus in corticocortical communication: A brief review. J. Anat. 187: 583–592.

Guinan, J.J. and Li, R.Y.-S. 1990. Signal processing in brainstem auditory neurons which receive giant endings (calyces of Held) in the medial nucleus of the trapezoid body of the cat. Hear. Res. 49: 321–334.

Gulyas, A.I., Görcs, T.J., and Freund, T.F. 1990. Innervation of different peptide-containing neurons in the hippocampus by GABAergic septal afferents. Neuroscience 37: 31–44.

Gustafsson, B. and Pinter, M.J. 1984. Relations among passive electrical properties of lumbar α-motoneurones of the cat. J. Physiol. (Lond.) 356: 401–431.

Guthrie, K.M., Anderson, A.J., Leon, M., and Gall, C. 1993. Odor-induced increases in c-*fos* mRNA expression reveal an anatomical 'unit' for odor processing in olfactory bulb. Proc. Natl. Acad. Sci. USA 90: 3329–3333.

Guthrie, K.M. and Gall, C.M. 1995. Odors increase Fos in olfactory bulb neurons including dopaminergic cells. NeuroReport 6: 2145–2149.

Guthrie, P., Segal, M., and Kater, S. 1991. Independent regulation of calcium revealed by imaging dendritic spines. Nature 354: 76–80.

Haberly, L.B. 1973. Unitary analysis of opossum prepyriform cortex. J. Neurophysiol. 36: 762–774.

Haberly, L.B. 1983. Structure of the piriform cortex of the opossum. I. Description of neuron types with Golgi methods. J. Comp. Neurol. 213: 163–187.

Haberly, L.B. 1985. Neuronal circuitry in olfactory cortex. Anatomy and functional implications. Chem. Senses 10: 219–238.

Haberly, L.B. 1990a. Comparative aspects of olfactory cortex. In: Cerebral Cortex, Vol. 8 (Jones, E.G. and Peters, A., eds.). New York: Plenum, pp. 137–166.

Haberly, L.B. 1990b. Olfactory cortex. In: Synaptic Organization of the Brain, 3rd ed. (Shepherd, G.M., ed.). New York: Oxford University Press, pp. 317–345.

Haberly, L.B. and Bower, J.M. 1982. Graphical methods for three-dimensional rotation of complex axonal arborizations. J. Neurosci. Methods 6: 75–84.

Haberly, L.B. and Bower, J.M. 1984. Analysis of association fiber system in piriform cortex with intracellular recording and staining methods. J. Neurophysiol. 51: 90–112.

Haberly, L.B. and Bower, J.M. 1989. Olfactory cortex. Model circuit for study of associative memory? Trends Neurosci. 12: 258–264.

Haberly, L.B. and Feig, S. 1983. Structure of the piriform cortex of the opossum. II. Fine structure of cell bodies and neuropil. J. Comp. Neurol. 216: 69–98.

Haberly, L.B., Hansen, D.J., Feig, S.L., and Presto, S. 1987. Distribution and ultrastructure of neurons in opposum displaying immunoreactivity to GABA and GAD and high affinity tritiated GABA uptake. J. Comp. Neurol. 266: 269–290.

Haberly, L.B. and Presto, S. 1986. Ultrastructural analysis of synaptic relationships of intracellularly stained pyramidal cell axons in piriform cortex. J. Comp. Neurol. 248: 464–474.

Haberly, L.B. and Price, J.L. 1977. The axonal projection patterns of the mitral and tufted cells of the olfactory bulb in the rat. Brain Res. 129: 152–157.

Haberly, L.B. and Price, J.L. 1978a. Association and commissural fiber systems of the olfactory cortex of the rat. I. Systems originating in the piriform cortex and adjacent areas. J. Comp. Neurol. 178: 711–740.

Haberly, L.B. and Price, J.L. 1978b. Association and commissural fiber systems of the olfactory cortex of the rat. II. Systems originating in the olfactory peduncle. J. Comp. Neurol. 181: 781–808.

Haberly, L.B. and Shepherd, G.M. 1973a. Current density analysis of opossum prepyriform cortex. J. Neurophysiol. 36: 789–802.

Haberly, L.B. and Shepherd, G.M. 1973b. Current-density analysis of summed evoked potentials in opossum prepyriform cortex. J. Neurophysiol. 36: 789–803.

Hablitz, J. and Langmoen, I. 1982. Excitation of hippocampal pyramidal cells by glutamate in the guinea-pig and rat. J. Physiol. (Lond.) 325: 317–331.

Hablitz, J. and Thalmann, R. 1987. Conductance changes underlying a late synaptic hyperpolarization in hippocampal neurons. J. Neurophysiol. 58: 160–179.

Hablitz, J.J. and Johnston, D. 1981. Endogenous nature of spontaneous bursts in hippocampal neurons. Cell. Mol. Neurobiol. 1: 325–334.

Hackett, J.T., Hou, S.M., and Cochran, S.L. 1979. Glutamate and synaptic depolarization of Purkinje cells evoked by climbing fibers. Brain Res. 170: 377–380.

Haglund, L., Swanson, L.W., and Köhler, C. 1984. The projection of the supramammillary nucleus to the hippocampal formation: An immunohistochemical and anterograde transport study with the lectin PHA-L in the rat. J. Comp. Neurol. 229: 171–185.

Halasy, K., Buhl, E.H., Lorinczi, Z., Tamas, G., and Somogyi, P. 1996. Synaptic target selectivity and input of GABAergic basket and bistratified interneurons in the CA1 area of the rat hippocampus. Hippocampus 6: 306–329.

Halasy, K., Miettinen, R., Szabat, E., and Freund, T.F. 1991. GABAergic interneurons are the major postsynaptic targets of median raphe afferents in the rat dentate gyrus. Eur. J. Neurosci. 4: 144–153.

Halasz, N. and Greer, C.A. 1993. Terminal arborizations of olfactory nerve fibers in the glomeruli of the olfactory bulb. J. Comp. Neurol. 337: 307–316.

Halasz, N., Ljungdahl, A., Hokfelt, T., Johannsson, O., Goldstein, M., Park, D., and Biberfeld, P. 1977. Transmitter histochemistry of the rat olfactory bulb. I. Immunohistochemical localization of monoamine-synthesizing enzymes. Brain Res. 455–474.

Halasz, N., Ljungdalh, A., and Hökfelt, T. 1978. Transmitter histochemistry of the rat olfactory bulb. II. Fluorescence histochemical, autoradiographic and electron microscopic localization of monoamines. Brain Res. 154: 253–271.

Halasz, N. and Shepherd, G.M. 1983. Neurochemistry of the vertebrate olfactory bulb. Neuroscience 10: 579–619.

Haldeman, S., Huffman, R., Marshall, K., and McLennan, H. 1972. The antagonism of the glutamate induced and synaptic excitations of the thalamic neurons. Brain Res. 39: 419–425.

Haldeman, S. and McLennan, H. 1972. The antagonistic action of glutamic acid diethylester toward amino-acid-induced and synaptic excitations of central neurons. Brain Res. 45: 393–400.

Hall, W.C. and Ebner, F.F. 1970. Thalamotelencephalic projections in the turtle (*Pseudemys scripta*). J. Comp. Neurol. 140: 101–122.

Halliwell, J.V. and Adams, P.R. 1982. Voltage-clamp analysis of muscarinic excitation in hippocampal neurons. Brain Res. 250: 71–92.

Halliwell, J.V. and Scholfield, C.N. 1984. Somatically recorded Ca-currents in guinea-pig hippocampal and olfactory cortex neurones are resistant to adenosine action. Neurosci. Lett. 50: 13–18.

Hamassaki-Britto, D.E., Hermans-Borgmeyer, I., Heinemann, S., and Hughes, T.E. 1993. Expression of glutamate receptor genes in the mammalian retina: The localization of GluR1 through GluR7 mRNAs. J. Neurosci. 13: 1888–1898.

Hamill, O.P., Bormann, J., and Sakmann, B. 1983. Activation of multiple-conductance state chloride channels in spinal neurones by glycine and GABA. Nature 305: 805–808.

Hamill, O.P., Huguenard, J., and Prince, D. 1991. Patch-clamp studies of voltage-gated currents in identified neurons of the rat cerebral cortex. Cereb. Cortex 1: 48–61.

Hamill, O.P., Marty, A., Neher, E., Sakmann, B., and Sigworth, F.J. 1981. Improved patch-clamp techniques for high-resolution current recordings from cells and cell-free membrane patches. Pflugers Arch. 391: 85–100.

Hamilton, K.A. and Kauer, J.S. 1985. Intracellular potentials of salamander mitral/tufted neurons in response to odor stimulation. Brain Res 338: 181–185.

Hamilton, K.A. and Kauer, J.S. 1988. Responses of mitral/tufted cells to orthodromic and antidromic electrical stimulation in the olfactory bulb of the tiger salamander. J. Neurophysiol. 59: 1736–1755.

Hamilton, K.A. and Kauer, J.S. 1989. Patterns of intracellular potentials in salamander mitral/tufted cells in response to odor stimulation. J. Neurophysiol. 62: 609–625.

Hamlyn, L.H. 1962. The fine structure of the mossy fibre endings in the hippocampus of the rabbit. J. Anat. 96: 112–120.

Hamori, J. and Mezey, E. 1977. Serial and triadic synapses in the cerebellar nuclei of the cat. Exp. Brain Res. 30: 259–273.

Hamori, J. and Szentagothai, J. 1966. Identification under the electron microscope of climbing fibers and their synaptic contacts. Exp. Brain Res. 1: 65–81.

Hamos, J.E., Van Horn, S.C., Rackowski, D., Uhlrich, D.J., and Sherman, S.M. 1985. Synaptic connectivity of a local circuit neurone in lateral geniculate nucleus of the cat. Nature 317: 618–621.

Hampson, E.C.G.M., Weiler, R., and Vaney, D.I. 1994. pH-gated dopaminergic modulation of horizontal cell gap junctions in mammalian retina. Proc. R. Soc. (Lond.) B 255: 67–72.

Hampson, E.C., Vaney, D.I., and Weiler, R. 1992. Dopaminergic modulation of gap junction permeability between amacrine cells in mammalian retina. J. Neurosci. 12: 4911–4922.

Hamrick, W.D., Wilson, D.A., and Sullivan, R.M. 1993. Neural correlates of memory for odor detection conditioning in adult rats. Neurosci. Lett. 163: 36–40.

Harlan, R.E., Shivers, B.D., Romano, G.J., Howells, R.D., and Pfaff, D.W. 1987. Localization of preproenkephalin mRNA in the rat brain and spinal cord by in situ hybridization. J. Comp. Neurol. 258: 159–184.

Harris, K.M., Jensen, F.E., and Tsao, B.H. 1989. Ultrastructure, development, and plasticity of dendritic spine synapses in area CA1 of the rat hippocampus: Extending our vision with serial electron microscopy and three-dimensional analyses. In: The Hippocampus—New Vistas. (Chan-Palay, V. and Köhler, C., eds.) New York: Alan R. Liss, pp. 33–52.

Harris, K.M. and Kater, S.B. 1994. Dendritic spines: Cellular specializations imparting both stability and flexibility to synaptic function. Annu. Rev. Neurosci. 17: 341–371.

Harris, K.M. and Stevens, J.K. 1988. Dendritic spines of rat cerebellar Purkinje cells: Serial electron microscopy with reference to their biophysical characteristics. J. Neurosci. 8: 4455–4469.

Harris, K.M. and Stevens, J.K. 1989. Dendritic spines of CA1 pyramidal cells in the rat hippocampus: Serial electron microscopy with reference to their biophysical characteristics. J. Neurosci. 9: 2982–2997.

Hartell, N. 1994. cGMP acts within cerebellar Purkinje cells to produce long-term depression via mechanisms involving PKC and PKG. NeuroReport 5: 833–836.

Hartell, N. 1996. Strong activation of parallel fibers produces localized calcium transients and a form of LTD that spreads to distant synapses. Neuron 16: 601–610.

Harting, J.K., Hashikawa, T., and Van Lieshout, D. 1986. Laminar distribution of tectal, parabigeminal and pretectal inputs to the primate dorsal lateral geniculate nucleus: Connectional studies in *Galago crassicaudatus*. Brain Res. 366: 358–363.

Hartzell, H.C. 1981. Mechanisms of slow postsynaptic potentials. Nature 291: 539–544.

Hasan, Z. and Stuart, D.G. 1984. Mammalian muscle receptors. In: Handbook of the Spinal Cord, Vol. 1: Physiology (Davidoff, R.E., eds.). New York: Marcel Dekker, pp. 559–608.

Hasselmo, M.E. 1994. Neuromodulation and cortical function. Modeling the physiological basis of behavior. Behav. Brain Res. 67: 1–27.

Hasselmo, M.E., Anderson, B.P., and Bower, J.M. 1992. Cholinergic modulation of cortical associative memory function. J. Neurophysiol. 67: 1230–1246.

Hasselmo, M.E. and Barkai, E. 1996. Cholinergic modulation of activity-dependent synaptic plasticity in the piriform cortex and associative memory function in a network biophysical simulation. J. Neurosci. 15: 6592–6604.

Hasselmo, M.E. and Bower, J.M. 1992. Cholinergic suppression specific to intrinsic not afferent fiber synapses in rat piriform (olfactory) cortex. J. Neurophysiol. 67: 1222–1229.

Hattori, T., Figbiger, H.C., McGeer, P.L., and Maller, L. 1973. Analysis of the fine structure of the dopaminergic nigrostriatal projection by electron microscopy. Exp. Neurol. 41: 599–611.

Hayashi, T. 1954. Effects of sodium glutamate on the nervous system. Keio J. Med. 302: 183–192.

Hebb, D.O. 1949. The Organization of Behavior. New York: John Wiley & Sons.

Heckman, C.J. and Binder, M.D. 1988. Analysis of effective synaptic currents generated by homonymous Ia afferent fibers in motoneurons of the cat. J. Neurophysiol. 60: 1946–1966.

Heckman, C.J. and Binder, M.D. 1993. Computer simulations of motoneuron firing rate modulation. J. Neurophysiol. 69: 1005–1008.

Heggelund, P. 1981. Receptive field organization of simple cells in cat striate cortex. Exp. Brain Res. 42: 89–98.

Heggelund, P. and Hartveit, E. 1990. Neurotransmitter receptors mediating excitatory input to cells in the cat lateral geniculate nucleus. I. Lagged cells. J. Neurophysiol. 63: 1347–1360.

Heimer, L. and Kalil, R. 1978. Rapid transneuronal degeneration and death of cortical neurons following removal of the olfactory bulb in adult rats. J. Comp. Neurol. 178: 559–619.

Hendrickson, A. and S. Hunt, J.-Y.W. 1981. Immunocytochemical localization of glutamic acid decarboxylase in monkey striate cortex. Nature 292: 605.

Hendry, A., Jones, E., DeFelipe, J., Schmechel, D., Brandon, C., and Emson, P. 1984. Neuropeptide-containing neurons of the cerebral cortex are also GABA-ergic. Proc. Natl. Acad. Sci. USA 81: 6526–6530.

Hendry, S.H.C. and Yoshioka, T. 1994. A neurochemically distinct third channel in the macaque dorsal lateral geniculate nucleus. Science 264: 575–577.

Henneman, E., Clamann, H.P., Gillies, J.D., and Skinner, R.D. 1974. Rank order of motoneurons within a pool: Law of combination. J. Neurophysiol. 37: 1338–1349.

Henneman, E., Lüscher, H.-R., and Mathis, J. 1984. Simultaneously active and inactive synapses of single Ia fibres on cat spinal motoneurones. J. Physiol. (Lond.) 352: 147–161.

Henneman, E. and Mendell, L.M. 1981. Functional organization of motoneuron pool and its inputs. In: Handbook of Physiology, Section I: The Nervous System, Vol. II: Motor Control, Part 1 (Brooks, V.B., eds.). Bethesda, MD: American Physiological Society, pp. 423–507.

Henneman, E. and Olson, C.B. 1965. Relations between structure and function in the design of skeletal muscles. J. Neurophysiol. 28: 581–598.

Henneman, E., Somjen, G., and Carpenter, D.O. 1965. Excitability and inhibitibility of motoneurons of different sizes. J. Neurophysiol. 28: 599–620.

Herkenham, M. 1978. The connections of the nucleus reuniens thalami: Evidence for a direct thalamo-hippocampal pathway in the rat. J. Comp. Neurol. 177: 589–610.

Herkenham, M. and Pert, C.B. 1981. Mosaic distribution of opiate receptors, parafascicular projections and acetylcholinesterase in the rat striatum. Nature 291: 415–418.

Herraras, O. 1990. Propagating dendritic actium potential mediates synaptic transmission in CA1 pyramidal cells in situ. J. Neurophysiol. 64: 1429–1441.

Herrling, P.L. and Hull, C.D. 1980. Iontophoretically applied dopamine depolarizes and hyperpolarizes the membrane of cat caudate neurons. Brain Res. 192: 441–462.

Hersch, S. and White, E. 1981. Quantification of synapses formed with apical dendrites of Golgi-impregnated pyramidal cells: Variability in thalamocortical inputs, but consistence in the ratios of asymmetrical to symmetrical synapses. J. Neurosci. 6: 1043–1051.

Hertz, J., Krogh, A., and Palmer, R.G. 1991. Introduction to the Theory of Neural Computation. Redwood City, CA: Addison-Wesley.

Hewitt, M.J. and Meddis, R. 1993. Regularity of cochlear nucleus stellate cells. A computational modeling study. J. Acoust. Soc. Am. 93: 3390–3399.

Hewitt, M.J., Meddis, R., and Shackleton, T.M. 1992. A computer model of a cochlear-nucleus stellate cell: Responses to amplitude-modulated and pure-tone stimuli. J. Acoust. Soc. Am. 91: 2096–2109.

Hicks, T.P., Lodge, D., and McLennan, H. eds. 1987. Excitatory Amino Acid Transmission. New York: Alan R. Liss. Hikosaka, O. and Wurtz, R.H. 1983. Visual and oculomotor functions of monkey substantia nigra pars reticulata. III. Memory-contingent visual and saccade responses. J. Neurophysiol. 49: 1268–1284.

Hildebrand, J.G. 1995. Analysis of chemical signals by nervous systems. Proc. Natl. Acad. Sci. USA 92: 67–74.

Hildebrand, J.G. 1996. Olfactory control of behavior in moths: Central processing of odor information and the functional significance of olfactory glomeruli. J. Comp. Physiol. A 178: 5–19.

Hildebrand, J.G. and Shepherd, G.M. 1997. Molecular mechanisms of olfactory discrimination: Converging evidence for common principles across phyla. Annu. Rev. Neurosci. 20: 595–631.

Hill, D. and Bowery, N. 1981. 3H-baclofen and H-GABA bind to bicuculine-insensitive $GABA_B$ sites in rat brain. Nature 290: 149–152.

Hille, B. 1992. Ionic Channels of Excitable Membranes (2nd ed.). Sunderland, MA: Sinauer Associates.

Hillman, D.E. and Chen, S.C. 1984. Reciprocal relationship between size of postsynaptic densities and their number. Constancy in contact area. Brain Res. 295: 325–343.

Hillman, D.E. and Chen, S.C. 1985a. Compensation in the number of presynaptic dense projections and synaptic vesicles in remaining parallel fibers follow cerebellar lesions. J. Neurocytol. 14: 673–687.

Hillman, D.E. and Chen, S.C. 1985b. Plasticity in the size of presynaptic and postsynaptic membrane specializations. In: Synaptic Plasticity (Cotman, C.W., ed.). New York: Guilford Press, pp. 39–76.

Hinds, J.W. 1970. Reciprocal and serial dendrodendritic synapses in the glomerular layer of the rat olfactory bulb. Brain Res. 17: 530–534.

Hirata, Y. 1964. Some observations on the fine structure of synapses in the olfactory bulb of the mouse, with particular reference to the atypical synaptic configurations. Arch. Histol. Jpn. 24: 303–317.

Hirsch, J., Alonso, J., and Reid, R.C. 1995. Visually evoked calcium action potentials in cat striate cortex. Nature 378: 612–616.

Hirsch, J. and Gilbert, C. 1991. Synaptic connections of horizontal connections in the cat's visual cortex. J. Neurosci. 11: 1800–1809.

Hirsch, J.A. and Oertel, D. 1988. Intrinsic properties of neurones in the dorsal cochlear nucleus of mice, *in vitro*. J. Physiol. (Lond.) 396: 535–548.

Hirsch, J.C., Fourment, A., and Marc, M.E. 1983. Sleep-related variations of membrane potential in the lateral geniculate body relay neurons of the cat. Brain Res. 259: 308–312.

Hjorth-Simonsen, A. and Jeune, B. 1972. Origin and termination of the hippocampal perforant path in the rat studied by silver impregnation. J. Comp. Neurol. 144: 215–232.

Hochstein, S. and Shapley, R.M. 1976. Linear and nonlinear spatial subunits in Y cat retinal ganglion cells. J. Physiol. (Lond.) 262: 265–284.

Hodgkin, A.L. and Huxley, A.F. 1952a. Currents carried by sodium and potassium ions through the membrane of the giant axon of Loligo. J. Physiol. (Lond.) 116: 449–472.

Hodgkin, A.L. and Huxley, A.F. 1952b. The components of membrane conductance in the giant axon of Loligo. J. Physiol. (Lond.) 116: 473–496.

Hodgkin, A.L. and Huxley, A.F. 1952c. The dual effect of membrane potential and sodium conductance in the giant axon of Loligo. J. Physiol. (Lond.) 116: 497–506.

Hodgkin, A.L. and Huxley, A.F. 1952d. A quantitative description of membrane current and its application to conduction and excitation in nerve. J. Physiol. (Lond.) 117: 500–544.

Hodgkin, A.L. and Katz, B. 1949. The effect of sodium ions on the electrical activity of the giant axon of the squid. J. Physiol. (Lond.). 108: 37–77.

Hoffer, B.J., Siggins, G.R., Oliver, A.P., and Bloom, F.E. 1973. Activation of the pathway from locus coeruleus to rat cerebellar Purkinje neurons. Pharmacological evidence of noradrenergic central inhibition. J. Pharmacol. Exp. Ther. 184: 553–569.

Hoffman, D., Magee, J.C., Colbert, C.M., and Johnston, D. 1997. Potassium channel regulation of signal propagation in dendrites of hippocampal pyramidal neurons. Nature (In press).

Hoffman, W.H. and Haberly, L.B. 1989. Bursting induces persistent all-or-none EPSPs by an NMDA-dependent process in piriform cortex. J. Neurosci. 9: 206–215.

Hoffman, W.H. and Haberly, L.B. 1991. Bursting induced epileptiform EPSPs in slices of piriform cortex are generated in deep cells. J. Neurosci. 11: 2021–2031.

Hoffman, W.H. and Haberly, L.B. 1993. Role of synaptic excitation in the generation of bursting-induced epileptiform potentials in the endopiriform nucleus and piriform cortex. J. Neurophysiol.

Hökfelt, T., Millhorn, D., Seroogy, K., Tsuruo, Y., Ceccatelli, S., Lindh, B., Meister, B., Melander, T., Schalling, M., and Bartfai, T. 1989. Coexistence of peptides with classical neurotransmitters. Experientia 56: 154–179.

Hollmann, M. and Heinemann, S. 1994. Cloned glutamate receptors. Annu. Rev. Neurosci. 17: 31–108.

Holmes, W.R. and Rall, W. 1992. Estimating the electrotonic structure of neurons with compartmental models. J. Neurophysiol. 68: 1438–1452.

Hongo, T., Jankowska, E., Ohno, T., Sasaki, S., Yamashita, M., and Yoshida, K. 1983. The same interneurones mediate inhibition of dorsal spinocerebellar tract cells and lumbar motoneurones in the cat. J. Physiol. (Lond.) 342: 161–180.

Honig, M.G., Collins, W.F., and Mendell, L.M. 1983. α-motoneuron EPSPs exhibit different frequency sensitivities to single Ia-afferent fiber stimulation. J. Neurophysiol. 49: 886–901.

Hoogland, P., Wouterlood, F.G., Welker, E., and van der Loos, H. 1991. Ultrastructure of giant and small thalamic terminals of cortical origin: A study of the projections from the barrel cortex in mice using *Phaseolus vulgaris* leuco-agglutinin (PHA-L). Exp Brain Res 87: 159–172.

Hoover, J.E. and Strick, P.L. 1993. Multiple output channels in the basal ganglia. Science 259: 819–821.

Hopfield, J.J. 1982. Neural networks and physical systems with emergent collective computational abilities. Proc. Natl. Acad. Sci. USA 79: 2554–2558.

Hopfield, J.J. 1984. Neurons with graded response have collective properties like those of two-state neurons. Proc. Natl. Acad. Sci. USA 81: 3088–3092.

Horikawa, K. and Armstrong, W.E. 1988. A versatile means of intracellular labeling injection of biocytin and its detection with avidin conjugates. J. Neurosci. Methods 25: 1–11.

Hornung, J. and Garey, L. 1981. The thalamic projection to cat visual cortex: Ultrastructure of neurons identified by golgi impregnation or retrograde horseradish peroxidase transport. Neurosci 6: 1053–1068.

Horton, J. and Hubel, D. 1981. A regular patchy distribution of cytochrome oxidase staining in primary visual cortex of the macaque monkey. Nature 292: 762–764.

Hotson, J.R. and Prince, D.A. 1980. A calcium-activated hyperpolarization follows repetitive firing in hippocampal neurons. J. Neurophysiol. 43: 409–419.

Hotson, J.R., Prince, D.A., and Schwartzkroin, P.A. 1979. Anomalous rectification in hippocampal neurons. J. Neurophysiol. 42: 889–895.

Houk, J.C. and Rymer, W.Z. 1981. Neural control of muscle length and tension. In: Handbook of Physiology, Section I: The Nervous System, Vol. II: Motor Control, Part 1 (Brooks, V.B., ed.). Bethesda, MD: American Physiological Society, pp. 257–323.

Hounsgaard, J., Hultborn, H., Jespersen, B., and Kiehn, O. 1988. Bistability of α-motoneurones in the decerebrate cat and in the acute spinal cat after intravenous 5-hydroxytryptophane. J. Physiol. (Lond.) 405: 345–367.

Hounsgard, J. and Kiehn, O. 1989. Serotonin-induced bistability of turtle motoneurones caused by a nifedipine-sensitive calcium plateau potential. J. Physiol. (Lond.) 414: 265–282.

Houser, C., Crawford, G., Salvaterra, P., and Vaugn, J. 1985. Immunocytochemical localization of choline acetyltransferase in rat cerebral cortex: A study of cholinergic neurons and synapses. J. Comp. Neurol. 234: 17–34.

Howe, A.R. and Surmeier, D.J. 1995. Muscarinic receptors modulate N-, P- and L-type Ca^{2+} currents in rat striatal neurons through parallel pathways. J. Neurosci. 15: 458–469.

Howell, G.A., Welch, M.G., and Frederickson, C.J. 1984. Simulation-induced uptake and release of zinc in hippocampal slices. Nature 308: 736–738.

Hsu, A., Tsukamoto, Y., Smith, R.G., and Sterling, P. 1997. Functional architecture of primate rod and cone axons. (Submitted).

Hu, B., Steriade, M., and Deschênes, M. 1989a. The effects of brainstem peribrachial stimulation on neurons of the lateral geniculate nucleus. Neuroscience 31: 13–24.

Hu, B., Steriade, M., and Deschênes, M. 1989b. The cellular mechanism of thalamic ponto-geniculo-occipital waves. Neuroscience 31: 25–35.

Hu, H., Tomasiewicz, H., Magnuson, T., and Rutishauser, U. 1996. The role of polysialic acid in migration of olfactory bulb interneuron precursors in the subventricular zone. Neuron 16: 735–743.

Hubel, D.H. and Wiesel, T.N. 1962. Receptive fields, binocular interaction and functional architecture in the cat's visual cortex. J. Physiol. (Lond.) 160: 106–154.

Hubel, D.H. and Wiesel, T.N. 1977. The functional architecture of the macaque visual cortex. Proc. R. Soc. Lond. B Biol. Sci. 198: 1–59.

Hudson, D.B., Valcana, T., Bean, G., and Timiras, P.S. 1976. Glutamic acid: A strong candidate as the neurotransmitter of the cerebellar granule cell. Neurochem. Res. 1: 73–81.

Huettner, J.E. and Baughman, R.W. 1988. The pharmacology of synapses formed by identified corticocollicular neurons in primary cultures of rat visual cortex. J. Neurosci. 8: 160–175.

Huguenard, J., Hamill, O., and Prince, D. 1989. Sodium channels in dendrites of rat cortical pyramidal neurons. Proc. Natl. Acad. Sci. USA 86: 2473–2477.

Huguenard, J.R. and McCormick, D.A. 1992. Simulation of the currents involved in rhythmic oscillations in thalamic relay neurons. J. Neurophysiol. 68: 1373–1383.

Huguenard, J.R. and McCormick, D.A. 1994. Electrophysiology of the Neuron. New York: Oxford University Press.

Hultborn, H., Jankowska, E., and Lindström, S. 1971a. Recurrent inhibition from motor axon collaterals of transmission in the Ia inhibitory pathway to motoneurones. J. Physiol. (Lond.) 215: 591–612.

Hultborn, H., Jankowska, E., and Lindström, S. 1971b. Recurrent inhibition of interneurones monosynaptically activated from group Ia afferents. J. Physiol. (Lond.) 215: 613–636.

Hultborn, H., Katz, R., and Mackel, R. 1988a. Distribution of recurrent inhibition within a motor nucleus. II. Amount of recurrent inhibition in motoneurones to fast and slow units. Acta Physiol. Scand. 134: 363–374.

Hultborn, H., Lipski, J., Mackel, R., and Wigström, H. 1988b. Distribution of recurrent inhibition within a motor nucleus. I. Contribution from slow and fast motor units to the excitation of Renshaw cells. Acta Physiol. Scand. 134: 347–361.

Humphrey, A.L. and Weller, R.E. 1988. Functionally distinct groups of X-cells in the lateral geniculate nucleus of the cat. J. Comp. Neurol. 268: 429–447.

Hunter, C., Petralia, R.S., Vu, T., and Wenthold, R.J. 1993. Expression of AMPA-selective glutamate receptor subunits in morphologically defined neurons of the mammalian cochlear nucleus. J. Neurosci. 13: 1932–1946.

Hyman, B.T., Van Hoesen, G.W., Damasio, A.R., and Barnes, C.L. 1984. Alzheimer's disease: Cell-specific pathology isolates the hippocampal formation. Science 225: 1168–1171.

Illert, M., Lundberg, A., and Tanaka, R. 1976. Integration in descending motor pathways controlling the forelimb in the cat. 2. Convergence on neurones mediating disynaptic corticomotoneuronal excitation. Exp. Brain Res. 26: 521–540.

Inagaki, N., Yamatodani, A., Ando-Yamamoto, M., Tohyama, M., Watanabe, T., and Wada, H. 1988. Organization of histaminergic fibers in the rat brain. J. Comp. Neurol. 273: 283–300.

Inagaki, S., Kubota, Y., Shinoda, K., Kawai, Y., and Tohyama, M. 1983. Neurotensin-containing pathway from the endopiriform nucleus and the adjacent prepiriform cortex to the dorsomedial nucleus in the rat. Brain Res. 260: 143–146.

Inagaki, S., Shiosaka, S., Takatsuki, K., Iida, H., Sakanaka, M., Senba, E., Hara, Y., Matsuzuki, T., Kawai, Y., and Tohyama, M. 1982. Ontogeny of somatostatin-containing neuron system of the rat cerebellum including its fiber connections: An experimental and immunohistochemical analysis. Dev. Brain Res. 3: 509–527.

Ingham, C.A., Hood, S.H., Taggart, P., and Arbuthnott, G.W. 1996. Synaptic plasticity in the rat neostriatum after unilateral 6-hydroxydopamine lesion of the nigrostriatal dopaminergic pathway. In: The Basal Ganglia V (Ohye, C., Kimura, M., and McKenzie, J.S., eds.). New York: Plenum, pp. 157–164.

Inoue, M., Matsuo, T., and Ogata, N. 1985a. Characterisation of pre- and postsynaptic actions of −baclofen in the guinea-pig hippocampus in vitro. Br. J. Pharmacol. 84: 843–853.

Inoue, M., Matsuo, T., and Ogata, N. 1985b. Possible involvement of conductance in action of gamma-aminobutyric acid in the guinea-pig hippocampus. Br. J. Pharmacol. 86: 515–524.

Inoue, M., Oomara, Y., Yakushiji, T., and Akaike, N. 1986. Intracellular calcium ions decrease the affinity of the GABA receptor. Nature 324: 156–158.

Iriki, A., Pavlides, C., Keller, A., and Asanuma, H. 1991. Long-term potentiation of thalamic input to the motor cortex induced by co-activation of thalamo-cortical afferents. J. Neurophysiol. 65: 1435–1441.

Irvin, G.E., Casagrande, V.A., and Norton, T.T. 1993. Center/surround relationships of magnocellular, parvocellular, and koniocellular relay cells in primate lateral geniculate nucleus. Vis. Neurosci. 10: 363–373.

Irvine, D.R.F. 1986. The Auditory Brainstem. Berlin: Springer-Verlag.

Isaac, J.T.R., Nicoll, R.A., and Malenka, R.C. 1995. Evidence for silent synapses: Implications for the expression of LTP. Neuron 15: 427–434.

Isayama, T., Berson, D.M., and Pu, M. 1997. The theta cell: A bistratified ganglion cell type in cat retina. Invest. Ophthalmol. Vis. Sci. Abstr. 38: S51.

Ishizuka, N., Cowan, W.M., and Amaral, D.G. 1995. A quantitative analysis of the dendritic organization of pyramidal cells in the rat hippocampus. J. Comp. Neurol. 362: 17–45.

Ishizuka, N., Mannen, H., Hongo, T., and Sasaki, S. 1979. Trajectory of group Ia afferent fibers stained with horseradish peroxidase in the lumbosacral spinal cord of the cat: Three-dimensional reconstructions from serial sections. J. Comp. Neurol. 186: 189–211.

Ishizuka, N., Weber, J., and Amaral, D.G. 1990. Organization of intrahippocampal projections originating from CA3 pyramidal cells in the rat. J. Comp. Neurol. 295: 580–623.

Israel, M. and Whittaker, V.P. 1965. The isolation of mossy fiber endings from the granular layer of the cerebellar cortex. Experientia 21: 325–326.

Ito, M., Sakurai, M., and Tongroach, P. 1982. Climbing fiber induced depression of both mossy fiber responsiveness and glutamate sensitivity of cerebellar Purkinje cells. J. Physiol. (Lond.) 113 134.

Ito, M., Yoshida, M., and Obata, K. 1964. Monosynaptic inhibition of the intracerebellar nuclei induced from the cerebellar cortex. Experientia 20: 575 576.

Itoh, K., Kamiya, H., Mitani, A., Yasui, Y., Takada, M., and Mizuno, N. 1987. Direct projection from the dorsal column nuclei and the spinal trigeminal nuclei to the cochlear nuclei in the cat. Brain Res. 400: 145–150.

Iversen, L., Mitchell, J., and Srinivasan, V. 1971. The release of gamma-aminobutyric acid during inhibition in the cat visual cortex. J. Physiol. (Lond.) 212: 519–534.

Izzo, P.N. and Bolam, J.P. 1988. Cholinergic synaptic input to different parts of spiny striatonigral neurons in the rat. J. Comp. Neurol. 269: 219–234.

Jack, J.J.B. 1979. Introduction to linear cable theory. In: The Neurosciences: Fourth Study Program (Schmitt, F.O. and Worden, F.G., eds.). Cambridge, MA: MIT Press, pp. 423–437.

Jack, J.J.B., Miller, S., Porter, R., and Redman, S.J. 1971. The time course of minimal excitatory post-synaptic potentials evoked in spinal motoneurons by group Ia afferent fibres. J. Physiol. (Lond.) 215: 353–380.

Jack, J.J.B., Noble, D., and Tsien, R.W. 1975. Electric Current Flow in Excitable Cells. Oxford: Oxford University Press.

Jack, J.J.B., Redman, S.J., and Wong, K. 1981a. The components of synaptic potentials evoked in cat spinal motoneurones by impulses in single group Ia afferents. J. Physiol. (Lond.) 321: 65–96.

Jack, J.J.B., Redman, S.J., and Wong, K. 1981b. Modifications to synaptic transmission at group Ia synapses on cat spinal motoneurones by 4-aminopyridine. J. Physiol. (Lond.) 321: 111–126.

Jackowski, A., Parnevalas, J.G., and Lieberman, A.R. 1978. The reciprocal synapse in the external plexiform layer of the mammalian olfactory bulb. Brain Res. 195: 17–28.

Jackson M.B. and Scharfman, H.E. 1996. Positive feedback from hilar mossy cells to granule cells in the dentate gyrus revealed by voltage-sensitive dye and microelectrode recording. J. Neurophysiol. 76: 601–616.

Jackson, M.B. and Yakel, J.L. 1995. The 5-HT$_3$ receptor channel. Annu. Rev. Physiol. 57: 447–468.

Jacobs, G.H. 1993. The distribution and nature of colour vision among the mammals. Biol. Rev. 68: 413–471.

Jacobson, M. 1978. Developmental Neurobiology, 2nd ed. New York: Plenum Press.

Jaeger, D., Kita, H., and Wilson, C.J. 1994. Surround inhibition among projection neurons is weak or nonexistent in the rat neostriatum. J. Neurophysiol. 72: 2555–2558.

Jaffe, D.B., Johnston, D., Lasser-Ross, N., Lisman, J.E., Miyakawa, H., and Ross, W.N. 1992. The spread of Na$^+$ spikes determines the pattern of dendritic Ca^{2+} entry into hippocampal neurons. Nature 357: 244–246.

Jahnsen, H. 1986a. Responses of neurons in isolated preparations of the mammalian central nervous system. Prog. Neurobiol. 27: 351–372.

Jahnsen, H. 1986b. Electrophysiological characteristics of neurones in the guinea-pig deep cerebellar nuclei in vitro. J. Physiol. (Lond.) 372: 129–147.

Jahnsen, H. and Llinás, R. 1984a. Electrophysiological properties of guinea-pig thalamic neurones: An in vitro study. J. Physiol. (Lond.) 349: 205–226.

Jahnsen, H. and Llinás, R. 1984b. Ionic basis for the electroresponsiveness and oscillatory properties of guinea-pig thalamic neurones in vitro. J. Physiol. (Lond.) 349: 227–247.

Jahr, C.E. and Nicoll, R.A. 1982a. An intracellular analysis of dendrodendritic inhibition in the turtle in vitro olfactory bulb. J. Physiol. (Lond.) 326: 213–34.

Jahr, C.E. and Nicoll, R.A. 1982b. Noradrenergic modulation of dendrodentritic inhibition in the olfactory bulb. Nature 297: 227–229.

Jahr, C.E. and Stevens, C.F. 1987. Glutamate activates multiple single channels conductances in hippocampal neurons. Nature 325: 522–525.

Jahr, C.E. and Yoshioka, K. 1986. Ia afferent excitation of motoneurones in the in vitro new-born rat spinal cord is selectively antagonized by kynurenate. J. Physiol. (Lond.) 370: 515–530.

Jameson, D. and Hurvich, L. 1959. Perceived color and its dependence on focal surrounding and preceding stimulus variables. J. Opt. Soc. Am. 49: 890–898.

Jami, L., Murthy, K.S.K., and Petit, J. 1982. A quantitative study of skeletofusimotor innervation on the cat peroneus tertius muscle. J. Physiol. (Lond.) 325: 125–144.

Jan, L.Y. and Jan, Y.N. 1990. How might the diversity of potassium channels be generated? Trends Neurosci. 13: 415–419.

Jankowska, E. 1992. Interneuronal relay in spinal pathways from proprioceptors. Prog. Neurobiol. 38: 335–378.

Jankowska, E. and Lindström, S. 1972. Morphology of interneurones mediating Ia reciprocal inhibition of motoneurones in the spinal cord of the cat. J. Physiol. (Lond.) 226: 805–823.

Jankowska, E. and Lundberg, A. 1981. Interneurones in the spinal cord. Trends Neurosci. 4: 230–233.

Jankowska, E., Lundberg, A., rudomin, P., and Sykova, E. 1977. Effects of 4-aminopyridine on transmission in excitatory and inhibitory synapses in the spinal cord. Brain Res. 136: 387–392.

Jankowska, E. and Roberts, W.J. 1972a. An electrophysiological demonstration of the axonal projections of single spinal interneurones in the cat. J. Physiol. (Lond.) 222: 597–622.

Jankowska, E. and Roberts, W.J. 1972b. Synaptic actions of single interneurons mediating reciprocal Ia inhibition of motoneurones. J. Physiol. (Lond.) 222: 623–642.

Jankowska, E. and Smith, D.O. 1973. Antidromic activation of Renshaw cells and their axonal projections. Acta Physiol. Scand. 88: 198–214.

Jansen, J. 1969. On cerebellar evolution and organization from the point of view of a morphologist. In: Neurobiology of Cerebellar Evolution and Development (Llinás, R., ed.). Chicago: American Medical Association, pp. 881–893.

Jasper, H., Khan, R., and Elliot, K. 1965. Amino acids released from the cerebral cortex in relation to its state of activation. Science 147: 1448–1449.

Jefferys, J.G.R., Traub, R.D., and Whittington, M.A. 1996. Neuronal networks for induced '40Hz' rhythms. Trends Neurosci. 19: 202–208.

Jensen, R.J. 1995. Receptive-field properties of displaced starburst amacrine cells change following axotomy-induced degeneration of ganglion cells. Vis. Neurosci. 12: 177–184.

Jessell, T.M. and Kandel, E.R. 1993. Synaptic transmission: A bidirectional and self-modifiable form of cell–cell communication. Neuron 10: 1–30.

Jiang, Z.G. and North, R.A. 1991. Membrane properties and synaptic responses of rat striatal neurones in vitro. J. Physiol. (Lond.) 443: 533–553.

Jimenez-Catellanos, J. and Graybiel, A.M. 1989. Compartmental origin of striatal efferent projections in the cat. Neuroscience 32: 297–321.

Johnson, D.H. 1980. The relationship between spike rate and synchrony in responses of auditory-nerve fibers to single tones. J. Acoust. Soc. Am. 68: 1115–1122.

Johnson, J.W. and Ascher, P. 1987. Glycine potentiates the NMDA response in cultured mouse brain neurons. Nature 325: 529–531.

Johnston, D. and Brown, T.H. 1981. Giant synaptic potential hypothesis for epileptiform activity. Science 211: 294–297.

Johnston, D. and Brown, T.H. 1983. Interpretation of voltage-clamp measurements in hippocampal neurons. J. Neurophysiol. 50: 464–486.

Johnston, D. and Brown, T.H. 1984a. Biophysics and microphysiology of synaptic transmission in hippocampus. In: Brain Slices (Dingledine, R., ed.). New York: Plenum Press, pp. 51–86.

Johnston, D. and Brown, T.H. 1984b. The synaptic nature of the paroxysmal depolarizing shift in hippocampal neurons. Ann. Neurol. 16: S65–S71.

Johnston, D. and Brown, T.H. 1984c. Mechanisms of neuronal burst generation. In: Electrophysiology of Epilepsy (Schwartzkroin, P.A. and Wheal, H., eds.). London: Academic Press, pp. 277–301.

Johnston, D. and Brown, T.H. 1986. Control theory applied to neural networks illuminates synaptic basis of interictal epileptiform activity. In: Basic Mechanisms of the Epilepsies Molecular and Cellular Approaches (Delgado-Escueta, A.V., Ward, A., Woodbury, D.M., and Porter, R.J., eds.). New York: Raven Press, pp. 263–274.

Johnston, D., Magee, J.C., Colbert, C.M., and Christie, B. 1996. Active properties of neuronal dendrites. Annu. Rev. Neurosci. 19: 165–186.

Johnston, D., Williams, S., Jaffe, D., and Gray, R. 1992. NMDA-receptor-independent long-term potentiation. Annu. Rev. Physiol. 54: 489–505.

Johnston, D. and Wu, S.M.-S. 1995. Foundations of Cellular Neurophysiology. Cambridge, MA: MIT Press.

Jonas, P., Major, G., and Sakmann, B. 1993. Quantal components of unitary EPSCs at the mossy fibre synapse on CA3 pyramidal cells of rat hippocampus. J. Physiol. (Lond.) 472: 615–663.

Jones, E.G. 1985. The Thalamus. New York: Plenum Press.

Jones, E.G. and Powell, T.P. 1968. The projection of the somatic sensory cortex upon the thalamus in the cat. Brain Res. 10: 369–391.

Jones, E.G., Powell, T.P. 1969a. Electron microscopy of synaptic glomeruli in the thalamic relay nuclei of the cat. Proc. R. Soc. Lond. B Biol. Sci. 172: 153–171.

Jones, E.G., Powell, T.P.S. 1969b. An electron microscopic study of the mode of termination of cortico-thalamic fibres within the sensory relay nuclei of the thalamus. Proc R. Soc Lond B Biol. Sci. 172: 173–185.

Jones, E.G. and Powell, T. 1969c. Morphological variations in the dendritic spines of the neocortex. J. Cell Sci. 5: 495–507.

Joris, P.X., Carney, L.H., Smith, P.H., and Yin, T.C.T. 1994. Enhancement of neural synchronization in the anteroventral cochlear nucleus. II: Responses in the tuning curve tail. J. Neurophysiol. 71: 1037–1051.

Jourdan, F. 1975. Ultrastructure de l'épithelium olfatif du rat: Polymorphisme des récepteurs. C.R. Séances Acad. Sci. [III] 280: 443–446.

Jourdan, F. 1982. Spatial dimension in olfactory coding: A representation of the 2-deoxyglucose patterns of glomerular labeling in the olfactory bulb. Brain Res. 240: 341–344.

Jung, M.W. and Larson, J. 1994. Further characteristics of long-term potentiation in piriform cortex. Synapse 18: 298–306.

Jung, M.W., Larson, J., and Lynch, G. 1990a. Long-term potentiation of monosynaptic EPSPs in rat piriform cortex in vitro. Synapse 6: 279–283.

Jung, M.W., Larson, J., and Lynch, G. 1990b. role of NMDA and non-NMDA receptors in synaptic transmission in rat piriform cortex. Synapse 82: 451–455.

Kaas, J.H. 1978. The organization of visual cortex in primates. In: Sensory Systems of Primates (Noback, C.R., ed.). New York: Plenum Press, pp. 151–179.

Kaba, H., Hayashi, Y., Higuchi, T., and Nakanishi, S. 1994. Induction of an olfactory memory by the activation of a metabotropic glutamate receptor. Science 265: 262–264.

Kaczmarek, L.K. and Levitan, I.B. 1987. Neuromodulation: The Biochemical Control of Neuronal Excitability. New York: Oxford University Press.

Kafitz, K.W. and Greer, C.A. 1997. Role of laminin in axonal extension from olfactory receptor cells. J. Neurobiol. 32: 298–310.

Kalil, R.E. and Chase, R. 1970. Corticofugal influence on activity of lateral geniculate neurons in the cat. J. Neurophysiol. 33: 459–474.

Kan, K.S.K., Chao, L.P., and Eng, L.F. 1978. Immunohistochemical localization of choline acetyltransferase in rabbit spinal cord and cerebellum. Brain Res. 146: 221–229.

Kan, K.S.K., Chao, L.P., and Forno, L.S. 1980. Immuno-histochemical localization of choline acetyltransferase in the human cerebellum. Brain Res. 193: 165–171.

Kanda, K., Burke, R.E., and Walmsley, B. 1977. Differential control of fast and slow twitch motor units in the decerebrate cat. Exp. Brain Res. 29: 57–74.

Kandel, E.R. and Spencer, W.A. 1961a. Electrophysiology of hippocampal neurons. II. Afterpotentials and repetitive firing. J. Neurophysiol. 24: 243–259.

Kandel, E.R. and Spencer, W.A. 1961b. Excitation and inhibition of single pyramidal cells during hippocampal seizure. Exp. Neurol. 4: 162–179.

Kane, E.C. 1973. Octopus cells in the cochlear nucleus of the cat: Heterotypic synapses upon homotypic neurons. Int. J. Neurosci. 5: 251–279.

Kane, E.C. 1974. Synaptic organization in the dorsal cochlear nucleus of the cat: A light and electron microscopic study. J. Comp. Neurol. 155: 301–329.

Kane, E.S. 1977. Descending inputs to the cat dorsal cochlear nucleus: An electron microscopic study. J. Neurocytol. 6: 583–605.

Kane, E.S., Puglisi, S.G., and Gordon, B.S. 1981. Neuronal types in the deep dorsal cochlear nucleus of the cat: I. Giant neurons. J. Comp. Neurol. 198: 483–513.

Kaneda, M., Hashimoto, M., and Kaneko, A. 1995. Neuronal nicotinic acetylcholine receptors of ganglion cells in the cat retina. Jpn. J. Physiol. 45: 491–508.

Kaneda, M. and Kaneko, A. 1991. Voltage-gated sodium currents in isolated retinal ganglion cells of the cat: Relation between the inactivation kinetics and the cell type. Neurosci. Res. 11: 261–275.

Kaneko, A. 1970. Physiological and morphological identification of horizontal, bipolar and amacrine cells in goldfish retina. J. Physiol. (Lond.) 207: 623–633.

Kanter, E.D. and Haberly, L.B. 1990. NMDA-dependent induction of long-term potentiation in afferent and association fiber systems of piriform cortex in vitro. Brain Res. 525: 175–179.

Kanter, E.D. and Haberly, L.B. 1993. Associative long-term potentiation in piriform cortex slices requires GABA$_A$ blockade. J. Neurosci. 13: 2477–2482.

Kanter, E.D., Kapur, A., and Haberly, L.B. 1996. A dendritic GABA$_A$-mediated IPSP regulates facilitation of NMDA-mediated responses to burst stimulation in piriform cortex. J. Neurosci. 16: 307–312.

Kaplan, E., Lee, B.B., and Shapley, R.M. 1990. New views of primate retinal function. In: Progress in Retinal Research (Osborne, N. and Chader, J., eds.). Oxford: Pergamon, pp. 273–336.

Kaplan, E. and Shapley, R.M. 1982. X and Y cells in the lateral geniculate nucleus of macaque monkeys. J. Physiol. (Lond.) 330: 125–143.

Kapur, A. and Haberly, L.B. 1991. Duration of LTP in piriform cortex in vivo is increased after epileptiform bursting. Soc. Neurosci. Abstr. 17: 386.

Kapur, A., Lytton, W.W., and Haberly, L.B. 1994. Simulation of the selective action of a slow dendritic GABA$_A$-mediated IPSC on the NMDA component of EPSPs in a pyramidal cell model. Soc. Neurosci. Abstr. 20: 652.

Kapur, A., Pearce, R.A., and Haberly, L.B. 1993. Regulation of an NMDA-mediated EPSP by a slow dendritic GABA$_A$-mediated IPSC in piriform cortex. Soc. Neurosci. Abstr. 19: 1521.

Karlsson, G., Pozzo, M., and Olpe, H.-R. 1988. Phaclofen: A GABA$_B$ blocker reduces long-duration inhibition in the neocortex. Eur. J. Pharmacol. 148: 485–486.

Katz, B. 1966. Nerve, Muscle, and Synapse. New York: McGraw-Hill.

Katz, L.C. 1987. Local circuitry of identified projection neurons in cat primary visual cortex brain slices. J. Neurosci. 7: 1223–1249.

Katz, L.C. and Shatz, C.J. 1996. Synaptic activity and the construction of cortical circuits. Science 274: 1133–1138.

Kauer, J.S. 1974. Response patterns of amphibian olfactory bulb neurones to odour stimulation. J. Physiol. 243: 695–715.

Kauer, J.S. and Shepherd, G.M. 1977. analysis of the onset phase of olfactory bulb unit responses to odour pulses in the salamander. J. Physiol. (Lond.) 272: 495–516.

Kauer, J.S. and Cinelli, A.R. 1993. Are there structural and functional modules in the vertebrate olfactory bulb? Microsc. Res. Tech. 24: 154–167.

Kauer, J.S. and Moulton, D.G. 1974. Responses of olfactory bulb neurones to odour stimulation of small nasal areas in the salamander. J. Physiol. (Lond.) 243: 717–737.

Kauer, J.S., Neff, S.R., Hamilston, K.A., Cinelli, A.R. 1993. The salamander olfactory pathway: Visualizing and modeling circuit activity. In: Olfaction: A Model for Computational Neuroscience (Eichenbaum, H. and Davis, J.L., eds.). Cambridge, MA: MIT Press, pp. 43–68.

Kaupmann, K., Huggel, K., Heid, J., Flor, P.J., Mickel, Bischoff, S., McMaster, G., Angst, C., Bittiger, H., Froestl, W., and Bettler, B. 1997. Expression cloning of GABA$_B$ receptors uncovers similarity to metabotropic glutamate receptors. Nature 386: 239–246.

Kawaguchi, Y. 1992. Large aspiny cells in the matrix of the rat neostriatum in vitro—Physiological identification, relation to the compartments and excitatory postsynaptic currents. J. Neurophysiol. 67: 1669–1682.

Kawaguchi, Y. 1993a. Groupings of nonpyramidal and pyramidal cells with specific physiological and morphological characteristics in layer II/III of rat frontal cortex. J. Neurosci. 69: 416–431.

Kawaguchi, Y. 1993b. Physiological, morphological and histochemical characterization of three classes of interneurons in rat neostriatum. J. Neurosci. 13: 4908–4923.

Kawaguchi, Y. 1995. Physiological subgroups of nonpyramidal cells with specific morphological characteristics in layer II/III of rat frontal cortex. J. Neurosci. 15: 2638–2655.

Kawaguchi, Y., Wilson, C.J., Augood, S.J., and Emson, P.C. 1995. Striatal interneurones—Chemical, physiological and morphological characterization. Trends Neurosci. 18: 527–535.

Kawaguchi, Y., Wilson, C.J., and Emson, P.C. 1989. Intracellular recording of identified neostriatal patch and matrix spiny cells in a slice preparation preserving cortical inputs. J. Neurophysiol. 62: 1052–1068.

Kawaguchi, Y., Wilson, C.J., and Emson, P.C. 1990. Projection subtypes of rat neostriatal matrix cells revealed by intracellular injection of biocytin. J. Neurosci. 10: 3421–3438.

Kawamura, H. and Provini, K. 1970. Depression of cerebellar Purkinje cells by microiontophoretic application of GABA and related amino acids. Brain Res. 24: 293–304.

Keller, A., Irki, A., and Asanuma, H. 1990. Identification of neurons producing long-term potentiation in the cat motor cortex: Intracellular recordings and labelling. J. Comp. Neurol. 300: 47–60.

Kelso, S.R., Ganong, A.H., and Brown, T.H. 1986. Hebbian synapses in hippocampus. Proc. Natl. Acad. Sci. USA 83: 5326–5330.

Kemp, J.A. and Sillito, A.M. 1982. The nature of the excitatory transmitter mediating X and Y cell inputs to the cat dorsal lateral geniculate nucleus. J. Physiol. (Lond.) 323: 377–391.

Kemp, J.M. and Powell, T. 1971a. The site of termination of afferent fibers in the caudate nucleus. Phil. Trans. Soc. Lond. [B] 262: 413–427.

Kemp, J.M. and Powell, T. 1971b. The synaptic organization of the caudate nucleus. Phil. Trans. Soc. Lond. [B] 262: 403–412.

Kennedy, H., Meissirel, C., and Dehay, C. 1991. Callosal pathways and their compliancy to general rules governing the organization of cortical connectivity. In: Vision and Visual Dysfunction, Vol. 3: Neuroanatomy of the Visual Pathways and Their Development (Dreher, B. and Robinson, S., eds.). London: Macmillan, pp. 324–359.

Kennedy, M.B. 1989. Regulation of neuronal function by calcium. Trends Neurosci. 12: 417–420.

Kernell, D. 1965a. The adaptation and the relation between discharge frequency and current strength of cat lumbrosacral motoneurones stimulated by long-lasting injected currents. Acta Physiol. Scand. 65: 65–73.

Kernell, D. 1965b. The limits of firing frequency in cat lumbrosacral motoneurones possessing different time course of afterhyperpolarization. Acta Physiol. Scand. 65: 87–100.

Kerr, D., Ong, J., Johnston, G., Abbenante, J., and Prager, R. 1988. 2-hydroxy-saclofen: An improved antagonist at central and peripheral GABA$_B$ receptors. Neurosci. Lett. 92.

Kerr, D., Ong, J., Prager, R., Gynther, B., and Curtis, D. 1987. Phaclophen: A peripheral and central baclophen antagonist. Brain Res. 405: 150–154.

Ketchum, K.L. and Haberly, L.B. 1991. Fast oscillations and dispersive propagation in olfactory cortex and other cortical areas a functional hypothesis. In: Olfaction. A Model System for Computational Neuroscience (Davis, J.L. and Eichenbaum, H., eds.). Cambridge, MA: MIT Press, pp. 69–100.

Ketchum, K.L. and Haberly, L.B. 1993a. Synaptic events that generate fast oscillations in piriform cortex. J. Neurosci. 13: 3980–3985.

Ketchum, K.L. and Haberly, L.B. 1993b. Membrane currents evoked by afferent fiber stimulation in rat piriform cortex. I. Current source-density analysis. J. Neurophysiol. 69: 248–260.

Ketchum, K.L. and Haberly, L.B. 1993c. Membrane currents evoked by afferent fiber stimulation in rat piriform cortex. II. Analysis with a system model. J. Neurophysiol. 69: 261–281.

Keverne, E.B. 1995. Olfactory learning. Curr. Opin. Neurobiol. 5: 482–488.

Kevetter, G.A. and Perachio, A.A. 1989. Projections from the sacculus to the cochlear nuclei in the Mongolian gerbil. Brain Behav. Evol. 34: 193–200.

Kiang, N.Y.S., Rho, J.M., Northrop, C.C., Liberman, M.C., and Ryugo, D.K. 1982. Hair-cell innervation by spiral ganglion cells in adult cats. Science 217: 175–177.

Kier, C.K., Buchsbaum, G., and Sterling, P. 1995. How retinal microcircuits scale for ganglion cells of different size. J. Neurosci. 15: 7673–7683.

Kim, D.O., Ghoshal, S., Khant, S.L., and Parham, K. 1994. A computational model with ionic conductances for the fusiform cell of the dorsal cochlear nucleus. J. Acoust. Soc. Am. 96: 1501–1514.

Kim, H. and Connors, B. 1993. Apical dendrites of the neocortex: Correlation between sodium- and calcium-dependent spiking and pyramidal cell morphology. J. Neurosci. 13: 5301–5311.

Kimura, F., Tsumoto, T., Nishigori, A., and Yoshimura, Y. 1990. Long-term depression but not potentiation is induced in Ca^{2+}-chelated visual cortex neurons. Neurosci. Rep. 1: 65–68.

Kimura, M., Raijkowski, J., and Evarts, E. 1984. Tonically discharging putamen neurons exhibit set-dependent responses. Proc. Natl. Acad. Sci. USA 81: 4998–5001.

Kincaid, A.E. and Wilson, C.J. 1996. Corticostriatal innervation of the patch and matrix in the rat neostriatum. J. Comp. Neurol. 374: 578–592.

Kingston, P.A., Barnstable, C.J., Shepherd, G.M., and Zufall, F. 1996. Expression of multiple cyclic nucleotide-gated channel genes in the rat olfactory bulb and cortex. Am. Chem. Soc. Abstr. XVIII: in press.

Kirkwood, A., Dudek, S., Gold, J., Aisenman, C., and Bear, M. 1993. Common forms of synaptic plasticity in hippocampus and neocortex in vitro. Science 260: 1518–1521.

Kirkwood, A., Lee, H.-K., and Bear, M. 1995. Co-regulation of long-term potentiation and experience-dependent synaptic plasticity in visual cortex by age and experience. Nature 375: 328–331.

Kirkwood, A., Rioutt, M., and Bear, M. 1996. Experience-dependent modification of synaptic plasticity in visual cortex. Nature 381: 526–528.

Kishi, K. 1987. Golgi studies on the development of granule cells of the rat olfactory bulb with reference to migration in the subependymal layer. J. Comp. Neurol. 258: 112–124.

Kishi, K., Mori, K., and Ojima, H. 1984. Distribution of local axon collaterals of mitral, displaced mitral and tufted cells in the rabbit olfactory bulb. J. Comp. Neurol. 225: 511–526.

Kishi, K., Stanfield, B.B., and Cowan, W.M. 1980. A quantitative EM autoradiographic study of the commissural and associational connections of the dentate gyrus in the rat. Anat. Embryol. 160. 173–186.

Kisvàrday, Z. 1992. GABAergic networks of basket cells in the visual cortex. Prog. Brain Res. 90: 385–405.

Kisvàrday, Z., Martin, K.A.C., Whitteridge, D., and Somogyi, P. 1985. Synaptic connections of intracellularly filled clutch neurons, a type of small basket neuron in the visual cortex of the cat. J. Comp. Neurol. 241: 111–137.

Kita, H. 1993. GABAergic Circuits of the Striatum. Oxford: Elsevier.

Kita, H. 1996. Glutamatergic and GABAergic postsynaptic responses of striatal spiny neurons to intrastriatal and cortical stimulation recorded in slice preparations. Neuroscience 70: 925–940.

Kita, H. and Kitai, S.T. 1987. Efferent projections of the subthalamic nucleus in the rat—Light and electron microscopic analysis with the PHA-L method. J. Comp. Neurol. 260: 435–452.

Kita, H. and Kitai, S.T. 1988. Glutamate decarboxylase immunoreactive neurons in rat neostriatum: Their morphological types and populations. Brain Res. 447: 346–352.

Kita, H., Kosaka, T., and Heizmann, C.W. 1990. Parvalbumin-immunoreactive neurons in the rat neostriatum: A light and electron microscopic study. Brain Res. 536: 1–15.

Kita, T., Kita, H., and Kitai, S.T. 1984. Passive electrical membrane properties of rat neostriatal neurons in an in vitro slice preparation. Brain Res. 300: 129–139.

Kitai, S.T. 1981. Electrophysiology of the corpus striatum and brain stem integrating systems. In: Section 1: The Nervous System, Vol. II: Motor Control, Part I: Handbook of Physiology (Brooks, V.B., ed.). Bethesda: American Physiological Society, pp. 997–1015.

Kitai, S.T., Kocsis, J.D., Preston, R.J., and Sugimori, M. 1976a. Monosynaptic inputs to caudate neurons identified by intracellular injection of horseradish peroxidase. Brain Res. 109: 601–606.

Kitai, S.T., Sugimori, M., and Kocsis, J.D. 1976b. Excitatory nature of dopamine in the nigro-caudate pathway. Exp. Brain Res. 24: 351–363.

Kleinfeld, D. 1986. Sequential state generation by model neural networks. Proc. Natl. Acad. Sci. USA 83: 9469–9473.

Klug, K., Herr, S., Esfahani, P., and Schein, S. 1997. Distribution of different cell types in a small region of the macaque fovea. (Submitted).

Knierim, J.J. and Van Essen, D.C. 1992. Visual cortex cartography, connectivity, and concurrent processing. Curr. Opin. Neurobiol. 2: 150–155.

Koch, C. 1985. Understanding the intrinsic circuitry of the cat's LGN electrical properties of the spine-triad arrangement. Proc. R. Soc. Lond. B Biol. Sci. 225: 365–390.

Koch, C. 1987. The action of the corticofugal pathway on sensory thalamic nuclei: A hypothesis. Neuroscience 23: 399–406.

Koch, C. 1997. Computation and the single neuron. Nature 385: 207–210.

Koch, C. and Poggio, T. 1983. A theoretical analysis of electrical properties of spines. Proc. R. Soc. Lond. B Biol. Sci. 218: 455–477.

Koch, C. and Poggio, T. 1987. Biophysics of computation: Neurons, synapses and membranes. In: Synaptic Function (Gall, W.E. and Cowan, W.M., eds.). New York: John Wiley, pp. 637–697.

Koch, C., Poggio, T., and Torre, V. 1982. Retinal ganglion cells: A functional interpretation of dendritic morphology. Phil. Trans. R. Soc. Lond. B 298: 227–263.

Koch, C., Poggio, T., and Torre, V. 1983. Nonlinear interactions in a dendritic tree: Localization, timing, and role of information processing. Proc. Natl. Acad. Sci. USA 80: 2799–802.

Koch, C. and Zador, A. 1993. The function of dendritic spines: Devices subserving biochemical rather than electrical compartmentalization. J. Neurosci. 13: 413–422.

Kocsis, J.D., Sugimori, M., and Kitai, S.T. 1976. Convergence of excitatory synaptic inputs to caudate spiny neurons. Brain Res. 124: 403–413.

Koerber, H.R., Druzinsky, R.E., and Mendell, L.M. 1988. Properties of somata of spinal dorsal root ganglion cells differ according to peripheral receptor innervated. J. Neurophysiol. 60: 1584–1596.

Kohler, C. 1985. A projection from the deep layers of the entorhinal area to the hippocampal formation in the rat brain. Neurosci. Lett. 56: 13–19.

Kohler, C., Chan-Palay, V., and Wu, J.Y. 1984. Septal neurons containing glutamic acid decarboxylase immuno-reactivity project to the hippocampal region in the rat brain. Anat. Embryol. 169: 41–44.

Kohler, C. and Steinbusch, H. 1982. Identification of serotonin and non-serotonin-containing neurons of the mid-brain raphe projecting to the entorhinal area and the hippocampal formation. A combined immunohistochemical and fluorescent retrograde tracing. Neuroscience 7: 951–975.

Kohler, C., Swanson, L.W., Haglund, L., and Wu, Y.Y. 1985. The cytoarchitecture, histochemistry, and projections of the tuberomammillary nucleus in the rat. Neuroscience 16: 85–110.

Kohonen, T. 1978. Associative Memory. Berlin: Springer-Verlag.

Kohonen, T., Lehtio, P., Hyvarinen, J., Bry, K., and Vainio, L. 1977. A principal of neural associative memory. Neuroscience 2: 1065–1076.

Kolb, H. 1970. Organization of the outer plexiform layer of the primate retina: Electron microscopy of Golgi-impregnated cells. Phil. Trans. R. Soc. (Lond.) B 258: 261–283.

Kolb, H. 1977. The organization of the outer plexiform layer in the retina of the cat: Electron microscopic observations. J. Neurocytol. 6: 131–153.

Kolb, H. 1994. The architecture of functional neural circuits in the vertebrate retina. Invest. Ophthalmol. Vis. Sci. 35: 2385–2404.

Kolb, H. and Dekorver, L. 1991. Midget ganglion cells of the parafovea of the human retina: A study by electron microscopy and serial section reconstructions. J. Comp. Neurol. 303: 617–636.

Kolb, H. and Famiglietti, E.V. 1974. Rod and cone pathways in the inner plexiform layer of cat retina. Science 186: 47–49.

Kolb, H. and Nelson, R. 1993. OFF-alpha and OFF-beta ganglion cells in cat retina: II. Neural circuitry as revealed by electron microscopy of HRP stains. J. Comp. Neurol. 329: 85–110.

Kolb, H., Nelson, R., and Mariani, A. 1981. Amacrine cells, bipolar cells and ganglion cells of the cat retina: A Golgi study. Vision Res. 21: 1081–1114.

Kolb, H. and West, R.W. 1977. Synaptic connections of the interplexiform cell in the retina of the cat. J. Neurocytol. 6: 155–170.

Komatsu, Y. and Iwakiri, M. 1993. Long-term modification of inhibitory synaptic transmission in developing visual cortex. Neurosci. Rep. 7: 907–910.

Komatsu, Y., Toyama, K., Maeda, J., and Sakaguchi, H. 1981. Long-term potentiation investigated in a slice preparation of striate cortex of young kittens. Neurosci. Lett. 26: 269–274.

Korn, H. and Faber, D.S. 1987. Regulation and significance of probabilistic release mechanisms at central synapses. In: Synaptic Functions (Edelman, G.M., Gall, W.E., and Cowan, W.M., eds.). New York: John Wiley, pp. 57–108.

Korn, H. and Faber, D.S. 1991. Quantal analysis and synaptic efficacy in the CNS. Trends Neurosci. 14: 439–445.

Kosel, K.C., Van Hoesen, G. W., and Rosene, D. L. (1983) A direct projection form the perirhinal cortex (area 35) to the subiculum in the rat. Brain Res. 269: 347–351.

Kosaka, T., Hama, K., and Wu, J.Y. 1984. GABAergic synaptic boutons in the granule cell layer of rat dentate gyrus. Brain Res. 293: 353–359.

Kosaka, T., Tauchi, M., and Dahl, J.L. 1988. Cholinergic neurons containing GABA-like and/or glutamic acid decarboxylase-like immunoreactivities in various brain regions of the rat. Exp. Brain Res. 70: 605–617.

Kosaka, T. 1983. Axon initial segments of the granule cell in the rat dentate gyrus: Synaptic contacts on bundles of axon initial segments. Brain Res. 274: 129–134.

Koulen, P., Sassoè-Pognetto, M., Grünert, U., and Wässle, H. 1996. Selective clustering of $GABA_A$ and glycine receptors in the mammalian retina. J. Neurosci. 16: 2127–2140.

Kouyama, N. and Marshak, D.W. 1992. Bipolar cells specific for blue cones in the Macaque retina. J. Neurosci. 12: 1233–1252.

Krettek, J.E. and Price, J.L. 1977a. Projections from the amygdaloid complex to the cerebral cortex and thalamus in the rat and cat. J. Comp. Neurol. 172: 687–722.

Krettek, J.E. and Price, J.L. 1977b. Projections from the amygdaloid complex and adjacent olfactory structures to the entorhinal cortex and to the subiculum in the rat and cat. J. Comp. Neurol. 172: 723–752.

Krettek, J.E. and Price, J.L. 1978. A description of the amygdaloid complex in the rat and cat, with observations on intra-amygdaloid axonal connections. J. Comp. Neurol. 178: 255–280.

Kriegstein, A.R. and Connors, B.W. 1986. Cellular physiology of the turtle visual cortex: Synaptic properties and intrinsic circuitry. J. Neurosci. 6: 178–191.

Krnjevic, K. 1981. Transmitters in motor systems. In: Handbook of Physiology, Section I: The Nervous System, Vol. II: Motor Control, Part 1 (Brooks, V.B., eds.). Bethesda: American Physiological Society, pp. 107–154.

Krnjevic, K. and Phillis, J.W. 1963. Acetylcholine sensitive cells in the cerebellar cortex. J. Physiol. (Lond.) 166: 296–327.

Krnjevic, K., Pumain, R., and Renaud, L. 1971. The mechanism of excitation by acetylcholine in the cerebral cortex. J. Physiol. (Lond.) 215: 247–268.

Krnjevic, K. and Schwartz, S. 1967. The action of γ-aminobutyric acid on cortical neurones. Exp. Brain Res. 3: 320–336.

Kröller, J. and Grüsser, O.-J. 1983. Convergence of muscle spindle afferents on single neurons of the cat dorsal spino-cerebellar tract and their synaptic efficacy. Brain Res. 253: 65–80.

Kubek, M.J., Knoblach, S.M., Sharif, N.A., Burt, D.R., Buterbaugh, G.G., and Fuson, K.S. 1993. Thyrotropin-releasing hormone gene expression and receptors are differentially modified in limbic foci by seizures. Ann. Neurol. 33: 70–76.

Kubota, Y. and Jones, E.G. 1992. Co-localization of two calcium binding proteins in GABA cell of rat piriform cortex. Brain Res. 600: 339–344.

Kubota, Y., and Kawaguchi, Y. 1993. Neostriatal GABAergic interneurones contain NOS, calretinin or parvalbumin. NeuroReport 5: 205–208.

Kuffler, S.W. Discharge patterns and functional organization of mammalian retina. 1953. J. Neurophysiol. 16: 37–68.

Kuhse, J., Becker, C.M., Schmieden, V., Hoch, W., Pribilla, I., Langosch, D., Malosio, M.L., Muntz, M., and Betz, H. 1991. Heterogeneity of the inhibitory glycine receptor. Ann. N.Y. Acad. Sci. 625: 129–135.

Kuhse, J., Betz, H., and Kirsch, J. 1995. The inhibitory glycine receptor: Architecture, synaptic localization and molecular pathology of a postsynaptic ion-channel complex. Curr. Opin. Neurobiol. 5: 318–323.

Kuno, M. 1964. Quantal components of excitatory synaptic potentials in spinal motoneurones. J. Physiol. (Lond.) 175: 81–99.

Kunzle, H. 1976. Thalamic projections from the precentral motor cortex in *Macaca* fascicularis, Brain Res. 105: 253–267.

Kwon, Y.H., Esguerra, M., and Sur, M. 1991. NMDA and non-NMDA receptors mediate visual responses of neurons in the cat's lateral geniculate nucleus. J. Neurophysiol. 66: 414–428.

Laatsch, R.H. and Cowan, W.M. 1967. Electron microscopic studies of the dentate gyrus of the rat. II. Degeneration of commissural afferents. J. Comp. Neurol. 130: 241–262.

Lacy, M.C., Mercuri, N.B., and North, R.A. 1987. Dopamine acts on D2 receptors to increase potassium conductance in neurons of the rat substantia nigra zona compacta. J. Physiol. (Lond.) 392: 397–416.

Lagerbäck, P. and Kellerth, J.-O. 1985. Light microscopic observations on cat Renshaw cells after intracellular staining with horseradish peroxidase. I. The axonal system. J. Comp. Neurol. 240: 359–367.

Lai, Y.C., Winslow, R.L., and Sachs, M.B. 1994. A model of selective processing of auditory-nerve inputs by stellate cells of the antero-ventral cochlear nucleus. J. Comput. Neurosci. 1: 167–194.

Lal, R. and Friedlander, M.J. 1989. Gating of retinal transmission by afferent eye position and movement signals. Science 243: 93–96.

Lamb, T.D. and Pugh, E.N.J. 1992. G-protein cascades: Gain and kinetics. Trends Neurosci. 15: 291–298.

Lamb, T.D. and Simon, E.J. 1976. The relation between intercellular coupling and electrical noise in turtle photoreceptors. J. Physiol. 263: 257–286.

Lambert, N., Borroni, A., Grover, L., and Teyler, T. 1991. Hyperpolarizing and depolarizing GABA$_A$ receptor mediated dendritic inhibition in area CA1 of the rat hippocampus. J. Neurophysiol. 66: 1538–1548.

Lancaster, B. and Adams, P.R. 1986. Calcium-dependent current generating the afterhyperpolarization of hippocampal neurons. J. Neurophysiol. 55: 1268–1282.

Lancet, D., Greer, C.A., Kauer, J.S., and Shepherd, G.M. 1982. Mapping of odor-related neuronal activity in the olfactory bulb by high-resolution 2-deoxyglucose autoradiography. Proc. Natl. Acad. Sci. USA 79: 670–674.

Land, E. 1959a. Color vision and the natural image. Part I. Proc. Natl. Acad. Sci. USA 45: 115–129.

Land, E. 1959b. Color vision and the natural image. Part II. Proc. Natl. Acad. Sci. USA 46: 36–44.

Land, E. 1983. Recent advances in retinex theory and some implications for cortical computations: Color vision and the natural image. Proc. Natl. Acad. Sci. USA 80: 5163–5169.

Land, L.J., Eager, R.P., and Shepherd, G.M. 1970. Olfactory nerve projections to the olfactory bulb in rabbit: Demonstration by means of a simplified ammoniacal silver degeneration method. Brain Res. 23: 250–254.

Land, L.J. and Shepherd, G.M. 1974. Autoradiographic analysis of olfactory receptor projections in the rabbit. Brain Res. 70: 506–10.

Landis, D.M.D. and Reese, T.S. 1983. Cytoplasmic organization in cerebellar dendritic spines. J. Cell. Biol. 97: 1169–1178.

Landmesser, L. 1978. The distribution of motoneurones supplying chick hind limb muscles. J. Physiol. (Lond.) 264: 371–389.

Lang, E., Sugihara, I., and Llinás, R. 1996. GABAergic modulation of complex spike activity by the cerebellar nucleolivary pathway in rat. J. Neurophysiol. 76: 255–275.

Langer, L.F. and Graybiel, A.M. 1989. Distinct nigrostriatal projection systems innervate striosomes and matrix in the primate striatum. Brain Res. 498: 344–350.

Langmoen, I.A. and Andersen, P. 1981. The hippocampal slice in vitro. A description of the technique and some examples of the opportunities it offers. In: Electrophysiology of Isolated Mammalian CNS Preparations (Kerkut, G.A. and Wheal, H.V., eds.). London: Academic Press, pp. 51–105.

Langner, G. 1992. Periodicity coding in the auditory system. Hear. Res. 60: 115–142.

Lankheet, M.J.M., Rowe, M.H., van Wezel, R.J.A., and van de Grind, W.A. 1996. Horizontal cell sensitivity in the cat retina during prolonged dark adaptation. Vis. Neurosci. 13: 885–896.

Lapper, S.R. and Bolam, J.P. 1992. Input from the frontal cortex and the parafascicular nucleus to cholinergic interneurons in the dorsal striatum of the rat. Neuroscience 51: 533–545.

Larkum, M.E., Rioult, M.G., and Lüscher, H.-R. 1996. Propagation of action potentials in the dendrites of neurons from rat spinal cord slice cultures. J. Neurophysiol. 75: 154–170.

Latorre, R., Oberhauser, A., Labarca, P., and Alvarez, O. 1989. Varieties of calcium-activated potassium channels. Annu. Rev. Physiol. 51: 385–399.

Läuger, P. 1991. Electrogenic Ion Pumps. Sunderland, MA: Sinauer.

Laughlin, S.B. 1994. Matching coding, circuits, cells, and molecules to signals: General principles of retinal design in the fly's eye. Prog. Retina Eye Res. 13: 165–196.

Laughlin, S.B. and de Ruyter van Steveninck, R.R. 1996. Measurements of signal transfer and noise suggest a new model for graded transmission at an adapting retinal synapse [Abstract]. J. Physiol. (Lond.) 494. p: 19.

Laughlin, S.B., Howard, J., and Blakeslee, B. 1987. Synaptic limitations to contrast coding in the retina of the blowfly Calliphora. Proc. R. Soc. (Lond.) B 231: 437–467.

Laurberg, S. and Sorensen, K.E. 1981. Associational and commissural collaterals of neurons in the hippocampal formation (hilus fasciae dentate and subfield CA3). Brain Res. 212: 287–300.

Laurent, G., Wehr, M., and Davidowitz, H. 1996. Temporal representations of odors in an olfactory network. J. Neurosci. 16: 3837–3847.

Lawrence, D.G., Porter, R., and Redman, S.J. 1985. Corticomotoneuronal synapses in the monkey: Light microscopic localization upon motoneurons of intrinsic muscles of the hand. J. Comp. Neurol. 232: 499–510.

Lee, K.H. and McCormick, D.A. 1995. Acetylcholine excites GABAergic neurons of the ferret perigeniculate nucleus through nicotinic receptors. J. Neurophysiol. 73: 2123–2127.

Lehky, S. and Sejnowski, T. 1988. Network model of shape from shading: Neural function arises from both receptive and projective fields. Nature 333: 452–454.

Lenn, N.J. and Reese, T.S. 1966. The fine structure of nerve endings in the nucleus of the trapezoid body and the ventral cochlear nucleus. Am. J. Anat. 118: 375–390.

LeVay, S. 1973. Synaptic patterns in the visual cortex of the cat and monkey. Electron microscopy of Golgi preparations. J. Comp. Neurol. 150: 53–86.

LeVay, S. and Gilbert, C. 1976. Laminar patterns of geniculocortical projection in the cat. Brain Res. 113: 1–19.

LeVay, S. and Sherk, H. 1981. The visual claustrum of the cat. J. Neurosci. 1: 956–980.

Leveteau, J. and MacLeod, P. 1966. Olfactory discrimination in the rabbit olfactory glomerulus. Science 175: 170–178.

Levey, A.I., Hallenger, A.E., and Wainer, B.H. 1987. Choline acetyltransferase immunoreactivity in the rat thalamus. J. Comp. Neurol. 257: 317–332.

Levine, M.S., Cepeda, C., Day, M., Altemus, K.L., and Li, Z. 1995. Dopaminergic modulation of responses evoked by activation of excitatory amino acid receptors in the neostriatum is dependent upon specific receptor subtypes. In: Molecular and Cellular Mechanisms of Neostriatal Function (Ariano, M.A. and Surmeier, D.J., eds.). Austin: R.G. Landes, pp. 217–228.

Lev-Tov, A., Fleshman, J.W., and Burke, R.E. 1983a. Primary afferent depolarization and presynaptic inhibition of monosynaptic group Ia EPSPs during post-tetanic potentiation. J. Neurophysiol. 50: 413–427.

Lev-Tov, A., Meyers, D.E.R., and Burke, R.E. 1988. Activation of type B γ-amino-butyric acid receptors in the intact mammalian spinal cord mimics the effects of reduced presynaptic Ca^{2+} influx. Proc. Natl. Acad. Sci. USA 85: 5330–5334.

Lev-Tov, A., Pinter, M.J., and Burke, R.E. 1983b. Post-tetanic potentiation of group Ia EPSPs: Possible mechanisms for differential distribution in the MG motor nucleus. J. Neurophysiol. 50: 379–398.

Levy, W.B. and Steward, O. 1979. Synapses as associative memory elements in the hippocampal formation. Brain Res. 175: 233–245.

Li, C.-L., Ortiz-Galvin, A., Chon, S., and Howard, S. 1960. Cortical intracellular potentials in response to stimulation of lateral geniculate body. J. Neurophysiol. 29: 367–381.

Li, X.-G., Somogyi, P., Ylinen, A., and Buzsaki, G. 1994. The hippocampal CA3 network: An in vivo intracellular labeling study. J. Comp. Neurol. 339: 181–208.

Liao, D., Hessler, N., and Malinow, R. 1995. Activation of postsynaptically silent synapses during pairing-induced LTP in CA1 region of hippocampal slice. Nature 375: 400–404.

Liberman, M.C. 1982. The cochlear frequency map for the cat: Labelling auditory-nerve fibers of known characteristic frequency. J. Acoust. Soc. Am. 72: 1441–1449.

Liberman, M.C. 1991. Central projections of auditory-nerve fibers of differing spontaneous rate. I. Anteroventral cochlear nucleus. J. Comp. Neurol. 313: 240–258.

Liberman, M.C. 1993. Central projections of auditory nerve fibers of differing spontaneous rate. II: Posteroventral and dorsal cochlear nuclei. J. Comp. Neurol. 327: 17–36.

Libri, V., Constanti, A., Calaminici, M., and Nistico, G. 1994. A comparison of the muscarinic response and morphological properties of identified cells in the guinea-pig olfactory cortex in vitro. Neuroscience 59: 331–347.

Liddell, E.G.T. and Sherrington, C.S. 1925. Recruitment and some other factors of reflex inhibition. Proc. R. Soc. Lond. B Biol. Sci. 97: 488–518.

Liesi, P. 1985. Laminin-immunoreactive glia distinguish regenerative adult CNS systems from non-regenerative ones. EMBO J. 4: 2505–2511.

Linberg, K.A. and Fisher, S.K. 1988. Ultrastructural evidence that horizontal cell axon terminals are presynaptic in the human retina. J. Comp. Neurol. 268: 281–297.

Linden, D.J. 1994. Long-term synaptic depression in the mammalian brain. Neuron 12: 457–472.

Linden, D.J. and Connor, J. 1991. Participation of postsynaptic PKC in cerebellar long-term depression in culture. Science 254: 1656–1659.

Linden, D.J. and Connor, J.A. 1993. Cellular mechanisms of long-term depression in the cerebellum. Curr. Opin. Neurobiol. 3: 401–406.

Linden, D.J. and Connor, J.A. 1995. Long-term synaptic depression. Annu. Rev. Neurosci. 18: 319–57.

Linden, D.J., Dawson, T.M., and Dawson, V.L. 1995. An evaluation of the nitric oxide/cGMP/cGMP-dependent protein kinase cascade in the induction of cerebellar long-term depression in culture. J. Neurosci. 15: 5098–5105.

Linden, D.J., Smeyne, M., and Connor, J.A. 1993. Induction of cerebellar long-term depression in culture requires postsynaptic action of sodium ions. Neuron 11: 1093–100.

Lindström, S. 1982. Synaptic organization of inhibitory pathways to principal cells in the lateral geniculate nucleus of the cat. Brain Res. 234: 447–453.

Linn, D.M., Blazynski, C., Redburn, D.A., and Massey, S.C. 1991. Acetylcholine release from the rabbit retina mediated by kainate receptors. J. Neurosci. 11: 111–122.

Linsenmeier, R.A., Frishman, L.J., Jakiela, H.G., and Enroth-Cugell, C. 1982. Receptive field properties of X and Y cells in the rat retina derived from contrast sensitivity measurements. Vision Res. 22: 1173–1183.

Liu, X.-B., Honda, C.N., and Jones, E.G. 1995. Distribution of four types of synapse on physiologically identified relay neurons in the ventral posterior thalamic nucleus of the cat. J. Comp. Neurol. 352: 69–91.

Livingstone, M. and Hubel, D.H. 1981. Effects of sleep and arousal on the processing of visual information in the cat. Nature 291: 554–561.

Ljungdahl, A., Hokfelt, T., and Nilsson, G. 1978. Distribution of substance P-like immunoreactivity in the central nervous system of the rat—I. Cell bodies and nerve terminals. Neuroscience 3: 861–943.

Llinás, R.R. 1981. Electrophysiology of the cerebellar networks. In: Handbook of Physiology, Section 1: The Nervous System, Vol. II: Motor Control, Part 2 (Brooks, V.B., eds.). Bethesda: American Physiological Society, pp. 831–876.

Llinás, R. 1985. Electrotonic transmission in the mammalian central nervous system. In: Gap Junctions (Bennett, M.V.L. and Spray, D.C., eds.). Cold Spring Harbor, NY: Cold Spring Harbor Laboratory, pp. 337–353.

Llinás, R. 1988. The intrinsic electrophysiological properties of mammalian neurons: Insights into central nervous system function. Science 242: 1654–1664.

Llinás, R. 1990. Intrinsic electrical properties of nerve cells and their role in network oscillation. Cold Spring Harb. Symp. Quant. 55: 933–938.

Llinás, R. and Hess, R. 1976. Tetrodotoxin-resistant dendritic spikes in avian Purkinje cells. Soc. Neurosci. Abstr. 2: 112.

Llinás, R. and Muhlethaler, M. 1988. An electrophysiological study of the in vitro, perfused brainstem-cerebellum of adult guinea pig. J. Physiol. (Lond.) 404: 215–240.

Llinás, R. and Nicholson, C. 1971. Electrophysiological properties of dendrites and somata in alligator Purkinje cells. J. Neurophysiol. 34: 532–551.

Llinás, R. and Nicholson, C. 1976. Reversal properties of climbing fiber potential in cat Purkinje cells: An example of a distributed synapse. J. Neurophysiol. 39: 311–323.

Llinás, R. and Sasaki, K. 1989. The functional organization of the olivo-cerebellar system as examined by multiple Purkinje cell recordings. Eur. J. Neurosci. 1: 587–602.

Llinás, R. and Sugimori, M. 1978. Dendritic calcium spiking in mammalian Purkinje cells: In vitro study of its function and development. Soc. Neurosci. Abstr. 4: 66.

Llinás, R. and Sugimori, M. 1980a. Electrophysiological properties of in vitro Purkinje cell somata in mammalian cerebellar slices. J. Physiol. (Lond.) 305: 171–195.

Llinás, R. and Sugimori, M. 1980b. Electrophysiological properties of in vitro Purkinje cell dendrites in mammalian cerebellar slices. J. Physiol. (Lond.) 305: 197–213.

Llinás, R., Sugimori, M., Hillman, D.E., and Cherksey, B. 1992. Distribution and functional significance of the P-type, voltage-dependent Ca^{2+} channels in the mammalian nervous system. Trends Neurosci. 15: 351–355.

Llinás, R. and Volkind, R.A. 1973. The olivo-cerebellar system: Functional properties as revealed by harmaline-induced tremor. Exp. Brain Res. 18: 69–87.

Llinás, R. and Welsh, J. 1993. On the cerebellum and motor learning. Curr. Opin. Neurobiol. 3: 958–965.

Llinás, R. and Yarom, Y. 1981a. Electrophysiological properties of mammalian inferior olivary cells in vitro: Different types of voltage-dependent conductances. J. Physiol. (Lond.) 315: 549–567.

Llinás, R. and Yarom, Y. 1981b. Properties and distribution of ionic conductances generating electroresponsiveness of mammalian inferior olivary neurones in vitro. J. Physiol. (Lond.) 315: 569–584.

Llinás, R. and Yarom, Y. 1986. Oscillatory properties of guinea pig inferior olivary neurons and their pharmacological modulation: An in vitro study. J. Physiol. (Lond.) 376: 163–182.

Lloyd, D.P.C. 1960. Spinal mechanisms involved in somatic activities. In: Handbook of Physiology, Section 1: Neurophysiology, Vol. II (Magoun, H.W., ed.). Bethesda: American Physiology Society, pp. 929–949.

Lo, F.-S., Lu, S.-M., and Sherman, S.M. 1991. Intracellular and extracellular in vivo recording of different response modes for relay cells of the cat's lateral geniculate nucleus. Exp. Brain Res. 83: 317–328.

Lois, C., Garcia-Verdugo, J.M., and Alvarez-Buylla, A. 1996. Chain migration of neuronal precursors. Science 271: 978–981.

Loren, I., Emson, P.C., Fahrenkrug, J., Bjorklund, A., Alumets, J., Hakanson, R., and Sundler, F. 1979. Distribution of vasoactive intestinal polypeptide in the rat and mouse brain. Neuroscience 4: 1953–1976.

Lorente de Nó, R. 1934. Studies on the structure of the cerebral cortex II. Continuation of the study of the ammonic system. J. Psychol. Neurol. 46: 113–177.

Lorente de Nó, R. 1981. The Primary Acoustic Nuclei. New York: Raven Press.

Loy, R., Koziell, D.A., Lindsey, J.D., and Moore, R.Y. 1980. Noradrenergic innervation of the adult rat hippocampal formation. J. Comp. Neurol. 189: 699–710.

Lu, S.-M., Guido, W., and Sherman, S.M. 1993. The brainstem parabrachial region controls mode of response to visual stimulation of neurons in the cat's lateral geniculate nucleus. Vis. Neurosci. 10: 631–642.

Lu, S.-M., Guido, W., Vaughan, J.W., and Sherman, S.M. 1995. Latency variability of responses to visual stimuli in cells of the cat's lateral geniculate nucleus. Exp. Brain Res. 105: 7–17.

Luchins, D.J. 1990. A possible role of hippocampal dysfunction in schizophrenic symptomatology. Biol. Psychiatry 28: 87–91.

Lund, J.S., Lund, R.D., Hendrickson, A.E., Bunt, A.H., and Fuchs, A.F. 1975. The origin of efferent pathways from the primary visual cortex, area 17, of the macaque monkey as shown by retrograde transport of horseradish peroxidase. J. Comp. Neurol. 164: 287–303.

Lundberg, A. 1969. Convergence of excitatory and inhibitory action on interneurones in the spinal cord. In: The Interneuron, UCLA Forum in Medical Sciences (Brazier, M.A.B., ed.). Berkely: University of California Press, pp. 231–265.

Lundberg, A. 1971. Function of the ventral spinocerebellar tract, a new hypothesis. Exp. Brain Res. 12: 317–330.

Lundberg, A. 1975. Control of spinal mechanisms from the brain. In: The Nervous System, Vol. 1: The Basic Neurosciences (Brady, R., eds.). New York: Raven Press, pp. 253–265.

Lundberg, A., Malmgren, K., and Schomburg, E.D. 1987. Reflex pathways from group II muscle afferents. 3. Secondary spindle afferents and the FRA: A new hypothesis. Exp. Brain Res. 65: 294–306.

Lundberg, A. and Weight, F.F. 1971. Functional organization of connexions to the ventral spinocerebellar tracts. Exp. Brain Res. 12: 295–316.

Luo, M., Pu, M., and Sterling, P. 1996. Volumes of beta and alpha cell dendritic arbors peak in different strata. Soc. Neurosci. Abstr. 26: 1603.

Lüscher, H.R. and Clamann, H.P. 1992. Relation between structure and function in information transfer in spinal monosynaptic reflex. Physiol. Rev. 72: 71–99.

Luskin, M.B. 1993. Restricted proliferation and migration of postnatally generated neurons derived from the forebrain subventricular zone. Neuron 11: 173–189.

Luskin, M.B. and Price, J.L. 1982. The distribution of axon collaterals from the olfactory bulb and the nucleus of the horizontal limb of the diagonal band to the olfactory cortex, demonstrated by double retrograde labeling techniques. J. Comp. Neurol. 209: 249–263.

Luskin, M.B. and Price, J.L. 1983a. The topographic organization of associational fibers of the olfactory system in the rat, including centrifugal fibers to the olfactory bulb. J. Comp. Neurol. 216: 264–291.

Luskin, M.B. and Price, J.L. 1983b. The laminar distribution of intracortical fibers originating in the olfactory cortex of the rat. J. Comp. Neurol. 216: 292–302.

Lynch, G. and Granger, R. 1991. Serial steps in mercury processing: Possible clues from studies of plasticity in the olfactory-hippocampal circuit. In: Olfaction: A Model System for Computational Neurosciences (Davis, J.L. and Eichenbaum, H., eds.). Cambridge: MIT Press, pp. 145–165.

MacDermott, A.B. and Dale, N. 1987. Receptors, ion channels and synaptic potentials underlying the integrative actions of excitatory amino acids. Trends Neurosci. 10: 280–284.

MacDermott, A.B., Mayer, M.L., Westbrook, G.L., Smith, S.J., and Barker, J.L. 1986. NMDA-receptor activation increases cytoplasmic calcium concentrations in cultured spinal cord neurones. Nature 321: 519–522.

Mackay-Sim, A. and Kesteven, S. 1994. Topographic patterns of responsiveness to odorants in the rat olfactory epithelium. J. Neurophysiol. 71: 150–160.

Macrides, F. and Davis, B.J. 1983. The olfactory bulb. In: Chemical Neuroanatomy (Emson, P.C., ed.). New York: Raven Press, pp. 391–426.

Macrides, F. and Schneider, S.P. 1982. Laminar organization of mitral and tufted cells in the main olfactory bulb of the adult hamster. J. Comp. Neurol. 208: 419–430.

Macrides, F., Schoenfeld, T.A., Marchand, J.E., and Clancy, A.N. 1985. Evidence for morphologically, neurochemically and functionally heterogeneous classes of mitral and tufted cells in the olfactory bulb. Chem. Senses 10: 175–202.

MacVicar, B.A. and Dudek, F.E. 1980. Local synaptic circuits in rat hippocampus interactions between pyramidal cells. Brain Res. 184: 220–223.

Madison, D.V., Malenka, R.C., and Nicoll, R.A. 1991. Mechanisms underlying long-term potentiation of synaptic transmission. Annu. Rev. Neurosci. 14: 379–397.

Madison, D.V. and Nicoll, R.A. 1984. Control of the repetitive discharge of rat CA1 pyramidal neurones in vitro. J. Physiol. (Lond.) 354: 319–331.

Madison, D.V. and Nicoll, R.A. 1986a. Actions of noradrenaline recorded intracellularly in rat hippocampal CA1 pyramidal neurones, in vitro. J. Physiol. (Lond.) 372: 221–244.

Madison, D.V. and Nicoll, R.A. 1986b. Cyclic adenosine 3′,5′-monophosphate mediates beta-receptor actions of noradrenaline in rat hippocampal pyramidal cells. J. Physiol. (Lond.) 372: 245–259.

Magee, J.C., Avery, R.B., Christie, B.R., and Johnston, D. 1996. Dihyropyridine-sensitive, voltage-gated Ca^{2+} channels contribute to the resting intracellular Ca^{2+} concentration of hippocampal CA1 pyramidal neurons. J. Neurophysiol. 76: 3460–3470.

Magee, J.C., Christofi, G., Miyakawa, H., Christie, B., Lasser-Ross, N., and Johnston, D. 1995. Subthreshold synaptic activation of voltage-gated Ca^{2+} channels mediates a localized Ca^{2+} influx into the dendrites of hippocampal pyramidal neurons. J. Neurophysiol. 74: 1335–1342.

Magee, J.C., Hoffman, D., Colbert, C.M., and Johnston, D. 1988. Electrical and Calcium Signaling in Dendrites of Hippocampal Pyramidal Neurons. Annu. Rev. Physiol. (In press).

Magee, J.C. and Johnston, D. 1995a. Characterization of single voltage-gated Na^+ and Ca^{2+} channels in apical dendrites of rat CA1 pyramidal neurons. J. Physiol. (Lond.) 487: 67–90.

Magee, J.C. and Johnston, D. 1995b. Synaptic activation of voltage-gated channels in the dendrites of hippocampal pyramidal neurons. Science 268: 301–304.

Magee, J.C. and Johnston, D. 1997. A synaptically controlled, associative signal for Hebbian plasticity in hippocampal neurons. Science 275: 209–213.

Magistretti, P.J., Dietl, M.M., Hof, P.R., Martin, J.-L., Palacios, J.M., Schaad, N., and Schorderet, M. 1988. Vasoactive intestinal peptide as a mediator of intercellular communication in the cerebral cortex: Release, receptors, actions, and interactions with norepinephrine. Ann. N. Y. Acad. Sci. 527: 110–129.

Mahowald, M. 1994. An Analog System for Stereoscopic Vision. Boston: Kluwer Academic Publishers.

Mainen, Z.F., Carnevale, N.T., Zador, A.M., Claiborne, B.J., and Brown, T.H. 1996. Electrotonic architecture of hippocampal CA1 pyramidal neurons based on three-dimensional reconstructions. J. Neurophysiol. 76: 1904–1923.

Mainen, Z.F. and Sejnowski, T. 1996. Influence of dendritic structure on firing pattern in model neocortical neurons. Nature 382: 362–366.

Major, G., Larkman, A.U., Jonas, P., Sakmann, B., and Jack, J.J.B. 1994. Detailed passive cable models of whole-cell recorded CA3 pyramidal neurons in rat hippocampal slices. J. Neurosci. 14: 4513–4638.

Majorossy, K. and Kiss, A. 1976a. Types of interneurons and their participation in the neuronal network of the medial geniculate body. Exp. Brain Res. 26: 19–37.

Majorossy, K. and Kiss, A. 1976b. Specific patterns of neuron arrangement and of synaptic articulation in the medial geniculate body. Exp. Brain. Res. 26: 1–17.

Makowski, L., Casper, D.L.D., Phillips, W.C., and Goodenough, D.A. 1977. Gap junction structure. II. Analysis of X-ray diffraction data. J. Cell Biol. 74: 629–645.

Malach, R. 1992. Dendritic sampling across processing streams in monkey striate cortex. J. Comp. Neurol. 315: 303–312.

Malenka, R.C. and Nicoll, R.A. 1993. NMDA-receptor-dependent synaptic plasticity: Multiple forms and mechanisms. Trends Neurosci. 16: 521–527.

Malinow, R. and Miller, J.P. 1986. Postsynaptic hyperpolarization during conditioning reversibly blocks induction of long-term potentiation. Nature 320: 529–530.

Malioso, M.-L., Marqueze-Pouey, B., Kuhse, J., and Betz, H. 1991. Widespread expression of glycine receptor subunit mRNAs in the adult and developing rat brain. EMBO J. 10: 2401–2409.

Mancillas, J., Siggins, G., and Bloom, F. 1986. Somatostatin selectively enhances acetylcholine-induced excitations in rat hippocampus and cortex. Proc. Natl. Acad. Sci. USA 83: 7518–7521.

Mangel, S.C. 1991. Analysis of the horizontal cell contribution to the receptive field surround of ganglion cells in the rabbit retina. J. Physiol. (Lond.) 442: 211–234.

Mangel, S.C. and Dowling, J.E. 1985. Responsiveness and receptive field size of carp horizontal cells are reduced by prolonged darkness and dopamine. Science 229: 1107–1109.

Manis, P.B. 1990. Membrane properties and discharge characteristics of guinea pig dorsal cochlear nucleus neurons studied *in vitro.* J. Neurosci. 10: 2338–2351.

Manis, P.B. and Marx, S.O. 1991. Outward currents in isolated ventral cochlear nucleus neurons. J. Neurosci. 11: 2865–2880.

Manis, P.B. and Molitor, S.C. 1996. *N*-methyl-D-aspartate receptors at parallel fiber synapses in the dorsal cochlear nucleus. J. Neurophysiol. 76: 1639–1656.

Manis, P.B., Spirou, G.A., Wright, D.D., Paydar, S., and Ryugo, D.K. 1994. Physiology and morphology of complex spiking neurons in the guinea pig dorsal cochlear nucleus. J. Comp. Neurol. 348: 261–276.

Marek, G.J. and Aghajanian, G.K. 1994. Excitation of interneurons in piriform cortex by 5-hydroxytryptamine blockade by MDL 100,907, a highly selective 5-HT$_{2A}$ receptor antagonist. Eur. J. Pharmacol. 259: 137–141.

Marek, G.J. and Aghajanian, G.K. 1995. Protein kinase C inhibitors enhance the 5-HT$_{2A}$ receptor-mediated excitatory effects of serotonin on interneurons in rat piriform cortex. Synapse 21: 123–130.

Margolis, F.L. 1985. Olfactory marker protein: From PAGE band to cDNA clone. Trends Neurosci. 8: 542–546.

Margolis, F.L., Kawano, T., and Grillo, M. 1986. Ontogeny of carnosine, olfactory marker protein and neurotransmitter enzymes in olfactory bulb and olfactory mucosa of the rat. In: Ontogeny of Olfaction (Breipohl, W., ed.). Berlin: Springer-Verlag, pp. 107–116.

Mariani, A.P. 1984. Bipolar cells in monkey retina selective for the cones likely to be blue-sensitive. Nature 308: 184–186.

Mariani, J., Crepel, F., Mikoshiba, K., Changeux, J.P., and Sotelo, C. 1977. Anatomical, physiological and biochemical studies of the cerebellum from Reeler mutant mouse. Trans. R. Soc. Lond [B] 281: 1–28.

Markham, J. and Fifkova, E. 1986. Actin filament organization within dendrites and dendritic spines during development. Brain Res. 392: 263–269.

Markram, H., Helm, P.J., and Sakmann, B. 1995. Dendritic calcium transients evoked by single back-propagating action potentials in rat neocortical pyramidal neurons. J. Physiol. (Lond.) 485: 1–20.

Markram, H., Lübke, J., Frotscher, M., and Sakmann, B. 1997. Regulation of synaptic efficacy by coincidence of postsynaptic APs and EPSPs. Science 275: 213–215.

Markram, H. and Sakmann, B. 1994. Calcium transients in apical dendrites evoked by single subthreshold excitatory post-synaptic potentials via low voltage-activated calcium channels. Proc. Natl. Acad. Sci. USA 91: 5207–5211.

Markram, H. and Tsodyks, M. 1996. Redistribution of synaptic efficacy between neocortical pyramidal neurons. Nature 382: 807–810.

Marr, D. and Poggio, T. 1979. A computational theory of human stereo vision. Proc. R. Soc. Lond. B. Biol. Sci. 204: 301–328.

Martin, A.R. 1977. Junctional transmission. II. Presynaptic mechanisms. In: Handbook of Physiology, Section I, The Nervous System, Vol. I: The Cellular Biology of Neurons (Kandel, E.R., ed.). Bethesda: American Physiological Society, pp. 329–355.

Martin, K. 1988. From single cells to simple circuits in the cerebral cortex. Q. J. Exp. Physiol. 73: 637–702.

Martin, P.R. 1986. The projection of different retinal ganglion cell classes to the dorsal lateral geniculate nucleus in the hooded rat. Exp. Brain Res. 62: 77–88.

Marty, A. and Llano, I. 1995. Modulation of inhibitory synapses in the mammalian brain. Curr. Opin. Neurobiol. 5: 335–341.

Masland, R.H. 1986. The functional architecture of the retina. Sci. Am. 254: 102–111.

Masland, R.H., Mills, J.W., and Cassidy, C. 1984. The functions of acetylcholine in the rabbit retina. Proc. R. Soc. (Lond.) B Biol. Sci. 223: 121–139.

Maslim, J. and Stone, J. 1986. Synaptogenesis in the retina of the cat. Brain Res. 373: 35–48.

Mason, A. and Larkman, A. 1990. Correlations between morphology and electrophysiology of pyramidal neurons in slices of rat visual cortex. J. Neurosci. 10: 1415–1428.

Mason, A., Nicoll, A., and Stratford, K. 1991. Synaptic transmission between individual pyramidal neurons of the rat visual cortex in vitro. J. Neurosci. 11: 72–84.

Massey, S.C. and Maguire, G. 1995. Excitatory amino acids and synaptic transmission. In: The Role of Glutamate in Retina Circuitry (Wheal, H.V. and Thomsin, A.M., eds.). London: Academic Press, pp. 201–227.

Massey, S.C. and Redburn, D.A. 1985. Light evoked release of acetylcholine in response to a single flash: Cholinergic amacrine cells receive ON and OFF input. Brain Res. 328: 374–377.

Masterton, R.B. and Granger, E.M. 1988. Role of the acoustic striae in hearing: Contribution of dorsal and intermediate striae to detection of noises and tones. J. Neurophysiol. 60: 1841–1860.

Masterton, R.B., Granger, E.M., and Glendenning, K.K. 1994. Role of acoustic striae in hearing—Mechanism for enhancement of sound detection in cats. Hear. Res. 73: 209–222.

Mastronarde, D.N. 1983. Correlated firing of cat retinal ganglion cells. II. Responses of X- and Y-cells to single quantal events. J. Neurophysiol. 49: 325–349.

Mastronarde, D.N. 1987. Two classes of single-input X-cells in cat lateral geniculate nucleus. I. Receptive field properties and classification of cells. J. Neurophysiol. 57: 357–380.

Mates, S. and Lund, J. 1983. Neuronal composition and development of lamina 4c of monkey striate cortex. J. Comp. Neurol. 221: 60–90.

Mathers, L.H. 1972. The synaptic organization of the cortical projection to the pulvinar of the squirrel monkey. J. Comp. Neurol. 146: 43–60.

Matsumoto, R. 1989. GABA receptors: Are cellular differences reflected in function. Brain Res. Revs. 14: 203–225.

Matthews, G. 1996. Neurotransmitter release. Annu. Rev. Neurosci. 19: 219–233.

Maturana, H.R., Lettvin, J.Y., McCulloch, W.S., and Pitts, W.H. 1960. Anatomy and physiology of vision in the frog (*Rana pipiens*). J. Gen. Physiol. 43: 129–175.

Matthews, M.A., Willis, W.D., and Williams, V. 1971. Dendrite bundles in lamina IX of cat spinal cord: A possible source for electrical interaction between motoneurons. Anat. Rec. 171: 313–327.

Matthews, P.B.C. 1972. Mammalian Muscle Receptors and Their Central Actions. London: Arnold.

Matthews, P.B.C. 1981. Muscle spindles: Their messages and their fusimotor supply. In: Handbook of Physiology, Section 1: The Nervous System, Vol. II: Motor Control, Part 1 (Brooks, V.B., ed.). Bethesda: American Physiological Society, pp. 189–228.

Maxwell, D.J., Christie, W.M., Ottersen, O.P., and Storm-Mathisen, J. 1990a. Terminals of group Ia primary afferent fibres in Clarke's column are enriched with L-glutamate-like immunoreactivity. Brain Res. 510: 346–350.

Maxwell, D.J., Christie, W.M., Short, A.D., and Brown, A.G. 1990b. Direct observations of synapses between GABA-immunoreactive boutons and muscle afferent terminals in lamina VI of the cat's spinal cord. Brain Res. 530: 215–222.

Mayer, M.L. and Westbrook, G.L. 1987. The physiology of excitatory amino acids in the vertebrate central nervous system. Prog. Neurobiol. 28: 197–276.

Mayer, M.L., Westbrook, G.L., and Guthrie, P.B. 1984. Voltage-dependent block by Mg^{2+} of NMDA responses in spinal cord neurones. Nature 309: 261–263.

McArdle, C.B., Dowling, J.E., and Masland, R.H. 1977. Development of outer segments and synapses in the rabbit retina. J. Comp. Neurol. 175: 253–274.

McBride, W.J., Aprison, M.H., and Kusano, K. 1976. Contents of several amino acids in the cerebellum, brainstem and cerebrum of the "staggerer", "weaver" and "nervous" neurologically mutant mice. J. Neurochem. 26: 867–870.

McCarley, R.W., Benoit, O., and Barrionuevo, G. 1983. Lateral geniculate nucleus unitary discharge in sleep and waking state- and rate-specific aspects. J. Neurophysiol. 50: 798–818.

McClurkin, J.W. and Marrocco, R.T. 1984. Visual cortical input alters spatial tuning in monkey lateral geniculate nucleus cells. J. Physiol. (Lond.) 348: 135–152.

McClurkin, J.W., Optican, L.M., and Richmond, B.J. 1994. Cortical feedback increases visual information transmitted by monkey parvocellular lateral geniculate nucleus neurons. Vis. Neurosci. 11: 601–617.

McCollum, J., Larson, J., Otto, T., Schottler, F., Granger, R., and Lynch, G. 1991. Short-latency single unit processing in olfactory cortex. J. Cogn. Neurosci. 3: 293–299.

McCormick, D. and Gray, C. 1996. Chattering cells: Superficial pyramidal neurons contributing to the generation of synchronous oscillations in the visual cortex. Science 274: 109–113.

McCormick, D.A. 1989a. Cholinergic and noradrenergic modulation of thalamocortical processing. Trends Neurosci. 12: 215–221.

McCormick, D.A. 1989b. GABA as an inhibitory neurotransmitter in the human cerebral cortex. J. Neurophysiol. 62: 1018–1027.

McCormick, D.A. 1990. Membrane properties and neurotransmitter actions. In: The Synaptic Organization of the Brain, 3rd ed. (Shepherd, G. ed.). New York: Oxford University Press, pp. 32–66.

McCormick, D.A. 1992. Neurotransmitter actions in the thalamus and cerebral cortex and their role in neuromodulation of thalamocortical activity. Prog. Neurobiol. 39: 337–388.

McCormick, D.A. and Bal, T. 1994. Sensory gating mechanisms of the thalamus. Curr. Opin. Neurobiol. 4: 550–556.

McCormick, D.A., Connors, B., Lighthall, J., and Prince, D. 1985. Comparative electrophysiology of pyramidal and sparsely spiny stellate neurons of the neocortex. J. Neurophysiol. 59: 782–806.

McCormick, D.A. and Feeser, H.R. 1990. Functional implications of burst firing and single spike activity in lateral geniculate relay neurons. Neuroscience 39: 103–113.

McCormick, D.A. and Huguenard, J.R. 1992. A model of the electrophysiological properties of thalamocortical relay neurons. J. Neurophysiol. 68: 1384–1400.

McCormick, D.A. and Pape, H.-C. 1988. Acetylcholine inhibits identified interneurons in the cat lateral geniculate nucleus. Nature 334: 246–248.

McCormick, D.A. and Pape, H.-C. 1990. Properties of a hyperpolarization-activated cation current and its role in rhythmic oscillation in thalamic relay neurones. J. Physiol. (Lond.) 431: 291–318.

McCormick, D.A. and Prince, D. 1985. Two types of muscarinic response to acetylcholine in mammalian cortical neurons. Proc. Natl. Acad. Sci. USA 82: 6344–6348.

McCormick, D.A., and Prince, D.A. 1986a. Acetylcholine induces burst firing in thalamic reticular neurones by activating a potassium conductance. Nature 319: 402–405.

McCormick, D.A. and Prince, D. 1986b. Mechanisms of action of acetylcholine in the guinea-pig cerebral cortex. J. Physiol. (Lond.) 375: 169–194.

McCormick, D.A. and Prince, D.A. 1987a. Actions of acetylcholine in the guinea-pig and cat medial and lateral geniculate nuclei, in vitro. J. Physiol. (Lond.) 392: 147–165.

McCormick, D.A. and Prince, D.A. 1987b. Acetylcholine causes rapid nicotinic excitation in the medial habenular nucleus of guinea pig, in vitro. J. Neurosci. 7: 742–752.

McCormick, D.A. and Von Krosigk, M. 1992. Corticothalamic activation modulates thalamic firing through glutamate "metabotropic" receptors. Proc. Natl. Acad. Sci. USA 89: 2774–2778.

McCormick, D.A. and Wang, Z. 1991. Serotonin and noradrenaline excite GABAergic neurones in the guinea-pig and cat nucleus reticularis thalami. J. Physiol. (Lond.) 442: 235–255.

McCormick, D.A., Wang, Z., and Huguenard, J. 1993. Neurotransmitter control of neocortical neuronal activity and excitability. Cereb. Cortex 3: 387–398.

McCormick, D.A. and Williamson, A. 1989. Convergence and divergence of neurotransmitter action in the human cerebral cortex. Proc. Natl. Acad. Sci. USA 86: 8098–8102.

McCurdy, M.L. and Hamm, T.M. 1992. Recurrent collaterals of motoneurons projecting to distal muscles in the cat hindlimb. J. Neurophysiol. 67: 1359–1366.

McGeer, P.L., McGeer, E.G., Sherer, U., and Sinh, K. 1977. A glutamatergic corticostriatal path? Brain Res. 128: 369–373.

McGinty, J.F., Henriksen, S.J., Goldstein, A., Terenius, L., and Bloom, F.E. 1983. Dynorphin is contained within hippocampal mossy fibers immunochemical alterations after kainic acid administration and colchicine. Proc. Natl. Acad. Sci. USA 80: 589–593.

McGuire, B.A., Stevens, J.K., and Sterling, P. 1984. Microcircuitry of bipolar cells in cat retina. J. Neurosci. 4: 2920–2938.

McHugh, T.J., Blum, K.I., Tsien, J.Z., Tonegawa, S., and Wilson, M.A. 1996. Impaired hippocampal representation of space in CA1-specific NMDAR1 knockout mice. Cell 87: 1339–1349.

McIlwain, J.T. 1966. Some evidence concerning the physiological basis of the periphery effect in the cat's brain. Exp. Brain Res. 1: 265–271.

McLaughlin, B.J., Woods, J.G., Saito, K., Barber, R., Vaughn, J.E., Roberts, E., and Wu, J. 1974. The fine structural localization of glutamate decarboxylase in synaptic terminals of rodent cerebellum. Brain Res. 76: 377–391.

McLennan, H. 1971. The pharmacology of inhibition of mitral cells in the olfactory bulb. Brain Res. 29: 177–187.

McLennan, H. 1983. Receptors for the excitatory amino acids in the mammalian central nervous system. Prog. Neurobiol. 20: 251–271.

McNaughton, B.L. 1982. Long-term synaptic enhancement and short-term potentiation in rat fascia dentata act through different mechanisms. J. Physiol. (Lond.) 324: 249–262.

Mead, C. 1990. Neuromorphic electronic systems. Proc. I.E.E.E. 78: 1629–1636.

Mehraein, P., Yamada, M., and Tarnowska-Dziduszko, E. 1975. Quantitative study on dendrites and dendritic spines in Alzheimer's disease and senile dementia. In: Advances in Neurology (Kreutzberg, G.W., ed.). New York: Raven Press, pp. 453–458.

Meister, M. 1996. Multineuronal codes in retinal signaling. Proc. Natl. Acad. Sci. USA 93: 609–614.

Meister, M., Pine, J., and Baylor, D.A. 1994. Multi-neuronal signals from the retina: Acquisition and analysis. J. Neurosci. Methods 51: 95–106.

Meister, M., Wong, R.O.L., Baylor, D.A., and Shatz, C.J. 1991. Synchronous bursts of action potentials in ganglion cells of the developing mammalian retina. Science 252: 939–943.

Mel, B. 1993. Synaptic integration in excitable dendritic trees. J. Neurophysiol. 70: 1086–1101.

Mendell, L.M. and Henneman, E. 1971. Terminals of single Ia fibers: Location, density, and distribution within a pool of 300 homonymous motoneurons. J. Neurophysiol. 34: 171–187.

Middlebrooks, J.C. and Green, D.M. 1991. Sound localization by human listeners. Annu. Rev. Psychol. 42: 135–159.

Midtgaard, J. 1994. Processing of information from different sources: Spatial synaptic integration in the dendrites of vertebrate CNS neurons. Trends Neurosci. 17: 166–173.

Milam, A.H., Dacey, D.M., and Dizhoor, A.M. 1993. Recoverin immunoreactivity in mammalian cone bipolar cells. Vis. Neurosci. 10: 1–12.

Miles, R. 1990. Variation in strength of inhibitory synapses in the CA3 region of guinea-pig hippocampus in vitro. J. Physiol. (Lond.) 431: 659–676.

Miles, R., Toth, K., Gulyas, A.I., Hajos, H., and Freund, T.F. 1996. Differences between somatic and dendritic inhibition in the hippocampus. Neuron 16: 815–823.

Miles, R. and Wong, R.K.S. 1984. Unitary inhibitory synaptic potentials in the guinea-pig hippocampus in vitro. J. Physiol. (Lond.) 356: 97–113.

Miles, R. and Wong, R.K.S. 1986. Excitatory synaptic interactions between CA3 neurones in the guinea-pig hippocampus. J. Physiol. (Lond.) 373: 397–418.

Miller, C. 1989. Genetic manipulation of ion channels: A new approach to structure and mechanism. Neuron 2: 1195–1205.

Miller, J.P., Rall, W., and Rinzel, J. 1985. Synaptic amplification by active membrane in dendritic spines. Brain Res. 325: 325–330.

Miller, R.F. and Bloomfield, S.A. 1983. Electroanatomy of a unique amacrine cell in the rabbit retina. Proc. Natl. Acad. Sci. USA 80: 3069–3073.

Mills, S.L. and Massey, S.C. 1991. Labeling and distribution of AII amacrine cells in the rabbit retina. J. Comp. Neurol. 304: 491–501.

Mills, S.L. and Massey, S.C. 1994. Distribution and coverage of A- and B-type horizontal cells stained with neurobiotin in the rabbit retina. Vis. Neurosci. 11: 549–560.

Mills, S.L. and Massey, S.C. 1995. Differential properties of two gap junctional pathways made by AII amacrine cells. Nature 377: 734–737.

Mintz, I.M. and Bean, B.P. 1993. GABA-B receptor inhibition of P-type Ca^{2+} channels in central neurons. Neuron 10: 889–898.

Misgeld, U. and Frotscher, M. 1986. Postsynaptic-GABAergic inhibition of non-pyramidal neurons in the guinea-pig hippocampus. Neuroscience 19: 193–206.

Mitchison, G. 1992. Axonal trees and cortical architecture. Trends Neurosci. 15: 122–126.

Mitzdorf, U. 1985. Current source-density method and application in cat cerebral cortex. Investigation of evoked potentials and EEG phenomena. Physiol. Rev. 65: 37–100.

Miyakawa, H., Ross, W.N., Jaffe, D., Callaway, J.C., Lasser-Ross, N., Lisman, J.E., and Johnston, D. 1992. Synaptically activated increases in Ca^{2+} concentration in hippocampal CA1 pyramidal cells are primarily due to voltage-gated Ca^{2+} channels. Neuron 9: 1163–1173.

Miyashita, C. and Chang, Y. 1988. Neuronal correlate of pictorial short-term memory in the primate temporal cortex. Nature 331: 68–70.

Miyashita, Y. 1988. Neuronal correlate of visual associative long-term memory in the primate temporal cortex. Nature 335: 817–820.

Mollon, J.D. and Bowmaker, J.K. 1992. The spatial arrangement of cones in the primate fovea. Nature 360: 677–679.

Molnar, C.E. and Pfeiffer, R.R. 1968. Interpretation of spontaneous spike discharge patterns of cochlear nucleus neurons. Proc. I.E.E.E. 56: 993–1004.

Mombaerts, P., Wang, F., Dulac, C., Chao, S.K., Nemes, A., Mendelsohn, M., Edmondson, J., and Axel, R. 1996. Visualizing an olfactory sensory map. Cell 87: 675–686.

Monaghan, D.T., Holets, V.R., Toy, D.W., and Cotman, C.W. 1983. Anatomical distributions of four pharmacologically distinct [^{3}H]-1-glutamate binding sites. Nature 306: 176–179.

Montero, V.M. 1987. Ultrastructural identification of synaptic terminals from the axon type 3 interneurons in the cat lateral geniculate nucleus. J. Comp. Neurol. 264: 268–283.

Montero, V.M. 1994. Quantitative immunogold evidence for enrichment of glutamate but not aspartate in synaptic terminals of retino-geniculate, geniculo-cortical, and cortico-geniculate axons in the cat. Vis. Neurosci. 11: 675–681.

Monti-Graziadei, G., Stanley, R., and Graziadei, P. 1980. The olfactory marker protein in the olfactory system of the mouse during development. Neuroscience 5: 1239–1252.

Moody, C.I. and Sillito, A.M. 1988. The role of the N-methyl-D-aspartate (NMDA) receptor in the transmission of visual information in the feline dorsal lateral geniculate nucleus (dLGN). J. Physiol. (Lond.) 396: 62P.

Moore, B.C.J. 1989. An Introduction to the Psychology of Hearing. London: Academic Press.

Moore, G.P., Segundo, J.P., Perkel, D.H., and Levitan, H. 1970. Statistical signs of synaptic interaction in neurons. Biophys. J. 10: 876–900.

Moore, R.Y. and Card, J.P. 1984. Noradrenaline-containing neuron systems. In: Handbook of Chemical Neuroanatomy, Vol. 2: Classical Transmitters in the CNS, Part I. (Bjorklund, A. and Hökfelt, T., eds.). Amsterdam: Elsevier, pp. 123–156.

Moran, D., Rowles, J., and Jafek, B. 1982. Electronmicroscopy of human olfactory epithelium reveals a new cell type: The microvillar cell. Brain Res. 253: 39–46.

Morest, D.K. 1975. Synaptic relationships of Golgi type II cells in the medial geniculate body of the cat. J. Comp. Neurol. 162: 157–193.

Mori, J., Kishi, K., and Ojima, H. 1983. Distribution of dendrites of mitral, displaced mitral, tufted, and granule cells in the rabbit olfactory bulb. J. Comp. Neurol. 219: 339–355.

Mori, K. 1987. Membrane and synaptic properties of identified neurons in the olfactory bulb. Prog. Neurobiol. 29: 274–320.

Mori, K., Mataga, N., and Imamura, K. 1992. Differential specificities of single mitral cells in rabbit olfactory bulb for a homologous series of fatty acid odor molecules. J. Neurophysiol. 67: 786–789.

Mori, K., Nowycky, M.C., and Shepherd, G.M. 1981a. Electrophysiological analysis of mitral cells in the isolated turtle olfactory bulb. J. Physiol. (Lond.) 314: 281–294.

Mori, K., Nowycky, M.C., and Shepherd, G.M. 1981b. Analysis of synaptic potentials in mitral cells in the isolated turtle olfactory bulb. J. Physiol. (Lond.) 314: 295–309.

Mori, K., Nowycky, M.C., and Shepherd, G.M. 1981c. Analysis of a long-duration inhibitory potential in mitral cells in the isolated turtle olfactory bulb. J. Physiol. (Lond.) 314: 311–320.

Mori, K., Nowycky, M.C., and Shepherd, G.M. 1982. Impulse activity in presynaptic dendrites: analysis of mitral cells in the isolated turtle olfactory bulb. J. Neurosci. 2: 497–502.

Mori, K. and Shepherd, G.M. 1994. Emerging principles of molecular signal processing by mitral/tufted cells in the olfactory bulb. Semin. Cell Biol. 5: 65–74.

Mori, K. and Yoshihara, Y. 1995. Molecular recognition and olfactory processing in the mammalian olfactory system. Prog. Neurobiol. 45: 585–619.

Morrison, J.H., Benoit, R., Magistretti, P.J., Ling, N., and Bloom, F.E. 1982. Immunohistochemical distribution of pro-somatostatin-related peptides in hippocampus. Neurosci. Lett. 34: 137–142.

Moruzzi, G. and Magoun, H.W. 1949. Brain stem reticular formation and activation of the EEG. Electroencephalogr. Clin. Neurophysiol. 1: 455–473.

Moschovakis, A.K., Burke, R.E., and Fyffe, R.E.W. 1991a. The size and dendritic structure of HRP-labeled gamma motoneurons in the cat spinal cord. J. Comp. Neurol. 311: 531–545.

Moschovakis, A.K., Sholomenko, G.N., and Burke, R.E. 1991b. Differential control of short latency cutaneous excitation in cat FDL motoneurons during fictive locomotion. Exp. Brain Res. 83: 489–501.

Mosko, S., Lynch, G., and Cotman, C.W. 1973. The distribution of septal projections to the hippocampus of the rat. J. Comp. Neurol. 152: 163–174.

Mott, D.D. and Lewis, D.V. 1991. Facilitation of the induction of long-term potentiation by $GABA_B$ receptors. Science 252: 1718.

Moyano, H.F., Cinelli, A.R., and Molina, J.C. 1985. Current generators and properties of early components evoked in rat olfactory cortex. Brain Res. Bull. 15: 237–248.

Mugnaini, E. and Oertel, W.H. 1981. Distribution of glutamate decarboxylase positive neurons in the rat cerebellar nuclei. Soc. Neurosci. Abstr. 7: 122.

Mugnaini, E., Oertel, W.H., and Wouterlood, F.F. 1984. Immunocytochemical localization of GABA neurons and dopamine neurons in the rat main and accessory olfactory bulbs. Neurosci. Lett. 47: 221–226.

Mugnaini, E., Osen, K.K., Dahl, A.L., Friedrich Jr., V.L., and Korte, G. 1980b. Fine structure of granule cells and related interneurons (termed Golgi cells) in the cochlear nuclear complex of cat, rat, and mouse. J. Neurocytol. 9: 537–570.

Mugnaini, E., Warr, W.B., and Osen, K.K. 1980a. Distribution and light microscopic features of granule cells in the cochlear nuclei of cat, rat, and mouse. J. Comp. Neurol. 191: 581–606.

Muhlethaler, M., de, C.M., Walton, K., and Llinás, R. 1993. The isolated and perfused brain of the guinea-pig in vitro. Eur. J. Neurosci. 5: 915–926.

Muir, R.B. and Porter, R. 1973. The effect of a preceding stimulus on temporal facilitation at corticomotoneuronal synapses. J. Physiol. (Lond.) 228: 749–763.

Mukherjee, P. and Kaplan, E. 1995. Dynamics of neurons in the cat lateral geniculate nucleus in vivo electrophysiology and computational modeling. J. Neurophysiol. 74: 1222–1243.

Müller, B. and Peichl, L. 1993. Horizontal cells in the cone-dominated tree shrew retina: Morphology, photoreceptor contacts, and topographical distribution. J. Neurosci. 13: 3628–3646.

Muller, W. and Connor, J. 1991. Dendritic spines as individual neuronal compartments for synaptic Ca^{2+} responses. Neuron 354: 73–76.

Mulligan, K. and Tork, I. 1988. Seratonergic innervation of the cat cerebral cortex. J. Comp. Neurol. 270: 86–110.

Mumford, D. 1994. Neuronal architectures for pattern theoretic problems. In: Large-Scale Neuronal Theories of the Brain (Koch, C. and Davis, J. eds.). Cambridge: MIT Press, pp. 125–152.

Murakami, M., Miyachi, E.-I., and Takahashi, K.-I. 1995. Modulation of gap junctions between horizontal cells by second messengers. In: Progress in Retinal and Eye Research. London: Elsevier Science, pp. 197–221.

Murphy, P.C. and Sillito, A.M. 1996. Functional morphology of the feedback pathway from area 17 of the cat visual cortex to the lateral geniculate nucleus. J. Neurosci. 16: 1180–1192.

Murthy, K.S.K., Ledbetter, W.D., Eidelberg, E., Cameron, W.E., and Petit, J. 1982. Histochemical evidence for the existence of skeletofusimotor (β) innervation in the primate. Exp. Brain Res. 46: 186–190.

Naegele, J. and Barnstable, C. 1989. Molecular determinants of GABAergic local circuit neurons in the cerebral cortex. Trends Neurosci. 12. 28–34.

Nafstad, P.H.J. 1967. An electron microscope study on the termination of the perforant path fibres in the hippocampus and the fascia dentata. Z. Zellforsch. 76: 532–542.

Nakamura, H., Gattass, R., Desimone, R., and Ungerleider, L.G. 1993. The modular organization of projections from areas V1 and V2 to areas V4 and TEO in macaques. J. Neurosci. 13: 3681–3691.

Nakamura, Y., McGuire, B.A., and Sterling, P. 1980. Interplexiform cell in cat retina: Identification by uptake of gamma-[^{3}H]aminobutyric acid and serial reconstruction. Proc. Natl. Acad. Sci. USA 77: 658–661.

Nakanishi, H., Kita, H., and Kitai, S.T. 1991. Intracellular study of rat entopeduncular nucleus neurons in an in vitro slice preparation response to subthalamic stimulation. Brain Res. 549: 285–291.

Nambu, A. and Llinás, R. 1994. Electrophysiology of globus pallidus neurons in vitro. J. Neurophysiol. 72: 1127–1139.

Narasimhan, K. and Linden, D.J. 1996. Defining a minimal computational unit for cerebellar long-term depression. Neuron 17: 333–41.

Nardone, A., Romano, C., and Schieppati, M. 1989. Selective recruitment of high-threshold human motor units during voluntary isotonic lengthening of active muscles. J. Physiol. (Lond.) 409: 451–471.

Nawy, S. and Jahr, C.E. 1990. Suppression by glutamate of cGMP-activated conductance in retinal bipolar cells. Nature 346: 269–271.

Nayeem, N., Green, T., I.M., and Barnard, E. 1994. Quaternary structure of the native GABA$_A$ receptor determined by electron microscopic image analysis. J. Neurochem. 62: 815–818.

Neer, E.J. 1995. Heterotrimeric G proteins: Organizers of transmembrane signals. Cell 80: 249–257.

Neher, E. 1971. Two fast transient current components during voltage clamp on snail neurons. J. Gen. Physiol. 58: 36–53.

Neher, E. and Sakmann, B. 1976. Single-channel currents recorded from membrane of denervated frog muscle fibers. Nature 260: 799–802.

Neher, E. and Sakmann, B. 1992. The patch clamp technique. Sci. Am. 266: 28–35.

Neitz, M., Neitz, J., and Jacobs, G.H. 1991. Spectral tuning of pigments underlying red-green color vision. Science 252: 971–974.

Nelken, I. and Young, E.D. 1994. Two separate inhibitory mechanisms shape the responses of dorsal cochlear nucleus type IV units to narrowband and wideband stimuli. J. Neurophysiol. 71: 2446–2462.

Nelson, P.G. 1966. Interaction between spinal motoneurons of the cat. J. Neurophysiol. 29: 275–287.

Nelson, P., Famiglietti, E.V., and Kolb, H. 1978. Intracellular staining reveals different levels of stratification for ON- and OFF-center ganglion cells of the cat retina. J. Neurophysiol. 41: 472–483.

Nelson, R. 1977. Cat cones have rod input: A comparison of the response properties of cones and horizontal cell bodies in the retina of the cat. J. Comp. Neurol. 172: 109–136.

Nelson, R. 1982. AII amacrine cells quicken time course of rod signals in the cat retina. J. Neurophysiol. 47: 928–947.

Nelson, R. and Kolb, H. 1983. Synaptic patterns and response properties of bipolar and ganglion cells in the cat retina. Vision Res. 23: 1183–1195.

Nelson, R. and Kolb, H. 1985. A17: A broad-field amacrine cell in the rod system of the cat retina. J. Neurophysiol. 54: 592–614.

Nernst, W. 1888. On the kinetics of substances in solution. [Translated from Z. Physik. Chemie 2.] In: Cell Membrane Permeability and Transport (Kepner, G.R., ed.). 1979 Stroudsburg, PA: Dowden, Itutchinsin and Ross pp. 613–622, 634–637.

Neveu, D. and Zucker, R. 1996. Postsynaptic levels of [Ca^{2+}]i needed to trigger LTD and LTP. Neuron 16: 619–629.

Newberry, N.R. and Nicoll, R.A. 1985. Comparison of the action of baclofen with gamma-aminobutyric acid on rat hippocampal pyramidal cells in vitro. J. Physiol. (Lond.) 360: 161–185.

Newman, E. and Reichenbach, A. 1996. The Müller cell: A functional element of the retina. Trends Neurosci. 19: 307–312.

Nicholls, J.G., Martin, A.R., and Wallace, B.G. 1992. From Neuron to Brain, 3rd ed. Sunderland, MA: Sinauer Associates.

Nickell, W.T., Behbehani, M.M., and Shipley, M.T. 1994. Evidence for GABA$_B$-mediated inhibition of transmission from the olfactory nerve to mitral cells in the rat olfactory bulb. Brain Res. Bull. 35: 119–123.

Nickell, W.T. and Shipley, M.T. 1993. Evidence for presynaptic inhibition of the olfactory commissural pathway by cholinergic agonists and stimulation of the nucleus of the diagonal band. J. Neurosci. 13: 650–659.

Nicoll, R.A. 1970. Recurrent excitation of secondary olfactory neurons: A possible mechanism for signal amplification. Science 171: 824–825.

Nicoll, R.A. 1971. Pharmacological evidence for GABA as the transmitter in granule cell inhibition in the olfactory bulb. Brain Res. 35: 137–149.

Nicoll, R.A. 1988. The coupling of neurotransmitter receptors to ion channels in the brain. Science 241: 545–551.

Nicoll, R.A., Alger, B.E., and Jahr, C.E. 1980a. Enkephalin blocks inhibitory pathways in the vertebrate CNS. Nature 287: 22–25.

Nicoll, R.A., Alger, B.E., and Jahr, C.E. 1980b. Peptides as putative excitatory neurotransmitters: Carnosine, enkephalin, substance P and TRH. Proc. R. Soc. Lond. B. Biol. Sci. 210: 133–149.

Nicoll, R.A., Kauer, J.A., and Malenka, R.C. 1988. The current excitement in long-term potentiation. Neuron 1: 97–103.

Nicoll, R.A. and Malenka, R.C. 1995. Contrasting properties of two forms of long-term potentiation in the hippocampus. Nature 377: 115–118.

Nicoll, R.A., Malenka, R.C., and Kauer, J.A. 1990. Functional comparison of neurotransmitter receptor subtypes in mammalian central nervous system. Physiol. Rev. 70: 513–565.

Nielsen, J. and Kagamihara, Y. 1993. Differential projection of the sural nerve to early and late recruited human tibialis anterior motor units: Change of recruitment gain. Acta Physiol. Scand. 147: 385–401.

Nielsen, J., Petersen, N., Deuschl, G., and Ballegaard, M. 1993. Task-related changes in the effect of magnetic brain-stimulation on spinal neurons in man. J. Physiol. (Lond.) 471: 223–243.

Nini, A., Fiengold, A., Slovin, H., and Bergman, H. 1995. Neurons in the globus pallidus do not show correlated activity in the normal monkey, but phase-locked oscillations appear in the MPTP model of Parkinsonism. J. Neurophysiol. 74: 1800–1805.

Nisenbaum, E.S. and Wilson, C.J. 1995. Potassium currents responsible for inward and outward rectification in rat neostriatal spiny projection neurons. J. Neurosci. 15: 4449–4463.

Nisenbaum, E.S., Wilson, C.J., Foehring, R.C., and Surmeier, D.J. 1996. Isolation and characterization of a persistent potassium current in neostriatal neurons. J. Neurophysiol. 76: 1180–1194.

Nishimura, Y. and Rakic, P. 1987a. Development of the rhesus monkey retina II. A three-dimensional analysis of the sequences of synaptic combinations in the inner plexiform layer. J. Comp. Neurol. 262: 290–313.

Nishimura, Y. and Rakic, P. 1987b. Synaptogenesis in primate retina proceeds from the ganglion cells towards the photoreceptors. Neurosci. Res. Suppl. 6: 253–268.

Nistri, A. 1983. Spinal cord pharmacology of GABA and chemically related mainoe acids. In: Handbook of the Spinal Cord, Vol. 1: Pharmacology (Davidoff, R.E., eds.). New York: Marcel Dekker, pp. 45–104.

Noda, H. 1975. Depression in the excitability of relay cells of lateral geniculate nucleus following saccadic eye movements in the cat. J. Physiol. (Lond.) 249: 87–102.

Nomura, A., Shigemoto, R., Nakamura, Y., Okamoto, N., Mizuno, N., and Nakanishi, S. 1994. Developmentally regulated postsynaptic localization of a metabotropic glutamate-receptor in rat rod bipolar cells. Cell 77: 361–369.

North, R.A. 1987. Receptors of individual neurones. Neuroscience 17: 899–907.

Nowycky, M.C., Fox, A.P., and Tsien, R.W. 1985. Three types of neuronal calcium channel with different calcium agonist sensitivity. Nature 316: 440–443.

Nowycky, M.C., Mori, K., and Shepherd, G.M. 1981a. GABAergic mechanisms of dendrodendritic synapses in isolated turtle olfactory bulb. J. Neurophysiol. 46: 693–648.

Nowycky, M.C., Mori, K., and Shepherd, G.M. 1981b. Blockade of synaptic inhibition reveals long-lasting synaptic excitation in isolated turtle olfactory bulb. J. Neurophysiol. 46: 649–658.

Nyakas, C., Luiten, P.G.M., Spencer, D.G., and Traber, J. 1987. Detailed projection patterns of septal and diagonal band efferents to the hippocampus in the rat with emphasis on innervation of CA1 and dentate gyrus. Brain Res. Bull. 18: 533–545.

Obata, K., Ito, M., Ochi, R., and Sato, N. 1967. Pharmacological properties of the postsynaptic inhibition by Purkinje cell axons and the action of gamma-aminobutyric acid on Dieters neurons. Exp. Brain Res. 4: 43–57.

Obata, K.T. and Shinozaki, H. 1970. Further study on pharmacological properties of the cere-
bellar-induced inhibition of Dieters neurones. Exp. Brain Res. 11: 327–342.

Oertel, D. 1983. Synaptic responses and electrical properties of cells in brain slices of the mouse
anteroventral cochlear nucleus. J. Neurosci. 3: 2043–2053.

Oertel, D., Wu, S.H., Garb, M.W., and Dizack, C. 1990. Morphology and physiology of cells in slice
preparations of the posteroventral cochlear nucleus of mice. J. Comp. Neurol. 295: 136–154.

Oertel, W.H., Schmechel, D.E., Mugnaini, E., Tappaz, M.L., and Kopin, I.J. 1981. Immunocytochemical localization of glutamate decarboxylase in rat cerebellum with a new antiserum.
Neuroscience 6: 2715–2735.

Oertel, W.H., Tappaz, M.L., Berod, A., and Mugnaini, E. 1982. Two-color immunohistochemistry for dopamine and GABA neurons in rat substantia nigra and zona incerta. Brain Res.
Bul. 9: 463–474.

Ogawa, T., Ito, S., and Kato, H. 1981. Membrane characteristics of visual cortical neurons in in
vitro slices. Brain Res. 226: 315–319.

Ogawa, T., Kato, H., and Ito, S. 1986. Studies on inhibitory neurotransmission in visual cortex
in vitro. In: Visual Neuroscience (Pettigrew, J., Sanderson, K., and Levick, W., eds.). Cambridge: Cambridge University Press, pp. 280–289.

Ogren, M.P. and Hendrickson, A.E. 1979. The morphology and distribution of striate cortex terminals in the inferior and lateral subdivisions of the Macaca monkey pulvinar. J. Comp.
Neurol. 188: 179–199.

Ohara, P.T. and Lieberman, A.R. 1985. The thalamic reticular nucleus of the adult rat experimental anatomical studies. J. Neurocytol. 14: 365–411.

Ohara, P.T., Lieberman, A.R., Hunt, S.P., and Wu, J.Y. 1983. Neural elements containing glutamic acid decarboxylase (GAD) in the dorsal lateral geniculate nucleus of the rat: Immunohistochemical studies by light and electron microscopy. Neuroscience 8: 189–211.

Ohtsuka, T. 1985. Relation of spectral types to oil droplets in cones of turtle retina. Science 229:
874–877.

Ojima, H., Mori, K., and Kishi, K. 1984. The trajectory of mitral cell axons in the rabbit olfactory cortex revealed by intracellular HRP injection. J. Comp. Neurol. 230: 77–87.

Okamato, K., Quastel, D.M.J., and Quastel, J.H. 1976. Action of amino acids and convulsants
on cerebellar spontaneous action potentials in vitro: Effects of deprivation of Cl^-, K^+ or
Na^+. Brain Res. 206: 371–386.

Okamato, K. and Sakai, Y. 1981. Inhibitory actions of taurocyamine, hypotaurine, homotaurine,
taurine and GABA on spike discharges of Purkinje cells, and localization of sensitive site,
in guinea pig cerebellar slices. Brain Res. 206: 371–386.

O'Keefe, J. 1979. A review of the hippocampal place cells. Prog. Neurobiol. 13: 419–439.

O'Leary, J.L. 1937. Structure of the primary olfactory cortex of the mouse. J. Comp. Neurol.
67: 1–31.

Oleskevich, S. and Decarries, L. 1990. Quantified distribution of the serotonin innervation in
adult rat hippocampus. Neuroscience 34: 19–33.

Oliver, D.L. and Huerta, M.F. 1992. Inferior and superior colliculi. In: The Mammalian Auditory Pathway: Neuroanatomy (Webster, D.B., Popper, A.N., and Fay, R.R., eds.). New York:
Springer-Verlag, pp. 168–221.

Olson, D. and Breckenridge, B. 1976. Calcium ion effects on guanylate cyclase of brain. Life
Sci. 18: 935–940.

O'Malley, D.M., Sandell, J.H., and Masland, R.H. 1994. Co-release of acetylcholine and GABA
by the starburst amacrine cells. J. Neurosci. 12: 1394–1408.

Ono, K., Tomasiewicz, H., Magnuson, T., and Rutishauser, U. 1994. N-CAM mutation inhibits
tangential neuronal migration and is phenocopied by enzymatic removal of polysialic acid.
Neuron 13: 595–609.

Oorschot, D.E. 1996. Total number of neurons in the neostriatal, pallidal, subthalamic, and substantia nigral neulei of the rat basal ganglia—A stereological study using the Cavalieri and optical disector methods. J. Comp. Neurol. 366: 580–599.

Örnung, G., Shupliakov, O., Ottersen, O.P., Storm-Mathisen, J., and Cullheim, S. 1994. Immunohistochemical evidence for coexistence of glycine and GABA in nerve terminals on cat spinal motoneurons: An ultrastructural study. NeuroReport 5: 889–892.

Orona, E., Rainer, E., and Scott, J. 1984. Dendritic and axonal organization of mitral and tufted cells in the rat olfactory bulb. J. Comp. Neurol. 226: 346–356.

Orona, E., Scott, J., and Rainer, E. 1983. Different granule cell populations innervate superficial and deep regions of the external plexiform layer in rat olfactory bulb. J. Comp. Neurol. 217: 227–237.

Osborn, C.E. and Poppele, R.E. 1993. Sensory integration by the dorsal spinocerebellar tract circuitry. Neuroscience 54: 945–956.

Osen, K.K. 1969. Cytoarchitecture of the cochlear nuclei in the cat. J. Comp. Neurol. 136: 453–482.

Osen, K.K. 1970a. Course and termination of the primary afferents in the cochlear nuclei of the cat. Arch. Ital. Biol. 108: 21–51.

Osen, K.K. 1970b. Afferent and efferent connections of three well-defined cell types of the cat cochlear nucleus. In: Excitatory Synaptic Mechanisms (Anderson, P. and Jansen, J.K.S., eds.). Oslo: Universitetsforlaget, pp. 295–300.

Osen, K.K. 1983. Orientation of dendritic arbors studied in Golgi sections of the cat dorsal cochlear nucleus. In: Mechanisms of Hearing (Webster, W.R. and Aitkin, L.M., eds.). Clayton: Monash University Press, pp. 83–89.

Osen, K.K., Ottersen, O.P., and Storm-Mathisen, J. 1990. Colocalization of glycine-like and GABA-like immunoreactivities. A semiquantitative study of individual neurons in the dorsal cochlear nucleus of cat. In: Glycine Neurotransmission (Ottersen, O.P. and Storm-Mathisen, J., eds.). New York: John Wiley & Sons, pp. 417–451.

Osen, K.K., Storm-Mathisen, J., Ottersen, O.P., and Dihle, B. 1995. Glutamate is concentrated in and released from parallel fiber terminals in the dorsal cochlear nucleus: A quantitative immunocytochemical analysis in guinea pigs. J. Comp. Neurol. 357: 482–500.

Ostapoff, E.M., Feng, J.J., and Morest, D.K. 1994. A physiological and structural study of neuron types in the cochlear nucleus. II. Neuron types and their structural correlation with response properties. J. Comp. Neurol. 346: 19–42.

Ostapoff, E.M. and Morest, D.K. 1991. Synaptic organization of globular bushy cells in the ventral cochlear nucleus of the cat: A quantitative study. J. Comp. Neurol. 314: 598–613.

Oyster, C.W., Takahashi, E.S., Cilluffo, M., and Brecha, N.C. 1985. Morphology and distribution of tyrosine hydroxylase-like immunoreactive neurons in the cat retina. Proc. Natl. Acad. Sci. USA 82: 6335–6339.

Packer, O., Hendrickson, A., and Curcio, C. 1989. Photoreceptor topography of the retina in the adult pigtail Macaque (*Macaca nemestrina*). J. Comp. Neurol. 288: 165–183.

Packer, O.S., Williams, D.R., and Bensinger, D.G. 1996. Photopigment transmittance imaging of the primate photoreceptor mosaic. J. Neurosci. 16: 2251–2260.

Palay, S.L. and Chan-Palay, V. 1974. Cerebellar Cortex: Cytology and Organization. New York: Springer-Verlag.

Palkovits, M. and Brownstein, M.J. 1985. Distribution of neuropeptides in the central nervous system using biochemical micromethods. In: Handbook of Chemical Neuroanatomy, Vol. 4: GABA and Neuropeptides in the CNS, Part I (Björklund, A. and Hökfelt, T., eds.). Amsterdam: Elsevier, pp. 1–71.

Palkovits, M., Mezey, E., Hamori, J., and Szentagothai, J. 1977. Quantitative histological analysis of the cerebellar nuclei in the cat. I. Numerical data on cells and on synapses. Exp. Brain Res. 28: 189–209.

Palmer, A.R., Jiang, D., and Marshall, D.H. 1996. Responses of ventral cochlear nucleus onset and chopper units as a function of signal bandwidth. J. Neurophysiol. 75: 780–794.

Palmer, L.A. and Davis, T.L. 1981. Receptive field structure in cat striate cortex. J. Neurophysiol. 46: 260–276.

Panico, J. and Sterling, P. 1995. Retinal neurons and vessels are not fractal but space filling. J. Comp. Neurol. 361: 479–490.

Papadopoulos, G., Parnevelas, J., and Buijs, R. 1987. Light and electron microscopic analysis of the noradrenaline innervation of the rat visual cortex. J. Neurocytol. 18: 1–10.

Pape, H.-C., Budde, T., Mager, R., and Kisvárday, Z.F. 1994. Prevention of Ca^{2+}-mediated action potentials in GABAergic local circuit neurones of rat thalamus by a transient K^+ current. J. Physiol. (Lond.) 478: 403–422.

Pape, H.-C. and Mager, R. 1992. Nitric oxide controls oscillatory activity in thalamocortical neurons. Neurons 9: 441–448.

Pape, H.-C. and McCormick, D.A. 1989. Noradrenaline and serotonin selectively modulate thalamic burst firing by enhancing a hyperpolarization-activated cation current. Nature 340: 715–718.

Pape, H.-C. and McCormick, D.A. 1995. Electrophysiological and pharmacological properties interneurons in the cat dorsal lateral geniculate nucleus. Neuroscience 68: 1105–1125.

Parent, A., Bouchard, C. and Smith, Y. 1984. The striatopallidal and striatonigral projections— two distinct fiber systems in primate. Brain Res. 303: 385–390.

Parham, K. and Kim, D.O. 1995. Spontaneous and sound-evoked discharge characteristics of complex-spiking neurons in the dorsal cochlear nucleus of the unanesthetized decerebrate cat. J. Neurophysiol. 73: 550–561.

Parnevelas, J. and Papadopoulos, G. 1989. The monoaminergic innervation of the cerebral cortex is not diffuse and nonspecific. Trends Neurosci. 12: 315–319.

Parsons, T.D., Lenzi, D., Almers, W., and Roberts, W.M. 1994. Calcium-triggered exocytosis and endocytosis in an isolated presynaptic cell: Capacitance measurements in saccular hair cells. Neuron 13: 875–883.

Passingham, R. 1982. The Human Primate. Oxford: W.H. Freeman.

Paternostro, M.A., Reyher, C.K.H., and Brunjes, P.C. 1995. Intracellular injections of Lucifer Yellow into lightly fixed mitral cells reveal neuronal dye-coupling in the developing rat olfactory bulb. Dev. Brain Res. 84: 1–10.

Patuzzi, R. 1996. Cochlear micromechanics and macromechanics. In: The Cochlea (Dallos, P., Popper, A.N., and Fay, R.R., eds.). New York: Springer-Verlag, pp. 186–257.

Paxinos, G. and Watson, C. 1986. The Rat Brain in Stereotaxic Coordinates. San Diego: Academic Press.

Pearce, G. and Watson, C. 1986. The Rat Brain in Stereotaxic Coordinates. San Diego: Academic Press.

Pearce, R.A. 1993. Physiological evidence for two distinct GABA-A responses in rat hippocampus. Neuron 10: 189–200.

Pedarzani, P. and Storm, J.F. 1993. PKA mediates the effects of monoamine transmitters on the K^+ current underlying the slow spike frequency adaptation in hippocampal neurons. Neuron 11: 1023–1035.

Pederson, P.E., Jastreboff, P.J., Stewart, W.B., and Shepherd, G.M. 1986. Mapping of an olfactory receptor population that projects to a specific region in the rat olfactory bulb. J. Comp. Neurol. 250: 93–108.

Pederson, P.L. and Carafoli, E. 1987. Ion motive ATPases. I. Ubiquity, properties, and significance to cell function. Trends Biochem. Sci. 12: 146–150.

Peichl, L. 1991. Alpha ganglion cells in mammalian retinae: Common properties, species differences, and some comments on other ganglion cells. Vis. Neurosci. 7: 155–169.

Peng, Y.-W., Blackstone, C.D., Huganir, R.L., and Yau, K.-W. 1995. Distribution of glutamate receptor subtypes in the vertebrate retina. Neuroscience 66: 483–497.

Peng, Y. and Frank, E. 1989a. Activation of GABA-B receptors causes presynaptic inhibition at synapses between muscle spindle afferents and motoneurons in the spinal cord of bullfrogs. J. Neurosci. 9: 1502–1515.

Peng, Y. and Frank, E. 1989b. Activation of GABA-A receptors causes presynaptic and postsynaptic inhibition at synapses between muscle spindle afferents and motoneurons in the spinal cord of bullfrogs. J. Neurosci. 9: 1516–1522.

Penn, A.A., Wong, R.O.L., and Shatz, C.J. 1994. Neuronal coupling in the developing mammalian retina. J. Neurosci. 14: 3805–3815.

Penny, G.R., Afsharpour, S., and Kitai, S.T. 1986. The glutamate decarboxylase immunoreactive, met-enkephalin-immunoreactive and substance P-immunoreactive neurons in the neostriatum of the rat and cat. Evidence for partial population overlap. Neuroscience 17: 1011–1045.

Perkel, D.H. and Perkel, D.J. 1985. Dendritic spines: Role of active membrane in modulating synaptic efficacy. Brain Res. 325: 331–335.

Perry, V.H., Oehler, R., and Cowey, A. 1984. Retinal ganglion cells that project to the dorsal lateral geniculate nucleus in the macaque monkey. Neuroscience 12: 1101–1123.

Peters, A. 1984. Chandelier cells. In: Cerebral Cortex: Cellular Components of the Cerebral Cortex (Peters, A. and Jones, E., eds.). New York: Plenum Press, pp. 361–380.

Peters, A. 1987. Number of neurons and synapses in the primary visual cortex. In: Cerebral Cortex, Vol. 6: Further Aspects of Cortical Functions Including Hippocampus (Jones, E. and Peters, A., eds.). New York: Plenum Press, pp. 267–294.

Peters, A. and Kaiserman-Abramof, I.R. 1970. The small pyramidal neuron of the rat cerebral cortex. The perikaryon, dendrites and spines. Am. J. Anat. 127: 321–356.

Peters, A. and Regidor, J. 1981. A reassessment of the forms of nonpyramidal neurons in area 17 of cat visual cortex. J. Comp. Neurol. 203: 685–716.

Peters, B.N. and Masland, R.H. 1996. Responses to light of starburst amacrine cells. J. Neurophysiol. 75: 469–480.

Peterson, G.E. and Barney, H.L. 1952. Control methods used in a study of the vowels. J. Acoust. Soc. Am. 24: 175–184.

Pettigrew, J. 1982. Pharmacological control of cortical plasticity. Retina 2: 360–372.

Pfeiffer, R.R. 1966a. Classification of response patterns of spike discharges for units in the cochlear nucleus: Tone burst stimulation. Exp. Brain Res. 1: 220–235.

Pfeiffer, R.R. 1966b. Anteroventral cochlear nucleus: Wave forms of extracellularly recorded spike potentials. Science 154: 667–668.

Pfeiffer, R.R. and Kim, D.O. 1975. Cochlear nerve fiber responses: Distribution along the cochlear partition. J. Acoust. Soc. Am. 58: 867–869.

Phelps, P.E., Houser, C.R., and Vaughn, J.E. 1985. Immunocytochemical localization of choline acetyltransferase within the rat neostriatum: A correlated light and electron microscopic study of cholinergic neurons and synapses. J. Comp. Neurol. 238: 286–307.

Phillips, C.G. 1959. Actions of antidromic pyramidal volleys on single Betz cells in the cat. Q. J. Exp. Physiol. 44: 1–25.

Phillips, C.G. 1969. Motor apparatus of the baboon's hand. Proc. R. Soc. Biol. 173: 141–174.

Phillips, C.G., Powell, T.P.S., and Shepherd, G.M. 1963. Responses of mitral cells to stimulation of the lateral olfactory tract in the rabbit. J. Physiol. (Lond.) 168: 65–88.

Phillis, J.W. 1968. Acetylcholinesterase in the feline cerebellum. J. Neurochem. 15: 691–698.

Phillis, J.W. and Wu, P.H. 1981. Catecholamines and the sodium pump in excitable cells. Prog. Neurobiol. 17: 141–184.

Piccolino, M. 1986. Cajal and the retina: A 100-year retrospective. Trends Neurosci. 9: 521–525.

Piccolino, M. 1995. Cross-talk between cones and horizontal cells through the feedback circuit. In: Neurobiology and Clinical Aspects of the Outer Retina. (Djamgoz, M.B.A., Archer, S., and Vallerga, S., eds.). London: Chapman & Hall, pp. 221–248.

Piccolino, M., Neyton, J., and Gerschenfeld, H.M. 1984. Decrease of gap-junction permeability induced by dopamine and cyclic adenosine $3',5'$-monophosphate in horizontal cells of turtle retina. J. Neurosci. 4: 2477–2488.

Pickles, J.O. 1988. An Introduction to the Physiology of Hearing. New York: Academic Press.

Pierce, J.P. and Mendell, L.M. 1993. Quantitative ultrastructure of Ia boutons in the ventral horn: Scaling and positional relationships. J. Neurosci. 13: 4748–4763.

Pierrot-Deseillegny, E. 1996. Transmission of the cortical command for human voluntary movement through cervical propriospinal premotoneurons. Prog. Neurobiol. 48: 489–517.

Pikel, V.M., Segal, M., and Bloom, F.E. 1974. A radioautographic study of the efferent pathways of the nucleus locus coeruleus. J. Comp. Neurol. 155: 15–42.

Pinching, A.J. 1971. Myelinated dendritic segments in the monkey olfactory bulb. Brain Res. 29: 133–138.

Pinching, A.J. and Powell, T.P.S. 1971a. The neuron types of the glomerular layer of the olfactory bulb. J. Cell Sci. 9: 305–345.

Pinching, A.J. and Powell, T.P.S. 1971b. The neuropil of the glomeruli of the olfactory bulb. J. Cell Sci. 9: 347–377.

Pinco, M. and Levtov, A. 1993. Synaptic excitation of alpha-motoneurons by dorsal root afferents in the neonatal rat spinal cord. J. Neurophysiol. 70: 406–417.

Pineda, J.C., Galarraga, E., Bargas, J., Cristancho, M., and Aceves, J. 1992. Charybdotoxin and apamin sensitivity of the calcium-dependent repolarization and the afterhyperpolarization in neostriatal neurons. J. Neurophysiol. 68: 287–294.

Pinsky, P. and Rinzel, J. 1994. Intrinsic and network rhythmogenisis in a reduced Traub model for Ca3 neurons. J. Comput. Neurosci 1: 39–60.

Pinter, M.J., Burke, R.E., O'Donovan, M.J., and Dum, R.P. 1982. Supraspinal facilitation of cutaneous polysynaptic EPSPs in cat medial gastrocnemius motoneurons. Exp. Brain Res. 45: 133–143.

Piredda, S. and Gale, K. 1985. A crucial epileptogenic site in the deep prepiriform cortex. Nature 317: 623–625.

Pollen, D. and Lux, H. 1966. Conductance changes during inhibitory postsynaptic potentials in normal and strychninized cortical neurons. J. Physiol. (Lond.) 29: 367–381.

Polyak, S.L. 1941. The Retina. Chicago: University of Chicago Press.

Porter, R. 1987. Corticomotoneuronal projections: Synaptic events related to skilled movement. Proc. R. Soc. Lond. B Biol. Sci. 231: 147–168.

Potts, A.M., Hodges, D., Shelman, C.B., Fritz, K.J., Levy, N.S., and Mangnall, Y. 1972. Morphology of the primate optic nerve. I. Method and total fiber count. Inv. Ophthalmol. Vis. Sci. 11: 980–988.

Pourcho, R.G. 1982. Dopaminergic amacrine cells in the cat retina. Brain Res. 252: 101–109.

Pourcho, R.G. and Goebel, D.J. 1987. Visualization of endogenous glycine in cat retina: An immunocytochemical study with Fab fragments. J. Neurosci. 7: 1189–1197.

Pourcho, R.G. and Owczarzak, M.T. 1989. Distribution of GABA immunoreactivity in the cat retina: A light- and electron-microscopic study. Vis. Neurosci. 2: 425–435.

Pourcho, R.G. and Owczarzak, M.T. 1991. Glycine receptor immunoreactivity is localized at amacrine synapses in cat retina. Vis. Neurosci. 7: 611–618.

Powell, T. 1981. Certain aspects of the intrinsic organisation of the cerebral cortex. In: Brain Mechanisms and Perceptual Awareness (Pompeiano, O. and Marsan, C.A., eds.). New York: Raven Press, pp. 1–19.

Powell, T. and B. Mountcastle, V. 1959. Some aspects of the functional organization of the cortex of the postcentral gyrus of the monkey: A correlation of findings obtained on a single unit analysis with cytoarchitecture. Bull. Johns Hopkins Hosp. 105: 133–162.

Pratt, C.A. and Jordan, L. 1987. Ia inhibitory interneurons and Renshaw cells as contributors to the spinal mechanisms of fictive locomotion. J. Neurophysiol. 57: 56–71.

Precht, W. and Yoshida, M. 1971. Blockage of caudate-evoked inhibition of neurons in the substantia nigra by picrotoxin. Brain Res. 32: 229–233.

Preuss, T.M., Beck, P.D., and Kaas, J.H. 1993. Areal, modular, and connectional organization of visual cortex in a prosimian primate, the slow loris (*Nycticebus coucang*). Brain Behav. Evol. 42: 321–335.

Price, J.L. 1973. An autoradiographic study of complementary laminar patterns of termination of afferent fibers to the olfactory cortex. J. Comp. Neurol. 150: 87–108.

Price, J.L. 1985. Beyond the primary olfactory cortex. Olfactory-related areas in the neocortex, thalamus and hypothalamus. Chem. Senses 10: 239–258.

Price, J.L. 1987. The central olfactory and accessory olfactory systems. In: Neurobiology of Taste and Smell (Finger, T.E. and Silver, W.L., eds.). New York: John Wiley & Sons, pp. 179–203.

Price, J.L., Carmichael, S.T., Carnes, K.M., Clugnut, M.C., Kuroda, M., and Ray, J.P. 1991. Olfactory input to the prefrontal cortex. In: Olfaction Model System for Computational Neuroscience (Davis, J.L. and Eichenbaum, H., eds.). Cambridge, MA: MIT Press, pp. 101–120.

Price, J.L. and Powell, T.P.S. 1970a. The morphology of granule cells of the olfactory bulb. J. Cell. Sci. 7: 91–123.

Price, J.L. and Powell, T.P.S. 1970b. The synaptology of the granule cells of the olfactory bulb. J. Cell. Sci. 7: 125–155.

Price, J.L. and Sprich, W.W. 1975. Observations on the lateral olfactory tract of the rat. J. Comp. Neurol. 162: 321–336.

Prince, D. and Huguenard, J. 1988. Functional properties of neocortical neurons. In: Neurobiology of the Neocortex (Rakic, P. and Singer, W., eds.). Chichester: John Wiley & Sons, pp. 153–176.

Pu, M. and Amthor, F.R. 1990. Dendritic morphologies of retinal ganglion cells projecting to the nucleus of the optic tract in the rabbit. J. Comp. Neurol. 302: 657–674.

Pugh, E.N.J. and Lamb, T.D. 1993. Amplification and kinetics of the activation steps in phototransduction. Biochim. Biophys. Acta 1141: 111–149.

Puil, E. 1983. Actions and interactions of S-glutamate in the spinal cord. In: Handbook of the Spinal Cord, Vol. 1: Pharmacology (Davidoff, R.A., ed.). New York: Marcel Dekker, pp. 105–169.

Purpura, D.P. 1974. Dendritic spine "dysgenesis" and mental retardation. Science 186: 1126–1128.

Rack, P.M.H. 1981. Limitations of somatosensory feedback in control of posture and movement. In: Handbook of Physiology, Section 1: The Nervous System, Vol. II: Motor Control, Part 1 (Brooks, V.B., ed.). Bethesda, American Physiological Society, pp. 229–256.

Rackowski, D. and Fitzpatrick, D. 1989. Organization of cholinergic synapses in the cat's dorsal lateral geniculate and perigeniculate nuclei. J. Comp. Neurol. 288: 676–690.

Radpour, S. and Thomson, A.M. 1991. Coactivation of local circuit NMDA receptor mediated epsps induces lasting enhancement of minimal Schaffer collateral EPSPs in slices of rat hippocampus. Eur. J. Neurosci. 3: 602–613.

Ragsdale, C.W.J. and Graybiel, A.M. 1991. Compartmental organization of the thalamostriatal connection in the cat. J. Comp. Neurol. 311: 134–167.

Rakic, P. (ed.). 1976a. Local Circuit Neurons. Cambridge, MA: MIT Press.

Rakic, P. 1976b. Prenatal genesis of connections subserving ocular dominance in the rhesus monkey. Nature 261: 467–471.

Rakic, P., Bourgeois, J.P., Eckenhoff, M.F., Zecevic, N., and Goldman-Rakic, P.S. 1986. Concurrent overproduction of synapses in diverse regions of the primate cerebral cortex. Science 232: 232–235.

Rakic, P. and Riley, K.P. 1983. Overproduction and elimination of retinal axons in the fetal rhesus monkey. Science 219: 1441–1444.

Rall, W. 1957. Membrane time constant of motoneurons. Science 126: 454–455.

Rall, W. 1959a. Dendritic current distribution and whole neuron properties. Naval Med. Res. Inst. Res. Report NM 01-05-00.01.01.

Rall, W. 1959b. Branching dendritic trees and notoneuron membrane resistivity. Exp. Neurol. 1: 491–527.

Rall, W. 1960. Membrane potential transients and membrane time constant of motoneurons. Exp. Neurol. 2: 503–532.

Rall, W. 1962. Electrophysiology of a dendritic neuron model. Biophys. J. 2: 145–167.

Rall, W. 1964. Theoretical significance of dendritic trees for neuronal input-output relations. In: Neural Theory and Modelling (Reiss, R.F., eds.). Stanford: Stanford University Press, pp. 73–97.

Rall, W. 1967. Distinguishing theoretical syanptic potentials computed for different soma-dendritic distributions of synaptic input. J. Neurophysiol. 30: 1138–1168.

Rall, W. 1970. Cable properties of dendrites and effects of synaptic location. In: Excitatory Synaptic Mechanisms (Andersen, P. and Jansen, J.K.S., eds.). Oslo: Universitetsforlag, pp. 175–187.

Rall, W. 1974a. Dendritic spines and synaptic potency. In: Studies in Neurophysiology (Porter, R., ed.). Cambridge: Cambridge University Press, pp. 203–209.

Rall, W. 1974b. Dendritic spines, synaptic potency in neuronal plasticity. In: Cellular Mechanisms Subserving Changes in Neuronal Activity (Woody, C.D., Brown, K.A., Crow, T.J., and Knispel, J.D., eds.). Los Angeles: Brain Information Service, pp. 13–21.

Rall, W. 1977. Core conductor theory and cable properties of neurons. In: The Nervous System, Vol. I: Cellular Biology of Neurons, Part 1 (Kandel, E.R., ed.). Bethesda: American Physiological Society, pp. 39–97.

Rall, W. 1989. Cable theory for dendritic neurons. In: Methods in Neuronal Modeling (Koch, C. and Segev, I., eds.). Cambridge, MA: MIT Press, pp. 9–62.

Rall, W., Burke, R.E., Holmes, W.R., Jack, J.J.B., Redman, S.J., and Segev, I. 1992. Matching dendritic neuron models to experimental data. Physiol. Rev. 72: S159–S186.

Rall, W., Burke, R.E., Nelson, P.G., Smith, T.G., and Frank, K. 1967. The dendritic location of synapses and possible mechanisms for the monosynaptic EPSP in motoneurons. J. Neurophysiol. 30: 1169–1193.

Rall, W. and Hunt, C.C. 1956. Analysis of reflex variability in terms of partially correlated excitability fluctuations in a population of motoneurons. J. Gen. Physiol. 39: 397–422.

Rall, W. and Rinzel, J. 1973. Branch input resistance and steady attenuation for input to one branch of a dendritic neuron model. Biophys. J. 13: 648–688.

Rall, W. and Segev, I. 1987. Functional possibilities for synapses on dendrites and on dendritic spines. In: Synaptic Function (Edelman, G.M., Gall, W.F., and Cowan, W.M., eds.). New York: John Wiley & Sons, pp. 605–636.

Rall, W. and Shepherd, G.M. 1968. Theoretical reconstruction of field potentials and dendro-dendritic synaptic interactions in olfactory bulb. J. Neurophysiol. 31: 884–915.

Rall, W., Shepherd, G.M., Reese, T.S., and Brightman, M.W. 1966. Dendrodendritic synaptic pathway for inhibition in the olfactory bulb. Exp. Neurol. 14: 44–56.

Ralston, H.J., III 1971. Evidence for presynaptic dendrites and a proposal for their mechanism of action. Nature 230: 585–587.

Ralston, H.J. 1983. The synaptic organization of the ventrobasal thalamus in the rat, cat, and monkey. In: Somatosensory Integration in the Thalamus (Macchi, G., Rustioni, A., and Spreafico, R., eds.). Amsterdam: Elsevier, pp. 241–250.

Ralston, H.J., III, Ohara, P.T., Ralston, D.D., and Chazal, G. 1988. The neuronal and synaptic organization of the cat and primate somatosensory thalamus. In: Cellular Thalamic Mechanisms (Bentivoglio, M. and Spreafico, R., eds.). Amsterdam: Elsevier, pp. 127–141.

Raman, I. and Trussell, L.O. 1992. The kinetics of the responses to glutamate and kainate in neurons of the avian cochlear nucleus. Neuron 9: 173–186.

Raman, I.M., Zhang, S., and Trussell, L.O. 1994. Pathway-specific variants of AMPA receptors and their contribution to neuronal signaling. J. Neurosci. 14: 4998–5010.

Ramoa, A., Campbell, G., and Shatz, C.J. 1988. Dendritic growth and remodeling of cat retinal ganglion cells during fetal and postnatal development. J. Neurosci. 8: 4239–4261.

Ramon-Cueto, A. and Valverde, F. 1995. Olfactory bulb ensheathing glia: A unique cell type with axonal growth-promoting properties. Glia 14: 163–173.

Ramón-Moliner, E. 1977. The reciprocal synapses of the olfactory bulb: Questioning the evidence. Brain Res. 128: 1–20.

Randall, A. and Tsien, R.W. 1995. Pharmacological dissection of multiple types of Ca^{2+} channel currents in rat cerebellar granule neurons. J. Neurosci. 15: 2995–3012.

Rao, R., Buchsbaum, G., and Sterling, P. 1992. Rod synapse geometry affects transmitter concentration at the bipolar cell. Soc. Neurosci. Abstr. 18: 837.

Rao, R., Buchsbaum, G., and Sterling, P. 1994a. Rate of quantal transmitter release at the mammalian rod synapse. Biophys. J. 67: 57–63.

Rao, R., Buchsbaum, G., and Sterling, P. 1994b. Minimum rate of transmitter release at a cone active zone. Invest. Ophthalmol. Vis. Sci. Abstr. 35: 2125.

Rao, R. and Sterling, P. 1991. Synaptic apparatus associated with transmission of a single photon event. Soc. Neurosci. [Abstr.]

Rao-Mirotznik, R., Buchsbaum, G., and Sterling, P. 1997. Functional architecture of the mammalian rod synapse. (Submitted).

Rao-Mirotznik, R., Harkins, A., Buchsbaum, G., and Sterling, P. 1995. Mammalian rod terminal: Architecture of a binary synapse. Neuron 14: 561–569.

Ratliff, F. 1965. Mach Bands: Quantitative Studies on Neural Networks in the Retina. San Francisco: Holden-Day.

Raviola, E. and Gilula, N.B. 1973. Gap junctions between photoreceptor cells in the vertebrate retina. Proc. Natl. Acad. Sci. USA 70: 1677–1681.

Ray, J.P. and Price, J.L. 1992. The organization of the thalamocortical connections of the mediodorsal thalamic nucleus in the rat, related to the ventral forebrain-prefrontal cortex topography. J. Comp. Neurol. 323: 167–197.

Reader, T., Ferron, A., Descarries, L., and Jasper, H. 1979. Modulatory role for biogenic amines in the cerebral cortex: Microiontophoretic studies. Brain Res. 160: 217–229.

Redman, S.J. 1973. The attenuation of passively propagating dendritic potentials in a motoneurone cable model. J. Physiol. (Lond.) 234: 637–664.

Redman, S.J. 190. Quantal analysis of synaptic potentials in neurons of the central nervous system. Physiol. Rev. 70: 165–198.

Redman, S.J. and Walmsley, B. 1983. Amplitude fluctuations in synaptic potentials evoked in cat spinal motoneurons at identified group Ia synapses. J. Physiol. (Lond.) 343: 135–145.

Reece, L.J. and Schwartzkroin, P.A. 1991. Effects of cholinergic agonists on two non-pyramidal cell types in rat hippocampal slices. Brain Res. 566: 115–126.

Reed, M.C. and Blum, J.J. 1995. A computational model for signal processing by the dorsal cochlear nucleus, I: Responses to pure tones. J. Acoust. Soc. Am. 97: 425–438.

Reep, R.L. and Winans, S.S. 1982. Efferent connections of dorsal and ventral agranular insular cortex in the hamster, *Mesocricetus auratus*. Neuroscience 7: 2609–2635.

Reese, B.E. 1988. 'Hidden lamination' in the dorsal lateral geniculate nucleus. The functional organization of this thalamic region in the rat. Brain Res. 472: 119–137.

Reese, T.S. and Brightman, M.W. 1970. Olfactory surface and central olfactory connections in some vertebrates. In: Taste and Smell in Vertebrates (Wolstenholme, G.E.W. and Knight, J., eds.). London: J & A Churchill, pp. 115–149.

Reese, T.S. and Shepherd, G.M. 1972. Dendro-dendritic synapses in the central nervous system. In: Structure and Function of Synapses (Pappas, G.D. and Purpura, D.P., eds.). New York: Raven Press, pp. 121–136.

Regehr, W.G. and Tank, D.W. 1992. Calcium concentration dynamics produced by synaptic activation of CA1 hippocampal pyramidal cells. J. Neurosci. 12: 4202–4223.

Regehr, W.G. and Tank, D.W. 1994. Dendritic calcium dynamics. Curr. Opin. Neurobiol. 4: 373–382.

Reh, T. and Constantine-Paton, M. 1984. Retinal ganglion cell terminals change their projection sites during larval development of *Rana pipiens*. J. Neurosci. 4: 442–457.

Reisine, T. and Bell, G.I. 1995. Molecular properties of somatostatin receptors. Neuroscience 67: 777–790.

Reithmeier, R.A.F. 1994. Mammalian exchangers and co-transporters. Curr. Opin. Cell Biol. 6: 583–594.

Ressler, K.J., Sullivan, S.L., and Buck, L.B. 1993. A zonal organization of odorant receptor gene expression in the olfactory epithelium. Cell 73: 597–609.

Ressler, K.J., Sullivan, S.L., and Buck, L.B. 1994. Information coding in the olfactory system: Evidence for a stereotyped and highly organized epitope map in the olfactory bulb. Cell 79: 1245–1255.

Rexed, B. 1952. The cytoarchitectonic organization of the spinal cord in the cat. J. Comp. Neurol. 96: 415–496.

Reyes, A.D., Rubel, E.W., and Spain, W.J. 1994. Membrane properties underlying the firing of neurons in the avian cochlear nucleus. J. Neurosci. 14: 5352–5364.

Reyher, C.K., Lubke, J., Larsen, W.J., Hendrix, G.M., Shipley, M.T., and Baumgarte, H.G. 1991. Olfactory bulb granule cell aggregates: Morphological evidence for interperikaryal electrotonic coupling via gap junctions. J. Neurosci. 11: 1485–1495.

Reymond, L. 1985. Spatial visual acuity of the eagle *Aquila audax:* A behavioural, optical and anatomical investigation. Vision Res. 25: 1477–1491.

Rhoades, B.K. and Freeman, W.J. 1990. Excitatory actions of GABA in the rat olfactory bulb. Soc. Neurosci. Abstr. 16: 403.

Rhode, W.S. and Greenberg, S. 1994. Encoding of amplitude modulation in the cochlear nucleus of the cat. J. Neurophysiol. 71: 1797–1825.

Rhode, W.S., Oertel, D., and Smith, P.H. 1983a. Physiological response properties of cells labeled intracellularly with horseradish peroxidase in cat ventral cochlear nucleus. J. Comp. Neurol. 213: 448–463.

Rhode, W.S. and Smith, P.H. 1986. Encoding timing and intensity in the ventral cochlear nucleus of the cat. J. Neurophysiol. 56: 261–286.

Rhode, W.S. and Smith, P.H., and Oertel, D. 1983b. Physiological response properties of cells labeled intracellulary with horseradish peroxidase in cat dorsal cochlear nucleus. J. Comp. Neurol. 213: 426–447.

Ribak, C.E. 1978. Aspinous and sparsely spinous stellate neurons in the visual cortex of rats contain glutamic acid decarboxylase. J. Neurocytol. 7: 461–478.

Ribak, C.E. and Seress, L. 1983. Five types of basket cell in the hippocampal dentate gyrus: a combined Golgi and electron microscopic study. J. Neurocytol. 12: 577–597.

Ribak, C.E., Seress, L., and Amaral, D.G. 1985. The development, ultrastructure and synaptic connections of the mossy cells of the dentate gyrus. J. Neurocytol. 14: 835–857.

Ribak, C.E., Vaughn, J.E., and Saito, K. 1978. Immunocytochemical localization of glutamic acid decarboxylase in neuronal somata following colchicine inhibition of axonal transport. Brain Res. 140: 315–332.

Ribak, C.E., Vaughn, J.E., Saito, K., Barber, R., and Roberts, E. 1977. Glutamate decarboxylase localization in neurons in the olfactory bulb. Brain Res. 126: 1–18.

Richardson, T.L., Turner, R.W., and Miller, J.J. 1987. Action-potential discharge in hippocampal CA1 pyramidal neurons current source-density analysis. J. Neurophysiol. 58: 981–996.

Richmond, B., Wurtz, R., and Sato, T. 1983. Visual responses of inferior temporal neurons in the awake rhesus monkey. J. Neurophysiol. 50: 1415–1432.

Rieke, F. and Schwartz, E.A. 1996. Asynchronous transmitter release: Control of exocytosis and endocytosis at the salamander rod synapse. J. Physiol. (Lond.) 493: 1–8.

Rihn, L.L. and Claiborne, B.J. 1990. Dendritic growth and regression in rat dentate granule cells during late postnatal development. Dev. Brain Res. 54: 115–124.

Ringham, G.L. 1971. Origin of nerve impulse in slowly adapting stretch receptor of crayfish. J. Neurophysiol. 34: 773–784.

Rinvik, E. 1972. Organization of thalamic connections from motor and somatosensory cortical areas in the cat. In: Corticothalamic Projections and Sensorimotor Activities (Frigyesi, T., Rinvik, E., Yahr, M.D., eds.). New York: Raven Press, pp. 57–90.

Rinzel, J. and Rall, W. 1974. Transient response in a dendritic neuronal model for current injected at one branch. Biophys. J. 14: 759–790.

Rivadulla, C., Rodriguez, R., Martinez-Conde, S., Acuña, C., and Cudeiro, J. 1996. The influence of nitric oxide on perigeniculate GABAergic cell activity in the anaesthetized cat. Eur. J. Neurosci. 8: 2459–2466.

Roberts, E., Chase, T.N., and Tower, D.B. 1976. GABA in Nervous System Function. New York: Raven Press.

Roberts, G.W., Woodhams, P.L., Polak, J.M., and Crow, T.J. 1982. Distribution of neuropeptides in the limbic system of the rat: The amygdaloid complex. Neuroscience 7: 99–131.

Roberts, P.J., Storm-Mathisen, J. and Johnston, G.A.R. 1981. Glutamate Transmission in the Central Nervous System. Chichester: John Wiley & Sons.

Robson, J.A. and Hall, W.C. 1977. The organization of the pulvinar in the grey squirrel (*Sciurus carolinensis*) II. Synaptic organization and comparisons with the dorsal lateral geniculate nucleus. J. Comp. Neurol. 173: 389–416.

Rockland, K.S. and Pandya, D.N. 1981. Cortical connections of the occipital lobe in the rhesus monkey. Interconnections between areas 17, 18, 19 and the superior temporal sulcus. Brain Res. 212: 249–270.

Rodieck, R.W. 1965. Quantitative analysis of cat retinal ganglion cell response to visual stimuli. Vision Res. 5: 583–601.

Rodieck, R.W. 1989. Starburst amacrine cells of the primate retina. J. Comp. Neurol. 285: 18–37.

Rodieck, R.W. and Brening, R.K. 1983. Retinal ganglion cells: Properties, types, genera, pathways and trans-species comparisons. Brain Behav. Evol. 23: 121–164.

Rodieck, R.W., Brening, R.K., and Watanabe, M. 1993. The origin of parallel visual pathways. In: Contrast Sensitivity (Shapley, R. and Lam, D.M.-K, eds.). Cambridge, MA: MIT Press, pp. 117–144.

Rodieck, R.W. and Watanabe, M. 1993. Survey of the morphology of macaque retinal ganglion cells that project to the pretectum, superior colliculus, and parvicellular laminae of the lateral geniculate nucleus. J. Comp. Neurol. 338: 289–303.

Rodriguez, R. and Haberly, L.B. 1989. Analysis of synaptic events in the opossum piriform cortex with improved current source density techniques. J. Neurophysiol. 61: 702–718.

Roffler, Tarlov, S. and Turey, M. 1982. The content of amino acids in the developing cerebellar cortex and deep cerebellar nuclei of granule cell deficient mutant mice. Brain Res. 247: 65–73.

Rohde, B.H., Rea, M.A., Simon, J.R., and McBride, W.J. 1979. Effects of X-irradiation induced loss of cerebellar granule cells on the synaptosomal levels and the high affinity uptake of amino acids. J. Neurochem. 32: 1431–1435.

Röhrenbeck, J., Wässle, H., and Boycott, B.B. 1989. Horizontal cells in the monkey retina: Immunocytochemical staining with antibodies against calcium binding proteins. Eur. J. Neurosci. 1: 407–420.

Roman, F.S., Chaillan, F.A., and Soumireu-Mourat, B. 1993. Long-term potentiation in rat piriform cortex following discrimination learning. Brain Res. 601: 265–272.

Roman, F.S., Staubli, U., and Lynch, G. 1987. Evidence for synaptic potentiation in a cortical network during learning. Brain Res. 418: 221–226.

Romanes, G.J. 1951. The motor cell columns of the lumbo-sacral spinal cord of the cat. J. Comp. Neurol. 94: 313–363.

Romer, A.S. 1969. Vertebrate history with special reference to factors related to cerebellar evolution. In: Neurobiology of Cerebellar Evolution and Development (Llinás, R., ed.). Chicago: American Medical Association, pp. 1–18.

Ropert, N., Miles, R., and Korn, H. 1990. Characteristics of miniature inhibitory postsynaptic currents in CA1 pyramidal neurones of rat hippocampus. J. Physiol. (Lond.) 428: 707–722.

Rose, A. 1973. Vision: Human and Electronic. New York: Plenum Press.

Rose, D. and Dobson, V.G. 1985. Models of the Visual Cortex. New York: John Wiley & Sons.

Rose, M. 1928. Die Inselrinde des Menschen und der Tiere. J. Psychol. Neurol. (Leipzig) 37: 467–624.

Rose, P.K. and Richmond, F.J.R. 1981. White-matter dendrites in the upper cervical spinal cord of the adult cat: A light and electron microscopic study. J. Comp. Neurol. 199: 191–203.

Ross, W.N. and Werman, J.R. 1986. Mapping calcium transients in the dendrites of Purkinje cells from the guinea-pig cerebellum in vitro. J. Physiol. (Lond.) 389: 319–336.

Rossi, D.J., Alford, S., Mugnaini, E., and Slater, N.T. 1995. Properties of transmission at a giant glutamatergic synapse in cerebellum: The mossy fiber-unipolar brush cell synapse. J. Neurophysiol. 74: 24–42.

Rossignol, S. and Dubuc, R. 1994. Spinal pattern generation. Curr. Opin. Neurobiol. 4: 894–902.

Rothman, J.S. and Young, E.D. 1996. Enhancement of neural synchronization in computational models of ventral cochlear nucleus bushy cells. Auditory Neurosci. 2: 47–62.

Rothman, J.S., Young, E.D., and Manis, P.B. 1993. Convergence of auditory nerve fibers onto bushy cells in the ventral cochlear nucleus: Implications of a computational model. J. Neurophysiol. 70: 2562–2583.

Rotter, A., Birdsall, N.J.M., Burgen, A.S.V., Field, P.M., Hulme, E.C., and Raisman, G. 1977. Muscarinic receptors in the central nervous system of the rat. I. Technique for autoradiographic localization of the binding of [3H] propylbenzilylcholine mustard and its distribution in the forebrain. Brain Res. Rev. 1: 141–165.

Rouiller, E.M., Cronin-Schreiber, R., Fekete, D.M., and Ryugo, D.K. 1986. The central projections of intracellularly labeled auditory nerve fibers in cats: An analysis of terminal morphology. J. Comp. Neurol. 249: 261–278.

Rouiller, E.M. and Ryugo, D.K. 1984. Intracellular marking of physiologically characterized cells in the ventral cochlear nucleus of the cat. J. Comp. Neurol. 225: 167–186.

Rousselot, P., Lois, C., and Alvarez-Buylla, A. 1995. Embryonic (PSA) N-CAM reveals chains of migrating neuroblasts between the lateral ventricle and the olfactory bulb of adult mice. J. Comp. Neurol. 351: 51–61.

Rudomin, P. 1990. Presynaptic inhibition of muscle spindle and tendon organ afferents in the mammalian spinal cord. Trends Neurosci. 13: 499–505.

Rudomin, P., Burke, R.E., Nunez, R., Madrid, J., and Dutton, H. 1975. Control of presynaptic correlation: A mechanism affecting information transmission from Ia fibers to motoneurons. J. Neurophysiol. 38: 267–284.

Rudy, B. 1988. Diversity and ubiquity of K$^+$ channels. Neuroscience 25: 729–749.

Rumelhart, D. and McClelland, J. 1986. Parallel Distributed Processing. Cambridge, MA: MIT Press.

Ruth, R.E., Collier, T.J., and Routtenberg, A. 1982. Topography between the entorhinal cortex and the dentate septotemporal axis in rats: I. Medial and intermediate entorhinal projecting cells. J. Comp. Neurol. 209: 69–78.

Ruth, R.E., Collier, T.J., and Routtenberg, A. 1988. Topographical relationship between the entorhinal cortex and the septotemporal axis of the dentate gyrus in rats: II. Cells projecting from lateral entorhinal subdivisions. J. Comp. Neurol. 270: 506–516.

Ryall, R.W., Piercey, M.F., and Polosa, C. 1971. Intersegmental and intrasegmental distribution of mutual inhibition of Renshaw cells. J. Neurophysiol. 34: 700–707.

Ryugo, D.K. 1992. The auditory nerve: Peripheral innervation, cell body morphology, and central projections. In: The Mammalian Auditory Pathway: Neuroanatomy (Webster, D.B., Popper, A.N., and Fay, R.R., eds.). New York: Springer-Verlag, pp. 23–65.

Ryugo, D.K. and Fekete, D.M. 1982. Morphology of primary axosomatic endings in the anteroventral cochlear nucleus of the cat: A study of the endbulbs of Held. J. Comp. Neurol. 210: 239–257.

Sachs, M.B. 1984. Speech encoding in the auditory nerve. In: Hearing Science, Recent Advances (Berlin, C.I., ed.). San Diego: College-Hill Press, pp. 263–307.

Sachs, M.B., Wang, X., and Molitor, S.C. 1993. Cross-correlation analysis and phase-locking in a model of the ventral cochlear nucleus stellate cell. In: The Mammalian Cochlear Nuclei: Organization and Function (Merchán, M.A., Juiz, M., and Godfrey, D.A., eds.). New York: Plenum Press, pp. 411–420.

Sachs, M.B. and Young, E.D. 1979. Encoding of steady-state vowels in the auditory nerve: Representation in terms of discharge rate. J. Acoust. Soc. Am. 66: 470–479.

Sagar, S.M. 1987. Somatostatin-like immunoreactive material in the rabbit retina: Immunohistochemical staining using monoclonal antibodies. J. Comp. Neurol. 266: 291–299.

Saint Marie, R.L., Benson, C.G., Ostapoff, E.M., and Morest, D.K. 1991. Glycine immunoreactive projections from the dorsal to the anteroventral cochlear nucleus. Hear. Res. 51: 11–28.

Saint Marie, R.L., Morest, D.K., and Brandon, C.J. 1989. The form and distribution of GABAergic synapses on the principal cell types of the ventral cochlear nucleus of the cat. Hear. Res. 42: 97–112.

Saito, H.-A. 1983. Morphology of physiologically identified X-, Y-, and W-type retinal ganglion cells of the cat. J. Comp. Neurol. 221: 279–288.

Saito, T., Kujiraoka, T., Yonaha, T., and Chino, Y. 1985. Reexamination of photoreceptor-bipolar connectivity patterns in carp retina: HRP-EM and Golgi-EM studies. J. Comp. Neurol. 236: 141–160.

Sakai, H.M. and Naka, K.-I. 1985. Novel pathway connecting the outer and inner vertebrate retina. Nature 315: 570–571.

Sakmann, B. 1992. Elementary steps in synaptic transmission revealed by currents through single ion channels. Science 256: 503–512.

Sakmann, B. and Creutzfeldt, O.D. 1969. Scotopic and mesopic light adaptation in the cat's retina. Pflügers Arch. 313: 168–185.

Salin, P.-A. and Bullier, J. 1995. Corticocortical connections in the visual system: Structure and function. Physiol. Rev. 75: 107–154.

Salkoff, L., Baker, K., Butler, A., Covarrubias, M., Pak, M.D., and Wei, A. 1992. An essential 'set' of K$^+$ channels conserved in flies, mice, and humans. Trends Neurosci. 15: 161–166.

Sallaz, M. and Jourdan, F. 1992. Apomorphine disrupts odour-induced patterns of glomerular activation in the olfactory bulb. Neuroreport 3: 833–836.

Sallaz, M. and Jourdan, F. 1993. C-*fos* expression and 2-deoxyglucose uptake in the olfactory bulb of odour-stimulated awake rats. Neuroreport 4: 55–58.

Salt, T.E. 1988. Electrophysiological studies of excitatory amino acid neurotransmitters in the ventrobasal thalamus. In: Cellular Thalamic Mechanisms (Macchi, G., Bentivoglio, M., and Spreafico, R., eds.). Amsterdam: Elsevier, pp. 297–310.

Salt, T.E. and Eaton, S.A. 1996. Functions of ionotropic and metabotropic glutamate receptors in sensory transmission in the mammalian thalamus. Prog. Neurobiol. 48: 55–72.

Salt, T.E. and Sillito, A. 1984. The action of somatostatin (SST) on the response properties of cells in the cat's visual cortex. J. Physiol. (Lond.) 350: 28P.

Salzman, C. and Newsome, W. 1994. Neural mechanisms for forming a perceptual decision. Science 264: 231–237.

Sandell, J.H. 1985. NADPH diaphorase cells in the mammalian inner retina. J. Comp. Neurol. 238: 466–472.

Sanderson, K.J. 1971. Visual field projection columns and magnification factors in the lateral geniculate nucleus of the cat. Exp. Brain Res. 13: 159–177.

Sandmann, D., Boycott, B.B., and Peichl, L. 1996. The horizontal cells of artiodactyl retinae: A comparison with Cajal's descriptions. Vis. Neurosci. 13: 735–746.

Sandoval, M.E. and Cotman, C.W. 1978. Evaluation of glutamate as a neurotransmitter of cerebellar parallel fibers. Neuroscience 3: 199–206.

Sanides, F. and Sanides, D. 1972. The "extraverted neurons" of the mammalian cerebral cortex. Z. Anat. Entwickl.-Gesch. 136: 272–293.

Sasaki, T. and Kaneko, A. 1996. L-glutamate-induced responses in OFF-type bipolar cells of the cat retina. Vision Res. 36: 787–795.

Sashihara, S., Greer, C.A., Oh, Y., and Waxman, S.G. 1996. Cell-specific differential expression of Na^+-channel B1-subunit mRNA in the olfactory system during postnatal development and after denervation. J. Neurosci. 16: 702–713.

Sassoè-Pognetto, M., Cantino, D., Panzanelli, P., Verdun Di Cantogno, L., Giustetto, M., Margolis, F.L., De Biasi, S., and Fasolo, A. 1993. Presynaptic co-localization of carnosine and glutamate in olfactory neurons. Neuroreport 5: 7–10.

Sassoè-Pognetto, M., Wässle, H., and Grünert, U. 1994. Glycinergic synapses in the rod pathway of the rat retina: Cone bipolar cells express the alpha-1 subunit of the glycine receptor. J. Neurosci. 14: 5131–5146.

Sato, T., Hirono, J., Tonoike, M., and Takebayashi, M. 1994. Tuning specificities to aliphatic odorants in mouse olfactory receptor neurons and their local distribution. J. Neurophysiol. 72: 2980–2989.

Satou, M., Mori, K., Tazawa, Y., and Takagi, S.F. 1982. Long-lasting disinhibition in pyriform cortex of the rabbit. J. Neurophysiol. 48: 1157–1163.

Satou, M., Mori, K., Tazawa, Y., and Takagi, S.F. 1983a. Neuronal pathways for activation of inhibitory interneurons in pyriform cortex of the rabbit. J. Neurophysiol. 50: 74–88.

Satou, M., Mori, K., Tazawa, Y., and Takagi, S.F. 1983b. Interneurons mediating fast postsynaptic inhibition in pyriform cortex of the rabbit. J. Neurophysiol. 50: 89–101.

Saul, A.B. and Humphrey, A.L. 1990. Spinal and temporal response properties of lagged and nonlagged cells in cat lateral geniculate nucleus. J. Neurophysiol. 64: 206–224.

Saul, A.B. and Humphrey, A.L. 1992. Evidence of input from lagged cells in the lateral geniculate nucleus to simple cells in cortical area 17 of the cat. J. Neurophysiol. 68: 1190–1208.

Savage, G.L. and Banks, M.S. 1992. Scotopic visual efficiency: Constraints by optics, receptor properties, and rod pooling. Vision Res. 32: 645–656.

Sayer, R., Schwindt, P., and Crill, W. 1992. Metabotropic glutamate receptor-mediated suppression of L-type calcium current in acutely isolated neocortical neurons. J. Neurophysiol. 68: 833–842.

Scatton, B., Simon, H., Moal, M.L., and Bischoff, S. 1980. Origins of dopaminergic innervation of the rat hippocampal formation. Neurosci. Lett. 18: 125–131.

Scharfman, H.E. 1994. EPSPs of dentate gyrus granule cells during epileptiform bursts of dentate hilar "mossy" cells and area CA3 pyramidal cells in disinhibited rat hippocampal slices. J. Neurosci. 14: 6041–6057.

Scharfman, H.E. 1995. Electrophysiological evidence that dentate hilar mossy cells are excitatory and innervate both granule cells and interneurons. J. Neurophysiol. 74: 179–194.

Scharfman, H.E., Kunkel, D.D., and Schwartzkroin, P.A. 1990a. Synaptic connections of dentate granule cells and hilar neurons: Results of paired intracellular recordings and intracellular horseradish peroxidase injections. Neuroscience 37: 693–707.

Scharfman, H.E., Lu, S.-M., Guido, W., Adams, P.R., and Sherman, S.M. 1990b. N-methyl-D-aspartate (NMDA) receptors contribute to excitatory postsynaptic potentials of cat lateral geniculate neurons recorded in thalamic slices. Proc. Natl. Acad. Sci. USA 87: 4548–4552.

Scharfman, H.E. and Sarvey, J. 1987. Responses to GABA recorded from identified rat visual cortical neurons. Neuroscience 23: 407–422.

Scharfman, H.E. and Schwartzkroin, P.A. 1988. Electrophysiology of morphologically identified mossy cells of the dentate hilus recorded in guinea pig hippocampal slices. J. Neurosci. 8: 3812–3821.

Scheibel, A.B. and Conrad, A.S. 1993. Hippocampal dysgenesis in mutant mouse and schizophrenic man—Is there a relationship? Schizophr. Bull. 19: 21–33.

Scheibel, M.E., and Scheibel, A.B. 1973. Hippocampal pathology in temporal lobe epilepsy. A Golgi survey. In: Epilepsy, Its Phenomena in Man (Brazier, M.A.B., ed.). New York: Academic Press, pp. 315–337.

Schein, S. 1988. Anatomy of macaque fovea and spatial densities of neurones in foveal representation. J. Comp. Neurol. 269: 479–505.

Schein, S.J. and de Monasterio, F.M. 1987. Mapping of retinal and geniculate neurons onto striate cortex of macaque. J. Neurosci. 7: 996–1009.

Schiller, P.H., Sandell, J.H., and Maunsell, J.H.R. 1986. Functions of the ON and OFF channels of the visual system. Nature 322: 824–825.

Schlaggar, B., Fox, K., and O'Leary, D. 1993. Postsynaptic control of plasticity in developing somatosensory cortex. Nature 364: 623–626.

Schmechel, D., Vickery, B., Fitzpatrick, D., and Elde, R. 1984. GABAergic neurons of mammalian cerebral cortex: Widespread subclass defined by somatostatin content. Neurosci Lett. 47: 227–232.

Schmidt, M., Humphrey, M.F., and Wässle, H. 1987. Action and localization of acetylcholine in the cat retina. J. Neurophysiol. 58: 997–1015.

Schmielau, F. and Singer, W. 1977. The role of visual cortex for binocular interactions in the cat lateral geniculate nucleus. Brain Res. 120: 354–361.

Schnapf, J.L., Nunn, B.J., Meister, M., and Baylor, D.A. 1990. Visual transduction in cones of the monkey *Macaca fascicularis*. J. Physiol. (Lond.) 427: 681–713.

Schneeweis, D.M. and Schnapf, J.L. 1995. Photovoltage of rods and cones in the macaque retina. Science 268: 1053–1056.

Schneider, S.P. and Fyffe, R.E.W. 1992. Involvement of GABA and glycine in recurrent inhibition of spinal motoneurons. J. Neurophysiol. 68: 397–406.

Schneider, S.P. and Macrides, F. 1978. Laminar distribution of interneurons in the main olfactory bulb of adult hamster. Brain Res. Bull. 3: 73–82.

Schneider, S.P. and Scott, J.W. 1983. Orthodromic response properties of rat olfactory bulb mitral and tufted cells correlate with their projection patterns. J. Neurophysiol. 50: 358–378.

Schoenbaum, G. and Eichenbaum, H. 1995. Information coding in the rodent prefrontal cortex. I. Single-neuron activity in orbitofrontal cortex compared with that in pyriform cortex. J. Neurophysiol. 74: 733–750.

Schoenfeld, T.A., Marchand, J.E., and Macrides, F. 1985. Topographic organization of tufted cell axonal projections in the hamster main olfactory bulb: An intrabulbar associational system. J. Comp. Neurol. 235: 503–518.

Schoepfer, R., Monyer, H., Sommer, B., Wisden, W., Sprengel, R., Kuner, T., Lomeli, H., Herb, A., Kohler, M., Burnashev, N., Gunther, W., Ruppersberg, P., and Seeburg, P. 1994. Molecular biology of glutamate receptors. Prog. Neurobiol. 42: 353–357.

Schoepp, D.D. and Conn, P.J. 1993. Metabotropic glutamate receptors in brain function and pathology. Trends Pharmacol. Sci. 14: 13–20.

Scholfield, C.N. 1978a. Electrical properties of neurones in the olfactory cortex slice in vitro. J. Physiol. (Lond.) 275: 535–546.

Scholfield, C.N. 1978b. A depolarizing inhibitory potential in neurones of the olfactory cortex in vitro. J. Physiol. (Lond.) 275: 547–557.

Schulz, P.E., Cook, E.P., and Johnston, D. 1994. Changes in paired-pulse facilitation suggest presynaptic involvement in long-term potentiation. J. Neurosci. 14: 5325–5337.

Schulz, P.E. and Fitzgibbons, J.C. 1997. Differing mechanisms of expression for short-term and long-term potentiation. J. Neurophysiol. 78 (In press).

Schuman, E.M. and Madison, D.V. 1991. A requirement for the intercellular messenger nitric oxide in long-term potentiation. Science 254: 1503–1506.

Schuman, E.M. and Madison, D.V. 1994. Nitric oxide and synaptic function. Annu. Rev. Neurosci. 17: 153–183.

Schwartz, E. 1987. Depolarization without calcium can release gamma-aminobutyric acid from a retinal neuron. Science 238: 350–355.

Schwartz, M.L., Dekker, J.J., and Goldman-Rakic, P.S. 1991. Dual mode of corticothalamic synaptic termination in the mediodorsal nucleus of the rhesus monkey. J. Comp. Neurol. 309: 289–304.

Schwartz, S.P. and Coleman, P.D. 1981. Neurons of origin of the perforant path. Exp. Neurol. 74: 305–312.

Schwartzkroin, P.A. 1975. Characteristics of CA1 neurons recorded intracellularly in the hippocampal in vitro slice preparation. Brain Res. 85: 423–436.

Schwartzkroin, P.A. 1977. Further characteristics of hippocampal CA1 cells in vitro. Brain Res. 128: 53–68.

Schwartzkroin, P.A. 1986. Regulation of excitability in hippocampal neurons. In: The Hippocampus (Isaacson, R.L. and Pribram, K.H., eds.). New York: Plenum Press, pp. 113–136.

Schwartzkroin, P.A. and Kunkel, D.D. 1985. Morphology of identified interneurons in the CA1 regions of guinea pig hippocampus. J. Comp. Neurol. 232: 205–218.

Schwartzkroin, P.A. and Mathers, L.H. 1978. Physiological and morphological identification of a nonpyramidal hippocampal cell type. Brain Res. 157: 1–10.

Schwartzkroin, P.A. and Slawsky, M. 1977. Probable calcium spikes in hippocampal neurons. Brain Res. 135: 157–161.

Schwindt, P. and Crill, W. 1980. Properties of a persistent inward current in normal and tea-injected motoneurons. J. Neurophysiol. 43: 1700–1724.

Schwindt, P. and Crill, W.E. 1977. A persistent negative resistance in cat lumbar motoneurons. Brain Res. 120: 173–178.

Schwindt, P., Spain, W., Foehring, R., Chubb, M., and Crill, W. 1988a. Slow conductances in neurons from cat sensorimotor cortex in vitro and their role in slow excitability changes. J. Neurophysiol. 59: 450–467.

Schwindt, P. 1992. Ionic currents governing input-output relations of Betz cells. In: Single Neuron Computation (McKenna, J.D.T. and Zornetzer, S., eds.). Orlando, FL: Academic Press, pp. 235–258.

Schwindt, P., Spain, W., Foehring, R., Stafstrom, C., Chubb, M., and Crill, W.E. 1988b. Multiple potassium conductances and their functions in neurons from cat sensorimotor cortex in vitro. J. Neurophysiol. 59: 424–449.

Schwob, J.E. 1992. The biochemistry of olfactory neurons: Stages of differentiation and neuronal subsets. In: Science of Olfaction (Serby, M.J. and Chobor, K.L., eds.). New York: Springer-Verlag, pp. 80–125.

Schwob, J.E. and Price, J.L. 1978. The cortical projection of the olfactory bulb: Development in fetal and neonatal rats correlated with quantitative variations in adult rats. Brain Res. 151: 369–374.

Scott, J.W. 1981. Electrophysiological identification of mitral and tufted cells and distributions of their axons in olfactory system of the rat. J. Neurophysiol. 46: 918–931.

Scott, J.W. and Harrison, T.A. 1987. The olfactory bulb: Anatomy and physiology. In: Neurobiology of Taste and Smell (Finger, T.E. and Silver, W.K., eds.). New York: John Wiley & Sons, pp. 151–178.

Scott, J.W., McBride, R.L., and Schneider, S.P. 1980. The organization of projections from the olfactory bulb to the piriform cortex and olfactory tubercle in the rat. J. Comp. Neurol. 194: 519–534.

Scoville, W.B. and Milner, B. 1957. Loss of recent memory after bilateral hippocampal lesions. J. Neurol. Psychiatry 20: 11–21.

Segev, I. 1995. Cable and compartmental models of dendritic trees. In: The Book of Genesis, Exploring Realistic Neural Models with the GEneral NEural SImulation System (Bower, J.M. and Beeman, D., eds.). New York: Springer-Verlag, pp. 53–82.

Segev, I., Fleshman, J.W., and Burke, R.E. 1989. Compartmental models of complex neurons. In: Methods in Neuronal Modeling: From Synapse to Network (Koch, C. and Segev, I., eds.). Cambridge, MA: MIT Press, pp. 63–93.

Segev, I., Fleshman, J.W., and Burke, R.E. 1990a. Computer simulation of group Ia EPSPs using morphologically realistic models of cat α-motoneurons. J. Neurophysiol. 64: 648–660.

Segev, I. and Rall, W. 1988. Computational study of an excitable dendritic spine. J. Neurophysiol. 60: 499–523.

Segev, I., Rinzel, J., and Shepherd, G.M. (eds.). 1995. The Theoretical Foundation of Dendritic Function. Cambridge, MA: MIT Press.

Sejnowski, T., Koch, C., and Churchland, P. 1988. Computational neuroscience. Science 241: 1299–1306.

Selemon, L.D. and Goldman-Rakic, P.S. 1985. Longitudinal topography and interdigitation of corticostriatal projections in the rhesus monkey. J. Neurosci. 5: 776–794.

Senaris, R.M., Humphrey, P.P., and Emson, P.C. 1994. Distribution of somatostatin receptors 1, 2 and 3 mRNA in rat brain and pituitary. Eur. J. Neurosci. 6: 1883–1896.

Sento, S. and Ryugo, D.K. 1989. Endbulbs of Held and spherical bushy cells in cats: Morphological correlates with physiological properties. J. Comp. Neurol. 280: 553–562.

Seress, L. and Ribak, C.E. 1984. Direct commissural connections to the basket cells of the hippocampal dentate gyrus: Anatomical evidence for feed-forward inhibition. J. Neurocytol. 13: 215–225.

Shadlen, M. and Newsome, W. 1996. Motion perception: Seeing and deciding. Proc. Natl. Acad. Sci. USA 93: 628–633.

Shannon, C.E. and Weaver, W. 1949. The Mathematical Theory of Communication. Urbana, IL: University of Illinois Press.

Shannon, R.V., Zeng, F.-G., Kamath, V., Wygonski, J., and Ekelid, M. 1995. Speech recognition with primarily temporal cues. Science 270: 303–304.

Shapley, R. and Lennie, P. 1985. Spatial frequency analysis in the visual system. Annu. Rev. Neurosci. 8: 547–583.

Shapley, R. and Perry, V.H. 1986. Cat and monkey retinal ganglion cells and their visual functional roles. Trends Neurosci. 9: 229–235.

Shapovalov, A.I. and Shiraev, B.I. 1980. Dual mode of junctional transmission at synapses between single primary afferent fibers and motoneurons in amphibian. J. Physiol. (Lond.) 306: 1–15.

Shapovalov, A.I. and Shiraev, B.L. 1982. Selective modulation of chemical transmission at a dual-action synapse (with special reference to baclofen). Gen. Physiol. Biophys. 1: 423–433.

Sharp, F.R., Kauer, J.S., and Shepherd, G.M. 1975. Local sites of activity-related glucose metabolism in rat olfactory bulb during olfactory stimulation. Brain Res. 98: 596–600.

Sharp, F.R., Kauer, J.S., and Shepherd, G.M. 1977. Laminar analysis of 2-deoxyglucose uptake in olfactory bulb and olfactory cortex of rabbit and rat. J. Neurophysiol. 40: 800–813.

Sharrard, W.J.W. 1955. The distribution of the permanent paralysis in the lower limb in poliomyelitis. J. Bone Joint Surg. 37: 540–558.

Sheldon, P.W. and Aghajanian, G.K. 1991. Excitatory responses to serotonin (5-HT) in neurons of the rat piriform cortex. Evidence for mediation by 5-HT1C receptors in pyramidal cells and 5-HT2 receptors in interneurons. Synapse 9: 208–218.

Shepherd, G.M. 1963. Responses of mitral cells to olfactory nerve volleys in the rabbit. J. Physiol. (Lond.) 89–100.

Shepherd, G.M. 1972a. The neuron doctrine: A revision of functional concepts. Yale J. Biol. Med. 45: 584–599.

Shepherd, G.M. 1972b. Synaptic organization of the mammalian olfactory bulb. Physiol. Rev. 52: 864–917.

Shepherd, G.M. 1974. The Synaptic Organization of the Brain (1st ed.). New York: Oxford University Press.

Shepherd, G.M. 1978. Microcircuits in the nervous system. Sci. Am. 238: 93–103.

Shepherd, G.M. 1979. The Synaptic Organization of the Brain (2nd ed.). New York: Oxford University Press.

Shepherd, G.M. 1988a. A basic circuit for cortical organization. In: Perspectives on Memory Research (Gazzaniga, M., ed.). Cambridge, MA: MIT Press, pp. 93–134.

Shepherd, G.M. 1988b. Studies of development and plasticity in the olfactory sensory neuron. J. Physiol. (Paris) 83: 240–245.

Shepherd, G.M. (ed.). 1990. The Synaptic Organization of the Brain (3rd ed.). New York: Oxford University Press.

Shepherd, G.M. 1991a. Computational structure of the olfactory system. In: Olfaction: A Model System for Computational Neuroscience (Davis, J.L. and Eichenbaum, H., eds.). Cambridge, MA: MIT Press, pp. 3–41.

Shepherd, G.M. 1991b. Foundations of the Neuron Doctrine. New York: Oxford University Press.

Shepherd, G.M. 1992. Modules for molecules. Nature 358: 457–458.

Shepherd, G.M. 1994a. Discrimination of molecular signals by the olfactory receptor neuron. Neuron 13: 771–790.

Shepherd, G.M. 1994b. Neurobiology (3rd ed.). New York: Oxford University Press.

Shepherd, G.M. 1996. The dendritic spine: A multifunctional integrative unit. J. Neurophysiol. 75: 2197–2210.

Shepherd, G.M. 1998. Information processing in complex dendrites. In: Fundamental Neuroscience (Zigmond, M., Bloom, F., Landis, S., Roberts, J., and Squire, L., eds.). New York: Academic Press, in press.

Shepherd, G.M. and Braun, J. 1989. The peak of electromechanical experimentation in physiology: A unique view through Walter Miles' "Report of a Visit to Foreign Laboratories" in 1920. Caduceus 5: 1–84.

Shepherd, G.M. and Brayton, R.K. 1979. Computer simulation of a dendrodendritic synaptic circuit for self- and lateral-inhibition in the olfactory bulb. Brain Res. 175: 377–382.

Shepherd, G.M. and Brayton, R.K. 1987. Logic operations are properties of computer-simulated interactions between excitable dendritic spines. Neuroscience 21: 151–166.

Shepherd, G.M., Brayton, R.K., Miller, J.F., Segev, I., Rinzel, J., and Rall, W. 1985. Signal enhancement in distal cortical dendrites by means of interactions between active dendritic spines. Proc. Natl. Acad. Sci. USA 82: 2192–2195.

Shepherd, G.M., Carnevale, N.T., and Woolf, T.B. 1989a. Comparisons between active properties of distal dendritic branches and spines: Implications for neuronal computations. J. Cogn. Neurosci. 1: 273–286.

Shepherd, G.M. and Firestein, S. 1991a. Making scents of olfactory transduction. Curr. Biol. 1: 204–206.

Shepherd, G.M. and Firestein, S. 1991b. Toward a pharmacology of odor receptors and the processing of odor images. J. Steroid Biochem. Mol. Biol. 39: 538–592.

Shepherd, G.M. and Greer, C.A. 1988. The dendritic spine: Adaptations of structure and function for different types of synaptic integration. In: Intrinsic Determinants of Neuronal Form and Function (Lassek, R., ed.). New York: Alan R. Liss, pp. 245–262.

Shepherd, G.M.G., Barres, B.A., and Corey, D.P. 1989b. "Bundle blot" purification and initial protein characterization of hair cell stereocilia. Proc. Natl. Acad. Sci. USA 86: 4973–4977.

Shepherd, G.M.G. and Corey, D.P. 1992. Sensational science. Sensory transduction: 45th annual symposium of the Society of General Physiologists, Marine Biological Laboratory, Woods Hole, MA, USA, September 5–8, 1991. New Biologist 4: 48–52.

Shepherd, G.M.G. and Corey, D.P. 1994. The extent of adaptation in bullfrog saccular hair cells. J. Neurosci. 14: 6217–6229.

Sherman, S.M. 1985. Functional organization of the W-, X-, and Y-cell pathways in the cat: A review and hypothesis. In: Progress in Psychobiology and Physiological Psychology (Sprague, J.M. and Epstein, A.N., eds.). Orlando: Academic Press, pp. 233–314.

Sherman, S.M. 1988. Functional organization of the cat's lateral geniculate nucleus. In: Cellular Thalamic Mechanisms (Macchi, G., Bentivoglio, M., and Spreafico, R., eds.). Amsterdam: Elsevier, pp. 163–183.

Sherman, S.M. 1993. Dynamic gating of retinal transmission to the visual cortex by the lateral geniculate nucleus. In: Thalamic Networks for Relay and Modulation (Minciacchi, D. Molinari, M., Macchi, G., and Jones, E.G., eds.). Oxford: Pergamon Press, pp. 61–79.

Sherman, S.M. 1995. Dual response modes in lateral geniculate neurons: Mechanisms and functions. Vis. Neurosci. 13: 205–213.

Sherman, S.M. and Friedlander, M.J. 1988. Identification of X versus Y properties for interneurons in the A-laminae of the cat's lateral geniculate nucleus. Exp. Brain. Res. 73: 384–392.

Sherman, S.M. and Guillery, R.W. 1996. The functional organization of thalamocortical relays. J. Neurophysiol. 76: 1367–1395.

Sherman, S.M. and Koch, C. 1986. The control of retinogeniculate transmission in the mammalian lateral geniculate nucleus. Exp. Brain. Res. 63: 1–20.

Sherman, S.M., and Spear P.D. (1982) Organization of visual pathways in normal and visually deprived cats. Physiol. Rev. 62: 738–855.

Sherrington, C. 1941. Man on His Nature. Cambridge: Cambridge University Press.

Shibuki, K. and Okada, D. 1991. Endogenous nitric oxide release required for long-term depression in the cerebellum. Nature 349: 326–328.

Shiells, R.A. and Falk, G. 1990. Glutamate receptors of rod bipolar cells are linked to a cyclic GMP cascade via a G-protein. Proc. R. Soc. (Lond.) B Biol. Sci. 242: 91–94.

Shinoda, Y., Ohgaki, T., and Futami, T. 1986. The morphology of single lateral vestibulospinal tract axons in the lower cervical spinal cord of the cat. J. Comp. Neurol. 249: 226–241.

Shinozaki, H. and Konishi, S. 1970. Actions of several athelmintics and insecticides on rat cortical neurones. Brain Res. 24: 368–371.

Shipley, M.T. 1974. Presubiculum afferents to the entorhinal area and the papez circuit. Brain Res. 67: 162–168.

Shipley, M.T. and Ennis, M. 1996. Functional organization of the olfactory system. J. Neurobiol. 30: 123–176.

Shupliakov, O., Örnung, G., Brodin, L., Ulfhake, B., Ottersen, O.P., Storm-Mathisen, J., and Culheim, S. 1993. Immunocytochemical localization of amino acid neurotransmitter candidates in the ventral horn of the cat spinal cord: A light microscopic study. Exp. Brain Res. 96: 404–418.

Siggins, G.R., Hoffer, B.J., and Bloom, F.E. 1971a. Studies on norepinephrine-containing afferents to Purkinje cells of rat cerebellum. III. Evidence for mediation of norepinephrine effects by cyclic 3',5-adenosine monophosphate. Brain Res. 25: 535–553.

Siggins, G.R., Hoffer, B.J., Oliver, A.P., and Bloom, F.E. 1971b. Activation of a central noradrenergic projection to the cerebellum. Nature 233: 481–483.

Siggins, G.R., Oliver, A.P., Hoffer, B.J., and Bloom, F.E. 1971c. Cyclic adenosine monophosphate and norepinephrine: Effects on transmembrane properties of cerebellar Purkinje cells. Science 171: 192–194.

Sik, A., Tamamaki, N., and Freund, T.F. 1993. Complete axon arborization of a single CA3 pyramidal cell in the rat hippocampus, and its relationship with postsynaptic parvalbumin-containing interneurons. Eur. J. Neurosci. 5: 1719–1728.

Siklos, L., Rickmann, M., Joo, F., Freeman, W.J., and Wolff, J.R. 1995. Chloride is preferentially accumulated in a subpopulation of dendrites and periglomerular cells of the main olfactory bulb in adult rats. Neuroscience 64: 165–172.

Silito, A.M., Kemp, J.A., Wilson, J.A., and Berardi, N. 1980. A re-evaluation of the mechanisms underlying simple cell orientation selectivity. Brain Res. 194: 517–520.

Sillito, A. 1975. The effectiveness of bicuculline as an antagonist of GABA and visually evoked inhibition in the cat's striate cortex. J. Physiol. (Lond.) 250: 287–304.

Sillito, A. and Kemp, J. 1983. Cholinergic modulation of the functional organization of the cat visual cortex. Brain Res. 289: 143–155.

Sillito, A.M., Cudeiro, J., and Murphy, P.C. 1993. Orientation sensitive elements in the corticofugal influence on centre-surround interactions in the dorsal lateral geniculate nucleus. Exp. Brain Res. 93: 6–16.

Sillito, A.M., Jones, H.E., Gerstein, G.L., and West, D.C. 1994. Feature-linked synchronization of thalamic relay cell firing induced by feedback from the visual cortex. Nature 369: 479–482.

Simon, S.M., Moal, M.L., and Calas, A. 1979. Efferents and afferents of the ventral tegmental-A-10-region studied after local injection of (^{3}H) leucine and horseradish peroxidase. Brain Res. 175: 1–23.

Singer, M.S., Oliveira, L., Vriend, G., and Shepherd, G.M. 1995a. Potential ligand-binding residues in rat olfactory receptors identified by correlated mutation analysis. Receptors & Channels 3: 89–95.

Singer, M.S., Shepherd, G.M., and Greer, C.A. 1995b. Olfactory receptors guide axons. Nature 377: 19–20.

Singer, M.S. and Shepherd, G.M. 1994. Molecular modeling of ligand-receptor interactions in the OR5 olfactory receptor. Neuroreport 5: 1297–1300.

Singer, W. 1977. Control of thalamic transmission by corticofugal and ascending reticular pathways in the visual system. Physiol. Rev. 57: 386–420.

Singer, W. 1994. Putative functions of temporal correlations in neocortical processing. In: Large-Scale Neuronal Theories of the Brain (Koch, C. and Davis, J. eds.). Cambridge: MA: Bradford Books, pp. 201–237.

Skaggs, W.E. and McNaughton, B.L. 1996. Replay of neuronal firing sequences in rat hippocampus during sleep following spatial experience. 271: 1870–1873.

Skeen, L.C. and Hall, W.C. 1977. Efferent projections of the main and accessory olfactory bulb in the tree shrew (*Tupaia glis*). J. Comp. Neurol. 172: 1–36.

Skou, J.C. 1988. Overview: The Na-K pump. Methods Enzymol. 156: 1–25.

Sloper, J. and R. Hiorns, T.P. 1979. A qualitative electron microscope study of the neurons in the primate motor and somatic sensory cortices. Phil. Trans. R. Soc. Lond. B 285: 141–171.

Sloper, J.J. and Powell, T.P.S. 1979a. An experimental electronmicroscopic study of afferent connections to the primate motor and somatic sensory cortices. Phil. Trans. R. Soc. Lond. B 285: 199–266.

Sloper, J.J. and Powell, T.P.S. 1979b. Ultrastructural features of the sensorimotor cortex of the primate. Phil. Trans. R. Soc. Lond. B 285: 123–139.

Sloviter, R.S., Dichter, M.A., Rachinsky, T.L., Dean, E., Goodman, J.H., Sollas, A.L., and Martin, D.L. 1996. Basal expression and induction of glutamate decarboxylase and GABA in excitatory granule cells of the rat and monkey hippocampal dentate gyrus. J. Comp. Neurol. 373: 593–618.

Smallman, H.S., MacLeod, D.I.A., He, S., and Kentridge, R.W. 1996. Fine grain of the neural representation of human spatial vision. J. Neurosci. 16: 1852–1859.

Smiley, J. and Goldman-Rakic, P. 1993. Heterogenous targets of dopamine synapses in monkey prefrontal cortex demonstrated by serial electron microscopy: A laminar analysis using the silver-enhanced diaminobenzidine sulfide (SEDS) immunolabling technique. Cereb. Cortex 3: 223–228.

Smirnakis, S.M., Berry, M.J., Warland, D.K., Bialek, W., and Meister, M. 1997. Adaptation of retinal processing to image contrast and spatial scale. Nature 386: 69–73.

Smith, J.L., Betts, B., Edgerton, V.R., and Zernicke, R.F. 1980. Rapid ankle extension during paw shakes: Selective recruitment of fast ankle extensors. J. Neurophysiol. 43: 612–620.

Smith, P.H. 1995a. Structural and functional differences distinguish principal from nonprincipal cells in the guinea pig MSO slice. J. Neurophysiol. 73: 1653–1667.

Smith, P.H., Joris, P.X., and Yin, T.C.T. 1993. Projections of physiologically characterized spherical bushy cell axons from the cochlear nucleus of the cat: Evidence for delay lines to the medial superior olive. J. Comp. Neurol. 331: 245–260.

Smith, P.H. and Rhode, W.S. 1985. Electron microscopic features of physiologically characterized, HRP-labeled fusiform cells in the cat dorsal cochlear nucleus. J. Comp. Neurol. 237: 127–143.

Smith, P.H. and Rhode, W.S. 1987. Characterization of HRP-labeled globular bushy cells in the cat anteroventral cochlear nucleus. J. Comp. Neurol. 266: 360–375.

Smith, P.H. and Rhode, W.S. 1989. Structural and functional properties distinguish two types of multipolar cells in the ventral cochlear nucleus. J. Comp. Neurol. 282: 595–616.

Smith, R.G. 1995b. Simulation of an anatomically-defined local circuit: The cone-horizontal cell network in cat retina. Vis. Neurosci. 12: 545–561.

Smith, R.G., Freed, M.A., and Sterling, P. 1986. Microcircuitry of the dark-adapted cat retina: Functional architecture of the rod-cone network. J. Neurosci. 6: 3505–3517.

Smith, R.G. and Sterling, P. 1990. Cone receptive field in cat retina computed from microcircuitry. Vis. Neurosci. 5: 453–461.

Smith, R.G. and Vardi, N. 1995. Simulation of the AII amacrine cell of mammalian retina: Functional consequences of electrical coupling and regenerative membrane properties. Vis. Neurosci. 12: 851–860.

Smith, T., Wuerker, R., and Frank, K. 1967. Membrane impedance changes during synaptic transmission in cat spinal motoneurons. J. Neurophysiol. 30: 1072–1096.

Smith, Y., Paré, D., Deschênes, M., Parent, A., and Steriade, M. 1988. Cholinergic and non-cholinergic projections from the upper brainstem core to the visual thalamus in the cat. Exp. Brain Res. 70: 166–180.

Smithson, K.G., Weiss, M.L., and Hatton, G.I. 1989. Supraoptic nucleus afferents from the main olfactory bulb. I. Anatomical evidence from anterograde and retrograde tracers in rat. Neuroscience 31: 277–287.

Snyder, S.H. 1992. Nitric oxide and neurons. Curr. Opin. Neurobiol. 2: 323–327.

Sofroniew, M.V., Campbell, P.E., Cuello, A.C., and Eckenstein, F. 1985. Central cholinergic neurons visualized by immunohistochemical detection of choline acetyltransferase. In: The Rat Nervous System, Vol. 1: Forebrain and Midbrain (Paxinos, G., ed.). Orlando: FL: Academic Press, pp. 471–485.

Somers, D. and Nelson, M. S. 1995. An emergent model of orientation selectivity in cat visual cortical simple cells. J. Neurosci. 15: 5448–5465.

Somogyi, G., Hajdu, F., and Tombol, T. 1978. Ultrastructure of the anterior ventral and anterior medial nuclei of the cat thalamus. Exp. Brain Res. 31: 417–431.

Somogyi, P. 1977. A specific 'axo-axonal' interneuron in the visual cortex of the rat. Brain Res. 136: 345–350.

Somogyi, P., Bolam, J.P., and Smith, A.D. 1981. Monosynaptic cortical input and local axon collaterals of identified striato nigral neurons. A light and electron microscopic study using the Golgi-peroxidase transport-degeneration procedure. J. Comp. Neurol. 195: 567–584.

Somogyi, P. and Cowey, A. 1981. Combined Golgi and electron microscope study on the synapses formed by double bouquet cells in the visual cortex of the cat and monkey. J. Comp. Neurol 195: 547–566.

Somogyi, P., Freund, T.F., and Cowey, A.D. 1982. The axo-axonic interneuron in the cerebral cortex of the rat, cat and monkey. Neuroscience 7: 2577–2607.

Somogyi, P., Freund, T.F., Hodgson, A.J., Somogyi, J., Berboukas, D., and Chubb, I.W. 1985. Identified axo-axonic cells are immunoreactive for GABA in the hippocampus and visual cortex of the cat. Brain Res. 332: 143–149.

Somogyi, P., Halasy, K., Somogyi, J., Storm-Mathisen, J., and Ottersen, O.P. 1986. Quantification of immunogold reveals enrichment of glutamate in mossy and parallel fiber terminals in cat cerebellum. Neuroscience 19: 1045–1050.

Somogyi, P., Hodgson, A., Smith, A.D., Nunzi, M., Gorio, A., and Wu, J.-Y. 1984. Differential populations of gabaergic neurons in the visual cortex and hippocampus of the cat contain somatostatin- or cholecystokinin-immunreactive material. J. Neurosci. 4: 2590–2603.

Somogyi, P., Kisvàrday, Z., Martin, K., and Whitteridge, D. 1983. Synaptic connections of morphologically identified and physiologically characterized large basket cells in the striate cortex of the cat. Neuroscience 10: 261–294.

Sonnhof, U., Richter, D.W., and Taugner, R. 1977. Electrotonic coupling between frog spinal motoneurons. An electrophysiological and morphological study. Brain Res. 138: 197–215.

Soriano, E. and Frotscher, M. 1989. A GABAergic axo-axonic cell in the fascia dentata controls the main excitatory hippocampal pathway. Brain Res. 503: 170–174.

Soriano, E. and Frotscher, M. 1993. Spiny nonpyramidal neurons in the CA3 region of the rat hippocampus are glutamate-like immunoreactive and receive convergent mossy fiber input. J. Comp. Neurol. 333: 435–448.

Soriano, E. and Frotscher, M. 1994. Mossy cells of the rat fascia dentata are glutamate-immunoreactive. Hippocampus 4: 65–69.

Sorra, K.E. and Harris, K.M. 1993. Occurrence and three-dimensional structure of multiple synapses between individual radiatum axons and their target pyramidal cells in hippocampal area CA1. J. Neurosci. 13: 3736–3748.

Sotelo, C., Gotow, T., and Wassef, M. 1986. Localization of glutamate acid-decarboxylase immunoreactive axon terminals in the inferior olive of the rat with special emphasis on anatomical relations between GABAergic synapses and dendrodendritic gap junctions. J. Comp. Neurol. 252: 32–50.

Sotelo, C., Hillman, D.E., Zamora, A.J., and Llinás, R. 1975. Climbing fiber deafferentiation: Its action on Purkinje cell dendritic spines. Brain Res. 98: 574–581.

Sotelo, C., Privat, A., and Drian, M. 1972. Localization of [³H]GABA in tissue culture of rat cerebellum using electron microscopy radioautography. Brain Res. 45: 302–308.

Spencer, W.A. and Kandel, E.R. 1961. Electrophysiology of hippocampal neurons. IV. Fast prepontentials. J. Neurophysiol. 24: 272–285.

Spirou, G.A., Brownell, W.E., and Zidanic, M. 1990. Recordings from cat trapezoid body and HRP labeling of globular bushy cell axons. J. Neurophysiol. 63: 1169–1190.

Spirou, G.A. and Young, E.D. 1991. Organization of dorsal cochlear nucleus type IV unit response maps and their relationship to activation by bandlimited noise. J. Neurophysiol. 65: 1750–1768.

Spoendlin, H. 1973. The innervation of the cochlear receptor. In: Basic Mechanisms in Hearing (Møller, A.R., ed.). New York: Academic Press, pp. 185–230.

Spreafico, R., Schmechel, D.E., Ellis, L.C., Jr., and Rustioni, A. 1983. Cortical relay neurons and interneurons in the n. ventralis posterolateralis of cats: A horseradish peroxidase, electron-microscopic Golgi and immunocytochemical study. Neuroscience 9: 491–509.

Spruston, N., Jaffe, D.B., and Johnston, D. 1994. Dendritic attenuation of synaptic potentials and currents: the role of passive membrane properties. Trends Neurosci. 17: 161–166.

Spruston, N. and Johnston, D. 1992. Perforated patch-clamp analysis of the passive membrane properties of three classes of hippocampal neurons. J. Neurophysiol. 67: 508–529.

Spruston, N., Lübke, J., and Frotscher, M. 1997. Interneurons in the stratum lucidum of the rat hippocampus: An anatomical and electrophysiological characterization. J. Comp. Neurol. (In press).

Spruston, N., Schiller, Y., Stuart, G., and Sakmann, B. 1995. Activity-dependent action potential invasion and calcium influx into hippocampal CA1 dendrites. Science 268: 297–300.

Srinivasan, M.V., Laughlin, S.B., and Dubs, A. 1982. Predictive coding: A fresh view of inhibition in the retina. Proc. R. Soc. (Lond.) B Biol. Sci. 216: 427–459.

Stafford, D.K. and Dacey, D. 1997. Physiology of the A1 amacrine: A spiking axon-bearing interneuron of the macaque monkey retina. Vis. Neurosci. 14: 507–522.

Stafstrom, C.E., Schwindt, P.C., Chubb, M.C., and Crill, W.E. 1985. Properties of persistent sodium conductance and calcium conductance of layer V neurons from cat sensorimotor cortex in vitro. J. Neurophysiol. 53: 153–170.

Stafstrom, C.E., Schwindt, P., and Crill, W. 1982. Negative slope conductance due to a persistent subthreshold sodium current in cat neocortical neurons in vitro. Brain Res. 236: 221–226.

Stafstrom, C.E., Schwindt, P., and Crill, W. 1984. Repetitive firing in layer v neurons from cat neocortex in vitro. J. Neurophysiol. 52: 264–277.

Staley, K.J., Otis, T.S., and Mody, I. 1992. Membrane properties of dentate gyrus granule cells: Comparison of sharp microelectrode and whole-cell recordings. J. Neurophysiol. 67: 1346–1358.

Staubli, U., Fraser, D., Kessler, M., and Lynch, G. 1986. Studies on retrograde and anterograde amnesia of olfactory memory after denervation of the hippocampus by entorhinal cortex lesions. Behav. Neural Biol. 46: 432–444.

Staubli, U., Thibault, O., DiLorenzo, M., and Lynch, G. 1989. Antagonism of NMDA receptors impairs acquisition but not retention of olfactory memory. Behav. Neurosci. 103: 54–60.

Stea, A., Soong, T.W., and Snutch, T.P. 1995. Voltage-gated calcium channels. In: Handbook of Receptors and Channels. Ligand- and Voltage-Gated Ion Channels (North, R.A., ed.). London: CRC Press, pp. 113–152.

Steinberg, R.H. 1969. Rod and cone contributions to S-potentials from the cat retina. Vision Res. 9: 1319–1329.

Steinberg, R.H., Reid, M., and Lacy, P.L. 1973. The distribution of rods and cones in the retina of the cat (*Felis domesticus*). J. Comp. Neurol. 148: 229–248.

Stengaard-Pedersen, K., Fredens, K., and Larsson, L.I. 1981. Enkephalin and zinc in the hippocampal mossy fiber system. Brain Res. 212: 230–233.

Stent, G.S. 1973. A physiological mechanism for Hebb's postulate of learning. Proc. Natl. Acad. Sci. USA 70: 997–1001.

Steriade, M. and Contreras, D. 1995. Relations between cortical and thalamic cellular events during transition from sleep patterns to paroxysmal activity. J. Neurosci. 15: 623–642.

Steriade, M., Datta, S., Paré, D., Oakson, G., and Curró Dossi, R. 1990a. Neuronal activities in brain-stem cholinergic nuclei related to tonic activation processes in thalamocortical systems. J. Neurosci. 10: 2541–2559.

Steriade, M., Domich, L., Oakson, G., and Deschênes, M. 1987. The deafferented reticular thalamic nucleus generates spindle rhythmicity. J. Neurophysiol. 57: 260–273.

Steriade, M., Jones, E.G., and Llinás, R. 1990b. Thalamic Oscillations and Signalling. New York: John Wiley & Sons.

Steriade, M. and Llinás, R. 1988. The functional states of the thalamus and the associated neuronal interplay. Physiol. Rev. 68: 649–742.

Steriade, M. and McCarley, R.W. 1990. Brainstem Control of Wakefulness and Sleep. New York: Plenum Press.

Steriade, M., McCormick, D.A., and Sejnowski, T.J. 1993. Thalamocortical oscillations in the sleeping and aroused brain. Science 262: 679–685.

Sterling, P. 1983. Microcircuitry of the cat retina. Annu. Rev. Neurosci. 6: 149–185.

Sterling, P. 1995. Tuning retinal circuits. Nature 377: 676–677.

Sterling, P., Calkins, D.J., Klug, K.J., Schein, S.J., and Tsukamoto, Y. 1994. Parallel pathways from primate fovea. Invest. Ophthalmol. Vis. Sci. Abstr. 35: 2001.

Sterling, P., Cohen, E., Freed, M.A., and Smith, R.G. 1987. Microcircuitry of the ON-beta ganglion cell in daylight, twilight and starlight. Neurosci. Res. (Suppl) 6: 5269–5285.

Sterling, P., Cohen, E., Smith, R.G,. and Tsukamoto, Y. 1992. Retinal circuits for daylight: Why ballplayers don't wear shades. In: Analysis and Modeling of Neural Systems (Eeckman, F.H., ed.). Boston: Kluwer Academic Publishers, pp. 143–162.

Sterling, P., Freed, M.A., and Smith, R.G. 1988. Architecture of the rod and cone circuits to the ON-beta ganglion cell. J. Neurosci. 8: 623–642.

Sterling, P., Smith, R.G., Rao, R., and Vardi, N. 1995. Functional architecture of mammalian outer retina and bipolar cells. In: Neurobiology and Clinical Aspects of the Outer Retina (Archer, S., Djamgoz, M.B.A., and Vallerga, S., eds.). London: Chapman & Hall, pp. 325–348.

Stevens, C.F. and Tsujimoto, T. 1995. Estimates for the pool size of releasable quanta at a single central synapse and for the time required to refill the pool. Proc. Natl. Acad. Sci. USA 92: 846–849.

Stevens, C.F. and Wang, Y. 1994. Changes in reliability of synaptic function as a mechanism for plasticity. Nature 371: 704–707.

Stevens, C.F. and Wang, Y. 1995. Facilitation and depression at single central synapses. Neuron 14: 795–802.

Stevens, J.R., Phillips, I., and Beaurepaire, R. 1988. γ-vinyl GABA in endopiriform area suppresses kindled amygdala seizures. Epilepsia 29: 404–411.

Steward, O. 1976. Topographic organization of the projections from the entorhinal area to the hippocampal formation of the rat. J. Comp. Neurol. 167: 285–314.

Steward, O. and Scoville, S.A. 1976. Cells of origin of entorhinal cortical afferents to the hippocampus and fascia dentata of the rat. J. Comp. Neurol. 169: 347–370.

Stewart, W.B., Kauer, J.S., and Shepherd, G.M. 1979. Functional organization of rat olfactory bulb analysed by the 2-deoxyglucose method. J. Comp. Neurol. 185: 715–734.

Stockman, A., Sharpe, L.T., Rüther, K., and Nordby, K. 1995. Two signals in the human rod visual system: A model based on electrophysiological data. Vis. Neurosci. 12: 951–970.

Stone, J. 1983. Parallel Processing in the Visual System. New York: Plenum Press.

Stone, J. and Fukuda, Y. 1974. Properties of cat retinal ganglion cells: a comparison of W-cells with X- and Y-cells. J. Neurophysiol. 37: 722–748.

Stone, T. and Taylor, D. 1977. Microiontophoretic studies of the effects of cyclic nucleotides on excitability of neurones in the rat cerebral cortex. J. Physiol. (Lond.) 266: 523–543.

Storm, J.F. 1990. Potassium currents in hippocampal pyramidal cells. Prog. Brain Res. 83: 161–187.

Storm-Mathisen, J. 1977. Localization of transmitter candidates in the brain: The hippocampal formation as a model. Prog. Neurobiol. 8: 119–181.

Storm-Mathisen, J. and Fonnum, F. 1972. Localization of transmitter candidates in the hippocampal region. Prog. Brain Res. 36: 41–58.

Stratford, K., Tarczy-Hornoch, K., Martin, K., Bannister, N., and Jack, J. 1996. Excitatory synaptic inputs to spiny stellate cells in cat visual cortex. Nature 382: 258–261.

Strettoi, E., Dacheux, R.F., and Raviola, E. 1990. Synaptic connections of rod bipolar cells in the inner plexiform layer of the rabbit retina. J. Comp. Neurol. 295: 449–466.

Stripling, J.S., Patneau, D.K., and Gramlich, C.A. 1992. Characterization and anatomical distribution of selective long-term potentiation in the olfactory forebrain. Brain Res. 542: 107–122.

Strotmann, J., Wanner, I., Krieger, J., Raming, K., and Breer, H. 1992. Expression of odorant receptors in spatially restricted subsets of chemsensory neeurones. Neuroreport 3: 1053–1056

Struble, R.G., Desmond, N.L., and Levy, W.B. 1978. Anatomical evidence for interlamellar inhibition in the fascia dentata. Brain Res. 152: 580–585.

Struble, R.G. and Wlaters, C.P. 1982. Light microscopic differentiation of two populations of rat olfactory bulb granule cells. Brain Res. 236: 237–251.

Stuart, G.J., Dodt, H.U., and Sakmann, B. 1993. Patch-clamp recordings from the soma and dendrites of neurones in brain slices using infrared video microscopy. Pflugers Arch. 423: 511–518.

Stuart, G.J. and Redman, S.J. 1992. The role of GABA-A and GABA-B receptors in presynaptic inhibition of Ia EPSPs in cat spinal motoneurones. J. Physiol. (Lond.) 447: 675–692.

Stuart, G.J. and Sakmann, B. 1994. Active propagation of somatic action potentials into neocortical pyramidal cell dendrites. Nature 367: 69–72.

Stuart, G.J. and Spruston, N. 1995. Probing dendritic function with patch pipettes. Curr. Opin. Neurobiol. 5: 389–394.

Stuart, G., Spruston, N., Sakmann, B., and Häusser, M. 1997. Action potential initiation and backpropagation in neurons of the mammalian CNS. Trends Neurosci. 20: 125–131.

Study, R. and Barker, J.L. 1981. Diazepam and (−)pentobarbital: Fluctuation analysis reveals different mechanisms for potentiation of gamma-amino-butyric acid responses in cultured neurons. Proc. Natl. Acad. Sci. USA 78: 7180–7184.

Suarez, H., Koch, C., and Douglas, R. 1995. Modeling direction selectivity of simple cells in striate visual cortex using the canonical microcircuit. J. Neurosci. 15: 6700–6719.

Sugimori, M., and Llinás, R. 1981. Localization of ionic conductances in soma-dendritic regions of Purkinje cells: An in vitro study of guinea pig cerebellar slices. Soc. Neurosci. Abstr. 7: 76.

Sugimori, M., Llinás, R., and Angelides, A. 1986. Fluorescence localization of tetrodotoxin receptors in mammalian cerebellar cortex in vitro. Soc. Neurosci. Abstr. 12: 463.

Sugimori, M., Preston, R.J., and Kitai, S.T. 1978. Response properties and electrical constants of caudate nucleus neurons in the cat. J. Neurophysiol. 41: 1662–1675.

Sur, M., Esguerra, M., Garraghty, P.E., Kritzer, M.F., and Sherman, S.M. 1987. Morphology of physiologically identified retinogeniculate X- and Y-axons in the cat. J. Neurophysiol. 58: 1–32.

Surmeier, D.J., Cantrell, A.R., and Carter-Russell, H. 1995. Dopaminergic and cholinergic modulation of calcium conductances in neostriatal neurons. In: Molecular and Cellular Mechanisms of Neostriatal Function (Ariano, M.A. and Surmeier, D.J., eds.). Austin: R.G. Landes, pp. 193–216.

Surmeier, D.J., Eberwine, J., Wilson, C.J., Cao, Y., Stefani, A., and Kitai, S.T. 1992. Dopamine receptor subtypes colocalize in rat striatonigral neurons. Proc. Natl. Acad. Sci. USA 89: 10178–10182.

Surmeier, D.J. and Kitai, S.T. 1993. D1 and D2 Dopamine Receptor Modulation of Sodium and Potassium Currents in Rat Neostriatal Neurons. Oxford: Elsevier.

Surmeier, D.J., Song, W.-J., and Yan, Z. 1996. Coordinated expression of dopamine receptors in neostriatal medium spiny neurons. J. Neurosci. 16: 6579–6591.

Svoboda, K., Denk, W., and Kleinfeld, D. 1997. *In vivo* dendritic calcium dynamics in neocortical pyramidal cells. Nature 385: 161–165.

Swanson, L.W. 1978. The anatomical organization of septo-hippocampal projections. In: Functions of the Septo-Hippocampal System (CIBA Foundation Vol. 58). Amsterdam: Elsevier North Holland, pp. 25–48.

Swanson, L.W. 1981. A direct projection from Ammon's horn to prefrontal cortex in the rat. Brain Res. 217: 150–154.

Swanson, L.W. 1982. The projections of the ventral tegmental area and adjacent regions: A combined fluorescent retrograde tracer and immunofluorescence study in the rat. Brain Res. Bull. 9: 321–353.

Swanson, L.W. and Cowan, W.M. 1975. Hippocampus-hypothalamic connections: Origin in subicular cortex, not ammon's horn. Science 25: 303–304.

Swanson, L.W. and Cowan, W.M. 1977. An autoradiographic study of the organization of the efferent connections of the hippocampal formation in the rat. J. Cmp. Neurol. 172: 49–84.

Swanson, L.W. and Hartman, B.K. 1975. The central adrenergic system. An immunofluorescence study of the location of cell bodies and their efferent connections in the rat utilizing dopamine-B-hydroxylase as a marker. J. Comp. Neurol. 163: 467–506.

Swanson, L.W., Köhler, C., and Björklund, A. 1987. The limbic region. I: The septohippocampal system. In: Handbook of Chemical Neuroanatomy, Vol. 5: Integrated Systems of the CNS, Part I (Björklund, A., Hökfelt, T., and Swanson, L.W., eds.). New York: Elsevier Science Publishing, pp. 125–227.

Swanson, L.W., Sawchenko, P.E., and Cowan, W.M. 1980. Evidence that the commissural, associational and septal projections of the regio inferior of the hippocampus arise from the same neurons. Brain Res. 197: 207–212.

Swanson, L.W., Wyss, J.M., and Cowan, W.M. 1978. An autoradiographic study of the organization of intrahippocampal association pathways in the rat. J. Comp. Neurol. 181: 681–716.

Swindale, N. 1981. Dendritic spines only connect. Trends Neurosci. 4: 240–241.

Switzer, R.C., de Olmos, J., and Heimer, L. 1985. Olfactory system. In: The Rat Nervous System Forebrain and Midbrain (Paxinos, G., ed.). Sydney: Academic Press, pp. 1–36.

Sypert, G.W. and Munson, J.B. 1984. Excitatory synapses. In: Handbook of the Spinal Cord, Vol. 1: Physiology (Davidoff, R.E., ed.). New York: Marcel Dekker, pp. 315–384.

Szél, A., Diamanstein, T., and Röhlich, P. 1988. Identification of the blue sensitive cones in the mammalian retina by anti-visual pigment antibody. J. Comp. Neurol. 273: 593–602.

Szél, A., Röhlich, P., Caffé, A.R., Juliussn, B., Aguirre, G., and Van Veen, T. 1992. Unique topographic separation of two spectral classes of cones in the mouse retina. J. Comp. Neurol. 325: 327–342.

Szentágothai, J. 1973. Synaptology of the visual cortex. In: Handbook of Sensory Physiology, Vol. VII/3: Central Processing of Visual Information, Part B: Visual Centers in the Brain (Jung, R., ed.). Berlin: Springer-Verlag.

Szentágothai, J. 1978. The neuron network of the cerebral cortex: A functional interpretation. Proc. R. Soc. Lond. B Biol. Sci. 201: 219–248.

Szot, P., Bale, T.L., and Dorsa, D.M. 1994. Distribution of messenger RNA for the vasopressin V1a receptor in the CNS of male and female rats. Mol. Brain Res. 24: 1–10.

Tachibana, M. and Kaneko, A. 1984. Gamma-aminobutyric acid acts at axon terminals of turtle photoreceptors: Difference in sensitivity among cell types. Proc. Natl. Acad. Sci. USA 81: 7961–7964.

Takagi, H., Somogyi, P., Somogyi, J., and Smith, A.D. 1983. Fine structural studies of a type of somatostatin-immunoreactive neuron and its synaptic connections in the rat neostriatum—A correlated light and electron microscopic study. J. Comp. Neurol. 214: 1–16.

Takagi, S.F. 1986. Studies on the olfactory nervous system in the old world monkey. Prog. Neurobiol. 27: 195–250.

Takeuchi, Y., Kumura, H., and Sano, Y. 1982. Immunohistochemical demonstration of serotonin-containing nerve fibers in the cerebellum. Cell Tissue Res. 226: 1–12.

Tamamaki, N., Abe, K., and Nijyo, Y. 1987. Columnar organization in the subiculum formed by axon branches originating from single CA1 pyramidal neurons in the rat hippocampus. Brain Res. 412: 156–160.

Tamamaki, N., Abe, K., and Nijyo, Y. 1988. Three-dimensional analysis of the whole axonal arbors originating from single CA2 pyramidal neurons in the rat hippocampus with the aid of a computer graphic technique. Brain Res. 452: 255–272.

Tamamaki, N., Uhlrich, D.J., and Sherman, S.M. 1994. Morphology of physiologically identified retinal X and Y axons in the cat's thalamus and midbrain as revealed by intra-axonal injection of biocytin. J. Comp. Neurol. 354: 583–607.

Tamamaki, N., Watanabe, K., and Nojyo, Y. 1984. A whole image of the hippocampal pyramidal neuron revealed by intracellular pressure-injection of horseradish peroxidase. Brain Res. 307: 336–340.

Tamura, T., Nakatani, K., and Yau, K.-W. 1991. Calcium feedback and sensitivity regulation in primate rods. J. Gen. Physiol. 98: 91–130.

Tanabe, T., Iino, M., and Takagi, S.F. 1975. Discrimination of odors in olfactory bulb, pyriform-amygdaloid areas, and orbitofrontal cortex of the monkey. J. Neurophysiol. 38: 1284–1296.

Tanaka, K., Saito, H.-A., Fukada, Y., and Moriya, M. 1991. Coding visual images of objects in the inferotemporal cortex of the macaque monkey. J. Physiol. (Lond.) 66: 170–189.

Tang, A.C. and Hasselmo, M.E. 1994. Selective suppression of intrinsic but not afferent fiber synaptic transmission by baclofen in the piriform (olfactory) cortex. Brain Res. 659: 75–81.

Tank, D.S., Sugimori, M., Connor, J.A., and Llinás, R. 1988. Spatially resolved calcium dynamics of mammalian Purkinje cells in cerebellar slices. Science 242: 773–777.

Tank, D.W. and Hopfield, J.J. 1987. Neural computation by concentrating information in time. Proc. Natl. Acad. Sci. USA 84: 1896–1900.

Tauchi, M. and Masland, R.H. 1984. The shape and arrangement of the cholinergic neurons in the rabbit retina. Proc. R. Soc. (Lond.) B Biol. Sci. 223: 101–119.

Taylor, C.P. and Dudek, F.E. 1984. Excitation of hippocampal pyramidal cells by electrical field effect. J. Neurophysiol. 52: 126–142.

Taylor, W.R. 1996. Response properties of long-range axon-bearing amacrine cells in the dark-adapted rabbit retina. Vis. Neurosci. 13: 599–604.

Taylor, W.R. and Wässle, H. 1995. Receptive field properties of starburst cholinergic amacrine cells in the rabbit retina. Eur. J. Neurosci. 7: 2308–2321.

Teicher, M.H., Stewart, W.B., Kauer, J.S., and Shepherd, G.M. 1980. Suckling pheromone stimulation of a modified glomerular region in the developing rat olfactory bulb revealed by the 2-deoxyglucose method. Brain Res. 194: 530–535.

ten Bruggencate, G. and Engberg, I. 1971. Iontophoretic studies in Deiters' nucleus of the inhibitory actions of GABA and related amino acids and the interactions of strychnine and picrotoxin. Brain Res. 25: 431–448.

Terenishi, T., Negishi, K., and Kato, S. 1984. Regulatory effect of dopamine on spatial properties of horizontal cells in carp retina. J. Neurosci. 4: 1271–1280.

Teyler, T.J., Cavus, I., Coussens, C., DiScenna, P., Grover, L., Lee, Y.P., and Little, Z. 1994. Multideterminant role of calcium in hippocampal synaptic plasticity. Hippocampus 4: 623–634.

Thalmann, R.H. 1988. Evidence that guanosine triphosphate (GTP)-binding proteins control a synaptic response in brain effect of pertussis toxin and GTPflS on the late inhibitory postsynaptic potential of hippocampal CA3 neurons. J. Neurosci. 8: 4589–4602.

Thomas, R.C. 1972. Electrogenic sodium pump in nerve and muscle cells. Physiol. Rev. 52: 563–594.

Thompson, S.M., Deisz, R.A., and Prince, D.A. 1988. Relative contributions of passive equilibrium and active transport to the distributin of chloride in mammalian cortical neurons. J. Neurophysiol. 60: 105–124.

Thomson, A., Deuchars, J., and West, D. 1993. Large, deep layer pyramid–pyramid single axon EPSPs in slices of rat motor cortex display paired pulse and frequency-dependent depression, mediated presynaptically and self-facilitation mediated postsynaptically. J. Neurosci 70: 2354–2369.

Thomson, A., Girdlestone, D., and West, D. 1988. Voltage-dependent currents prolong single axon postsynaptic potentials in layer pyramidal neurons in rat neocortical slices. J. Neurophysiol. 6: 1896–1907.

Thurbon, D., Field, A., and Redman, S. 1994. Electronic profiles of interneurons in stratum pyramidale of the CA1 region of rat hippocampus. J. Neurophysiol. 71: 1948–1958.

Tigges, J. and Tigges, M. 1985. Subcortical sources of direct projections to visual cortex. In: Cerebral Cortex, Vol. 3 (Peters, A. and Jones, E., eds.). New York: Plenum Press, pp. 351–378.

Tolbert, L.P. and Morest, D.K. 1982. The neuronal architecture of the anteroventral cochlear nucleus of the cat in the region of the cochlear nerve root: Golgi and Nissl methods. Neuroscience 7: 3013–3030.

Toth, K. and Freund, T.F. 1992. Calbindin D_{28k}-containing nonpyramidal cells in the rat hippocampus: Their immunoreactivity for GABA and projection to the medial septum. Neuroscience 49: 793–805.

Townes-Anderson, E., Dacheux, R.F., and Raviola, E. 1988. Rod photoreceptors dissociated from the adult rabbit retina. J. Neurosci. 8: 320–331.

Townes-Anderson, E., MacLeish, P.R., and Raviola, E. 1985. Rod cells dissociated from mature salamander retina: Ultrastructure and uptake of horseradish peroxidase. J. Cell Biol. 100: 175–188.

Toyama, K., Matsunami, K., Ohno, T., and Tokashiki, S. 1974. An intracellular study of neuronal organization in the visual cortex. Exp. Brain Res. 21: 45–66.

Traub, R.D. and Llinás, R. 1977. The spatial distribution of ionic conductances in normal and axotomized motoneurons. Neuroscience 2: 829–849.

Traub, R.D. and Llinás, R. 1979. Hippocampal pyramidal cells' significance of dendritic ionic conductances for neuronal function and epileptogenesis. J. Neurophysiol. 42: 476–496.

Traub, R.D. and Miles, R. 1991. Neuronal Networks of the Hippocampus. Cambridge: Cambridge University Press.

Traub, R.D., Miles, R., and Wong, R.K.S. 1989. Model of the origin of rhythmic population oscillations in the hippocampal slice. Science 243: 1319–1325.

Traub, R.D. and Wong, R.K.S. 1981. Penicillin-induced epileptiform activity in the hippocampal slice a model of synchronization of CA3 pyramidal cell bursting. Neuroscience 6: 223–230.

Treloar, H., Walters, E., Margolis, F., and Key, B. 1996. Olfactory glomeruli are innervated by more than one distinct subset of primary sensory olfactory neurons in mice. J. Comp. Neurol. 367: 550–562.

Trombley, P.Q. 1992. Norepinephrine inhibits calcium currents and EPSPs via a G-protein-coupled mechanism in olfactory bulb neurons. J. Neurosci. 12: 3992–3998.

Trombley, P.Q. and Shepherd, G.M. 1993. Synaptic transmission and modulation in the olfactory bulb. Curr. Opin. Neurobiol. 3: 540–547.

Trombley, P.Q. and Shepherd, G.M. 1994. Glycine exerts potent inhibitory actions on mammalian olfactory bulb neurons. J. Neurophysiol. 71: 761–767.

Trombley, P.Q. and Shepherd, G.M. 1997. The olfactory bulb. In: Encyclopedia of Neuroscience (Edelman, G. and Smith, B., eds.). Amsterdam: Elsevier, (In press).

Tsai, K.Y., Carnevale, N.T., Caliborne, B.J., and Brown, T.H. 1994. Efficient mapping from neuroanatomical to electrotonic space. Network 5: 21–46.

Tseng, G.-F. and Haberly, L.B. 1988. Characterization of synaptically mediated fast and slow inhibitory processes in piriform cortex in an in vitro slice preparation. J. Neurophysiol. 59: 1352–1376.

Tseng, G.-F. and Haberly, L.B. 1990a. Deep neurons in piriform cortex. I. Morphology and synaptically evoked responses including a unique high amplitude paired shock facilitation. J. Neurophysiol. 62: 369–385.

Tseng, G.-F. and Haberly, L.B. 1989b. Deep neurons in piriform cortex. II. Membrane properties that underlie unusual synaptic responses. J. Neurophysiol. 62: 386–400.

Tsien, R.W., Ellinor, P.T., and Horne, W.A. 1991. Molecular diversity of voltage-dependent Ca^{2+} channels. Trends Pharmacol. Sci. 12: 349–354.

Tsien, R.W., Lipscombe, D., Madison, D.V., Bley, K.R., and Fox, A.P. 1988. Multiple types of neuronal calcium channels and their selective modulation. Trends Neurosci. 11: 431–438.

Tsubokawa, H. and Ross, W.N. 1996. IPSPs modulate spike backpropagation and associated $[Ca^{2+}]_i$ changes in the dendrites of hippocampal CA1 pyramidal neurons. J. Neurophysiol. 76: 2896–2906.

Tsukamoto, Y., Smith, R.G., and Sterling, P. 1990. "Collective coding" of correlated cone signals in the retinal ganglion cell. Proc. Natl. Acad. Sci. USA 87: 1860–1864.

Tsukamoto, Y. and Sterling. P. 1991. Spatial summation by ganglion cells: Some consequences for the efficient encoding of natural scenes. Neurosci. Res. Suppl. 15: S185–S198.

Tsukamoto, Y. Masarachia, P. Schein, S.J., Sterling, P. 1992. Gap junctions between the pedicles of macaque foveal cones. Vision Res. 32: 1809–1815.

Tsumoto, T., Eckart, W., and Creutzfeld, O. 1979. Modifications of orientation sensitivity of cat visual cortex neurons by removal of GABA-mediated inhibition. Exp. Brain Res. 46: 157–169.

Tsumoto, T. and Suda, K. 1979. Cross-depression: An electrophysiological manifestation of binocular competition in developing visual cortex. Brain Res. 168: 190–194.

Tsumoto, T. and Suda, K. 1980. Three groups of cortico-geniculate neurons and their distribution in binocular and monocular segments of cat striate cortex. J. Comp. Neurol. 193: 223–236.

Turner, C.P. and Perez-Polo, J.R. 1993. Expression of p75NGFR in the olfactory system following peripheral deafferentation. Neuroreport 4: 1023–1026.

Turner, R.W., Meyers, D.E.R., Richardson, T.L., and Barker, J.L. 1991. The site for initiation of action potential discharge over the somatodendritic axis of rat hippocampal CA1 pyramidal neurons. J. Neurosci. 11: 2270–2280.

Uchiyama, H. and Barlow, R.B. 1994. Centrifugal inputs enhance responses of retinal ganglion cells in the Japanese quail without changing their spatial coding properties. Vision Res. 34: 2189–2194.

Uchiyama, Y. and Ito, H. 1993. Target cells for the isthmo-optic fibers in the retina of the Japanese quail. Neurosci. Lett. 154: 35–38.

Uhlrich, D.J., Cucchiaro, J.B., Humphrey, A.L., and Sherman, S.M. 1991. Morphology and axonal projection patterns of individual neurons in the cat perigeniculate nucleus. J. Neurophysiol. 65: 1528–1541.

Uhlrich, D.J., Manning, K.A., and Pienkowski, T.P. 1993. The histaminergic innervation of the lateral geniculate complex in the cat. Vis. Neurosci. 10: 225–235.

Ulfhake, B., Arvidsson, U., Cullheim, S., Hökfelt, T., Brodin, E., Verhofstad, A., and Visser, T. 1987. An ultrastructural study of 5-hydroxytryptamine-, thrytropin-releasing hormone- and substance P-immunoreactive axonal boutons in the motor nucleus of spinal cord segments L7-S1 in the adult cat. Neuroscience 23: 917–929.

Updyke, B.V. 1977. Topographic organization of the projections from cortical areas 17, 18, and 19 onto the thalamus, pretectum and superior colliculs in the cat. J. Comp. Neurol. 173: 81–122.

Usrey, W.M. and Fitzpatrick, D. 1996. Specificity in the axonal connections of layer VI neurons in three shrew striate cortex: Evidence for distinct granular and supragranular systems. J. Neurosci. 16: 1203–1218.

Valcana, T., Hudson, D., and Timiras, P.S. 1972. Effects of X-irradiation on the content of amino acids in the developing rat cerebellum. J. Neurochem. 19: 2229–2232.

Valverde, F. 1965. Studies on the Piriform Lobe. Cambridge, MA: Harvard University Press.

Valverde, F. and Lopez-Mascaraque, L. 1991. Neuroglial arrangements in the olfactory glomeruli of the hedgehog. J. Comp. Neurol. 307: 658–674.

van Daal, J.H.H.M., Zanderink, H.E.A., Jenks, B.G., and van Abellen, J.H.F. 1989. Distribution of dynorphin B and methionine-enkephalin in the mouse hippocampus: Influence of genotype. Neurosci. Lett. 97: 241–244.

van den Pol, A.N. and Gorcs, T. 1988. Glycine and glycine receptor immunoreactivity in brain and spinal cord. J. Neurosci. 8: 472–492.

Vandermaelen, C.P. and Aghajanian, G.K. 1983. Electrophysiological and pharmacological characterization of serotonergic dorsal raphe neurons recorded extracellularly and intracellularly in rat brain slices. Brain Res. 289: 109–119.

van Eden, C., Hoorneman, E., Buijs, R., Matthijssen, M., Geffard, M., and Uylings, H. 1987. Immunocytochemical localization of dopamine in the prefrontal cortex of the rat at light and electron microscopic level. Neuroscience 22: 849–862.

Van Essen, D.C. 1985. Functional organization of primate visual cortex. In: Cerebral Cortex (Peters, A., and Jones, E.G., eds.). New York: Plenum Press, pp. 259–329.

Van Essen, D.C., Anderson, C.H., and Felleman, D.J. 1992. Information processing in the primate visual system: An integrated systems perspective. Science 255: 419–423.

Van Essen, D.C., Felleman, D.J., DeYoe, E.A., Olvarria, J., and Knierim, J.J. 1990. Modular and hierarchical organization of extrastriate visual cortex in the macaque monkey. Cold Spring Harbor Symp. Quant. Biol. 55: 679–696.

Van Essen, D.C. and Maunsell, J.H.R. 1983. Hierarchical organization and functional streams in the visual cortex. Trends Neurosci. 6: 370–375.

Vaney, D.I. 1985. The morphology and topographic distribution of AII amacrine cells in the cat retina. Proc. R. Soc. (Lond.) B Biol. Sci. 224: 475–488.

Vaney, D.I. 1990. The mosaic of amacrine cells in mammalian retina. In: Progress in Retinal Research (Osborne, N. and Chader, J., eds.). Oxford: Pergamon Press, pp. 49–100.

Vaney, D.I. 1993. The coupling pattern of axon-bearing horizontal cells in the mammalian retina. Proc. R. Soc. (Lond.) B Biol. Sci. 252: 93–101.

Vaney, D.I. 1994a. Patterns of neuronal coupling in the retina. Prog. Retina & Eye Res. 13: 301–355.

Vaney, D.I. 1994b. Territorial organization of direction-selective ganglion cells in rabbit retina. J. Neurosci. 14: 6301–6316.

Vaney, D.I. and Collin, S.P. 1989a. Dendritic relationships between cholinergic amacrine cells and direction-selective retinal ganglion cells. In: Neurobiology of the Inner Retina (Weiler, R. and Osborne, N.N., eds.). Berlin: Springer-Verlag, pp. 157–168.

Vaney, D.I., Gynther, I.C., and Young, H.M. 1991. Rod-signal interneurons in the rabbit retina: 2. AII amacrine cells. J. Comp. Neurol. 310: 154–169.

Vaney, D.I., Whitington, G.E., and Young, H.M. 1989b. The morphology and topographic distribution of substance-P-like immunoreactive amacrine cells in the cat retina. Proc. R. Soc. (Lond.) B Biol. Sci. 237: 471–488.

Vaney, D.I. and Young, H.M. 1988. GABA-like immunoreactivity in NADPH-diaphorase amacrine cells of the rabbit retina. Brain Res. 474: 380–385.

Van Groen, T. and Wyss, J.M. 1990. Extrinsic projections from area CA1 of the rat hippocampus. Olfactory, cortical, subcortical and bilateral hippocampal formation projections. J. Comp. Neurol. 302: 515–528.

van Harteren, J.H. 1992. A theory of maximizing sensory information. Biol. Cybern. 68: 23–29.

Van Horn, S.C., Erişir, A., and Sherman, S.M. 1997. Re-evaluation of relative distribution of synaptic terminals in the LGN of cats. Soc. Neurosci. Abstr. (In Press).

Van Keulen, L. 1981. Autogenetic recurrent inhibition of individual spinal motoneurones of the cat. Neurosci. Lett. 21: 297–300.

Van Tasell, D.J., Soli, S.D., Kirby, V.M., and Widin, G.P. 1987. Speech waveform envelope cues for consonant recognition. J. Acoust. Soc. Am. 82: 1152–1161.

Vardi, N. 1997a. Localization of G_{olf} and adenylyl cyclase type III in mammalian retina. (Submitted).

Vardi, N. 1997b. The alpha subunit of G_o localizes in the dendritic tips of ON bipolar cells. (Submitted).

Vardi, N. and Auerbach, P. 1995. Specific cell types in cat retina express different forms of glutamic acid decarboxylase. J. Comp. Neurol. 351: 374–384.

Vardi, N., Kaufman, D.L., Sterling, P. 1994. Horizontal cells in cat and monkey retina express different isoforms of glutamic acid decarboxylase. Vis Neurosci 11: 135–142.

Vardi, N., Masarachia, P., and Sterling, P. 1989. Structure of the starburst amacrine network and its association with alpha ganglion cells. J. Comp. Neurol. 288: 601–611.

Vardi, N., Masarachia, P., and Sterling, P. 1992. Immunoreactivity to $GABA_A$ receptor in the outer plexiform layer of the cat retina. J. Comp. Neurol. 320: 394–397.

Vardi, N., Matesic, D.F., Manning, D.R., Liebman, P.A., Sterling, P. 1993 Identification of a G-protein in depolarizing rod bipolar cells. Vis. Neurosci. 10: 473–478.

Vardi, N., Morigiwa, K. 1997. ON cone bipolar cells in rat express the metabotropic receptor mGluR6. Vis. Neurosci. (In press).

Vardi, N. and Shi, Y.-J. 1996. Identification of GABA containing bipolar cells in cat retina. Invest. Ophthalmol. Vis. Sci. Abstr. S418.

Vardi, N. and Smith, R.G. 1996. The AII amacrine network: Coupling can increase correlated activity. Vision Res. 36: 3743–3757.

Vardi, N. and Sterling, P. 1994. Subcellular localization of $GABA_A$ receptor on bipolar cells in macaque and human retina. Vision Res. 34: 1235–1246.

Vasilaki, A., Hatzilaris, E., Liapakis, G., Georgoussi, Z., and Thermos, K. 1996. Somatostatin receptor subtypes (SSTR2) in the rabbit retina. Soc. Neurosci. Abstr. 22: 180.

Vassar, R., Chao, S.K., Sitcheran, R., Nunez, J.M., Vosshall, L.B., and Axel, R. 1994. Topographic organization of sensory projections to the olfactory bulb. Cell 79: 981–991.

Vassar, R., Ngai, J., and Axel, R. 1993. Spatial segregation of odorant receptor expression in the mammalian olfactory epithelium. Cell 74: 309–318.

Verney, C., Alvarez, C., Geffard, M., and Berger, B. 1990. Ultra-structural double-labelling study of dopamine terminals and GABA-containing neurons in rat anteromedial cerebral cortex. Eur. J. Neurosci. 2: 960.

Veruki, M.L. and Wässle, H. 1996. Immunohistochemical localization of dopamine D1 receptors in rat retina. Europ. J. Neurosci. 8: 2286–2297.

Vittala, J., Korpimäki, E., Palokangas, P., and Koivula, M. 1995. Attraction of kestrels to vole scent marks visible in ultraviolet light. Nature 373: 425–427.

Vincent, S.R. and Kimura, H. 1992. Histochemical mapping of nitric oxide synthase in the rat brain. Neuroscience 46: 755–784.

Vincent, S.R., Satoh, K., Armstrong, D., and Fibiger, H. 1983a. Substance p in the ascending cholinergic reticular system. Nature 306: 688–691.

Vincent, S.R., Johansson, O., Hökfelt, T., Skirboll, L., Elde, R.P., Terenius, L., Kimmel, J., and Goldstein, M. 1983b. NADPH-diaphorase—A selective histochemical marker for striatal neurons containing both somatostatin- and avian pancreatic polypeptide (APP)-like immunoreactivities. J. Comp. Neurol. 217: 252–263.

Vogel, M. 1978. Postnatal development of the cat's retina. Adv. Anat. Embryol. Cell Biol. 54: 7–64.

Voigt, H.F. and Young, E.D. 1980. Evidence of inhibitory interactions between neurons in the dorsal cochlear nucleus. J. Neurophysiol. 44: 76–96.

Voigt, H.F. and Young, E.D. 1990. Cross-correlation analysis of inhibitory interactions in dorsal cochlear nucleus. J. Neurophysiol. 64: 1590–1610.

Voight, T. and Wässle, H. 1987. Dopaminergic innervation of AII amacrine cells in mammalian retina. J. Neurosci. 7: 4115–4128.

von der Malsburg, C. 1981. The correlation theory of brain function. Intern. Rep. 81: 2.

von Gersdorff, H. and Matthews, G. 1994. Dynamics of synaptic vesicle fusion and membrane retrieval in synaptic terminals. Nature 367: 735–739.

von Gersdorff, H., Vardi, E., Matthews, G., and Sterling, P. 1996. Evidence that vesicles on the synaptic ribbon of retinal bipolar neurons can be rapidly released. Neuron 16: 1221–1227.

von Krosigk, M., Bal, T., and McCormick, D.A. 1993. Cellular mechanisms of a synchronized oscillation in the thalamus. Science 261: 361–364.

Voogd, J. and Bigare, F. 1980. Topographical distribution of olivary and corticonuclear fibers in the cerebellum: A review. In: The Inferior Olivary Nucleus (Courville, J., de Montigny, C., and Lamarre, Y., eds.). New York: Raven Press, pp. 207–234.

Wada, E., Wada, K., Boulter, J., Deneris, E., Heinemann, S., Patrick, J., and Swanson, L.W. 1989. Distribution of alpha$_2$, alpha$_3$, alpha$_4$, and beta$_2$ neuronal nicotinic receptor subunit mRNAs in the central nervous system—A hybridization histochemical study in the rat. J. Comp. Neurol. 284: 314–335.

Wainer, B.H., Levey, A.I., Rye, D.B., Mesulam, M.M., and Mufson, E.J. 1985. Cholinergic and non-cholinergic septohippocampal pathways. Neurosci. Lett. 54: 45–52.

Walmsley, B. 1991. Central synaptic transmission: Studies at the connection between primary afferent fibres and dorsal spinocerebellar tract (DSCT) neurones in Clarke's column of the spinal cord. Prog. Neurobiol. 36: 391–423.

Walmsley, B. and Bolton, P.S. 1994. An *in vivo* pharmacological study of single group Ia fibre contacts with motoneurones in the cat spinal cord. J. Physiol. (Lond.) 481: 731–741.

Walmsley, B. and Edwards, F.R. 1988. Nonuniform release probabilities underlie quantal synaptic transmission at a mammalian excitatory central synapse. J. Neurophysiol. 60: 889–908.

Walmsley, B., Hodgson, J.A., and Burke, R.E. 1978. Forces produced by medial gastrocnemius and soleus muscles during locomotion in freely moving cats. J. Neurophysiol. 41: 1203–1216.

Walmsley, B. and Tracey, D.J. 1981. An intracellular study of Renshaw cells. Brain Res. 223: 170–175.

Walmsley, B., Wieniawa-Narkiewicz, E., and Nicol, M.J. 1985. The ultrastructural basis for synaptic transmission between primary muscle afferents and neurons in Clarke's column of the cat. J. Neurosci. 5: 2095–2106.

Wan, H. and Cahc, P. 1995. The effects of 1-ap4 and 1-serine-o-phosphate on inhibition in primary somatosensory cortex of the adult rat in vivo. Neuropharmacology 34: 1053–1062.

Wang, J.H. and Kelly, P.T. 1996. Regulation of synaptic facilitation by postsynaptic Ca^{2+}/CaM pathways in hippocampal CA1 neurons. J. Neurophysiol. 76: 276–286.

Wang, X.Y., McKenzie, J.S., and Kemm, R.E. 1996. Whole-cell K^+ currents in identified olfactory bulb output neurones of rat. J. Physiol. (Lond.) 490: 63–77.

Wang, X.Y. and Sachs, M.B. 1993. Neural encoding of single-formant stimuli in the cat: I. Responses of auditory nerve fibers. J. Neurophysiol. 70: 1054–1075.

Wang, X.Y. and Sachs, M.B. 1994. Neural encoding of single-formant stimuli in the cat. II. Responses of anteroventral cochlear nucleus neurons. J. Neurophysiol. 71: 59–78.

Wang, X.Y. and Sachs, M.B. 1995. Transformation of temporal discharge patterns in a ventral cochlear nucleus stellate cell model: Implications for physiological mechanisms. J. Neurophysiol. 73: 1600–1616.

Wang, Z. and McCormick, D. 1993. Control of firing mode of corticotectal and corticopontine layer V burst-generating neurons by norepinephrine, acetylcholine and 1s, 3r-ACPD. J. Neurosci. 13: 2199–2216.

Wässle, H. and Boycott, B.B. 1991. Functional architecture of the mammalian retina. Physiol. Rev. 71: 447–480.

Wässle, H., Boycott, B.B., and Illing, R.B. 1981a. Morphology and mosaic of ON and OFF beta cells in the cat retina and some functional considerations. Proc. R. Soc. B (Lond.) Biol. Sci. 212: 177–195.

Wässle, H., Boycott, B.B., and Peichl, L. 1978a. Receptor contacts of horizontal cells in the retina of the domestic cat. Proc. R. Soc. B (Lond.) Biol. Sci. 203: 247–267.

Wässle, H. and Chun, M.H. 1989. GABA-like immunoreactivity in the cat retina: Light microscopy. J. Comp. Neurol. 279: 43–54.

Wässle, H., Grünert, U., Chun, M.-H., and Boycott, B.B. 1995. The rod pathway of the macaque monkey retina: Identification of AII-amacrine cells with antibodies against calretinin. J. Comp. Neurol. 361: 537–551.

Wässle, H., Grünert, U., Martin, P.R., and Boycott, B.B. 1994. Immunocytochemical characterization and spatial distribution of midget bipolar cells in the macaque monkey retina. Vision Res. 34: 561–579.

Wässle, H., Grünert, U., Röhrenbeck, J., and Boycott, B.B. 1989. Cortical magnification factor and the ganglion cell density of the primate retina. Nature 341: 643–646.

Wässle, H., Peichl, L., and Boycott, B.B. 1978b. Topography of horizontal cells in the retina of the domestic cat. Proc. R. Soc. (Lond.) B Biol. Sci. 203: 269–291.

Wässle, H., Peichl, L., and Boycott, B.B. 1981b. Dendritic territories of cat retinal ganglion cells. Nature 292: 344–345.

Wässle, H., Peichl, L., and Boycott, B.B. 1981c. Morphology and topography of ON- and OFF-alpha cells in the cat retina. Proc. R. Soc. B (Lond.) Biol. Sci. 212: 157–175.

Wässle, H., and Riemann, H.J. 1978. The mosaic of nerve cells in the mammalian retina. Proc. R. Soc. B (Lond) 200: 441–461.

Wässle, H., Yamashita, M., Greferath, U., Grünert, U., and Müller, F. 1991. The rod bipolar cell of the mammalian retina. Vis. Neurosci. 7: 99–112.

Watanabe, M. and Rodieck, R.W. 1989. Parasol and midget ganglion cells of the primate retina. J. Comp. Neurol. 289: 434–454.

Waterhouse, B., Azizi, B.R., and Woodward, S.A.D. 1990. Modulation of rat cortical area 17. Neuronal responses to moving visual stimuli during norepinephrine and serotonin microiontophoresis. Brain Res. 514: 276–292.

Waterhouse, B., Lin, C.-S., Burne, R., and Woodward, D. 1983. The distribution of neocortical projection neurons in the locus coeruleus. J. Comp. Neurol. 217: 418–431.

Watkins, J.C. and Olverman, H.J. 1987. Agonists and antagonists for excitatory amino acid receptors. Trends Neurosci. 10: 265–272.

Weedman, D.L., Pongstaporn, T., and Ryugo, D.K. 1996. Ultrastructural study of the granule cell domain of the cochlear nucleus in rats: Mossy fiber endings and their targets. J. Comp. Neurol. 369: 345–360.

Weedman, D.L. and Ryugo, D.K. 1996. Projections from auditory cortex to the cochlear nucleus in rats: Synapses on granule cell dendrites. J. Comp. Neurol. 371: 311–324.

Wehr, M. and Laurent, G. 1996. Odour encoding by temporal sequences of firing in oscillating neural assemblies. Nature 384: 161–164.

Weinberg, R.J. and Rustioni, A. 1987. A cuneocochlear pathway in the rat. Neuroscience 20: 209–219.

Wellis, D.P. and Kauer, J.S. 1993. GABA$_A$ and glutamate receptor involvement in dendrodendritic synaptic interactions from salamander olfactory bulb. J. Physiol. (Lond.) 469: 315–339.

Wellis, D.P. and Scott, J.W. 1987. Intracellular recordings of odor-induced responses in the rat olfactory bulb. Chem. Senses 12: 707.

Wenthold, R.J. 1991. Neurotransmitters of brainstem auditory nuclei. In: Neurobiology of Hearing: The Central Auditory System (Altschuler, R.A., Bobbin, R.P., Clopton, B.M., and Hoffman, D.W., eds.). New York: Raven Press, pp. 121–139.

Wenthold, R.J., Huie, D., Altschuler, R.A., and Reeks, K.A. 1987. Glycine immunoreactivity localized in the cochlear nucleus and superior olivary complex. Neuroscience 22: 897–912.

Wenthold, R.J., Parakkal, M.H., Oberdorfer, M.D., and Altschuler, R.A. 1988. Glycine receptor immunoreactivity in the ventral cochlear nucleus. J. Comp. Neurol. 276: 423–435.

Werblin, F.S. and Dowling, J.E. 1969. Organization of the retina of the mudpuppy, *Necturus maculosus*. II. Intracellular recording. J. Neurophysiol. 32: 339–355.

Westbrook, G.L. 1994. Glutamate receptor update. Curr. Opin. Neurobiol. 4: 337–346.

Westenbroek, R.E., Ahlijanian, M.K., and Catterall, W.A. 1990. Clustering of L-type Ca^{2+} channels at the base of major dendrites in hihppocampal pyramidal neurons. Nature 347: 281–284.

Westenbroek, R.E., Westrum, L.E., Hendrickson, A.E., and Wu, J.-Y. 1987. Immunocytochemical localization of cholecystokinin and glutamic acid decarboxylase during normal development in the prepyriform cortex of rats. Dev. Brain Res. 34: 191–206.

Wheeler, D.B., Randall, A., and Tsien, R.W. 1994. Roles of N-type and Q-type Ca^{2+} channels in supporting hippocampal synaptic transmission. Science 264: 107–111.

White, C.A., Chalupa, L.M., Johnson, D., and Brecha, N.C. 1990a. Somatostatin-immunoreactive cells in the adult cat retina. J. Comp. Neurol. 293: 134–150.

White, E.L. 1972. Synaptic organization in the olfactory glomerulus of the mouse. Brain Res. 37: 69–80.

White, E.L. 1989. Cortical Circuits. Boston: Burkhauser.

White, E.L. and Rock, M. 1980. Three-dimensional aspects and synaptic relationships of a Golgi-impregnated spiny stellate cell reconstructed from serial thin sections. J. Neurocytol. 9: 615–636.

White, G., Levy, W.B., and Steward, O. 1990b. Spatial overlap between populations of synapses determines the extent of their associative interaction during the induction of long-term potentiation and depression. J. Neurosci. 64: 1186–1198.

White, J.A., Young, E.D., and Manis, P.B. 1994. The electrotonic structure of regular-spiking neurons in the ventral cochlear nucleus may determine their response properties. J. Neurophysiol. 71: 1774–1786.

Wickens, J.R., Begg, A.J., and Arbuthnott, G.W. 1996. Dopamine reverses the depression of rat cortico-striatal synapses which normally follows high frequency stimulation of cortex in vitro. Neuroscience 70: 1–5.

Wickesberg, R.E. and Oertel, D. 1988. Tonotopic projection from the dorsal to the anteroventral cochlear nucleus of mice. J. Comp. Neurol. 268: 389–399.

Wickesberg, R.E. and Oertel, D. 1990. Delayed, frequency-specific inhibition in the cochlear nuclei of mice: A mechanism for monaural echo suppression. J. Neurosci. 10: 1762–1768.

Wightman, F.L. and Kistler, D.J. 1992. The dominant role of low-frequency interaural time differences in sound localization. J. Acoust. Soc. Am. 91: 1648–1661.

Wigstrom, H. and Gustafsson, B. 1983. Facilitated induction of hippocampal long-lasting potentiation during blockade of inhibition. Nature 301: 603–604.

Wigstrom, H., Gustafsson, B., Huang, Y.Y., and Abraham, W.C. 1986. Hippocampal long-term potentiation is induced by pairing single afferent volleys with intracellularly injected depolarizing current pulses. Acta Physiol. Scand. 126: 317–319.

Williams, D.R. 1992. Photoreceptor sampling and aliasing in human vision. In: Tutorials in Optics (Moore, D.T., ed.). Optical Society of America, Rochester, NY: pp. 15–27.

Williams, D.R., MacLeod, D.I.A., and Hayhoe, M.M. 1981. Punctate sensitivity of the blue-sensitive mechanism. Vision Res. 21: 1357–1375.

Williams, D,R., Sekiguchi, N., and Brainard, D. 1993b. Color, contrast sensitivity, and the cone mosaic. Proc. Natl. Acad. Sci. USA 90: 9770–9777.

Williams, J.T., North, R.A., Shefner, S.A., Nishi, S., and Egan, T.M. 1984. Membrane properties of rat locus coeruleus neurones. Neuroscience 13: 137–156.

Williams, R.W., Bastiani, M.J., and Chalupa, L. 1983. Loss of axons in the cat optic nerve following fetal unilateral enucleation: An electron microscopic analysis. J. Neurosci. 3: 133–144.

Williams, R.W., Bastiani, M.J., Lia, B., and Chalupa, L.M. 1996. Growth cones, dying axons, and developmental fluctuations in the fiber population of the cat's optic nerve. J. Comp. Neurol. 246: 32–69.

Williams, R.W., Cavada, C., and Reinoso-Suárez, F. 1993a. Rapid evolution of the visual system: A cellular assay of the retina and dorsal lateral geniculate nucleus of the Spanish wildcat and the domestic cat. J. Neurosci. 13: 208–228.

Williams, R.W. and Herrup, K. 1988. The control of neuron number. Annu. Rev. Neurosci. 11: 423–453.

Williams, S.H. and Johnston, D. 1993. Muscarinic cholinergic inhibition of glutamatergic transmission. In: Presynaptic Receptors in the Mammalian Brain (Dunwiddie, T.V. and Lovinger, D.M., eds.). Boston: Burkhauser, pp. 27–41.

Williams, S.H. and Johnston, D. 1996. Actions of endogenous opioids on NMDA receptor-independent long-term potentiation in area CA3 of the hippocampus. J. Neurosci. 16: 3652–3660.

Wilson, C.J. 1986a. Postsynaptic potentials evoked in spiny neostriatal projection neurons by stimulation of ipsilateral or contralateral neocortex. Brain Res. 367: 201–213.

Wilson, C.J. 1986b. Three-dimensional analysis of dendritic spines by means of HVEM J. Electron Microsc. 35(Suppl.): 1151–1155.

Wilson, C.J. 1987. Morphology and synaptic connections of crossed corticostriatal neurons in the rat. J. Comp. Neurol. 263: 567–580.

Wilson, C.J. 1988. Cellular mechanisms controlling the strength of synapses. J. Electron Microsc. Tech. 10: 293–313.

Wilson, C.J. 1992. Dendritic morphology, inward rectification and the functional properties of neostriatal neurons. In: Single Neuron Computation (McKenna, T., Davis, J. and Zornetzer, S.F., eds.). San Diego: Academic Press, pp. 141–171.

Wilson, C.J. 1993. Generation of natural firing patterns in neostriatal neurons. In: Chemical Signaling in the Basal Ganglia. Progress in Brain Research (Arbuthnott, G.W. and Emson, P.C., eds.). Oxford: Elsevier, pp. 227–297.

Wilson, C.J., Chang, H.T., and Kitai, S.T. 1983a. Origins of postsynaptic potentials evoked in spiny neostriatal projection neurons by thalamic stimulation in the rat. Exp. Brain Res. 51: 217–226.

Wilson, C.J., Chang, H.T., and Kitai, S.T. 1990. firing patterns and synaptic potentials of identified giant aspiny interneurons in the rat neostriatum. J. Neurosci. 10: 508–519.

Wilson, C.J. and Groves, P.M. 1980. Fine structure and synaptic connections of the common spiny neuron of the rat neostriatum. J. Comp. Neurol. 194: 599–615.

Wilson, C.J. and Groves, P.M. 1981. Spontaneous firing patterns of identified spiny neurons in the rat neostriatum. Brain Res. 22: 67–80.

Wilson, C.J., Groves, P.M., Kitai, S.T., and Linder, J.C. 1983b. Three-dimensional structure of dendritic spines in the rat neostriatum. J. Neurosci. 3: 383–398.

Wilson, C.J. and Kawaguchi, Y. 1996. The origins of two-state spontaneous membrane potential fluctuations of neostriatal spiny neurons. J. Neurosci. 16: 2397–2410.

Wilson, D.A. 1997. Bi-naral interactions in rat piriform cortex J. Neurophysiol. (In press).

Wilson, D.A. and Leon, M. 1987a. Abrupt decrease in synaptic inhibition in the postnatal rat olfactory bulb. Brain Res. 430: 134–138.

Wilson, D.A. and Leon, M. 1987b. Evidence of lateral synaptic interactions in olfactory bulb output cell responses to odors. Brain Res. 417: 175–180.

Wilson, J.R., Friedlander, M.J., and Sherman, S.M. 1984. Fine structural morphology of identified X- and Y-cells in the cat's lateral geniculate nucleus. Proc. R. Soc. Lond. B Biol. Sci. 221: 441–436.

Wilson, M.A. and Bower, J.M. 1988. A computer simulation of olfactory cortex with functional implications for storage and retrieval of olfactory information. In: Neural Information Processing Systems (Anderson, D.Z., ed.). New York: American Institute of Physics, pp. 114–126.

Wilson, M.A. and McNaughton, B.L. 1993. Dynamics of the hippocampal ensemble code for space. Science 261: 1055–1058.

Wilson, M.A. and McNaughton, B.L. 1994. Reactivation of hippocampal ensemble memories during sleep. Science 265: 676–679.

Winter, I.M. and Palmer, A.R. 1995. Level dependence of cochlear nucleus onset unit responses and facilitation by second tones or broadband noise. J. Neurophysiol. 73: 141–159.

Witkovsky, P., Nicholson, C., Rice, M.E., and Bohmaker, K. 1993. Extracellular dopamine concentration in the retina of the clawed frog, *Xenopus laevis*. Proc. Natl. Acad. Sci. USA 90: 5667–5671.

Witter, M.P. and Groenewegen, H. 1992. Organizational principles of hippocampal connections. In: The Temporal Lobes and the Limbic System (Trimble, M. and Bolwig, T., eds.). Wrightson Biomedical Publishing, pp. 37–60.

Witter, M.P., Ostendorf, R.H., and Groenewegen, H.J. 1990. Heterogeneity in the dorsal subiculum of the rat. Distinct neuronal zones project to different cortical and subcortical targets. Eur. J. Neurosci. 2: 718–725.

Wong, R. and Watkins, D. 1982. Cellular factors influencing GABA responses in hippocampal pyramidal cells. J. Neurophysiol. 48: 938–951.

Wong, R.K.S. and Prince, D.A. 1978. Participation of calcium spikes during intrinsic burst firing in hippocampal neurons. Brain Res. 159: 385–390.

Wong, R.K.S., Prince, D.A., and Basbaum, A.I. 1979. Intradendritic recordings from hippocampal neurons. Proc. Natl. Sci. USA 76: 986–990.

Wong, R.O.L., Chernjavsky, A., Smith, S.J., and Shatz, C.J. 1995. Early functional neural networks in the developing retina. Nature 374: 716–718.

Wong, R.O.L., Herrmann, K., and Shatz, C.J. 1991. Remodeling of retinal ganglion cell dendrites in the absence of action potential activity. J. Neurobiol. 22: 685–697.

Wong-Riley, M. and Carroll, E. 1984. Quantitative light and electron microscopic analysis of cytochrome oxidase-rich zones in v11 prestriate cortex of the squirrel monkey. J. Comp. Neurol. 222: 18–37.

Woo, C.C., Coopersmith, R., and Leon, M. 1987. Localized changes in olfactory bulb morphology associated with early olfactory learning. J. Comp. Neurol. 263: 113–125.

Woolf, T.B. and Greer, C.A. 1994. Local communication within dendritic spines: Models of second messenger diffusion in granule cell spines of the mammalian olfactory bulb. Synapse 17: 247–267.

Woolf, T.B., Shepherd, G.M., and Greer, C.A. 1988. Models of local electrical interactions within spiny dendrites of granule cells in mouse olfactory bulb. Soc. Neurosci. Abstr. 14: 620.

Woolf, T.B., Shepherd, G.M., and Greer, C.A. 1991a. Local information processing in dendritic trees: Subsets of spines in granule cells of the mammalian olfactory bulb. J. Neurosci. 11: 1837–1854.

Woolf, T.B., Shepherd, G.M., and Greer, C.A. 1991b. Serial reconstructions of granule cell spines in the mammalian olfactory bulb. Synapse 7: 181–192.

Woolley, D.E. and Timiras, P.S. 1965. Prepyriform electrical activity in the rat during high altitude exposure. Electroencephalogr. Clin. Neurophysiol. 18: 680–690.

Woolsey, T. and Van der Loos, H. 1970. The structural organization of layer IV in the somatosensory region (S1) of mouse cortex. The description of a cortical field composed of discrete cytoarchitectonic units. Brain Res. 17: 205–242.

Wouterlood, F.G. and Mugnaini, E. 1984. Cartwheel neurons of the dorsal cochlear nucleus. A Golgi-electron microscopic study in the rat. J. Comp. Neurol. 227: 136–157.

Wouterlood, F.G., Mugnaini, E., Osen, K.K., and Dahl, A.-L. 1984. Stellate neurons in rat dorsal cochlear nucleus studied with combined Golgi impregnation and electron microscopy: Synaptic connections and mutual coupling by gap junctions. J. Neurocytol. 13: 639–664.

Wouterlood, F.G., Saldana, E., and Witter, M.P. 1990. Projection from the nucleus reuniens thalami to the hippocampal region: Light and electron microscopic tracing study in the rat with the antrograde tracer Phaseolus vulgaris-0leucoagglutinin. J. Comp. Neurol. 296: 179–203.

Wright, D.D. and Ryugo, D.K. 1996. Mossy fiber projections form the cuneate nucleus to the dorsal cochlear nucleus of rat. J. Comp. Neurol. 365: 159–172.

Wu, S.H. and Oertel, D. 1984. Intracellular injection with horseradish peroxidase of physiologically characterized stellate and bushy cells in slices of mouse anteroventral cochlear nucleus. J. Neurosci. 4: 1577–1588.

Wu, S.M. 1992. Feedback connections and operation of the outer plexiform layer of the retina. Curr. Opin. Neurobiol. 2: 462–468.

Wyss, J.M., Swanson, L.W., and Cowan, W.M. 1979a. Evidence for an input to the molecular layer and the stratum granulosum of the dentate gyrus from the supramammillary region of the hypothalamus. Anat. Embryol. 156: 165–176.

Wyss, J.M., Swanson, L.W., and Cowan, W.M. 1979b. A study of subcortical afferents to the hippocampal formation in the rat. Neuroscience 4: 463–476.

Xiang, M., Zhou, L., and Nathans, J. 1996. Similarities and differences among inner retinal neurons revealed by the expression of reporter transgenes controlled by Brn-3a, Brn-3b, and Brn-3c promoter sequences. Vis. Neurosci. 13: 955–962.

Xiang, Z., Greenwood, A.C., Kairiss, E.W., and Brown, T.H. 1994. Quantal mechanism of long-term potentiation in hippocampal mossy-fiber synapses. J. Neurophysiol. 71: 2552–2556.

Xie, C.W. and Lewis, D.V. 1995. Endogenous opioids regulate long-term potentiation of synaptic inhibition in the dentate gyrus of rat hippocampus. J. Neurosci. 15: 3788–3795.

Xu, Z.C., Wilson, C.J., and Emson, P.C. 1991. Restoration of thalamostriatal projections in rat neostriatal grafts: An electron microscopic analysis. J. Comp. Neurol. 303: 22–34.

Yang, G. and Masland, R.H. 1992. Direct visualization of the dendritic and receptive fields of directionally selective retinal ganglion cells. Science 258: 1949–1952.

Yau, K.-W. 1994. Phototransduction mechanism in retinal rods and cones. Invest. Ophthalmol. Vis. Sci. 35: 9–32.

Yeckel, M.F. and Berger, T.W. 1990. Feedforward excitation of the hippocampus by afferents from the entorhinal cortex redefinition of the role of the tryisynaptic pathway. Proc. Natl. Acad. Sci. USA 87: 5832–5836.

Yeckel, M.F. and Berger, T.W. 1995. Monosynaptic excitation of hippocampal CA1 pyramidal cells by afferents from the entorhinal cortex. Hippocampus 5: 108–114.

Yeterian, E.H. and Hoesen, G. 1978. Cortico-striate projections in the rhesus monkey. The organization of certain cortico-caudate connections. Brain Res. 139: 43–63.

Yokoi, M., Mori, K., and Nakanishi, S. 1995. Refinement of odor molecule tuning by dendro-dendritic synaptic inahibition in the olfactory bulb. Proc. Natl. Acad. Sci. USA 92: 3371–3375.

Yoshimura, R., Kiyama, H., Kimura, T., Araki, T., Maeno, H., Tanizawa, O., and Tohyama, M. 1993. Localization of oxytocin receptor messenger ribonucleic acid in the rat brain. Endocrinology 133: 1239–1246.

Young, A.B. and Macdonald, R.L. 1983. Glycine as a spine cord neurotransmitter. In: Handbook of the Spinal Cord, Vol. 1: Pharmacology (Davidoff, R.E., ed.). New York: Marcel Dekker, pp. 1–43.

Young, A.B., Oster-Granite, M.L., Herndon, R.M., and Snyder, S.H. 1974. Glutamic acid: Selective depletion by viral induced granule cell loss in hamster cerebellum. Brain Res. 73: 1–13.

Young, E.D. 1980. Identification of response properties of ascending axons from dorsal cochlear nucleus. Brain Res. 200: 23–38.

Young, E.D. and Brownell, W.E. 1976. Responses to tones and noise of single cells in dorsal cochlear nucleus of unanesthetized cats. J. Neurophysiol. 39: 282–300.

Young, E.D., Nelken, I., and Conley, R.A. 1995. Somatosensory effects on neurons in dorsal cochlear nucleus. J. Neurophysiol. 73: 743–765.

Young, E.D., Rice, J.J., and Tong, S.C. 1996. Effects of pinna position on head-related transfer functions in the cat. J. Acoust. Soc. Am. 99: 3064–3076.

Young, E.D., Robert, J.M., and Shofner, W.P. 1988. Regularity and latency of units in ventral cochlear nucleus: Implications for unit classification and generation of response properties. J. Neurophysiol. 60: 1–29.

Young, E.D. and Voigt, H.F. 1981. The internal organization of the dorsal cochlear nucleus. In: Neuronal Mechanisms of Hearing (Syka, J. and Aitkin, L. eds.). New York: Plenum Press, pp. 127–133.

Young, E.D. and Voigt, H.F. 1982. Response properties of type II and type IV units in dorsal cochlear nucleus. Hear. Res. 6: 153–169.

Young, H.M. and Vaney, D.I. 1991. Rod-signal interneurons in the rabbit retina: 1. Rod bipolar cells. J. Comp. Neurol. 310: 139–153.

Young, M.P. 1992. Objective analysis of the topological organization of the primate cortical visual system. Nature 358: 152–155.

Young, M.P. and Yamane, S. 1992. Sparse population coding of faces in the inferotemporal cortex. Science 256: 1327–1331.

Young, W.S., III, Alheid, G.F., and Heimer, L. 1984. The ventral pallidal projection to the mediodorsal thalamus. A study with fluorescent retrograde tracers and immunohistofluorescence. J. Neurosci. 4: 1626–1638.

Youngentob, S.L., Kent, P.F., Schwob, J.E., Tzoumaka, E. 1995. Mucosal inerent activity patterns in the rat: Evidence from voltage-sensitive dyes. J. Neurophysiol. 73: 387–398.

Youngentob, S.L., Mozell, M.M., Sheehe, P.R., and Hornung, D.E. 1987. A quantitative analysis of sniffing strategies in rats performing odor detection tasks. Physiol. Behav. 41: 59–69.

Yuan, B., Morrow, T.J., and Casey, K.L. 1986. Corticofugal influences of S1 cortex on ventrobasal thalamic neurons in the awake rat. J. Neurosci. 6: 3611–3617.

Yung, K., Smith, A.D., Levey, A.I., and Bolam, J.P. 1996. Synaptic connections between spiny neurons of the direct and indirect pathways in the neostriatum of the rat—Evidence from dopamine receptor and neuropeptide staining. Eur. J. Neurosci. 8: 861–869.

Yuste, R. and Denk, W. 1995. Dendritic spines as basic functional units of neuronal integration. Nature 375: 682–684.

Yuste, R., Gutnick, M., Saar, D., Delaney, K., and Tank, D. 1994. Calcium accumulations in dendrites from neocortical neurons: An apical band and evidence for functional compartments. Neuron 13: 23–43.

Yuste, R. and Tank, D.W. 1996. Dendritic integration in mammalian neurons, a centruy after Cajal. Neuron 16: 701–716.

Zador, A. and Koch, C. 1994. Linearized models of calcium dynamics: Formal equivalence to the cable equation. J. Neurosci. 14: 4705–4715.

Zador, A., Koch, C., and Brown, T. 1990. Biophysical model of a hebbian synapse. Proc. Natl. Acad. Sci. USA 87: 6718–6722.

Zarbin, M.A., Innis, R.B., Wamsley, J.K., Snyder, S.H., and Kuhar, M.J. 1983. Autoradiographic localization of cholecystokinin receptors in rodent brain. J. Neurosci. 3: 877–906.

Zeki, S. and Shipp, S. 1988. The functional logic of cortical connections. Nature 335: 311–317.

Zengel, J.E., Reid, S.A., Sypert, G.W., and Munson, J.B. 1985. Membrane electrical properties and prediction of motor-unit type of cat medial gastrocnemius motoneurons in the cat. J. Neurophysiol. 53: 1323–1344.

Zhang, S. and Oertel, D. 1993a. Cartwheel and superficial stellate cells of the dorsal cochlear nucleus of mice: Intracellular recordings in slices. J. Neurophysiol. 69: 1384–1397.

Zhang, S. and Oertel, D. 1993b. Giant cells of the dorsal cochlear nucleus of mice: Intracellular recordings in slices. J. Neurophysiol. 69: 1398–1408.

Zhang, S. and Oertel, D. 1993c. Tuberculoventral cells of the dorsal cochlear nucleus of mice: Intracellular recordings in slices. J. Neurophysiol. 69: 1409–1421.

Zhang, S. and Oertel, D. 1994. Neuronal circuits associated with the output of the dorsal cochlear nucleus through fusiform cells. J. Neurophysiol. 71: 914–930.

Zhao, H.Q., Firestein, S., and Greer, C.A. 1994. NADPH-diaphorase localization in the olfactory system. Neuroreport 6: 149–152.

Zheng, L.M. and Jourdan, F. 1988. Atypical olfactory glomeruli contain original olfactory axon terminals: An ultrastructural horseradish peroxidase study in the rat. Neuroscience 26: 367–378.

Zhou, L., Yoshioka, T., and Nathans, J. 1996. Retina-derived POU-domain factor-1: A complex POU-domain gene implicated in the development of retinal ganglion and amacrine cells. J. Neurosci. 16: 2261–2274.

Zhou, Q., Godwin, D.W., Bickford, M.E., Sherman, S.M., and Adams, P.R. 1994. Relay cells and local GABAergic cells contribute to responses mediated by metabotropic glutamate receptors in cat LGN. Soc. Neurosci. Abstr. 20: 133.

Zipp, F., Nitsch, R., Soriano, E., and Frotscher, M. 1989. Entorhinal fibers form synaptic contacts on parvalbumin-immunoreactive neurons in the rat fascia dentata. Brain Res. 495: 161–166.

Zipser, D. and Andersen, R. 1988. A back-propagation programmed network that simulates response properties of a subset of posterior parietal neurons. Nature 331: 679–684.

Zola-Morgan, S., Squire, L.R., and Amaral, D.G. 1986. Human amnesia and the medial temporal region: Enduring memory impairment following a bilateral lesion limited to field CA1 of the hippocampus. J. Neurosci. 6: 2950–2967.

Zucker, C.L. and Dowling, J.E. 1987. Centrifugal fibres synapse on dopaminergic interplexiform cells in the teleost retina. Nature 330: 166–168.

INDEX